W9-CMZ-888

Geriatric Audiology

Geriatric Audiology

Barbara E. Weinstein, Ph.D.
Professor
Speech and Theatre
Lehman College, CUNY and
Graduate School and University Center, CUNY
Bronx, New York

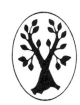

2000
Thieme
New York • Stuttgart

Thieme New York
333 Seventh Avenue
New York, NY 10001

Editor: Andrea Seils
Editorial Assistant: Michelle Carini
Developmental Manager: Kathleen P. Lyons
Director, Production and Manufacturing: Anne Vinnicombe
Production Editor: David Stewart
Marketing Director: Phyllis Gold
Sales Manager: Ross Lumpkin
Chief Financial Officer: Seth S. Fishman
President: Brian D. Scanlan
Compositor: Compset
Printer: Maple-Vail Book Manufacturing Group

Library of Congress Cataloging-in-Publication Data is available from the publisher.

Important note: Medical knowledge is ever-changing. As new research and clinical experience broaden our knowledge, changes in treatment and drug therapy may be required. The authors and editors of the material herein have consulted sources believed to be reliable in their efforts to provide information that is complete and in accord with the standards accepted at the time of publication. However, in view of the possibility of human error by the authors, editors, or publisher of the work herein, or changes in medical knowledge, neither the authors, editors, publisher, nor any other party who has been involved in the preparation of this work, warrants that the information contained herein is in every respect accurate or complete, and they are not responsible for any errors or omissions or for the results obtained from use of such information. Readers are encouraged to confirm the information contained herein with other sources. For example, readers are advised to check the product information sheet included in the package of each drug they plan to administer to be certain that the information contained in this publication is accurate and that changes have not been made in the recommended dose or in the contraindications for administration. This recommendation is of particular importance in connection with new or infrequently used drugs.

Some of the product names, patents, and registered designs referred to in this book are in fact registered trademarks or proprietary names even though specific reference to this fact is not always made in the text. Therefore, the appearance of a name without designation as proprietary is not to be construed as a representation by the publisher that it is in the public domain.

Printed in the United States of America

5 4 3 2 1

TNY ISBN 0-86577-701-2
GTV ISBN 3-13-108111-2

Contents

Section I. Aging: Normal and Abnormal Aspects

Section II. The Aging Auditory System

Section III. Rehabilitative Considerations

Section IV. Health Care Delivery

Contributors

Jaynee H. Calder, Ph.D.
Coordinator, Balance Function Laboratory
Department of Otolaryngology, Head & Neck Surgery
Henry Ford Hospital
Detroit, Michigan

Craig W. Newman, Ph.D.
Director of Audiology
Department of Otolaryngology & Communicative
*   Disorders*
The Cleveland Clinic Foundation
Cleveland, Ohio

Sharon A. Sandridge, Ph.D.
Audiologist
Department of Otolaryngology
The Cleveland Clinic Foundation
Cleveland, Ohio

Foreword

The viability of audiology as an independent, self-sustaining profession has been questioned for as long as I've been in the field. We always seem to be at a "crossroads," with our future being determined by the path we take (Ross & Giolas, 1977; Hardick, 1977). This uncertainty can be traced to the way we were conceived shortly after World War II. As the profession emerged from the amalgamation of the specialists mobilized by the army and navy to rehabilitate men with service-connected hearing loss, two major roles characterized our "scope of practice." In one role, we worked as technical support persons for otolaryngologists. The audiometric test results we provided them in our "technicians" role were used for medical/diagnostic purposes, but this same information was also applicable for planning and implementing a comprehensive aural rehabilitation (AR) program, our second role. In this latter function, we selected and fit hearing aids, conducted speechreading and auditory training classes, counseled the patients, and generally tried to help them understand and cope with their hearing losses. How autonomously we functioned depended upon the role we assumed. In one we were technicians, in the other case managers. This early duality bedevils us still. Do we define ourselves as a profession whose primary function is that of providing technical support for physicians, or do we have a role in which we have independent, and unique, responsibilities?

The short answer, at least in my judgment, is that both are necessary for a well-rounded profession. In the last 50 years, audiologists have devised or learned how to administer and interpret an impressive armamentarium of auditory tests. But no matter how sophisticated our test battery, or how skilled our interpretation of the results, if this activity becomes our raison d'etre, then we basically remain technical support persons for the medical profession. It is when we practice the second role, as the professional responsible for evaluating and managing the communication handicap imposed by a hearing loss, that we fully come into our own.

This is not a new insight. Jerger made the same point in 1960 and again in 1996: "If we want to have a unique profession it must be founded on the non-medical management of hearing disorder, not on ABR or ENG or Intraoperative monitoring, or anything else that places us in the role of technician supplying helpful information to a member of a different profession" (Jerger, 1996, personal communication). The same point was made even earlier, when the profession was in its infancy, with the following definition of audiology by Hallowell Davis in 1947 (the term had been coined by Carhart and Canfield several years earlier):

> We shall use it (Audiology) in a very broad sense. For some purposes, it may be helpful to speak more specifically of "Medical Audiology" when medical aspects of impaired hearing are our primary concern. It (the term, Audiology) is particularly useful here, however, because it indicates an interest in the *function* and not only in the *diseases* of the ear. The diseases of the ear, the recognized province of *Otology* may be a threat to life, and hearing then becomes secondary. Audiology considers the ear as an *aid* to life. (Emphasis in the original.)

This is not a bad distinction to make—one that I think the profession can happily live with. But the history of our professional activities (actual, as opposed to laudatory, but unrealistic "scope of practice" statements) subsequent to World War II has not shown an equal emphasis on the two tracks. The practice and progression of AR was not comparable to the growth of the medical/diagnostic role when the field moved into academia and into the world at large after World War II. There are undoubtedly many reasons for this, including but not limited to the rewards system in universities and the demands and influence of the marketplace on our activities. The consequence of this change in focus is that from a core and defining activity, AR moved into the periphery. Academically, it was relegated to one, or at the most two, courses in speechreading and auditory training, and clinically, assigned to the lowest-status professionals in the department.

During these years, research on AR was sparse and rather superficial. Except for a few centers, notably some Veterans Administration clinics, and the various Leagues for the Hard-of-Hearing, few professionals provided AR, even with its initial restrictive definition as primarily speechreading and auditory training. It was in response to this trend that Jack Rosen, in a widely quoted article, wrote: "The drift from aural rehabilitation has been so extensive that it represents a change in the basic direction of the field. The audiologist who voluntarily chooses the role of rehabilitation worker must be truly dedicated, for he runs the danger of being considered incompetent for other functions by his peers" (Rosen 1967).

Not that audiology ever explicitly abandoned AR. It remained, and remains, a significant element in our self-definition; all audiological curricula, including the ones proposed for the Au.D. include AR courses, and when it becomes necessary for us to justify our existence as a unique profession to various health, education, and governmental agencies, we never fail to claim this activity as our own. We just don't do it (Schow, Balsara, Smedley, & Whitcomb, 1993), or value it very much (Malinoff, Kisiel, Kisiel, & Dygert, 1990).

Why am I taking this excursion into our history? Because every time I despair over the future of audiology, when I think we've been so beguiled by the new array of diagnostic technology available that we've lost sight of "the communication needs of human beings resulting from impaired hearing" (Jerger, 1960), something comes along to reassure me that the profession does indeed have a future. My most recent reassurance occurred when I looked at the scope of the book titled "Geriatric Audiology."

As I have followed the debates on the Au.D., and as I look at some of the curricula meant to train Au.D. candidates, I've often felt that we're losing balance, that too much stress has been placed upon the diagnostic and medical aspects of the profession. In this book, however, we can see the balance, how information on rehabilitation of older adults leads from, and requires a basic understanding of the audiological and psychological correlates of the aging process. The progression from basic areas to management conveys the necessary notion that we cannot effectively fit an older person with amplification or other assistive devices without appreciating the psychosocial and neurological consequences of the aging brain. AR, then, is the goal, the culmination of our efforts. It is the reason that we need to understand the comprehensive impact of a hearing loss upon older hard-of-hearing adults. Being concerned with AR, then, does not imply overlooking or minimizing the medical/diagnostic implications of a hearing loss—these are indeed vital—only that their major significance for us comes when this information is employed to reduce the handicap imposed by a hearing loss.

What the content and organization of this book suggest is that, in truth, there need be no conflict in roles—as long as in the profession (as a profession, not necessarily every individual practitioner), AR receives equal billing and equal emphasis to our technical support role. AR is not an afterthought, not something that "would be nice to do," if we had the time or if we could generate the necessary funding. As Erdman, Wark, and Montano (1994) eloquently point out: "To assume the position that change is not possible because of time constraints or reimbursement constraints when we know that change is indicated is indefensible. Ultimately, when we make time, when our services are defensible, and when we are truly accountable, reimbursement will not be a concern." AR, then, should be seen not only as an integral component of our efforts with patients, but also as its logical conclusion.

But there are other reasons why we must continue to make AR an integral component of our clinical activities. First of all, they work. Time and time again AR programs have been shown to be effective, to reduce the handicap imposed by a hearing loss (Hardick, 1977; Abrahamson, 1991; Kricos & Lesner, 1995). And secondly, if audiologists don't take this task on, it won't get done.

There is no other professional group that has the requisite training to conduct AR programs designed for adults. Not that we can't use some refinement in our training programs. As I examined the curricula of four of the existing and current Au.D. programs, none offered what I could consider an adequate background in understanding and managing the psychosocial implications of a hearing loss. None included courses on personal counseling techniques or how to act as a group facilitator. Not enough of the balance we should be seeking in our clinical activities are reflected in these curricula. Nevertheless, in spite of these shortcomings, (which should not be difficult to correct), there is still no profession more qualified than ours to conduct AR programs with adults. And there doesn't seem to be any better resource on the market to help audiologists carry on this function than this book, which is designed to help us both understand and deal with "Geriatric Audiology."

Mark Ross, Ph.D.

REFERENCES

ABRAHAMSON, J. (1991). Teaching coping strategies: a client education approach. *Journal of the Academy of Rehabilitative Audiology*, 14: 43–54.

DAVIS, H. (1947). *Hearing and Deafness.* New York: Rinehart & Company.

ERDMAN, S.A., WARK, D.J., & MONTANO, J.J. (1994). Implications of service delivery models in audiology. *Journal of the Academy of Rehabilitative Audiology*, 27: 45–60.

HARDICK, E.J. (1977). Aural rehabilitation programs for the aged can be successful. *Journal of the Academy of Rehabilitative Audiology*, 10(1): 51–67.

JERGER, J. (1960). Our professional future. Remarks at the 1960 American Speech and Hearing Convention. Los Angeles. In: *Tejas*, Summer, 1976: 25.

KRICOS, P.B., & LESNER, S.A. (Eds.). (1995). *Hearing Care for Older Adults.* Boston: Butterworth-Heinemann.

MALINOFF, R., KISIEL, D., KISIEL, S., DYGERT, P.K. (1990). The dispensing of hearing instruments: a study of industry structure and trends. *Hearing Instruments,* 42(5): 12–16.

ROSEN, J. (1967). Distortions in the training of audiologists. *American Speech-Language-Hearing Association,* 9: 171–174.

ROSS, M., & GIOLAS, T.M. (1977). Audiologists at the crossroads (again)? *Tejas,* 3: 19–22.

SCHOW, R.L., BALSARA, N.R., SMEDLEY, T.C., & WHITCOMB, C.J. (1993). Aural rehabilitation by ASHA audiologists: 1980–1990. *American Journal of Audiology,* 2(3): 28–37.

Preface

When I was first approached to write this textbook I was at a very different stage in my life than I am now. My grandparents' memory was very vivid in my mind . . . they both had lived a very rich life, aging quite successfully. My mother had just passed away at the age of 67 years, having had the opportunity to enjoy three of her grandchildren. She too exemplified for me the joy of aging. More recently, after completing the writing of the text, I came to appreciate what life's challenge truly was. My twin sister lost her three year struggle with cancer at the young age of 45. She had just barely begun to enjoy middle age. One of her biggest regrets was that she would not have the chance to experience old age and the opportunities it offers. To me one of the greatest challenges of life is to age and to do so successfully!

Getting older is no longer what it used to be. Aging successfully is the operative phrase for the 34 million adults aged 65 or over. More than 70% of Americans now live to the traditional age of retirement, namely 65 years of age. Most seniors plan to spend their post career years starting new activities, including some form of volunteer work. The keys to successful aging, according to The MacArthur Foundation Study are: (1) avoiding disease and disability; (2) maintaining high mental and physical function; and (3) continuing to engage actively in life through strong interpersonal relationships. In my view, the fourth key is the ability to hear and understand family members, and age cohorts, as well.

Audiologists have an important role to play, and it is my hope that this text will empower them to help older adults age successfully. This is why I agreed to write a textbook on geriatric audiology. My entire professional career has been devoted to unraveling some of the mysteries of the aging process and how it impacts on the hearing impaired. Along the way I have tried to convey to audiologists the importance of identifying the psychosocial consequences of hearing loss on the elderly, encouraging early identification of hearing loss and ensuring that older adults obtain hearing aids and benefit from them adequately. As Dr. Mark Ross so eloquently states, "audiology is a unique profession if its members seize the opportunity to manage as well as evaluate older adults with impaired hearing."

As we enter the next millenium we are armed with research findings which can help us to help older adults. These findings are exciting and have considerable implications for audiologists and older adults. The following are some illustrative data which impact on audiology as a profession:

- The brain appears to generate a daily stream of new cells that migrate into the cerebral cortex, the area responsible for higher intellectual functions. The notion that new cells continue to be formed in the adult brain has implications for the brain's mechanism for learning.
- Researchers are gaining a better understanding of what promotes cell growth and cell death.
- Within 20 years age-related hearing loss may be correctable with medication, according to researchers at the International Center for Hearing and Speech Research housed at the National Technical Institute for the Deaf. They have found that, in addition to damage to the inner ear, hearing loss is caused by miscommunication within the brain linked to chemical reactions that change with age. Specifically, the researchers, led by Robert Frisina, Ph.D., contend that the inability to discriminate speech from background noise appears to be related to a chemical (i.e., calcium) imbalance in the brain.

- Amazingly while only 500,000 adults use devices for the visually impaired, over 4.5 million adults use some type of "auditory" assistive listening device, such as an amplified telephone, closed captioned television and other devices for the hearing impaired.
- A guided consumer education reading program, using a textbook titled "The Consumer Handbook on Hearing Loss and Hearing Aids: A Bridge to Healing", helped to reduce the hearing aid return for credit rate reported by dispensing audiologists, which in turn led to greater customer satisfaction. These findings underline the value of counseling-based intervention with hearing aid users.
- According to a recent large scale survey conducted by the National Council on Aging in cooperation with the Hearing Industries Association, hearing aid nonusers are more likely than hearing aid users with similar self-reported hearing loss to report being sad, depressed, anxious, and insecure. Irrespective of hearing loss severity, older adults do not seek out audiologic services because they feel their hearing is not bad enough and that they can get along without amplification. Some things never change!

It is my hope that the information contained in this text will raise awareness among audiologists and health care professionals regarding a number of pertinent issues. These include the prevalence of hearing loss and balance problems; the consequences of untreated hearing loss and speech understanding problems; the value of audiologic interventions in terms of their impact on the individual and families; and the role audiologists can play in helping older adults cope with one of the many losses sustained by some fortunate enough to have the gift of longevity. The positive thing about age related hearing loss is that it *can* be treated and available treatments do have a positive impact. This is a message we cannot, and tend not to, emphasize enough.

In closing I would like to emphasize the goals I had in mind when I embarked on this project. It is important not only to see rehabilitation with hearing aids as the mainstream of geriatric audiology, but also to bring more geriatrics into audiologic rehabilitation.

Barbara E. Weinstein, Ph.D.

Dedication

This text is dedicated to my children, Michael, 13 years, Benjamin, 11 years, and Rachel Bernstein, 7 years. From their perspective this text took a lifetime to write. To my husband, Louis Bernstein whose love, respect, admiration, and support enabled me to overlook the domestic front and stay focused on my family, my career, and my writing obligations. To my parents, who barely reached their golden years but instilled in me the ability to continue along a path devoted to educating and helping others less fortunate than I.

This text is also specially dedicated to my twin sister, Robin, who never even made it through middle age. "It is not the quantity of years on earth, but the quality . . . we had joy, we had fun, we had seasons in the sun. . . ." Thanks for the 45 years of wonderful memories which I will carry with me forever.

A portion of the proceeds from this text will be donated to research conducted to find a cure for sarcoma, a rare form of cancer to which my sister succumbed too early in life.

Acknowledgments

Many thanks to the efforts of David Stewart, Production Editor, and Andrea Seils, Senior Medical Editor; and to the inspiration of Ira M. Ventry, Ph.D., my mentor.

Aging: Normal and Abnormal Aspects

Chapter 1

The Demography and Epidemiology of Aging

It is now proved beyond a doubt that aging is one of the leading causes of statistics.

—How and Why We Age

In the twenty-first century, the only age group that will experience a significant increase in numbers will be people over age fifty-five. . . . Growing old is a phenomenon that affects all of us whatever our age.

—How and Why We Age

Middle aged and older people today can expect to spend more time caring for their parents than they did caring for their children.

—Charles Schewe

LEARNING OBJECTIVES

After reading this chapter, you should be able to:

- Outline the demographic revolution, which is taking place as we move into the 21st century, as it pertains to your client list.
- Explain how the aging of the population will influence caseloads and audiologic practice.

SIZE AND GROWTH OF THE OLDER POPULATION

One of the most significant demographic facts affecting America's present and future course is the aging of its population. The demographic curve poses great challenges for society in general and health care professionals in particular. The absolute and relative growth in numbers of the elderly in this country is noteworthy. Since the turn of the century, we have moved from a situation where fewer than 1 in 10 Americans was age 55+ and only 1 in 25 was 65+, to a situation where, at present, approximately 1 in 5 Americans is 55+ years and 1 in 8 is at least 65 years. By the year 2040, 1 in 5 persons in the United States will be over 65 years of age. Estimates of the elderly population in the United States suggest that, whereas in 1900 the population over 65 represented 4% of the total U.S. population and in 1995 they constituted 12.8% of the population, by 2020 this age group will represent 16.6% and by 2040 20.7% of the U.S. population. Thus, as is depicted in Table 1–1, in 1990 more than 31 million Americans were 65+, in 1995 more than 33 million persons were over 65 years, and by the year 2040 the over 65 population will exceed 75 million, well over double what it was in 1990. By the year 2050, people over 65 will account for 20% of the population. The most rapid increase in the 65+ population is expected between the years 2010 and 2030 when the baby boom generation reaches age 65.

SPECIAL CONSIDERATION

In the year 2000, 34.7 million persons in the U.S. will be 65+ (AOA, 1998).

The relative rate of growth within the over 65 population has increased substantially within this past century. The fact that the older population itself is getting older is apparent from the growth within selected age groups. In 1990, the 65 to 74 year age group was eight times larger, the 75 to 84 group 13 times larger, and the 85+ group 24 times larger than in 1900. The 85+ age group, oftentimes termed the oldest old, is the most rapidly growing subgroup of older persons (Abrams, Beers, & Berkow, 1995). Between 1960 and 1994 their numbers rose 274% as compared to a 100% rise for the elderly population in general (U.S. D.H.H.S., 1997). While at present the 85+ population represents 10% of the elderly population, around 2050 they will constitute over 20% of the 65+ population. In fact, people over 85 will become the fastest growing age group by the middle of the next century, representing about 4.6% of the total population by the year 2050. Figure 1–1 captures the projection that the 65+ population will constitute over one-fifth of the elderly around the middle of the 21st century.

SPECIAL CONSIDERATION

The growth of the 85+ population, a major outgrowth of improved disease prevention/health promotion activities and health care, will have a marked impact on the health care system and accordingly implications for hearing health care.

3

TABLE 1–1 Total Population and Number of Persons 65+ (in millions): 1960 to 2040

Year	Total population	Number	Percentage of total
1960	226	16.7	9.2
1990	249	31.2	12.5
1995	262	33.5	12.8
2000	275	34.9	12.7
2020	323	53.6	16.6
2040	364	75.6	20.7

Source: Adapted from U.S. Bureau of the Census. Current Population Reports, Special Studies, 123–178, Sixty-five Plus in America. Washington, DC: U.S. Government Printing Office, 1992.

PEARL

Within the older population, the fastest growing segment is the oldest old, a group with greater needs in all areas of health care. The oldest old will number 19 million in 2050.

The changing age distribution of the American population is rather dramatic. The projected growth in the older population is expected to raise the median age of the U.S. population to 36 years by the year 2000 and to 43 years by the year 2050. Figure 1–1 depicts the shift in the proportion of persons 65+ and under 18 years. In 1900 persons under

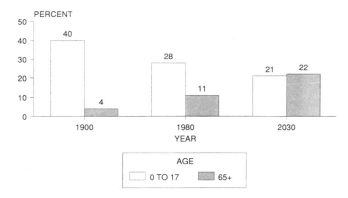

Figure 1–1 Percent of children and elderly in the population: 1900, 1980, and 2030. (Sources: 1900 figures, which exclude Alaska, Hawaii, and Armed Forces overseas: U.S. Bureau of the Census. "Estimates of the Population of the United States, by Single Years of Age, Color, and Sex: 1900 to 1959." *Current Population Reports* Series P-25, no. 311 (July 1965). 1980 and 2030 figures: U.S. Bureau of the Census. "Projections of the Population of the United States, by Age, Sex, and Race: 1988 to 2080," by Gregory Spencer. *Current Population Reports* Series P-25, no. 1018 [January 1989].)

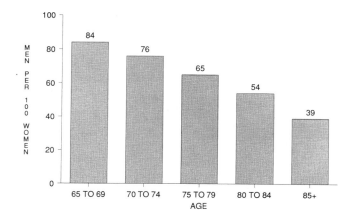

Figure 1–2 Number of men per 100 women by age group: 1989. (Source: U.S. Bureau of the Census. "U.S. Population Estimates, by Age, Sex, Race, and Hispanic Origin: 1989," by Frederick W. Hollman. *Current Population Reports* Series P-25, no. 1057 [March 1990].)

the age of 18 years constituted 40% and persons 65+ constituted 4% of the total U.S. population. It is projected that by the year 2030, the proportion of the population under 18 will be comparable to that of 65+. That is by the year 2030, 21% of the U.S. population will be under 17 years and 22% will be over 65 years.

Life Expectancy

Changes in life expectancy have been dramatic with the decline in mortality among middle-aged and older persons. Average life expectancy has increased substantially since 1900 such that a person born in 1995 could expect to live 75.8 years, and a baby born in 1997 could expect to live 76 years in the United States, 76 years in Japan, and 64 years in Russia.

PEARL

In 1996, a women reaching 65 had an average life expectancy of an additional 19 years and a male an additional 15.5 years.

Thus, in 1997 persons reaching age 65 had an average life expectancy about 28 years longer than a baby born in 1900. Projected life expectancy varies somewhat with age, gender, and race. For example, a male who reached his 65th birthday in 1990 could expect to live another 15 years, whereas a female could expect to live another 19.4 years. It is projected that by the year 2050 a male who reaches his 65th birthday can expect to live an additional 17.7 years and a women 22.7 more years. Survival rates to age 85 have also increased dramatically. Of those born in 1987, 41% of White women and 21% of White males are projected to survive to 85 years. The pattern is similar for Noncaucasian males and females. Noncaucasian women (32%) and Noncaucasian males (16%)

born in 1987 are projected to survive to 85 years. It is apparent that, overall, women live longer than men, and, at birth, life expectancy for Whites is about 6 to 8 years longer than for Blacks (Abrams, Beers, & Berkow, 1995).

The mortality rate for women has declined more rapidly

PEARL

We now live in a society where over one-third of females can expect to celebrate their 85th birthday (Grundy, 1998).

---

than that for men over the past several decades. Thus, females live longer than males, older women outnumber older men, and women are more likely to live alone (Abrams, Beers, & Berkow, 1995). In 1989, there were 18.3 million women and only 12.6 million men. It is estimated that elderly women outnumber elderly men by 3 to 2. As is shown quite dramatically in Figure 1–2, the number of men per 100 women declines sharply from 65 to 85 years. In 1989, there were 84 men between 65 and 69 for every 100 women and among those 85+ there were 39 men for every 100 women. In 1997, for every 100 women over 65, there were only 77 men. This gender gap is expected to narrow in the next century as more men live longer.

The difference in mortality rates among men and women influences family composition, marital status, and living arrangements. Overall, about one-third of noninstitutionalized elderly persons live alone, with the very old and women being the most likely to do so. In 1994, about 19% of older men and 42% of older women lived alone or with a nonrelative. The majority of older noninstitutionalized persons, however, did live in a family setting in 1994. According to a 1995 report, about 82% of men aged 65+ lived with their spouse or other family members compared with 58% of women in this age group. Among women aged 75+, less than half lived with spouses or family. Whereas among men in this age group, more than 70% reported living with a spouse or other relatives. Living arrangements of older adults vary by race and origin. Whites and Hispanics are more likely to live with a spouse, Blacks are most likely to live alone, and Blacks and Hispanics are more likely than Whites to live with other relatives (U.S. Bureau of the Census, 1990). Trends in living arrangements are of relevance to audiologists when attempting to gauge the impact of hearing loss on the individual and family members and when deciding about candidacy for hearing aids or assistive listening devices.

SPECIAL CONSIDERATION

It is critical that audiologists appreciate that living alone brings with it a series of nonmedical needs including poverty and loneliness. The ability to hear can ease the burden of loneliness for some.

Geographic Considerations— a Cross-National Perspective

Worldwide, the older population is growing at a rate of 2.4% per year, which is much faster than the overall population. Between 1975 and 2025, the percentage of persons greater than 60 years old is projected to increase by 224%, compared with only 102% for the general population. In 1990, 28 countries had more than 2 million people aged 65 and 12 countries had more than 5 million 65+ (U.S. Senate, 1991). In 1990, The United States had the second largest elderly population (31,560,000), after China which reported a 65+ population of 63,398,000. In that same year the United States reported the second largest oldest-old population, also behind the more populous China. In 1990, the United States reported the over 80 population to be approximately 7,716,000. Despite its very large older population, the United States is considered one of the younger of the developed countries. Table 1–2 presents estimates of the proportion of persons over 65 and projections for the year 2050. It is evident that Sweden has the highest proportion (17.9%) of older adults as compared to the United States, Canada, and other industrialized countries. It is projected that by the year 2025, Japan and Italy will have the largest proportion of older adults whereas the United States will rank the lowest among the eight countries with the largest older adult population. Although the relative number of older persons is higher in developed countries, the number of those in less developed countries is growing quite rapidly such that by the year 2025, more than two-thirds of the world's older citizens will be living in poorer geographic regions (Abrams, Beers, & Berkow, 1995). Asia will contribute nearly 50% of the world's population of older individuals by the year 2000. It is of interest, as well, that worldwide the older population is growing at a much faster rate than the overall population.

Within the United States more than half of persons 65+ lived in one of nine states in 1997. As would be expected, the most populous states are also the ones with the largest numbers of elderly. The states with the largest number of older

TABLE 1–2   Percentage of Population Age 65+ in Selected Countries: 1990 and 2025

Country	Year 1990	Year 2025
Sweden	17.9%	23.7%
United Kingdom	15.6	21.9
Germany	15.0	24.4
Italy	14.7	25.1
France	14.1	21.8
United States	12.6	20.0
Japan	11.8	26.3
Canada	11.5	21.8

Source: Modified from U.S. Senate, 1991.

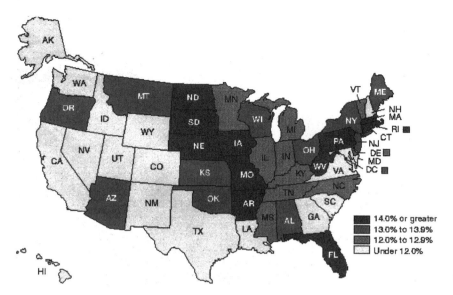

Figure 1–3 Percentage of 65+ population by state: 1993.

Map legend:
- 14.0% or greater
- 13.0% to 13.9%
- 12.0% to 12.9%
- Under 12.0%

adults in rank order include: California (3.5 million), Florida (2.7 million), New York, Pennsylvania, Texas, Illinois, Ohio, Michigan, and New Jersey (AOA, 1998). While the most populous state, California, has the largest number of persons 65+, Florida has the highest (19%) proportion of residents over 65 years of age. In contrast, Alaska has the lowest number and proportion of individuals over 65 years. States wherein older adults constituted 14% or more of the total population in 1995 were: Florida, Pennsylvania, Rhode Island, West Virginia, Iowa, Arkansas, North Dakota, South Dakota, Connecticut, and Massachusetts.

> ## PEARL
>
> **The states with the greatest proportion of older adults are different from those with the greatest number. California has the largest number of elderly whereas Florida has the greatest proportion.**

In the 1980s, the number of older persons in all states increased dramatically (Abrams, Beers, & Berkow, 1995). Also notable has been the proportional increase in the elderly population in the 1980s in selected regions, and the projected increase in proportion of older adults residing in selected states between 1989 and 2010. The states projected to have the largest percent increase in the over 65 population during that time frame include: Hawaii, Alaska, Arizona, and Georgia whereas those with the smallest increase include: North Dakota, Iowa, and Montana. By the year 2010 California's elderly population will increase by 52% to more than 4.7 million, maintaining its rank as the state with the largest number of older adults. Florida will continue to have the largest percentage of older adults rising to nearly 20% of their population as we move into the next century. It is projected that by the year 2020, 32 states will have more than 16% of their population over 65 years of age. These states are highlighted in Figure 1–3. These demographic changes have implications for the demand for hearing health care services. In short, these "retirement areas" will need hearing health care services as their populations reach the oldest ages.

Growth of the Minority Population

The number and percentage of White, Black, and Hispanic older adults is displayed in Table 1–3. It is evident that the proportion of older adults in the white population is larger than Nonwhites with the Hispanics having the lowest representation. In 1997, 15% of persons 65+ were minorities (AOA, 1998). However, population projections suggest that between 1990 and 2030 the older White population will grow by 92%, the older Black population will grow by 257%, and the older Hispanic population will grow by 395%. It is noteworthy that between 1980 and 1990, the older population of Native Americans already increased by close to 85%. In addition to ethnic variations in the growth rate of the

TABLE 1–3 65+ Population by Age and Race: 1989

Age	Race (in thousands)			
	White	Black	Hispanic	Other*
65+	27,822	2,555	1,073	607
85+	2,761	236	91	44

Age	Percent of population			
	White	Black	Hispanic	Other*
65+	13%	8%	5%	7%
85+	1	1	0	1

*Native American and Asian/Pacific Islanders.
Source: Modified from U.S. Senate, 1991.

older populations there are variations within these groups in educational attainment (Shadden & Warnick, 1994). In 1987, only 5% of White males and 4.3% of older White females had less than 5 years of education, as compared to 24.8% of older African American males and 16% of older African American females (Shadden & Warnick, 1994). Similarly, 31% of older Hispanic males and 32% of older Hispanic females had less than 5 years of education according to a 1987 report (Shadden & Warnick, 1994). The more rapid increase in the minority older adult population and the disparity in educational level has implications for delivery of health care services in general and hearing health care services in particular. Audiologists must make every attempt to insure that members of all ethnic groups have access to audiology services.

PEARL

Minority populations are projected to represent 25% of the elderly population in 2030, an increase of 13% from 1990.

Economic Status

The economic resources and status of older adults must be considered in terms of noncash and cash resources. In general, the elderly have substantially lower average cash incomes than do the nonelderly. However, when lifetime accumulations of wealth, government in-kind transfers, real estate, etc., are taken into account some of the differences in economic status are obliterated. Specifically, in 1994 the major income sources for persons 65+ include Social Security (42%), public and private pensions (19%), earnings (18%), asset income (18%), and all other sources (3%). Income from Social Security, the most important source of income for the elderly, has been the major source of income for the elderly since 1976.

If one were to judge economic status on money income, it is clear that older Americans have a lower economic status than do younger adults.

SPECIAL CONSIDERATION

However, it is notable that in 1997, the median income for men and women over 65 rose more than 170% from 1947 to 1995 whereas the median income for the overall population in the same time span rose 49%.

In 1989, the median income of families whose head of the household was between 25 and 64 years was $36,058 versus $22,806 for those families where the head was 65+. These figures were slightly higher in 1996 where households containing families headed by persons 65+ reported a median income of $28,983, with incomes for Whites ($29,470) higher than for Blacks ($21,328) and Hispanics ($21,068). In 1995, the median income of older persons was $16,684 for males

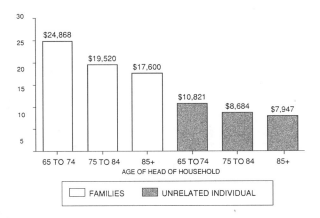

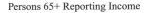

Figure 1–4 Median income of older families by age group-1989. (Source: *Current Population Survey.* March 1990. Data prepared by the Congressional Research Service.)

and $9,626 for females. Within the over 65 population, the oldest old have the lowest family incomes. In 1989, the median cash income of families age 85+ was $17,600 versus $24,868 for families whose head of the household was 65 to 74 years (Figure 1–4). For all older persons reporting income in 1997 (31.4 million), the median income was $13,049 with only 6% reporting incomes more than $50,000 (Figure 1–5).

In 1995, approximately 3.7 million persons 65+ had incomes below the poverty level. The numbers are decreasing such that in 1996 3.4 million older adults lived below the poverty level (U.S. D.H.H.S., 1997). A greater proportion of the elderly live near poverty and are likely to have incomes below the poverty level. In fact, the poverty rate for persons 65+ was 10.5%, slightly less than the rate for persons 18 to 64 years. The oldest elderly are the most likely to have incomes below poverty level. The proportion of all people 65 or older

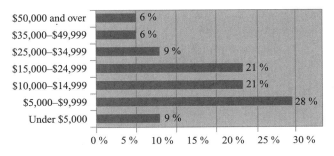

$13,049 median for 31.4 million persons 65+ reporting income

Figure 1–5 Percent of elderly with incomes ranging from under $5,000 to over $50,000: 1998. (Source: Based on data from *Current Population Reports,* "Consumer Income," P60-200, issued September, 1998, by the U.S. Bureau of the Census.)

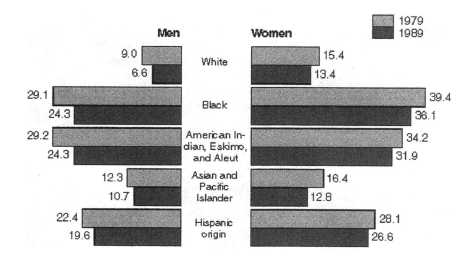

Figure 1–6 Poverty rate of elderly by selected characteristics: 1989. (Source: Persons of Hispanic origin may be of any race. This graph is based on 1980 and 1990 census sample data.)

living in poverty has dropped from 35% in 1959 to the present rate of 11%. Similarly, in 1965, 63% of Blacks 65 or older lived below the poverty level versus approximately 25% today. Figure 1–6 depicts the poverty rate as a function of ethnicity and race.

Income status is influenced by a number of factors including living arrangement, gender, marital status, and race. As is evident from Figure 1–7, overall the median income of elderly men is higher than that of elderly women. It is of interest that married women had the lowest income according to the 1990 population survey, presumably due to dependence on the income of a husband (U.S. D.H.H.S., 1991). Overall the median income of Whites is higher than

that of Blacks and Hispanics. The lowest median income is for older Hispanic women (Table 1–4). Consumption

PEARL

The major source of income for older persons in 1996 was Social Security (AOA, 1998).

patterns of the elderly relative to the nonelderly are most revealing. People 65+ spend the bulk of their economic resources on essentials, more so than persons under 65 years. With the exception of health care, for each category of ex-

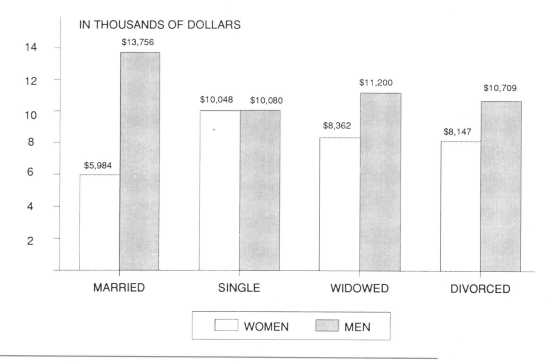

Figure 1–7 Median income of older men and women by marital status: 1990. (Source: *Current Population Survey,* March 1990. Data prepared by the Congressional Research Service.)

TABLE 1–4 Median Income of People Age 65+ by Age, Race, Hispanic Origin, and Sex: 1989

Race and Hispanic Origin	Both sexes			Men			Women		
	65+	65 to 69	70+	65+	65 to 69	70+	65+	65 to 69	70+
All races	9,420	10,722	8,936	13,024	15,273	12,022	7,508	7,584	7,476
White	9,838	11,323	9,305	13,391	15,680	12,410	7,816	7,977	7,756
Black	5,772	6,552	5,517	8,192	10,464	7,224	5,059	5,235	5,032
Hispanic*	5,978	6,664	5,715	8,469	10,240	6,816	4,992	4,640	5,112

*Hispanic people may be of any race.
Source: Unpublished data from the *Current Population Survey,* March 1990.

penditures persons under 65 spend more in actual dollars. The major health care expenditure for the elderly in 1988 was health insurance. Older adults spent twice as much as their younger counterparts on health insurance. Further, persons over 65 spent over twice as much on prescription drugs and medical supplies than did persons under 65 years. Benefits from government programs, including Medicare, Medicaid, and others cover a significantly larger proportion of health expenditures for older persons as compared to persons under 65 (AARP, 1996). In light of their health care expenditures, older adults are likely to spend money on hearing health care if they can see that the benefit justifies the expense. Outcome measures demonstrating actual benefit and satisfaction can be valuable as patients make informal cost-benefit analyses. Minority populations with their limited income are an underserved population and should be targeted for screening and outcome studies.

Health Status

The growth in the older population results from improvements in medical care, changes in lifestyle patterns (e.g., exercise), and living conditions. The gain in life expectancy brings with it changes in patterns of illness, a decrease in mobility, an increase in dependency, and an increase in the utilization of health services. Chronic rather than acute conditions predominate (Figure 1–8).

> **SPECIAL CONSIDERATION**
>
> As people age, acute conditions become less frequent and the likelihood of experiencing one or more chronic conditions increases.

In contrast to acute conditions, the clinical consequences of chronic conditions are usually long term.

> **SPECIAL CONSIDERATION**
>
> 80% of persons 65+ experience at least one chronic condition.

The high prevalence of chronic conditions and the increased prevalence of chronic disease with age lead to the cooccur-rence of chronic conditions or comorbidity of chronic disease in large numbers of older adults. Specifically, 49% of persons 60 and over have two or more chronic conditions, 23% have three or more, and 8% have four or more (Guralnik, LaCroix, Everett, & Kovar, 1989). The prevalence of comorbidity of disease increases with age, and among the oldest old comorbidity occurs in most people (Abrams, Beers, & Berkow, 1995). As would be expected, the prevalence of disability increases with age, number, and comorbidity of chronic conditions (Abrams, Beers, & Berkow, 1995). In 1995, 37% of older adults reported that they were limited in their activity by chronic conditions (AOA, 1998).

> **PEARL**
>
> Women are more likely than men to experience multiple chronic conditions.

A recent U.S. national study of the comorbidity of chronic disease revealed that 70% of the women and 53% of the men had two or more chronic conditions (Guralnik et al, 1989).

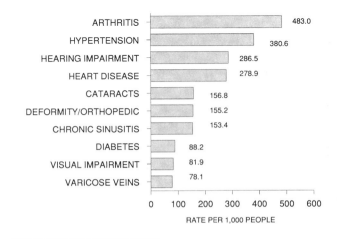

Figure 1–8 Prevalence of chronic conditions in the 65+ population in the United States: 1989. (Source: National Center for Health Statistics. Current Estimates from the National Health Interview Survey, 1989. *Vital and Health Statistics* Series 10, no. 176 [October 1990].)

TABLE 1–5 Prevalence of Selected Chronic Conditions per 1000 Persons over 65 Years of Age (1991)

Condition	≥65	65 to 74 years	≥75 years
Arthritis	484.8	425.6	575.2
Hypertension	372.2	376.6	365.5
Hearing impairment	295.2	256.4	354.3
Heart disease	320.5	266.2	403.6
Deformity or orthopedic impairment	177.5	167.1	193.3
Cataracts	173.0	127.6	242.3
Sinusitis	139.5	156.4	113.7
Diabetes	99.3	103.8	92.6
Tinnitus	82.4	95.3	62.6
Visual impairment	79.2	56.8	113.3

Source: Adams and Benson, 1991.

SPECIAL CONSIDERATION

The three most prevalent chronic conditions include arthritis, hypertension, and hearing impairment. These conditions have remained the most prevalent for several years.

Table 1–5 displays the ten most prevalent chronic conditions among persons 65+ in the United States according to the 1991 National Health Interview Survey. Note that the prevalence of hearing impairment among persons 65 and over, 295.2/1000 persons, is demonstrably higher than visual impairment, which was reportedly the tenth most prevalent chronic condition. Note also that tinnitus was reportedly the ninth most prevalent chronic condition affecting older adults responding to the survey. This hierarchy of chronic conditions is similar, albeit not identical, for persons 75+. However, the prevalence of each condition increases dramatically among those over 75 years (Adams & Benson, 1991). The prevalence data in Table 1–5 differ slightly from those in Figure 1–8, yet hearing impairment is stable as the third most prevalent condition.

For example, the prevalence of hearing impairment among persons 75+ rises to 354.3/1000 while the prevalence of visual impairment rises to 113.3/1000 persons. The prevalence of these chronic conditions tends to vary somewhat with race. As is evident in Table 1–6, the prevalence of hearing impairment was higher among Whites than Blacks whereas the prevalence of hypertension was higher among Blacks than Whites in the 1989 National Health Interview Survey. According to a 1994 report issued by the U.S. Department of Health and Human Services, overall more than 22 million Americans experience chronic hearing impair-

ment with the rate increasing with age such that 6,563,000 people under 45 years of age experience chronic hearing impairment with it affecting 6,952,000 persons between 45 and 64 years of age, and rising dramatically to 8,886,000 persons 65 years and older.

TABLE 1–6 Ten Most Prevalent Chronic Conditions by Race: 1989 (Number per 1000 Persons)

Condition	Race White	Black
Arthritis	483.2	522.6
Hypertension	367.4	517.7
Hearing impairment	297.4	174.5
Heart disease	286.5	220.5
Cataracts	160.7	139.8
Deformity or orthopedic impairment	156.2	150.8
Chronic sinusitis	157.1	125.2
Diabetes	80.2	165.9
Visual impairment	81.1	77.0
Varicose veins	80.3	64.0

Source: National Center for Health Statistics. Current Estimates from the National Health Interview Survey, 1989. *Vital and Health Statistics* Series 10, no. 176 (October, 1990).

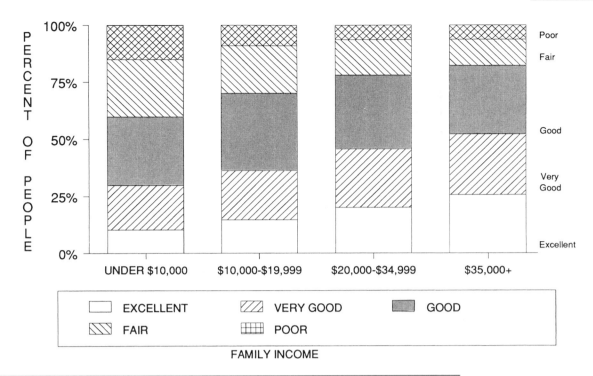

Figure 1–9 Self-reported health status by family income level: 1989. (Source: National Center for Health Statistics. Current Estimates from the National Health Interview Survey, 1989. *Vital and Health Statistics* Series 10, no. 176 [October 1990].)

Despite the prevalence of chronic conditions, older adults tend to rate their health positively. In 1994, nearly 72% of older adults living in the community self-rated their health status as excellent, very good, or good. Only 28% perceived their health status to be fair or poor compared to 10% of all persons (AARP, 1996). Self-reported health status does vary with family income. According to Figure 1–9, approximately 26% of older persons with incomes in excess of $35,000 rated their health as excellent versus 10% of persons with incomes under $10,000. Gender does not appear to influence self-reported health status. Similarly, self-reported health status varies with race; older Blacks are more likely to rate their health as fair or poor than older Whites.

Mental health problems are prevalent among older adults, influencing quite dramatically the course of acute and chronic medical conditions. Alzheimer's disease and other cognitive impairments affect 10% of persons 65+, rising to nearly 50% among persons 85+. The prevalence of cognitive impairment is much higher among the institutionalized, as it is the major reason for institutionalization among persons 65+. Symptoms of depression have been reported in as many as 15% of older persons who live in the community. The suicide rate among the elderly is quite high, making it a more frequent cause of death among the elderly than any other age group. Older White males have the highest suicide rate, over two and one-half times that of older Black males and nearly six times the rate for older White females.

Older adults use health care services more frequently than do younger adults and their health care costs are corre-

spondingly higher. Health care utilization is highest among the oldest old. One important indicator of health service utilization is use of physician services. Persons 65 and older made over 150 million visits to physicians' offices in 1989, representing 22% of all visits (Abrams, Beers, & Berkow, 1995). The average number of physician contacts for persons 45 to 64 years was 6.1 in 1989, versus 8.2 contacts for persons 65 to 74 years and 9.9 for persons 85+. Given the high prevalence of chronic conditions, the elderly use more prescription drugs, dental care services, vision aids, hearing aids, and medical equipment than do younger adults. In 1987, the 65+ population accounted for 36% of total personal health care expenses. These expenditures totaled $162 billion, averaging $5360 per year for each older person, which is more than four times the $1290 spent for younger persons (AARP, 1996). Approximately 37% of health care expenditures were through direct payments to providers or through premiums for insurance.

SPECIAL CONSIDERATION

In light of the high number of physician visits among older adults, it is incumbent on audiologists to educate physicians about hearing loss in older adults, its consequences, and devices available to help overcome the handicap resulting from hearing impairment.

Workforce and Retirement Trends

The increase in longevity in this century brings with it an increase in the amount of time spent in all major activities, including work and retirement. Cross-sectional data reveal that participation in the labor force declines with age for Caucasians and Blacks of both genders. It is projected that by the year 2000, workers 65+ will constitute 2.5% of the total labor force, which is comparable to the rate in 1988. However, in a 1997 survey, the proportion of men 65 or older who work full time has dropped dramatically, from 46% in 1950 to 16% in 1993. Interestingly, the proportion of women the same age who were working in 1993 (8%) was slightly less than in 1950 (10%). An interesting trend for the next decade is the opportunity for part-time work among persons 65+. In recent decades, there has been a dramatic increase in the proportion of part-time workers over 65 years. In 1960, 30% of men and 44% of women 65+ were on part-time schedules. This is in contrast to 1989 when 48% of men and 59 percent of women were working part time. The educational level of the older population is increasing, as well. The proportion of older adults with at least a high-school education will increase in the coming decades as will the proportion of older adults with a bachelor's degree.

SPECIAL CONSIDERATION
These educational and workforce trends would suggest that hearing health care interventions will take on increasing importance as the ability to hear and understand is typically viewed as essential to job performance.

The "future elderly" come from a generation with higher expectations, demanding greater access to services and, of course, better results (Shadden & Toner, 1997).

Nursing Home Use

The United States has more than 16,000 nursing homes with approximately 1.9 million beds, an insufficient number to meet the increased demographic demand (Abrams, Beers, & Berkow, 1995). Approximately 5% of the elderly are institutionalized in nursing homes, yet, at any one point, approximately 35% of older adults will require nursing home care. Nursing home projections indicate that 43% of persons who turned 65 in 1990 will spend some time in a nursing home before they die and and an even greater proportion of those admitted, 50%, will spend at least a year in a home (Murtaugh, Kemper, & Spillman, 1990; Ouslander, 1998). The probability of nursing home placement within a person's

lifetime is closely related to age as is nursing home utilization. The nursing home utilization rate for persons 65 to 74 years is approximately 3% versus 22% for those 85 years and older (U.S. D.H.H.S., 1991). In 1985, 45% of persons 85+ resided in a nursing home versus 7.6% living in the community. Similarly, only 16% of persons 65 to 74 years lived in a nursing home versus 62% living in the community.

The average resident of a nursing home is over 75 years of age, is White, widowed, has several chronic conditions, and was hospitalized prior to admission (U.S. D.H.H.S., 1991). In 1990, 75% of nursing home residents were women, 16% were age 65 to 74 years, 39% were 75 to 84 years, and 45% were over 85 years (Abrams, Beers, & Berkow, 1995). The majority of nursing home residents are disoriented or have impaired memory and require assistance with routine activities including bathing, dressing, and using the toilet. Close to half are confined to a wheelchair or bed. Need for assistance increases with age and cognitive status. It is likely that the nursing home population will rise with increasing longevity. Projections indicate that the nursing home population will increase from 1.5 in 1990 to 2.6 million in 2020.

PEARL
In light of the fact that the majority of nursing home residents are over 75 years of age, the prevalence of significant hearing loss is rather high, necessitating the need for hearing aids or, more appropriately, assistive listening devices.

Use of Community Services

Older adults tend to use community services to a large extent and this is likely to increase in the coming decades. Use of community services varies dramatically with level of impairment. During 1990 about 5.2 million unimpaired and 1.5 million impaired older adults used some type of community service at least once. It is projected that by the year 2020, 8.6 million unimpaired and 2.4 million impaired older adults will use some type of community service. The most widely used of the community services are senior centers and home food service programs. Visiting nurse or home health aide programs were used by 11% of older adults with activity limitations whereas only 1% of unimpaired older adults took advantage of home health services. Use of senior centers was comparable for the impaired (13%) and unimpaired (16%) older adult. Changes in health care delivery systems and emphasis on health promotion programs are likely to influence use of community services such that more older adults will use the services of home health agencies and senior citizen centers. In fact, a mandate of Healthy People 2000, a set of national health objectives in the area of health promotion and disease prevention for the year 2000, is to increase use of community-based programs by older adults (U.S. D.H.H.S., 1990).

Specific objectives of Healthy People 2000 in the area of community service include the following: (1) to increase to at least 80% the proportion of people 65+ who receive home food services because they have difficulty preparing their own meals; (2) to increase to at least 90% the proportion of people aged 65 and older who participate in at least one organized health promotion program through a senior center, lifecare facility, or other community-based setting that serves the elderly; and (3) to establish community health promotion programs that address at least three of the priorities targeted by Healthy People 2000 including reduction in prevalence of hearing loss among older adults and increasing the proportion of primary care physicians who screen for hearing loss (U.S. D.H.H.S., 1990). Screening protocols should be innovative, based in large part on the settings in which they will take place.

IMPLICATIONS OF THE DEMOGRAPHIC CHANGES FOR HEARING HEALTH CARE PROFESSIONALS

We are about to enter an era where there will be more older adults than ever before with significant chronic conditions including hearing loss.

SPECIAL CONSIDERATION

Audiologists must be cognizant of the demographic changes and the characteristics of this large subsample of the total U.S. population that will impact on the demand for hearing health care services.

These demographic imperatives are as follows:

- The older population will continue to grow in the future, with the most rapid increase taking place between the years 2010 and 2030.
- By 2030 there will be about 70 million older persons, representing 20% of the population.
- Minority populations are projected to represent 25% of the elderly population in 2030, with the growth rate being greatest for Hispanics.
- The number of older adults will exceed the number of children 0 to 17 years by the year 2030.
- The 85+ population is expected to triple in size between 1980 and 2030.
- The prevalence of hearing loss will rise dramatically with the increase in the absolute and relative proportion of older adults.
- The elderly spend more in dollars than do the nonelderly on health care including services and products.

- The proportion of life spent in retirement has increased dramatically and is projected to increase further as we move into the 21st century.
- The number of persons 55+ in the work force by the year 2000 will increase dramatically by the year 2000.
- The use of physician services is more widespread among older adults than younger persons.

The increase in the number and proportion of older adults who are 65+ coupled with the high prevalence of hearing loss in this age group is likely to expand the ranks of persons requiring hearing health care services. Shifting demographics will impact on the proportion of persons 65+ occupying the audiologist's caseload. At present persons between 65 to 84 years constitute 26% and persons 85+ 6.78% of the audiologist's caseload. In contrast, persons birth to 2 years constitute 11%, persons 3 to 5 years constitute 14.57%, and persons 6 to 17 years 17% of the audiologist's caseload. Many of these individuals will be healthier and will be spending a good deal of time retired. Many will be better educated, and gainfully employed through their ninth decade. Their sense of hearing and the ability to communicate on all levels with all media will become even more critical. Tomorrow's old people will probably expect more in terms of service and will want control over what happens to them (Kane, 1994).

SPECIAL CONSIDERATION

In delivering hearing health care services to older adults, the professional must be cognizant of their social, physical, and psychological characteristics, as they will impact on the nature of our services.

Older adults will look toward hearing health care professionals to restore a lost sense that is interfering with their ability to function on a variety of levels in a very dynamic world. They will demand that the services provide tangible benefits to themselves and family members enhancing or allowing them to maintain an adequate quality of life. Living well—not merely living longer—and making productive use of the years that have been added to their lives will be the goal for healthy older adults surviving into the 21st century (Friedan, 1993). Audiologists should be the professional of choice to ensure adequate hearing health care for the aging adult.

REFERENCES

ADMINISTRATION ON AGING (1998). *A Profile of Older Americans.* Available at: http://www.aoa.dhhs.gov/aoa/stats/profile/default.htm.

AARP. (1996). *A Profile of Older Americans.* Washington, DC: AARP and AOA.

ABRAMS, W., BEERS, M., & BERKOW, R. (1995). *The Merck Manual of Geriatrics.* 2d ed. Rahway, NJ: Merck & Co., Inc.

ADAMS, P., & BENSON, V. (1991). Current estimates from the National Health Interview Survey. National Center for Health Statistics. *Vital Health Statistics*, 10: 184.

FRIEDAN, B. (1993). *The Fountain of Age*. New York: Simon & Schuster.

GRUNDY, E. (1998). The epidemiology of aging. In: R. Tallis, H. Fillit, & J. Brocklehurst (Eds.), *Brocklehurst's Textbook of Geriatric Medicine and Gerontology*. London: Churchill Livingstone.

GURALNIK, J., LaCROIX, A., EVERETT, D., & KOVAR, M. (1989). Aging in the eighties: The prevalence of comorbidity and association with disability. Advance data from *Vital and Health Statistics*, No. 170. Hyattsville, MD: National Center for Health Statistics.

HAYFLICK, L. (1994). *How and Why We Age*. New York: Ballantine Books.

KANE, R. (1994). Looking toward the next millenium. *ASHA*, 36: 34–35.

KANE, R., OUSLANDER, J., & ABRASS, I. (1994). *Essentials of Clinical Geriatrics*. 3d ed. New York: McGraw-Hill.

MURTAUGH, C., KEMPER, P., & SPILLMAN, B. (1990). The risk of nursing home use in later life. *Medical Care*, 10: 28.

NATIONAL CENTER FOR HEALTH STATISTICS (1990). Current Estimates from the National Health Interview Survey, 1989. *Vital and Health Statistics*, 10: 176.

OUSLANDER, J. (1998). The American nursing home. In: R. Tallis, H. Fillit, & J. Brocklehurst (Eds.), *Brocklehurst's Textbook of Geriatric Medicine and Gerontology*. London: Churchill Livingstone.

SHADDEN, B., & TONER, M. (1997). *Aging and Communication: For Clinicians by Clinicians*, Vol. 9. Austin, TX: Pro-Ed.

SHADDEN, B., & WARNICK, P. (1994). Multicultural aspects of aging. *ASHA*, 36: 45–46.

U.S. BUREAU OF THE CENSUS. (1990). Marital status and living arrangements: March, 1989. *Current Population Reports Series*, 445: 20.

U.S. DEPARTMENT OF HEALTH AND HUMAN SERVICES. (1990). Public Health Service, Publication No. (PHS) 91–50212. In: *Healthy People 2000: National Health Promotion and Disease Prevention Objectives*, p. 1002. Boston: Jones and Bartlett Publishers.

———. (1997).Profile of Older Americans. Prepared by the Program Resources Department, American Association of Retired Persons (AARP), and the Administration on Aging (AOA).

U.S. SENATE SUBCOMMITTEE ON AGING, AMERICAN ASSOCIATION OF RETIRED PERSONS, FEDERAL COUNCIL ON AGING AND U.S. ADMINISTRATION ON AGING. (1991). *Aging America: Trends and Projections*. DHHS Publ. No. (FCoA)91-28001. U.S. Department of Health and Human Services.

Chapter 2

The Biology of Aging

Age is a question of mind over matter. If you don't mind, it doesn't matter.

—Satchel Paige

LEARNING OBJECTIVES

After reading this chapter, you should be able to:

- Become familiar with the theories of aging and the distinction between normal aging and disease.
- Apply your knowledge of the physical changes in the organ systems to your audiologic practice.
- Understand the implications of these changes for audiologic interventions.

WHAT IS AGING?

The terms *aging* and *senescence* are often used interchangeably when referring to the condition of being old. For the purposes of this text, the term *senescence* is restricted to the state of old age characteristic of the later years of the life span, whereas *aging* is a more global biologic term that refers to the process of growing old, regardless of chronologic age (Timiras, 1988). The latter term will be used throughout the text. Further, "older adult" or "older person" will be used to refer to individuals over 65 years. Three forms of aging have been described: intrinsic, extrinsic, and normal. Intrinsic aging refers to characteristics and processes that occur universally with aging in all members of a particular gender within a given species (Peterson, 1994). In contrast, extrinsic aging refers to outside factors, such as lifestyle or environmental factors that influence the varying degree and rate at which people age. Normal aging can be conceived of as the sum of intrinsic and extrinsic aging plus idiosyncratic or genetic variables unique to each individual (Peterson, 1994). In contrast, Busse (1969) distinguished between primary and secondary aging. He defined the former as a time-related biological process that was not contingent on stress, trauma, or disease. Secondary or pathological aging refers to decrements in function associated with chronic disease or trauma. The focus of this chapter will be on intrinsic or primary aging. However, the influence of extrinsic or secondary aging is acknowledged throughout.

The normal biological aging process has several features which distinguish it. First, the aging process is ubiquitous, universal, and developmental, occurring to some extent in everyone after maturation (Evans, 1994). It is an individualized and variable process such that organ systems within individuals age at different rates and thus, as people get older the less alike they actually become (Lewis, 1990; Peterson, 1994; Williams, 1994). Yet aging is characterized by a predictable, inevitable evolution and maturation until death (Williams, 1994). It is progressive such that the probability of developing age-related conditions increases with time. Further, normal biological aging processes cause irreversible changes in cells or organs and permanently increase the probability that a given individual will suffer from harmful consequences (Peterson, 1994). Similarly, there is an increased vulnerability to disease with increasing age and a reduced ability to adapt to environmental change (Cristofalo, 1990). According to Cristofalo (1990, p. 6), "aging is a process which is quite distinct from disease, the fundamental changes of aging can be thought of as providing the substratum in which the age-associated diseases can flourish."

PEARL

It appears that age changes can be attributed to a host of factors including normal development, environmental factors, genetic traits, disease, and an inborn aging process (Harman, 1998).

THEORIES OF AGING

Currently, there are a multiplicity of theories used to classify the aging process. Many have been rejected, others considered plausible, yet others still under scrutiny. The theories derive from changes within selected organ systems, and are cellular system or population based. Abrams, Beers, and Berkow (1995) classified the theories as stochastic or nonstochastic. Stochastic theories posit that aging events occur randomly and accumulate with time whereas nonstochastic theories hold that aging is predetermined. The nonstochastic theories are organ-system based whereas the stochastic theories include the error catastrophe theory, crosslinking theory, and the free radical theory.

Geriatric Audiology. B.E. Weinstein. Thieme Medical Publishers, Inc., New York © 2000

The Nonstochastic or Organ System-Based Theories

Organ system–based theories of aging relate aging to changes in certain organ systems. These theories suppose that certain organs or organ systems (e.g., the immune and endocrine systems) are intrinsic pacemakers of the aging process, genetically programmed to fail at specific times during the life cycle. This programmed senescence is hypothesized to affect the aging of the entire organism (Abrams, Beers, & Berkow, 1995).

The Immune System Theory

The immune system theory of aging was described in depth by Walford (1969).

PEARL
The immune system theory of aging is based on the changes within the immune system with age, which are frequently associated with immunodeficiency and defective host defense mechanisms that can increase the chances of developing infectious disease and associated morbidity and mortality (Adler & Nagel, 1994).

It has its basis in biologists' understanding of the normal immune system. The immune system provides a crucial mechanism for the individual's interaction with the environment. It is the body's line of defense against foreign substances entering the body, producing antibodies to foreign proteins or chemicals introduced from outside the body (Hayflick, 1994). The immune system comprises several cell types, which form a network of interacting elements (Abrams, Beers, & Berkow, 1995). These interacting elements work together to generate cell-mediated immunity (T lymphocytes or T cells), humoral immunity (B lymphocytes or B cells), and nonspecific immunity (monocytes and polymorphonuclear neutrophil leukocytes) (Abrams, Beers, & Berkow, 1995). The thymus plays an important role in cell-mediated immunity because it is the gland that provides the site for T-cell precursors from the bone marrow to mature and differentiate (Abrams, Beers, & Berkow, 1995). The thymus gland involutes in middle age with the loss of thymic mass beginning at age 30 and continuing until age 50. By age 50, only about 5 to 10% of thymic mass remains (Abrams, Beers, & Berkow, 1995). However, the total number of T and B cells in circulation does not appear to change with age. But T-cell functional capacity does decline. The term *functional capacity* refers to the ability of the immune system to produce the appropriate antibodies in adequate numbers. The decline in functional capacity as one ages leads to a deficiency in cell-mediated immunity as these cells are integral to the body's ability to fight disease (Hayflick, 1994). It has been reported that only 25% of older persons have no decline in T-cell function, while 50% have a moderate decline and 25% a marked decline (Abrams, Beers, & Berkow, 1995). Associated with the decline in the function of T cells with age, there is an increase in autoimmune disease and reduced resistance to disease with age.

SPECIAL CONSIDERATION
Although plausible, there are some inherent flaws in the immune system theory of aging. Most notable are its lack of universality, the large interpopulation variability in levels of immune function among individuals, and the fact that a faulty immune system leads to disease that is pathological, rather than normal (Hayflick, 1994).

The Neuroendocrine Theory

The neuroendocrine theory of aging is based on functional changes in the neuroendocrine system. The neuroendocrine system comprises the hypothalamus, the thyroid, and the pituitary and adrenal glands. Endocrine glands secrete hormones that regulate early development, growth, puberty, reproduction, protein synthesis, metabolism, and, in part, the activities of the major organ systems in the body (Cristofalo, 1990). In short, the hormones produced by the endocrine system are in large part responsible for the maintainence of normal life processes. Accordingly, functional changes within the system are accompanied by or regulate functional decrements throughout the organism (Cristofalo, 1990). The neuroendocrine theory proposes that changes in the endocrine glands, such as age-related decline in the release of selected hormones, can accelerate selected aging processes (Hayflick, 1994). However, according to Cristofalo (1990), the changes in the neuroendocrine system, although fundamental and occurring in all tissues of the body, are not universal. Cristofalo (1990) and others have reasoned,

SPECIAL CONSIDERATION
Although the study of aging in the neuroendocrine system is revealing about the aging of the organism, it falls short of accounting for aging at the most fundamental level.

therefore, that as with the immune system theory, the role of the endocrine theory in the regulation of aging remains to be determined.

The Rate of Living Theory

The rate of living theory holds that humans are born with a limited amount of important, life sustaining substances, which upon becoming expended lead to aging and death. Genetic factors largely determine life span, with the factors differing for each species (Abrams, Beers, & Berkow, 1995). There is no solid evidence supporting this theory, as the substance or entity that becomes depleted has not yet been isolated (Hayflick, 1994).

Stochastic or Cellular-Based Theories

Stochastic or cellular-based theories reason that aging is caused by the accumulation of insults from the environment that ultimately reach a level that is destructive to life (Cristofalo, 1990). Thus, stochastic theories hold that aging events occur at random, tending to accumulate over time. The theories described in this section are among the most prominent.

The Error Catastrophe Theory

The error catastrophe theory was first detailed by Orgel (1963) of the Salk Institute. It is based in part on the assumption that proteins, molecules that are designed by DNA, are essential to almost all of a cell's vital processes, the cell being the fundamental living unit. Similarly, protein molecules are integral to a number of bodily functions such as holding tissues together. Protein molecules are manufactured in cells with the assistance of enzymes that are proteins as well (Hayflick, 1994). According to this theory, if an error occurs in an enzyme used to manufacture proteins, then the protein molecules produced in cells and manufactured by the enzyme might exhibit certain structural alterations.

SPECIAL CONSIDERATION

If the error containing protein is involved in the synthesis of genetic material or in the protein synthesizing material, then these molecules could potentially produce further errors, increasing the number of error-containing protein molecules. If sufficient errors in the protein molecules accumulate, the end result could be an aging crisis.

The error catastrophe theory, or the idea that error accumulation is responsible for age changes, has not been supported by subsequent research, which has demonstrated that, despite the presence of altered proteins in aging cells and tissues, there is no evidence of age-dependent missynthesis (Cristofalo, 1990). Hayflick (1994) acknowledged that accumulation of errors in proteins may contribute to aging. In sum, this theory holds that over time an accumulation of errors in protein synthesis results in impaired cell function (Abrams, Beers, & Berkow, 1995).

The Somatic Mutation Theory

The error catastrophe and the somatic mutation theory are interrelated cellular-based theories. The somatic mutation theory, or the genetic mutation theory, is based on biologists' understanding of mutations, which are changes that occur in genes and are fundamental to life (Hayflick, 1994). It states that genetic damage or mutations are radiation induced. The resulting mutations will accumulate, ultimately leading to functional failure and death (Cristofalo, 1990).

CONTROVERSIAL POINT

Despite experimental evidence that exposure to ionizing radiation shortens life, there are ample data to the contrary. Further, life span shortening by exposure to radiation is not necessarily related to the mechanism of normal aging (Cristofalo, 1990).

The Free Radical Theory

The free radical theory of aging is one of the oldest and still the most popular mechanistic theory of aging (Ashock & Ali, 1999). Having originated in radiation biology, the seed for the free radical theory was first planted by Gerschman in 1954; however, Denham Harman is the chief proponent of this theory of aging (Hayflick, 1994). There has been a flurry of research over the past decade documenting the role of oxidants on reactive oxgen species in aging (Beckman & Ames, 1998). It holds that aging occurs because of damage caused by free radicals, which are unstable molecular fragments formed by complex chemical reactions (Cristofalo, 1990; Hayflick, 1994; Martin, 1992). The free radicals are highly reactive elements, which contain an unpaired electron or are missing an electron from the outer shell. They are capable of and eager to react or pair with available molecules from any part of the cell, including DNA, protein, and lipids (Martin, 1992).

PEARL

The most common free radical in cells is superoxide and the molecules caused by its interactions (Cristofalo, 1990).

Free radicals can quickly be destroyed by protective enzyme systems, yet according to the free-radical theory, some escape destruction and cause damage in important biological structures (Cristofalo, 1990). Upon uniting with neighboring molecules free radicals can create considerable destruction because the molecules to which they attach are prevented from performing their designated function in the cell (Martin, 1992). This accumulation of damage, which ultimately interferes with function, can cause death.

Examples of the damage created by free radicals includes the accumulation of lipofuscin, an "age pigment" that accumulates in aging cells, such as those in the inner ear, or the formation of the neuritic plaques characteristic of dementia of the Alzheimer's type (Hayflick, 1994). Evidence in support of the free radical theory of aging is the observation that chemicals, known as antioxidants, can inhibit the formation of free radicals by preventing unpaired oxygen electrons from attaching to susceptible molecules (Hayflick, 1994). Antioxidants, such as vitamins E and C, are produced by the human body and can be taken orally in the form of vitamins.

Additional evidence in support of the free radical theory is the fact that metabolic rate is directly related to free radical production and inversely proportional to life span. As such, it has been hypothesized that free radical generation is related in some way to life span determination (Cristofalo, 1990). While the free radical theory enjoys considerable popularity it has not been proven categorically to be a major cause of age changes (Hayflick, 1994).

Population-Based Theories

Population-based theories are of two varieties. Type I theories imply that aging is an inherent, fundamental property of biological systems whereas the Type II theories assume that aging is the result of collagen cross-linking.

The Rate of Living Theory

The rate of living theory holds that humans are born with a limited amount of important, life-sustaining substances that, upon becoming expended, lead to aging and death. There is no solid evidence supporting this theory, as the substance or entity that becomes depleted has not yet been isolated (Hayflick, 1994).

The Cross-Linking Theory

The cross-linking theory proposed by Kohn (1978) and Bjorksten (1974) holds that selected molecules, including proteins such as collagen, elastin, and nucleic acids, which are abundant in the human body, increasingly cross-link because of the action of selected chemicals in the body. Cross-linking is a natural process of maturation that can potentially interfere with basic physiologic and metabolic processes (Hayflick, 1994). Many of the molecules that cross-link serve basic human functions. Thus cross-linking of molecules at certain sites may lead to improved function while at other sites it may lead to impaired function (Cristofalo, 1990). Nucleic acids are the molecules that constitute our genes whereas collagen and elastin are proteins that help to hold cells together. Nearly one-third of all the protein in the human body is made up of collagen, which is found in tendons, ligaments, bone, cartilage, and skin (Hayflick, 1994). Collagen is essentially the glue that holds soft tissue together. It is composed of parallel molecules, held together by cross-links, which are analogous to rungs that hold the legs of a ladder together (Hayflick, 1994). In animals, small numbers of adjacent molecules cross-link yet the collagen remains pliable enough to allow for movement of the molecules. As animals age, there is an increase in the number of molecules that cross-link with one another, leading to stiffness and shrinkage of tissue. In general, with increasing age, this theory postulates that many molecules within the human body become increasingly cross-linked, interfering with basic physiologic processes, including the passage of nutrients and wastes into and out of cells. As errors occur over time in different molecules due to cross-linking, age changes are thought to occur (Hayflick, 1994). In sum, this theory posits that the cross-linking of protein and other substances leads to age dependent disease and disorders.

CONCLUDING REMARKS

Hayflick (1994) suggested that perhaps no one theory or mechanism can account for why humans and animals age. In fact, one of the most fascinating aspects of aging remains how different the process is from individual to individual (Christensen, 1999). In considering the possible causes of aging, Strehler (1977) proposed that to be a contender, the theories should meet the following set of criteria:

1. The theory must explain why the process is deleterious or why losses in physiological function occur.
2. The process must be gradual.
3. The phenomenon must be intrinsic and unable to be corrected.
4. The theory must be universal, applying to all species.

According to the conditions established by Strehler (1977), Table 2–1 summarizes the status of each of the aging theories. Based on the review of aging theories, it appears safe to conclude the following: (1) aging is a series of biological changes associated with the passage of time, which occurs in biological as well as nonbiological systems; (2) there is no one theory that explains "why" or "how" we age; (3) aging is unavoidable, universal, and has many causes; (4) aging is an extremely variable phenomenon across biological, cognitive, personality, and social characteristics; and (5) the aging process is progressive and deleterious (Blass, Cherniack, & Weiss, 1992). Further, most scientists would agree that gerontology as a science is considered to be in an early stage, with research necessary and, in many cases underway, to unravel the mechanism(s) of aging (Hayflick, 1994). The discussion that follows outlines recent findings on changes in the human organism due to intrinsic aging. I have attempted to describe only the changes that are viewed as part of normal biological aging processes and/or normal physiologic aging. Minimal attention has been devoted to diseases that show increasing incidence with increasing age, diseases that are aging processes themselves, or diseases

TABLE 2–1 Theories of Aging

Theory	Status*
Organ System-Based Theories	
Immune System Theory	No experimental evidence
Neuroendocrine System Theory	No experimental evidence
Stochastic or Cellular-Based Theories	
Orgel's Error Catastrophe Theory	Refuted
Somatic Mutation Theory	Refuted
Free Radical Theory	Popular—still under study
Population-Based Theories	
Rate of Living Theory	No evidence
Crosslinking Theory	Currently disfavored

*As of this writing.

that have more serious consequences with increasing age (Peterson, 1994).

CHANGES ASSOCIATED WITH AGING

A number of changes in organ systems occur gradually as people age. Many of the changes can be explained on the basis of the theories of aging previously discussed. Most of the

SPECIAL CONSIDERATION

For the most part, aging changes are highly specific to the individual and the organ system, and thus the rate of decline or failure varies dramatically across individuals (Hayflick, 1994).

data derive from cross-sectional studies of cohorts of older adults and to a lesser extent from ongoing longitudinal studies. While several thousands of age changes have been identified, the discussion will focus on morphologic changes in the systems and those functional implications that may have a potential impact on hearing status and/or the delivery of comprehensive audiologic services to older adults.

Body Configuration and Composition

As humans age there are a number of changes taking place that contribute to declines in body systems. Most notable is the loss of body water or decline in the proportion of body weight attributable to water. Water makes up two-thirds of the body weight and is found in extracellular and intracellular compartments, and in the form of plasma, lymph fluid, and spinal fluid. Accordingly, changes in water metabolism contribute to a number of changes within organ systems (Morley, 1990). Further, aging is associated with reductions in lean body mass; declines in protein synthesis and in pro-

tein degradation rates; and a decrease in the amount of potassium in the human body (Morley, 1990). On average, by age 75, the number of cells in the human body may have declined by as much as 30% exacting a toll on major systems. These changes have implications for appearance, size of selected body parts, structure, and function.

Appearance

Overall, there is a gradual decrease in height in both genders as we age, along with a decrease in weight after age 55. Reductions in height are attributable to changes in the skeleton, including calcification of tendons and ligaments; thinning of vertebral discs associated with osteoporosis; and weakening and shrinkage of muscle groups (Tideiksaar & Silverton, 1989). Characteristically, as people age they assume a more stooped posture with the head and neck bent slightly forward and the hips and knees flexed. It is likely that normal aging changes in height contribute to instability and an increased prevalence of falls among older adults.

Declines in weight are due to a decline in lean tissue mass, decrease in total body water, decline in muscle mass, and bone loss (Kane, Ouslander, & Abrass, 1994). Whereas slight weight loss is common with increasing age, significant weight loss may be symptomatic of an active disease process. For example, it is well recognized that weight loss is common in individuals who are undernourished, have Alzheimer's disease, suffer from depression, undergo drug–nutrient interactions, and have cancer. The changes in body composition can have a significant effect on level of function.

PEARL

An audiologist's index of suspicion should be aroused when a hearing-impaired client suffers from a dramatic weight loss, and the appropriate referral should be made.

The Skin

Human skin has several major roles. It serves as a protective barrier against mechanical, thermal, or chemical injuries and from loss of fluid; as an interface with the external environment; as a thermoregulator; and as a window through which the body reveals its internal pathology (Kaminer & Gilchrest, 1994). Specialized mechanoreceptors in the skin register pressure, touch, and vibration (Despopoulos & Silbernagl, 1991; Frick, Leonhardt, & Starck, 1991). The skin also participates in immunobiological defense reactions. In general, the skin shows dramatic changes with age. In fact, some of the changes in the skin lining the external ear canal are of particular relevance to audiologists during selected procedures (e.g., cerumen management; earmold/hearing aid impressions; and diagnostic tests including immittance testing and otoacoustic emissions). A brief overview of skin anatomy will facilitate the discussion.

The skin is composed of several interrelated functional layers that tend to undergo changes with age. The layers include the epidermis, the dermis, the subcutaneous fat, and the cutaneous appendages (Balin, 1990). The layers are shown in Figure 2–1. The epidermis is the outer or most superficial layer of the skin. It serves as the cutaneous surface of the skin. It comprises several layers and functions primarily to protect the deeper tissues from drying, invasion by organisms, and trauma. The epidermis is composed primarily of keratinocytes, which are constantly being reproduced after being pushed to the surface, replacing other keratinocyte cells that have died and are subsequently shed (Kaminer & Gilchrest, 1994). It takes approximately 28 days for the turnover of keratinocyte cells to take place. The turnover time of these epidermal cells is reduced dramatically as people age (Kaminer & Gilchrest, 1994). As a result of these age-related changes, there is a decrease in the rate at which wounds heal. In addition to keratinocytes, the epidermis contains melanocytes and Langerhans cells. The melanocytes contain melanin, which is responsible for defining skin color and serves as the body's protection against solar radiation (Kaminer & Gilchrest, 1994). There is a steady decrease in melanocytes with each decade, which occurs in both sun-protected and sun-exposed skin. Graying of hair, for example, is a manifestation of loss of function of the melanocytes (Balin, 1990). The Langerhans cells, which derive from the bone marrow, are important for antigen recognition. With age, there is a dramatic decrease in the number of Langerhans cells. This decrease is greatest in photoaged skin.

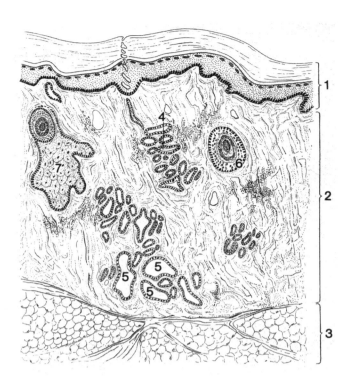

Figure 2–1 Functional layers of the skin: 1, epidermis; 2, dermis; 3, subcutaneous connective tissue; 4, sweat gland; 5, apocrine sweat gland; 6, hair root sheath; 7, sebaceous gland with hair root sheath. (From Frick, Leonhardt, and Starck, 1991. Reprinted by permission.)

PEARL

The decline in the number of Langerhans cells is associated with delayed hypersensitivity reactions. Accordingly, older adults have a diminished capacity to manifest characteristic reactions when exposed to known allergens.

The dermis or inner layer of skin lies beneath the epidermis. It contains blood vessels, nerves, lymphatics, and such cellular components as collagen and elastin, which are produced by fibroblasts and provide the skin with its tensile strength and elasticity (Kaminer & Gilchrest, 1994). With few exceptions, throughout the body the dermis contains hair follicles and the major sensory fibers that help humans distinguish between pain, touch, heat, and cold. Sebaceous glands, such as those located in the outer third of the ear canal, are located in the dermis. These glands have primary responsibility for protecting the skin against dryness through the production of an oily substance known as sebum. Sweat glands, which produce perspiration, allowing for the elimination of water and electrolytes, are also found in the dermis (Falvo, 1991). The dermis has an extensive microvasculature network that contributes to thermoregulation and the inflammatory response of the skin (Kaminer & Gilchrest, 1994). The dermis undergoes significant anatomic and physiologic change with age, which may impact considerably on audiologic practice. Overall, there is an approximate 20% loss in dermal thickness with age that can account for the paper thin appearance of the skin of some older adults (Kaminer & Gilchrest, 1994). The most pertinent anatomic and physiologic changes are displayed in Table 2–2. The reduced vascular response of old skin to chemical irritants and microbial invasion can mute inflammatory reactions. Further, the diminished tensile strength of the dermis, which is produced by the decrease in collagen, and the re-

TABLE 2–2   Age-Related Anatomic and Physiologic Changes within the Dermis

Anatomic:
1. Decrease in number of cells
2. Decrease in elasticity
3. Decrease in thickness
4. Reduction in microvasculature
5. Decrease in amount of fibroblasts, collagen, and elastin
6. Loss of efficiency of nerve cells

Physiologic:
1. Decreased sensitivity to pain and pressure
2. Increase in the size of sebaceous glands and decrease in sebum output
3. Skin more easily damaged
4. Altered thermal regulation
5. Decreased sweating
6. Decreased wound healing
7. Muted inflammatory reactions
8. Decreased sensation

Source: Balin (1990).

duction in microvasculature, account in part for diminished wound healing in older adults (Kaminer & Gilchrest, 1994). Another consequence of changes in the dermis is that the cutaneous end organs responsible for pressure, vibration, and light touch sensation decrease to about one-third of their density with advancing age, leading to an increase in pain threshold and resulting susceptibility to skin injury (Kaminer & Gilchrest, 1994).

SPECIAL CONSIDERATION

Audiologists who engage in cerumen management, who take earmold impressions, and who dispense completely-in-the-canal (CIC) hearing aids, must keep in mind the aforementioned dematological concerns and should be ever vigilant about cutaneous pathology.

Finally, the subcutaneous fat layer below the dermis undergoes change with age interfering with its protective and insulation functions (Kaminer & Gilchrest, 1994). The cutaneous appendages are eccrine glands, apocrine glands, and pilosebaceous units composed of hair follicles and sebaceous glands. Sebacous glands increase dramatically in size in the elderly. However, there is a 40 to 60% decrease in sebum production with age (Kaminer & Gilchrest, 1994). The implications for cerumen production are discussed in Chapter 4.

In sum, with aging the epidermis undergoes an overall thinning and a decrease in the size and proliferation rate of keratinocytes. Similarly, the thickness, density, and cellularity of the dermis decrease leading to a thin feeling to the skin. Further, collagen fibers become thicker and corre-

spondingly less flexible resulting in increased susceptibility to tear. Finally, there is a loss of vascularity of the skin.

SPECIAL CONSIDERATION

The above changes in older skin often affect the skin that lines structures of the ear, making it more sensitive to trauma, disorders, and compromised wound healing relative to younger adults.

Cutaneous disorders with a predilection for the ear include pruritus, or itching; seborrheic dermatitis, a chronic superficial inflammatory disorder of the skin; seborrheic keratoses, a benign lesion of the skin; and basal or squamous cell carcinoma. Dermatologic pathology warrants referral to the dermatologist.

THE NERVOUS SYSTEM

The nervous system serves as the command center, or as a relayer of information, for a variety of body functions. It coordinates and controls behavioral activities throughout the body in response to the internal and external environment by sending, receiving, and sorting electrical impulses (Falvo, 1991). The major functional unit of the nervous system is the neuron that transmits neural impulses. The component parts of the neuron are shown in Figure 2–2. The nervous system is composed of the central and peripheral nervous systems. Figure 2–3 displays the central nervous system. The brain and spinal cord make up the central nervous system, while the nerves that extend from the brain and spinal cord make up the peripheral nervous system. The brain contains approximately one hundred billion nerve cells and billions of supporting or glial cells. At its peak (age 20), the brain weighs approximately three pounds (Hayflick, 1994). Lipids account for more than half of the dry weight of the brain and the protein content is high as well (Poirier & Finch, 1994). The nerves within the peripheral nervous system that bring information toward the central nervous system from other parts of the body constitute the afferent division of the peripheral nervous system. Those nerves that carry impulses from the central nervous system to other parts of the body make up the efferent division of the peripheral nervous system. The neurons in the brain are postmitotic cells that do not duplicate or replicate themselves following cell death. The cells of the auditory sense organ and neural pathways are nonmitotics. That is, after specialized function has been established, they too pursue the course of aging and dying.

SPECIAL CONSIDERATION

The brain is plastic such that remaining neurons tend to sprout new connections and "repair or compensate for the short or broken circuits that occur when a neighboring neuron dies" (Hayflick, 1994, p. 163).

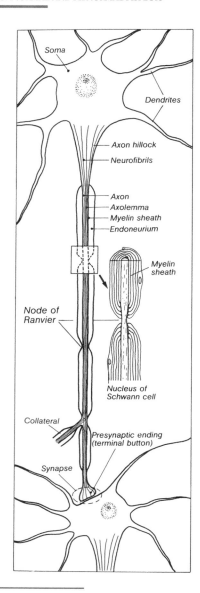

Figure 2–2 Component parts of the neuron. (From Despopoulos and Silbernagl, 1991. Reprinted by permission.)

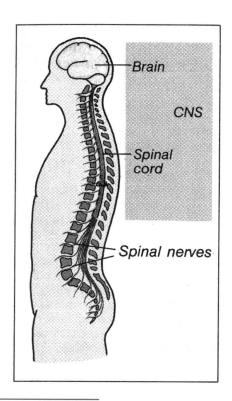

Figure 2–3 The central nervous system. (From Despopoulos and Silbernagl, 1991. Reprinted by permission.)

leased by the axons enable nerve impulses to be transmitted between neurons. Examples of neurotransmitters within the brain include dopamine, norepinephrine, epinephrine, serotonin, and acetylcholine. Enzymes such as acetyltransferase or acetylcholinesterase work with the neurotransmit-

When the brain is sectioned, gray brown regions known as gray matter can be distinguished from glistening white areas known as white matter (Frick, Leonhardt, & Starck, 1991). The distribution of white and gray matter in the central nervous system is shown in Figure 2–4. The white matter of the central nervous system, which makes up the inner part of the brain and the outer part of the spinal cord, is composed of myelinated fibers that conduct nerve messages. The white appearance of the nerve fibers is due to the glial cells, which form a fatty insulation around the axons. Gray matter or nonmyelinated nerve fibers make up the outer portion of the brain and the inner part of the spinal cord. The gray matter of the brain is responsible for receiving, sorting, and processing nerve messages, whereas the gray matter of the spinal cord serves as a center for reflexive actions (Falvo, 1991). Neurotransmitters or chemicals re-

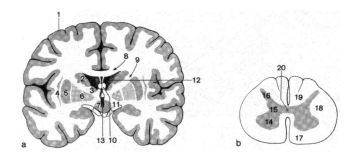

Figure 2–4 Distribution of white and gray matter in the central nervous system: (a) frontal section through the brain, section surface viewed from behind; (b) cross section through the spinal chord. 1, cerebrum; 2, caudate nucleus; 3, thalamus; 4, claustrum; 5, putamen; 6, globus pallidus; 7, hypothalmic nuclei; 8, corpus callosum; 9, inner capsule; 10, fornix; 11, optic tract; 12, lateral ventricle; 13, third ventricle; 14, anterior column; 15, lateral column; 16, posterior column; 17, anterior funiculus; 18, lateral funiculus; 19, posterior funiculus; 20, central canal. (From Frick, Leonhardt, and Starck, 1991. Reprinted by permission.)

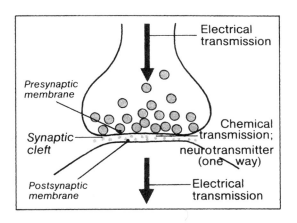

Figure 2–5 The synapse. (From Despopoulos and Silbernagl, 1991. Reprinted by permission.)

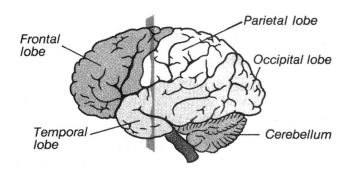

Figure 2–6 Lateral surface of the brain. (From Despopoulos and Silbernagl, 1991. Reprinted by permission.)

ters to enable neurons to communicate with each other. Figure 2–5 displays the synapse where signals are transmitted from the axon of one neuron to axon, dendrite, or soma of another.

The nervous system undergoes anatomic and physiologic changes with age that underlie some of the behavioral changes to be discussed in subsequent chapters. With age the human brain undergoes a considerable decrement in weight such that at age 90 it weighs nearly 10% less than it did at age 20 (Hayflick, 1994). The decrease in weight is associated in part with the loss of chemical constituents of the brain including loss of selected proteins and lipids, which occurs with aging (Poirier & Finch, 1994). In light of the weight loss, the brain also undergoes a change in shape especially on its surface with a narrowing of the gyri/convolutions and a widening of the sulci/grooves between the gyri. During aging there is reportedly a change in the neurotransmitter system including a decrease in the amount of chemical associated with neurotransmitter activity and corresponding loss in the synthetic ability of certain catecholaminergic and serotoninergic neurons (Poirier & Finch, 1994).

The number of nerve cells decreases with normal aging as well. Neuronal loss within the brain is quite variable between regions of the brain and among individuals. Nerve cell loss is minimal in the brainstem nuclei yet neuron death is considerable in the cerebral cortex (Abrams, Beers, & Berkow, 1995). In general, neuronal loss ranges from 10 to 60%. With respect to the auditory system, it has been reported that the superior temporal gyrus may lose as much

as 55% of its neuronal content whereas the tip of the temporal lobe may show only a 10 to 35% loss (Poirier & Finch, 1994). Figure 2–6 shows the lateral surface of the brain including the temporal lobe, and Figure 2–7 shows the superior temporal gyrus. Neurons that remain tend to accumulate lipofuscin, or aging pigment, which is most pronounced in the cell body. In certain individuals the accumulation of lipofuscin contributes to the development of neurofibrillary tangles upon which metals such as aluminum may deposit. In the extreme case, the appearance of neurofibrillary tangles is associated with senile dementia of the Alzheimer's type. Although plaques and tangles are a hallmark of Alzheimer's disease, they also appear, albeit in lesser numbers, in the brains of older persons without clinical evidence of the disease (Abrams, Beers, & Berkow, 1995). Finally, the amount of sheath surrounding the axons of peripheral nerves decreases with age, perhaps contributing to a reduction in neural conduction time. These changes in the nerve fibers explain in part the decrease in the speed with which action potentials travel with age in both the afferent and the efferent systems.

PEARL

The behavioral implications of the changes in the nervous system include a slowing of central processing, which may manifest as slowed psychomotor responses, decreased motor reaction time, increased motor response time, and decreased performance on selected intellectual tasks including a slowing in the ability to learn new information, and noncritical forgetfulness (Abrams, Beers, & Berkow, 1995).

However, in persons free of brain disease, overall intellectual performance tends to be maintained well into the 80s (Abrams, Beers, & Berkow, 1995). It is important to note that as the brain has a surplus of brain cells, it is not the number of cells lost that accounts for behavioral changes, but rather the location of the brain cell loss and the ability of cells in

PEARL

The histological changes that are universal in the aging brain include accumulation of lipofuscin and the appearance of neurofibrillary tangles in mesial temporal structures (Mrak, Griffin, & Graham, 1997).

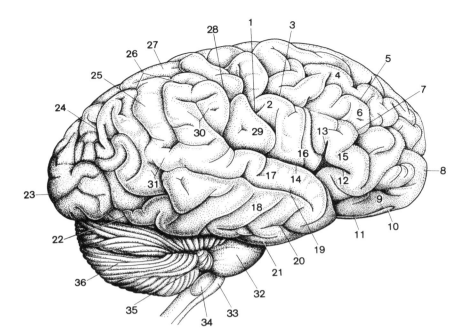

Figure 2–7 View of the superior temporal gyrus. 1, central sulcus; 2, precentral gyrus; 3, precentral sulcus; 4, superior frontal gyrus; 5, superior frontal sulcus; 6, middle frontal gyrus; 7, inferior frontal sulcus; 8, frontal pole; 9, orbital gyri; 10, olfactory bulb; 11, olfactory tract; 12, anterior ramos; 13, ascending ramus; 14, posterior ramos; 15, frontal operculum; 16, frontoparietal operculum; 17, superior temporal gyrus; 18, middle temporal gyrus; 19, superior temporal sulcus; 20, inferior temporal sulcus; 21, inferior temporal gyrus; 22, preoccipital notch; 23, occipital pole; 24, transverse occipital sulcus; 25, inferior parietal lobule; 26, intraparietal sulcus; 27, superior parietal lobule; 28, postcentral sulcus; 29, postcentral gyrus; 30, supramarginal gyrus; 31, angular gyrus; 32, pons; 33, pyramid; 34, olive; 35, flocculus; 36, cerebellar hemisphere. (From Frick, Leonhardt, and Starck, 1991. Reprinted by permission.)

that region to make new connections with remaining neurons. Further, certain properties of the brain including its redundancy, the availability of compensatory mechanisms, and plasticity at the level of the nerve cell, may mitigate some of the adverse effects of age-related changes in the brain (Abrams, Beers, & Berkow, 1995). For example, recent studies have shown that the gradual deterioration and dying off of nerve cells may be accompanied by compensatory lengthening and an increasing number of dendrites in the remaining nerve cells. Thus, possible new connections within the dendritic tree may make up for fewer cells (Abrams, Beers, & Berkow, 1995).

PEARL

The changes in response time have implications for pure-tone testing. The slowing in the ability to learn new information impacts on aspects of audiologic rehabilitation. The fact that overall intellectual performance is maintained well into the 80s underlines the importance of treating the older adult as an intelligent human being deserving of respect and support.

Modifications in the test battery due to changes in the nervous system consist of the following:

- Respect the patient.
- Do not be condescending.
- Do not infantilize.
- Allow extra time in schedule.
- Provide extra pacing between stimulus presentations and patient responses.
- Repeat instructional set.

- Verify that the patient understands the response task required.
- Use facilitatory strategies to make sure that the patient learns new tasks.
- Repeat or review material from previous section before moving on to next lesson in the lesson plan.
- Write down important information at end of each section.
- Use all modalities to ensure or promote recall of new information.

The Musculoskeletal System

The skeletal system is made of 206 bones, which support the framework of the body. Bone is metabolically active and its structural integrity relies on the metabolic processes of its bony tissue (Abrams, Beers, & Berkow, 1995). The skeletal system supports the surrounding tissues and assists in movement, providing leverage and attachment of muscles. Bones store calcium and other mineral salts and along with ligaments, tendons, and cartilage are connective tissue, which support and connect other tissue and tissue parts. Tendons, made of cells and macromolecules (e.g., collagen), are bands of connective tissue that connect muscle to bone, enabling muscle movement. Collagen makes up most of the weight of tendons. Collagen fibers form the main supportive protein in skin, tendon, bone, cartilage, and connective tissue and provide the necessary rigidity and strength. Ligaments are tough bands of tissue that connect bones at the joint site and provide stability during movement. Bones are bound together at joints, of which there are several different varieties. Thus, a joint is the place where two or more bones come together. *Articulation* is the term that defines the coming together of two bones at a joint. Joints are classified according to different criteria depending for the most part on

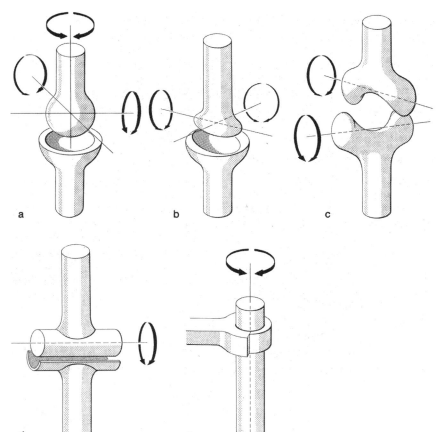

Figure 2–8 Forms of joints: (a) ball-and-socket joint; (b) ellipsoid joint; (c) saddle joint; (d) hinge joint; (e) pivot joint. The arrows indicate the direction in which skeletal elements can be moved around respective axis. (From Frick, Leonhardt, and Starck, 1991. Reprinted by permission.)

the number of skeletal elements articulating at a joint cavity (Frick, Leonhardt, & Starck, 1991). Some joints are synovial or freely movable, others are ball and socket and allow for circular movements. Some joints are fibrous or fixed and still others are cartilaginous allowing for slight movements.

SPECIAL CONSIDERATION

The middle ear contains a number of joints of different varieties that are susceptible to age-related change.

Figure 2–8 shows five different forms of joints classified according to the shape of their joint surfaces. Cartilage is a dense type of connective tissue that can withstand considerable tension. It is typically found covering the ends of bone, and is composed primarily of water and secondarily of chondrocytes and macromolecules. There are several types of cartilage in the human body including elastic cartilage, which is found in the external ear; fibrocartilage, located between the vertebral disks of the spine; articular cartilage; hyaline cartilage; and annular cartilage. Articular cartilage, which is avascular, forms the lining of the articular surfaces of bone. It is encircled by a fibrous articular capsule that is lined by the synovial membrane. The latter produces syno-

vial fluid, a lubricant that allows for smooth articulation of bone. Thus, articular cartilage receives its nourishment from synovial fluid helping it to absorb shock associated with joint movement. Figure 2–9 shows the auricular (elastic) cartilage of the pinna and the cartilage surrounding a portion of the eustachian tube.

The body comprises several different types of muscles. Some muscles such as the smooth muscle in the digestive tract are involuntary, working automatically, while others such as striated or skeletal muscle are under voluntary control (Falvo, 1991). Muscles are surrounded by a muscle sheath of connective tissue containing blood vessels and nerve fibers. Muscles produce movement by the contraction of opposite muscle groups and always maintain a partial state of contraction because of continuous muscle stimulation. Figure 2–10 shows a pennate type muscle (i.e., stapedius muscle) that is unique in light of the oblique attachments of the muscle fibers to the tendons.

In general, the skeleton undergoes dramatic change with age. After age 30, there is a 15% turnover of the skeleton annually, which results in an increase in bone density (Abrams, Beers, & Berkow, 1995). Turnover refers to events at the cellular level responsible for bone constantly being formed and resorbed. However, the rate of resorption exceeds the rate of formation after age 30 such that there is a gradual net loss of bone density with age. This is accelerated

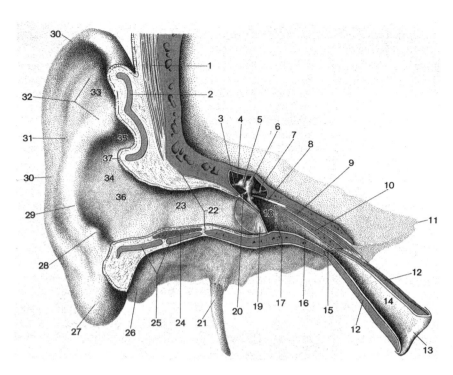

Figure 2–9 Auricular cartilage of the pinna, and cartilage surrounding a portion of the eustachian tube. 1, temporalis muscle; 2, auricular cartilage; 3, posterior ligament of incus; 4, epitympanic recess; 5, body of incus with superior ligament; 6, head of malleus with superior ligament of malleus; 7, stapes; 8, tendon of sensor tympani, attachment at manubrium of malleus; 9, tensor tympani in semicanal for tensor tympani; 10, septum of musculotubal canal; 11, apex of petrous part of temporal bone; 12, cartilage; 13, pharyngeal opening; 14, cartilaginous part; 15, isthmus; 16, bony part; 17, tympanic opening; 18, tympanic cavity; 19, tympanic membrane; 20, lateral ligament of malleus; 21, styloid process of temporal bone; 22, opening of external acoustic meatus; 23, external acoustic meatus; 24, ceruminous glands; 25, cartilaginous portion of external auditory meatus; 26, mastoid process; 27, lobule; 28, antitragus; 29, anthelix; 30, helix; 31, scaphoid fossa; 32, crura of anthelix; 33, triangular fossa; 34, concha; 35, cymba conchae; 36, cavity of concha; 37, crus of helix. (From Frick, Leonhardt, and Starck, 1991. Reprinted by permission.)

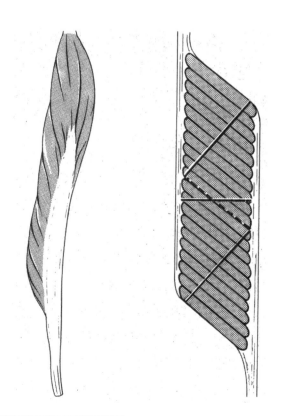

Figure 2–10 Pennate type muscle. (From Frick, Leonhardt, and Starck, 1991. Reprinted by permission.)

in women because of hormonal changes of menopause (Abrams, Beers, & Berkow, 1995). Thus, overall, normal aging produces a loss of bone tissue beginning at age 50, proceeding at a more rapid rate for women than men, such that women lose about 30% and men about 17% of their bone mass with age (Hayflick, 1994). *Senile osteopenia* is a term that refers to normal age-associated bone loss. In contrast, osteoporosis is a metabolic bone disorder wherein the structural integrity of bone tissue is compromised (Boskey, 1990). It is a pathologic state characterized by a gradual decline in bone mass with decreasing bone density increasing one's susceptibility to fractures.

Collagen becomes irregular in shape, bound more tightly together, and more rigid with age. Further, the fibers are less likely to be in a uniform parallel formation. As noted earlier in this chapter, less collagen is degraded and less is synthesized with age. The changes in collagen tissue are in part responsible for decreased mobility in the body's tissue with advancing age (Lewis & Bottomley, 1990). When collagen in the fibers surrounding joints undergoes age-related changes, joints become stiff and their range of motion limited. In addition, cartilage becomes less pliable with age. The tissue water content of normal-aged cartilage decreases with age. However osteoarthritis, a disorder of hyaline cartilage and subchondrial bone, which is a leading cause of physical disability in persons over 65, is associated with an increase in tissue water content (Fife, 1994).

Additionally, as people age, muscle fiber is replaced by fatty tissue, which leads to a decrease in muscle mass. Aging is also associated with a decrease in the size and number of available muscle fibers, and a decline in the number of muscle motor units. The speed of muscle contraction, muscular strength, endurance, and muscle mass tend to decrease with age (Tideiksaar, 1989; Lewis & Bottomley, 1990). As a consequence, grip strength tends to decline with age as do exercise tolerance and performance. However, physically active older adults often have exercise capacities equivalent to younger active people (Hayflick, 1994).

In sum, the musculoskeletal system undergoes a number of changes as individuals age. Musculoskeletal disease is a leading cause of functional impairment in older adults. The disabling functional sequelae of musculoskeletal disease are often chronic, considerably altering an individual's lifestyle. However, musculoskeletal disease is considered a disease process rather than an inevitable consequence of aging (Abrams, Beers, & Berkow, 1995).

The Visual System

The visual system is quite complex. The aging process has a number of effects on the eye, some of which have variable effects on vision. Further, there are a number of ocular diseases that are quite prevalent in the elderly. A brief overview of the anatomy and physiology of the eye will facilitate the discussion. The visual organ consists of a globe and its adnexa (Hollwich, 1985). The important anatomical landmarks of the eye are contained in Figure 2–11. The globe has three coats and is embedded in the adnexa. The coats of the globe

include the outer fibrous layer, namely the cornea and sclera; the middle layer or tunica vasculosa, which includes the uvea, which consists of the iris, ciliary body, and choroid; and the inner layer consisting of the retina and pigment epithelium (Hollwich, 1985). The adnexa are the upper and lower lids including the eyelashes, the eyebrows, the muscles that open and close the lids, the lacrimal glands, and the lacrimal drainage system.

The retina, the innermost of the three ocular coats, is a thin, semitransparent, netlike membrane. The retina, which comprises 10 layers of tissue, is continuous with the optic nerve. The retina contains two kinds of photoreceptors, namely the rods and cones, which are the antennae of the visual system. The color-sensitive cones are concerned with visual acuity and color discrimination whereas the rods are concerned with peripheral vision, especially when a room is dim (Tabbara, 1989). The rods are sensitive to differences in degree of illumination and function with reduced illumination responsible for dark adaptation (Hollwich, 1985). The macula, an oval, yellowish spot in the center of the retina, is the key focusing area of the retina, and is responsible for central vision. The macula is the area of sharpest vision. The major functions of the retina are to receive visual images, to partly analyze the visual image, and to send the latter information to the brain.

The outer coat of the visual organ consists of the cornea and the sclera, which together provide a tough resistant coat and capsule for the globe, a highly mobile structure that moves in all directions (Hollwich, 1985). The cornea is a transparent avascular tissue that inserts into the sclera. It has a high water content. It functions as a protective membrane and a window through which light rays pass on their way to the retina. The sclera is the dense, white, opaque, outer coat of the eye that is continuous with the cornea. It prevents scattered light from entering the eye so that the optical pathway through the pupil is not disturbed (Hollwich, 1985).

The middle ocular coat contains a number of important structures. The uvea is spongy and blood-filled and divided into three parts, namely the choroid lining of the sclera, the iris, and the ciliary body. The iris is a colored circular membrane that is suspended behind the cornea and immediately in front of the lens. The round aperture in the center of the iris is the pupil. The pupil located within the iris controls the amount of light entering the eye. The iris contains fibers that constrict to control the pupil, regulating pupillary size and reaction to light. The ciliary body in conjunction with the ciliary muscle and ciliary processes alters the tension of the lens helping it to focus on near and distant objects. The central portion of the eye is filled with vitreous humor. The vitreous is a clear, avascular gelatinous body constituting two-thirds of the volume and weight of the eye. It helps maintain the shape and transparency of the eye (Tabbara, 1989). Finally, the lens, whose sole purpose is to focus light on the retina, is an avascular, colorless, transparent structure that is suspended behind the iris.

The eye undergoes a number of morphologic and functional changes as an individual ages (Rumney, 1998). The physiological changes within the eye and their functional correlates are listed in Table 2–3. The lens of the eye undergoes a host of changes. It tends to thicken, becoming rigid

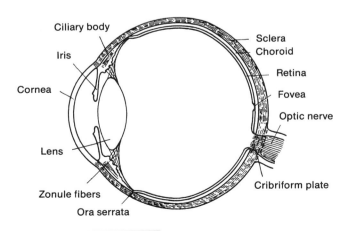

Figure 2–11 Section through the globe.

TABLE 2–3 Physiological Changes and Functional Implications in the Aging Eye

Physiological changes	Functional implications
Lens:	
Increased stiffness	Reduced ability to focus on nearby objects
	Decreased depth perception
	Reduced visual acuity
Yellowing	Decreased color sensitivity
Pupil:	
Narrowing of the pupil's dilation	Slowed dark and light adaptation
Visual Field:	
Reduced visual field	Loss of peripheral vision
Retina:	
Decreased function of the rods and cones	Decreased visual acuity

and inelastic hence limited in its ability to change shape. These changes interfere with visual accommodation or the ability to shift focus from distant to near objects. As a result, the majority of individuals become farsighted as they age as exhibited by the tendency to hold things at arm's length for greater clarity. Presbyopia, or the diminished ability to focus clearly on objects at a normal distance, is the most apparent of the visual changes associated with aging. The lens tends to yellow and become more opaque with age causing the cooler colors to be filtered out whereas the warm colors (e.g., red, yellow, orange) remain more easily seen. Therefore, it becomes difficult to distinguish between blues and greens. Finally, the aging lens develops pinpoint opacities, which produces dazzle from sources of bright light.

The iris becomes more rigid and there is a corresponding decrease in the size of the pupil with age. Further, aging is associated with an impaired ability to increase pupillary diameter. That is, pupillary diameter decreases and direct and consensual reaction to light tends to be reduced. As a result, far less light reaches the retina in older adults than in young adults. In fact, the retina of a 60-year-old receives only one-third of the light received by a 20-year-old. This explains, in part, why older adults require more illumination for reading and to get around safely indoors. The ability to adjust to abrupt changes in illumination is decreased as a result of changes in the pupil. That is, both light and dark adaptation require greater time with age. This difficulty in adjusting when moving from a light to a dark area has implications for speech reading ability. Older adults may complain that objects are not bright because a small pupil allows less light to enter the eye.

Table 2–4 lists the normal visual changes with age that result from the above structural changes along with suggestions for minimizing their functional effects. By far the most common age-related eye problem is presbyopia, which explains why by age 55, nearly all persons have great diffi-

culty focusing on objects at close range without glasses. Presbyopia occurs in 42% of people aged 52 to 64, in 73% of people aged 65 to 74 and in 92% of people aged 75 and over (Hayflick, 1994). The normal visual changes with age include decreased contrast sensitivity, decreases in dark/light adaptation, and delayed glare recovery (Carter, 1994). Each of these may impact on speech reading ability. Contrast sensitivity, which refers to the ability to discern the difference between an object and its background, decreases with age due to a decrease in retinal sensitivity, retinal luminance, and central nervous system changes with age (Carter, 1994). The major complaint of individuals with decreased contrast sensitivity is that they do not see well under conditions of poor lighting or contrast. A partial solution is to increase illumination, to wear amber-tinted lenses indoors, and to use a handheld magnifier to enhance functioning. Dark/light adaptation decreases because the retinal rod photosensitive discs are not replaced efficiently with age, resulting in an inability of the eye to respond to changes in light intensity. The best solution is to wear sunglasses on sunny days and to allow time for adaptation when entering or exiting a dark room (Carter, 1994). Finally, older adults often suffer from delayed glare recovery, which interferes with optimal visual function. Glare arises when scatter from bright lights does not form part of the retinal image.

PEARL

When communicating with older adults audiologists should attempt to avoid poor sources of light such as fluorescent lights, a major source of light scatter. Use of incandescent bulbs decreases disturbing glare, as does use of antireflective coatings on the surface of eyeglasses (Carter, 1994).

TABLE 2–4   Solutions to Age-Related Visual Changes which may Impact on Assessment, Audiologic Rehabilitation, and Communication Ability

Visual change	Diagnosis and management implication
Decrease in visual acuity	Increase illumination without increasing glare; increase contrast during interactions with patient, use large print materials and large images on written instructions and when performing paper-pencil evaluations; establish eye contact and position yourself in the person's line of vision.
Presbyopia	Increase illumination, advise use of corrective lenses to focus the light especially during audiologic rehabilitation.
Decrease in contrast sensitivity	Use magnifiers, good illumination, use bright colors (e.g. red and yellow); add a contrast between colors; (e.g. dark image on a light surface); colors used for identification and locating information should be contrasting such as yellow and blue. This is especially important when highlighting hearing aid controls.
Decrease in dark adaptation	Take a moment to dark/light adapt; use sunglasses to facilitate speechreading ability; avoid abrupt changes in light.
Delayed recovery from glare	Less fluorescent lighting, use of hats and visors can both promote better speechreading ability; light should be even and from multiple sources to insure adequate light levels without glare; curtains or blinds should be adjusted to diffuse sunlight and to prevent direct illumination; shiny surfaces, reflective fixtures or waxed floors add to the problems created by glare.

The information contained in Table 2–4 should be reviewed with older adults with hearing impairment who are instructed to use visual cues to supplement audition. Some of the suggestions can enhance the amount of information derived from vision.

A number of ocular diseases, prevalent among older adults, cause abnormal visual changes. In particular four eye diseases, namely cataracts, glaucoma, macular degeneration, and diabetic retinopathy, account for about 98% of visual loss in persons over 70 years of age (Wainapel, 1994). Table 2–5 provides a brief description of each of these diseases. Audiologists should be familiar with the diseases listed in Table 2–5 as more than 2 million individuals over 65 years are classified as having low vision resulting from one or more of these conditions. These conditions will influence speech reading ability and the environment in which hearing-aid orientation and group counseling sessions should be designed to maximize auditory-visual communication. The term *low vision* refers to persons with corrected visual acuity between 20/70 and 20/200 (acuity measurements are based on the Snellen eye chart with optimal acuity rated at 20/20 and reduced vision indicated by a higher number in the denominator). The diagnosis of low vision is made when vision cannot be fully corrected by lenses, medical treatment, or surgery. According to the World Health Organization (WHO), persons with moderate low vision have corrected acuity between 20/70 and 20/160 in the better eye whereas persons with severe low vision have corrected acuity between 20/200 and 20/400 or a visual field of 20 degrees or less in the better eye (Wainapel, 1994). A low vision loss can be central (reduced visual acuity) or peripheral (reduced visual field). Loss of peripheral or side vision can result from glaucoma or stroke. The major functional implication of a central loss is difficulty with detail discrimination (e.g., reading positive and negative on hearing-aid battery doors, reading volume control numbers) whereas the major functional implication of a peripheral problem is

TABLE 2–5 Age-Related Ocular Diseases

Condition	Etiology	Functional consequence
Macular Degeneration	Residue of intracelluar digestion is deposited on the macular region between the retinal pigment epithelial cells and Bruch's membrane. The hard drusen appears as dots of yellow or white lying below retinal vessels.	Difficulty reading and identifying faces.
Open-Angle Glaucoma	Occurs when a sustained increase in the intraocular pressure damages the retinal nerve fibers.	Decreased ability to function in dim light, decreased dark adaptation, glare disability, and gradual loss of visual fields.
Cataracts	Opacity of the lens.	Decreased visual acuity, contrast sensitivity, and color perception.
Diabetic Retinopathy	Retinopathy associated with diabetes mellitus.	Glare disability, decreased acuity, and decreased dark/light adaptation.

Source: Adapted from Carter (1994).

difficulty in orientation and mobility. In older adults, the most frequent type of vision loss is central, as a result of macular degeneration (Fletcher, 1994).

In sum, vision impairment is a major health issue for older adults: 3.1 million people between 65 and 74 years and 3.5 million people 75 years and older report a vision impairment (Lighthouse, Inc., 1995). This translates into a prevalence of self-reported visual impairment of 17% among persons 65 to 74 years, rising to 26% for persons over 75 years of age (Lighthouse, Inc., 1995). Half of all people with impaired vision report that their vision problem interferes to some degree with routine activities. However, as with hearing loss, people with impaired vision underutilize both vision rehabilitation services and high- and low-tech adaptive devices. In light of the above demographics, audiologists are likely to have contact with large numbers of older adults who accept vision and hearing loss as a normal consequence of old age and are reluctant to intervene in either area.

SPECIAL CONSIDERATION

It is incumbent on audiologists to make every effort to maximize the sense of hearing in persons with visual impairment as these individuals are likely to be suffering from an already diminished quality of life.

Similarly, audiologists must make every effort to insure that vision acuity is maximized during counseling sessions by using, for example, handheld or stand magnifiers to demonstrate the function of various hearing aid controls, appropriate lighting, large print reading materials, and raised-dot markings on hearing aids to help in locating particular controls. Audiologists should refer clients with low-vision problems to the appropriate professional for evaluation and management. Table 2–6 lists some strategies for promoting communication with older adults with hearing, as well as visual, impairments.

PEARL

Nearly every person will experience changes in vision with age. As with hearing loss, the impact of the changes will vary considerably.

The Somatosensory System

In general, aging is accompanied by a microscopic loss of the number and integrity of peripheral receptors most notable in the lower extremities and a lower concentration of touch corpuscles in the skin. Further, as was noted earlier, nerve conduction velocity slows with age, and the latency period for sensory and motor nerves increases. As a result of

TABLE 2–6   Strategies for Promoting Communication for People with Visual Problems

Improving Verbal Communication
- Introduce yourself by name
- Let the patient know when you enter or leave the room
- Speak before touching the person
- Approach the patient on the side of his or her better eye
- Allow the person with visual loss to speak for themselves, talk directly to the person with the visual impairment
- Let the person with visual loss do as much as possible, this builds confidence

Making Text More Legible for Persons with Visual Impairment and Low Vision
- Keep in mind that text should be printed with the highest possible contrast light against dark
- Keep in mind that printed material is most readable in black and white
- Use wide spacing between letters
- Use extra-wide margins especially for bound material, makes it easier to use on a flat surface
- Use large fonts, 16–18 point
- Use ordinary typeface, upper and lower case, and/or bold face print
- Do not use paper with glossy finish

Telephone Features for Patients with Visual Impairments
- Telephones with large buttons
- Telephones with good color contrasts
- A paging feature
- Memory and redial features

these alterations, aging is associated with a decrease in response to tactile stimuli; an increase in the threshold for vibration sense; and a decline in sensitivity to light touch, to deep pain perception, to position sense, and to pinprick sensation. These changes can impact on hearing-aid fittings with older adults.

The Metabolic System

Metabolism is the sum of all of the numerous and complex chemical events taking place in the human body (Hayflick, 1994). *Metabolic rate* is a term that refers to the rate at which the substances that run our body are utilized to provide energy for the physiological activities in which humans engage. Protein tissue is the most metabolically active body compartment. Additional energy sources within our body include fat tissue, which is metabolized as we exercise, and carbohydrates. The basal metabolic rate (BMR) tends to be expressed as energy expenditure per total body mass, thus the latter is a key determinant of BMR. Age is associated with a reduction in total body protein. Further, protein, or lean body mass, and BMR tend to decline with age. The mass of fat stored within the body tends to increase. Further, as people age, less energy is required to maintain metabolically active body mass (Chernoff, 1990). Chernoff (1990) cautioned that these changes occur in all people as they age, albeit at different rates. Chronic disease states, exercise, and nutritional status may influence the rate at which they occur. The metabolic changes that occur with age may account for some of the age-related changes occurring in the auditory system.

Physiological Changes in Remaining Systems

A number of other systems undergo physiological changes with age. These include the kidneys, the respiratory system, the cardiovascular system, the immune system, and the endocrine system. The basic changes are listed below along with the implications of the changes for audiologists.

The Renal System

The ordinary function of the renal system is to remove wastes and to adequately regulate the volume and content of extracellular fluid. A substantial reduction in renal function accompanies normal aging due for the most part to age-related anatomic and physiologic changes within the kidneys. The changes in renal function reduce the older adult's ability to respond to a variety of physiologic and pathologic stresses with substantial implications for overall function (Abrams, Beers, & Berkow, 1995). The size and weight of the kidneys tend to decline with age, with weight decreasing from 250 to 270 g in young adulthood to 180 to 200 g in the eighth decade of life. Further, there is a decrease in the number and functioning of glomeruli and tubules. The role of the kidney is to maintain the internal environment of the body by eliminating many of the products of metabolism and regulating the body's water content. A well-known end product of metabolism is creatinine. Kidney function, measured by the ability to clear nitrogenous wastes from the blood, declines with age. Further, creatinine clearance has been shown to decrease with increasing age. The tendency for, or capacity of, the kidney to hypertrophy is lost and blood flow is reduced with aging (Kenney, 1988). In general, the functional changes in the kidney leave the older adult more vulnerable to a variety of environmental or drug-induced stresses, but do not generally lead to disease or disability (Kenney, 1988).

The kidney has primary responsibility for clearance of drugs. Renal drug clearance decreases with increasing age and this effect is exaggerated when older adults do not receive the correct dosing of medications. In older adults, the doses of drugs excreted by the kidneys (e.g., aminoglycocides, antibiotics, digoxin preparations) require adjustment to compensate for age-related changes in renal function. If not, older adults will be vulnerable to drug overdose. It is often the case that drugs that are misprescribed and do not clear properly are toxic to the auditory and/or vestibular system. The latter can have vestibulotoxic (balance problems), ototoxic (hearing problems) or combined otovestibulotoxic effects. Aminoglycoside antibiotics, furosemides, and digoxin, commonly prescribed drugs for the elderly, require dosage adjustments based on gender and

---

SPECIAL CONSIDERATION

Older adults with renal insufficiency and/or high blood pressure are frequently prescribed medications that are oto- or vestibulotoxic. Monitoring of hearing status is important in these individuals.

---

age-adjusted creatinine clearance values to prevent toxicity associated with age-related changes in renal drug clearance. Finally, audiologists should familiarize themselves with the chronic diseases prevalent among older adults and the medications used to treat these diseases, as large enough doses of some of the medications can be ototoxic. A familiar example is arthritis for which large doses of salicylates may be prescribed, resulting in temporary hearing loss and possibly tinnitus.

PEARL

In light of age-related changes in pharmacodynamics, professionals should be attuned to possible drug-induced causes of hearing and balance problems. Similarly, audiologists should be familiar with the names of medications commonly prescribed for the elderly and associated with oto- and vestibulotoxic effects.

The Endocrine System

The endocrine system consists of a number of glands, cells, and tissues scattered throughout the body that produce hormones. Some of the glands of the endocrine system are autonomous, secreting hormones in response to chemical changes within the blood, whereas others do so through such endocrine organs as the pituitary gland and the hypothalamus. Neuroendocrine function, neurotransmitter regulation, and the hypothalamic-pituitary-adrenal axis all fall

into this system. The endocrine system, which affects virtually all cells of the body, undergoes changes with age that may in fact reduce the physiological reserve of tissues and organ systems (Hayflick, 1994). The major age-related change in this system is a decrease in production and secretion of hormones that control many essential bodily functions. For example, the production and secretion of testosterone, insulin, androgens, aldosterone, thyroid, and growth hormones decrease with normal aging. Further, the ability of the blood to maintain a normal level of glucose declines with age. Hayflick (1994) suggested that the latter age-related hormonal changes may erode the body's responsivity to stresses and hence interfere with such variables as healing, recovery from trauma, and adaptation to heat and cold.

The Immunologic System

The role of the immune system is protective and defensive. It consists of a group of mechanisms that detect, inactivate, and remove foreign materials and pathogens from the body. The thymus gland, which contains lymphocytes, is integral to the performance of the immune system (Hayflick, 1994). T cells are thymus-derived lymphocytes that circulate in the peripheral blood and in the lymph channel (Adler & Nagel, 1994). In addition to T lymphocytes, immune reactions are coordinated by the interaction among B lymphocytes and antigen presenting cells. The immune system performs these duties primarily through the release of a class of proteins known as antibodies, which come in different varieties and are uniquely tailored to combat particular microorganisms or foreign cells. For the most part, the immune system develops antibodies that detect and deactivate foreign protein bodies and to a lesser extent "self" proteins essential to vital life processes (Hayflick, 1994).

As people age there is a decline in the mass of the thymus, and the proportion of lymphocytes within the thymus changes as well. Whereas it is generally accepted that T-cell function declines with age, there is no consensus on the effects of age on the B-cell response (Miller, 1990; Adler & Nagel, 1994). As we age, "self" proteins undergo some minor changes and the antibodies produced by the immune system may attack as foreign what is really a slightly changed "self" protein (Hayflick, 1994). The end result of this phenomenon is the development of autoimmune diseases, which tend to increase in prevalence as people age. Examples of autoimmune diseases prevalent in older adults include some forms of arthritis and some forms of lupus. In sum, the immune system undergoes some significant functional changes with age including a decline in the ability to produce antibodies to foreign substances, an increase in the tendency to produce antibodies to self-proteins, and a general decline in the ability to mount an immune response against pathogens. The decline in protective immune reactions with age increases the susceptibility of older adults to infection and neoplasia (Miller, 1990). It is also important to emphasize the large individual variability that characterizes the age changes within the immune system, and that behavioral or lifestyle variables also influence immunosenescence. The pharmacologic management of individuals with autoimmune disease has implications for audiologists as some of the medication is potentially ototoxic or vestibulo-toxic.

The Cardiovascular System

The size of a fist in shape, and resembling a cone lying on its side, the normal heart acts as a pump circulating blood throughout the body (Frick, Leonhardt, & Starck, 1991). While in males, the healthy heart weighs about 300g, its size and weight vary with body size and degree of physical activity (Frick, Leonhardt, & Starck, 1991). The relative heart weight of females tends to be less and, partly due to a reduction in physical activity, there is a decrease in heart size in older adults (Frick, Leonhardt, & Starck, 1991). Located somewhat to the left of the center of the chest, the heart is a combined suction and pressure pump. The heart muscle, which requires oxygen and nutrients to survive, is composed of muscle that contracts continuously with only brief periods of rest between contractions. Blood carries oxygen and nutrients to all parts of the body. Arteries convey blood from the heart; thus, coronary arteries are vessels that carry the blood with oxygen and nutrients to the myocardial muscle. The contraction phase of the heart's work is called the systole whereas the time when the heart is relaxed and the chambers are filled is called diastole. Blood pressure is the ratio between these two pressures. The amount of pressure produced varies with the force with which the heart pumps and the degree to which the blood vessels resist blood flow (Falvo, 1991).

The heart undergoes some structural changes with age that can lead to some significant changes in cardiac function. The muscular mass of the normal adult heart, known as the myocardium, tends to enlarge with age. Further, although the heart itself demonstrates little change in chamber size with age, heart weight tends to increase because of increased ventricular wall thickness, especially in the area of the left ventricle. The aorta and its valves tend to undergo an increase in rigidity/stiffness and a decrease in elasticity. In general, there is also an increase in elastic and collagenous tissue in all parts of the conduction system of the heart and increased arterial stiffening with age. Arterial stiffening is due in part to a thickening of the innermost tissue constituting the arterial pipeline that leads to a narrowing of the diameter of the artery and increased rigidity (Hayflick, 1994). The structural changes that occur with aging (e.g., change in collagen and elastin in vessel walls) are qualitatively similar but quantitatively different from those changes observed in older adults with heart disease.

Cardiovascular function results from an interaction among a number of different variables. Thus, in discussing the age effects, the individual factors that tend to regulate cardiovascular performance will be isolated. There is widespread agreement that aging is associated with an increase in peak systolic blood pressure, but diastolic pressure does not seem to change (Hayflick, 1994). In general, aging is associated with a diminished maximum heart rate in the sitting position, decreased myocardial contractility, and a decrease in stroke volume or the volume of blood pumped during each contraction (Lakatt, 1990). There seems to be little agreement on the effect of age on resting cardiac output (i.e., the amount of blood pumped by the heart to the rest of the body each minute). Although most studies suggest a decline in cardiac output with age some suggest that resting cardiac output does not change with age in healthy active individuals. Decreased cardiac output can lead to reductions in cerebral blood flow and cardiac syncope; thus the area continues to be investigated. There is general agreement that the heart's ability to respond to stress declines with age as does the maximum heart rate achieved during exercise (Lakatt, 1990). Further, the amount of oxygen delivered to and used by muscles (i.e., maximum oxygen consumption) progressively declines with age, with the decline modifiable with certain lifestyle changes. The reduced ability of the cardiovascular system to deliver raw materials (e.g., proteins) to working muscles changes the chemical composition of muscle fibers, contributing in part to a generalized decline in muscular strength and function with age. Further, the decline in pumping ability of the aging heart under stress can lead to limited endurance, easy and early fatigability, compromised ability to maintain prolonged sustained activity, and reduced exercise tolerance (Roth, 1991). Additionally, there is general agreement that with increasing age, there is an increase in workload on the heart as it has the job of pumping blood against less compliant arteries. It is important to emphasize that, although there is a high prevalence of hypertension and coronary artery disease in older adults, neither of these disease entities is a normal consequence of aging (Kane, Ouslander, & Abrass, 1994). It is noteworthy that coronary artery or ischemic heart disease is the most common disease in individuals over the age of 60 and heart disease remains the most common cause of death in older adults in the United States. As is discussed in Chapter 5, a number of cardiovascular risk factors for hearing loss have recently been identified.

The Respiratory System

The respiratory system has two major components: (1) the pulmonary system, which consists of the lungs and the lower airways, including the bronchioles and associated tissue, and (2) the chest wall, which consists of the rib cage and the diaphragm-abdomen (Rochet, 1991). The lungs lie within the thoracic cavity. In general, the lungs assume the gross shape of the chest wall, and as the dimensions of the chest wall change so do the lungs. The left lung tends to be smaller than the right due in part to the left displacement of the apex of the heart (Frick, Leonhardt, & Starck, 1991). The lungs provide an interface between the atmosphere with which the body exchanges gases, and the blood that transports gases to and from active cells where oxygen is used and carbon dioxide produced (Kenney, 1988). In essence, the primary task of the lungs is respiration, however they play a role in metabolism as well (Despopoulos & Silbernagl, 1991).

The overall function of the respiratory system is gaseous exchange between the human organism and the environment. In short, the respiratory system transports oxygen, inspired from the air, in the blood to the tissues. In turn the carbon dioxide, a waste product of tissue metabolism, moves in the opposite direction (Despopoulos & Silbernagl, 1991). The respiratory gases are thus alternately transported over distances. Abnormal functioning of the respiratory system adversely affects every system of the body by diminishing the oxygen supply (Falvo, 1991). The functioning of the respiratory system is closely linked to proper function of the neuromuscular and cardiovascular systems, thus anatomic changes in the latter systems may result in functional changes in the pulmonary system. In general, lung structure and function reach their maximum level of development and efficiency early in the second decade of life, declining slowly thereafter (Saltzman, 1992).

Selected parts of the respiratory system undergo structural and functional changes with age. The shape of the chest wall changes, becoming more barrel shaped with age. The joints of the thorax become more rigid, the cartilage becomes calcified, the rib cage stiffens, and, correspondingly, chest wall compliance decreases. Further, medium and small airways, which are composed primarily of smooth muscle, tend to narrow due to a decrease in elasticity. Similarly, changes in elastin and collagen structures within the lung lead to a gradual increase in lung compliance with age (Saltzman, 1992). The latter changes in compliance may account in part for the alteration in pulmonary function with aging. Examples of changes in pulmonary function include a decline in vital capacity, a decrease in total lung capacity, decrease in elastic recoil, increased airflow resistance, and a potential decrease in forced expiratory volume (Saltzman, 1992). Respiratory muscle strength and mass decrease with age interfering in part with exercise tolerance (Saltzman, 1992). The principal muscle of respiration, the diaphragm, tends to flatten as a consequence of the age-related changes in lung compliance and hyperinflation of the chest wall (Dean, 1994). Similarly, there is a weakening of intercostal and abdominal muscles with age. The latter changes contribute to decreased elasticity of the lung. Further, the tissues of the respiratory system undergo changes with age. The alveolar sacs and ducts enlarge progressively with age and join together with adjacent alveoli. Further, the pulmonary vessels undergo an increase in internal fibrosis and thickening of the vessel walls. A notable functional change in the respiratory system associated with age is a decrease in lung function and reserve especially during stress. Maximal ventilation, which is the process of moving air from the environment to the alveoli during inspiration, and from the alveoli to the environment during expiration, tends to decline with age. Aging is associated with alterations in respiratory defense mechanisms. Specifically, there is a decrease in ciliary action and secretory immunoglobulin of nasal and respiratory passages, which can in some cases neutralize viral activities (Abrams, Beers, & Berkow, 1995).

SPECIAL CONSIDERATION

As otitis media often arises in the face of upper respiratory disease (URI), older adults at risk for URI should be closely monitored for middle ear disease.

In sum, changes in pulmonary structure and progressive declines in pulmonary function have been noted with aging. In general, the reduced pulmonary function with age can be translated into the fact that smaller amounts of air are expelled from the lungs with each breath. Further, older adults may inhale more often in an attempt to supply the organ systems throughout the body with the necessary oxygen (Burzynski, 1987). The extent to which the latter changes have functional implications depends in large part on alterations in related systems especially the cardiovascular and neuromuscular systems.

The Vocal Mechanism (Laryngeal Cavity)

The vocal mechanism or laryngeal cavity consists of the glottis, the supraglottis, and the subglottis. The glottis is formed by the true vocal cords that include the vocal ligament, the vocalis muscle, and the mucosal covering. The supraglottis comprises the epilarynx and the vestibule whereas the subglottic space extends into the lower border of the cricoid cartilage (Becker, Naumann, & Pfaltz, 1989). The joints and muscles of the larynx adjust the position and tension of the vocal chords, with efficient joint production depending on intact respiratory and vocal mechanisms. The human voice, an organ of communication, can be viewed as a wind instrument. In short, air from the lungs, bronchi, and trachea (the wind space) is driven past a narrow slit (vocal chords) causing vibration, whose character is influenced by the chest and oronasal cavity (i.e., the resonance chamber) (Despopoulos & Silbernagl, 1991). The structure and action of the larynx is shown in Figure 2–12.

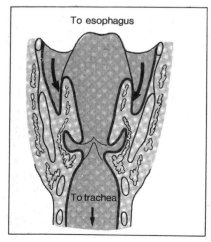

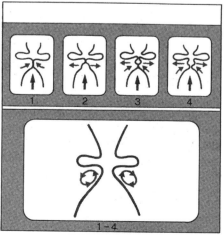

Figure 2–12 Structure of the larynx (left); motion of the vocal chords (right). (From Despopoulos and Silbernagl, 1991. Reprinted by permission.)

The laryngeal system undergoes a number of changes with age, which tend to have implications for voice production. As the vocal mechanism is truly a system of cartilage, glands, joints, nerves, ligaments, and muscles, many of the changes are predictable from the aforementioned discussions. In general, the laryngeal cartilage calcifies and ossifies. The latter occurs earlier in males than in females. The true vocal folds undergo fatty degeneration and atrophy. The laryngeal muscles atrophy and undergo degeneration, as well. The laryngeal ligaments in many cases stiffen, and thinning and breakdown have been observed in some of the joints, most notably the cricoarytenoid (Kahane & Beckford, 1991). These changes have been attributed to a reduction in blood supply to the laryngeal muscles. The laryngeal nerves undergo changes with age by virtue of the thickening of the capillary walls and reduction in diameter of the vessels.

As a result of these physiological changes, the aging voice is characterized by slight hoarseness, increased variability in pitch, declines in pitch control and pitch range, and a decrease in loudness (Kahane & Beckford, 1991). The latter vocal changes can interfere with communication, especially when hearing loss is present. Once again, it is important to emphasize that there is large individual variability among older persons in vocal characteristics, due to the highly variable rate in the onset and progression of physiological aging in the vocal mechanism (Burzynski, 1987). The rehabilitative implications of changes in the laryngeal system as they pertain to audiologists primarily derive from the fact that older voices can be difficult for the hearing impaired to hear and understand.

SPECIAL CONSIDERATION

A voice amplifier, similar to the pocket talker, can be used with older adults whose vocal intensity is so weak as to interfere with expressive communication. Voice amplifiers are helpful with individuals who can produce voice consistently, yet at a reduced loudness level (Yorkston & Garrett, 1997). Amplifiers are especially helpful during group hearing-aid orientation or counseling sessions.

The Gastrointestinal System

The gastrointestinal (GI) system includes the stomach, liver, esophagus, mouth, colon, small intestine, and pancreas. Each of these systems undergoes structural and functional changes with age. For the most part, the great functional reserve of the digestive tract reduces the clinical impact of age-related changes. The sense of taste is subserved by selected structures within the GI system, specifically the mouth within the oral cavity. The mouth has an intricate sensory control system with receptors for pain, taste, texture, and temperature. Taste receptors are collected in the taste bud located on the tongue and palate. Four basic taste qualities are recognized, namely salt, sour, bitter, and sweet. As is shown in Figure 2–13, these receptors are unevenly distributed over the tongue. The sense of taste is mediated in part by three nerves including the chorda tympani, the greater superficial petrosal, and the glossopharyngeal, which innervate various parts of the tongue. The chorda tympani, a branch of the seventh cranial nerve, which passes across the eardrum en route to the brain, innervates a portion of the front of the tongue. The greater superficial petrosal, also a branch of the seventh cranial nerve, innervates taste buds on the palate. Age is associated with decreased sensation of taste due to a progressive loss of taste buds predominantly on the anterior tongue. Aging is primarily associated with a decrease in detection of sweet and salty taste. Further, space-occupying lesions on selected cranial nerves may also alter taste sensation. Professionals working with older adults must ask case history questions that enable them to distinguish between changes in gustation related to age from changes associated with head trauma, surgical trauma, disease, or pathology such as an acoustic tumor.

Age-related changes in the jaw and temporomandibular joints may also be of relevance to audiologists. The temporomandibular joint (TMJ) is located between the maxillary glenoid fossa and the condylar process of the mandible (Abrams, Beers, & Berkow, 1995). It is essential to all articulated maxillary and mandibular functions. In general, the structures constituting the TMJ undergo degenerative changes, which are similiar to changes in the joints throughout the body (Baum & Ship, 1994). TMJ disorders, which may include osteoarthritis, displacement of the TMJ disk, and myofascial pain in the masseter and temporal muscles, are often associated with otalgia, neck pain, and pain re-

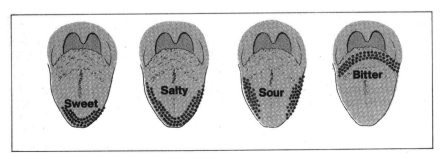

Figure 2–13 Localization of taste qualities on the tongue. (From Despopoulos and Silbernagl, 1991. Reprinted by permission.)

ferred to healthy teeth (Abrams, Beers, & Berkow, 1995). Joint noises such as a click are often present in persons with TMJ dysfunction.

PEARL

Joint noises may be mistaken for tinnitus, a common symptom experienced by older adults, and TMJ dysfunction should be ruled out as a cause of tinnitus in older adults.

FUNCTIONAL IMPLICATIONS OF AGE-RELATED CHANGES WITHIN THE ORGAN SYSTEMS

Older adults tend to overestimate their healthiness or underestimate the significance of given age-related change in the function of organ systems and associated medical condition(s). The latter tends to cause delay in their seeking medical assistance for potentially grave diseases and for potentially reversible conditions (Besdine, 1990). A major reason for the tendency to underreport symptoms relates to "ageism." Older adults come to expect that the aging process is associated with irremediable physiologic and functional declines as well as selected chronic conditions and disease processes. Accordingly, they regard the changes they experience as conditions they must accept and live with. So, too, do health care professionals lacking familiarity with the normal aging process. To the contrary, normal old age is increasingly characterized by good health and independence. The latter being components of successful aging according to Rowe and Kahn (1998).

> Although decline in some biologic functions accompanies normal human aging, these declines and their functional impact are gradual, and their impact is further softened by the decades over which they occur and by remaining, if shrinking, physiologic reserve. Major functional decline occurring abruptly in an already aged person should be assumed to be caused by disease, not aging.
>
> —Besdine, 1990, p. 177

Another characteristic of the aging process is the presence of multiple disease processes or chronic conditions. The prevalence of chronic conditions and the potential for co-occurring diseases is directly proportional to age. The oldest and frailest adults, especially residents of nursing facilities may have multiple diseases (Besdine, 1990). Similarly, whereas 80% of Americans over 65 have at least one chronic condition, a significant proportion of those over 80 have multiple chronic conditions. A final unique characteristic of older adults is the role of functional disability rather than acute disease. In light of the poor correlation between the type and severity of functional disability, age-related changes

in organ systems, and disease, a complete examination of older adults entails a comprehensive functional assessment as well as a thorough medical evaluation. The major premise underlying this recommendation is that as we age a number of organ systems undergo changes that in isolation or in combination have functional implications for older adults. Often the client's perception of the functional impact of age-related changes in selected organ systems guides referral and management. That is, the functional consequences of disease often take priority over the medical consequences, assuming the change is not life threatening.

The clinical assessment of older adults must by virtue of the changes associated with age be multidimensional, interdisciplinary, and above all functional (Williams, 1994). A multidimensional approach entails quantifying the older adult's medical, psychosocial, and functional capabilities (Brockelhurst & Williams, 1989). An interdisciplinary approach implies collaboration between health professionals and health agencies. Members of the team might include a nurse, social worker, psychologist, audiologist, nutritionist, and, of course, a physician. A functional approach implies that the physician's reality, namely the etiologic and anatomic-pathophysiologic diagnoses, is supplemented by the patient's reality, namely the functional diagnosis (Kane, Ouslander, & Abrass, 1994). The information that emerges from a comprehensive functional assessment assists in determining overall health, well-being, need for health and social services, and, ultimately, quality of life. Similarly, the audiologic history of an older adult should have a functional basis. Self-assessment scales are used to obtain information about the functional implications of age-related changes in the auditory system.

IMPLICATIONS OF AGE-RELATED CHANGES FOR AUDIOLOGICAL ASSESSMENT

In addition to impacting on the questions asked during the case history, the functional implications of changes in the organ systems influence procedures during the routine diagnostic assessment, as well as aspects of audiologic rehabilitation. Table 2–7 summarizes the functional decline and its impact on aspects of assessment and intervention. Keep the test modifications in mind as they will increase the reliability and validity of test results.

CONCLUDING REMARKS

The human body undergoes dramatic changes with the normal aging process. Hence, aging can be conceived of as the "accumulation of diverse adverse changes that hasten the probability of death" (Harman, 1998). There is great variation in the rate of decline for each organ system, and a decline in function in one organ system does not necessarily imply a similar decline in other organ systems. It is important to emphasize that environment and lifestyle influence to a great extent the actual and perceived effects of aging on the individual, contributing to the individual variations in the rate at which organ systems age. Further, while physiologic reserve diminishes with aging, it often remains adequate unless disease intervenes. Emphasis in this chapter was placed on age-related changes distinct from disease, as detection of a disease or disorder depends on an understanding of that which is normal for a given person's age. The age-related changes discussed in this chapter do not necessarily lead to illness nor do they necessarily have major implications for function.

SPECIAL CONSIDERATION

The response to age-related changes in structure and function is variable and is essential to management decisions. Audiologists should be cognizant of normal age-related changes to the extent that they may impact on the evaluation process, on the formulation of an effective rehabilitative approach, and on the client's response to management.

TABLE 2–7 Implications of Age-Related Changes in Organ Systems for Assessment and Intervention

Age-related change	Modification	Age-related change	Modification
Intellectual performance maintained into the 80's	Do not be condescending, do not infantilize	Confusion associated with Alzheimer's Disease	Do not correct incorrect responses. If patient can not answer questions during the case history, assuming the clinician is sure that the question was heard, do not get angered or lose patience. This strategy will avoid emotional responses to failure and catastrophic reactions that can worsen performance on selected tasks
Performing tasks may take longer	Allow extra time in schedule for hearing aid fitting and post fitting. Allow enough time between stimulus presentations and patient response		
More difficulty in learning new tasks	Repeat instructional set. Verify that patient understands response tasks. Verify that patient understands material presented during the hearing aid orientation and counseling sessions. Use facilitatory strategies to make sure patient learns tasks required	Decrease in recall	During hearing aid orientation review material learned at previous session before moving on to new procedures. Use all modalities to insure or promote recall of new information
More plasticity at the nerve cell level	Fitting a previously unamplified ear may result in recovery of speech understanding ability	Decreased visual acuity	Make sure test-suite and management rooms have adequate illumination
Motor reaction time decreases	Evaluate different response patterns during pure-tone test (e.g. yes/no versus hand-raising or button pushing)		Handouts from audiologic rehabilitation sessions should have enlarged print, with highest possible contrast. Printed material is best in black and white

REFERENCES

ABRAMS, W., BEERS, M., & BERKOW, R. (1995). *The Merck Manual of Geriatrics.* 2d ed. Whitehouse Station, NJ: Merck & Co., Inc.

ADLER, W., & NAGEL, J. (1994). Clinical immunology and aging. In: W. Hazzard, E. Bierman, J. Blass, W. Ettinger, & J. Halter (Eds.), *Principles of Geriatric Medicine and Gerontology.* 3d ed. New York: McGraw-Hill.

ASHOK, B., & ALI, R. (1999). The aging paradox: Free radical theory of aging. *Experimental Gerontology, 34:* 293–303.

BALIN, A. (1990). Aging of human skin. In: W. Hazzard, R. Andres, E. Bierman, & J. Blass (Eds.), *Principles of Geriatric Medicine and Gerontology.* New York: McGraw-Hill.

BAUM, B., & SHIP, J. (1994). The oral cavity. In: W. Hazzard, E. Bierman, J. Blass, W. Ettinger, & J. Halter (Eds.), *Principles of Geriatric Medicine and Gerontology,* 3d ed. New York: McGraw-Hill.

BECKER, W., NAUMANN, H., & PFALTZ, C. (1989). *Ear, Nose and Throat Diseases—A Pocket Reference.* Stuttgart: Georg Thieme Verlag.

BECKMAN, K., & AMES, B. (1998). The free radical theory of aging matures. *Physiological Review, 78:* 547–581.

BESDINE, R. (1990). Clinical evaluation of the elderly patient. In: W. Hazzard, R. Andres, E. Bierman, & J. Blass (Eds.), *Principles of Geriatric Medicine and Gerontology.* New York: McGraw-Hill.

BJORKSTEN, J. (1974). Cross linkage and the aging process. In: M. Rothstein (Ed.), *Theoretical Aspects of Aging.* New York: Academic Press.

BLASS, J., CHERNIACK, P., & WEISS, M. (1992). In: E. Calkins, A. Ford, & P. Katz (Eds.), *Practice of Geriatrics.* 2d ed. Philadelphia: W.B. Saunders Company.

BOSKEY, A. (1990). Bone mineral and matrix: Are they altered in osteoporosis? *Orthopedic Clinics of North America, 21:* 19.

BROCKELHURST, J., & WILLIAMS, T. (1989). Multidisciplinary health assessment of the elderly. *Danish Med. Bulletin, Gerontology Special Supplement, 7.*

BURZYNSKI, C. (1987). The voice. In: H.G. Mueller & V. Geoffrey (Eds.), *Communication Disorders in Aging.* Washington, DC: Gallaudet University Press.

BUSSE, E. (1969). Theories of aging. In: E. Busse & E. Pfeiffer (Eds.), *Behavior and Adaptation in Late Life.* Boston: Little Brown.

CARTER, T. (1994). Age-related vision changes: A primary guide. *Geriatrics, 49:* 37–45.

CHERNOFF, R. (1990). Nutritional rehabilitation and the elderly. In: *Aging: The Health Care Challenge.* 2d ed. Philadelphia: F.A. Davis.

CHRISTENSEN, K. (1999). Why do we age so differently? *Ugesk Laeger, 161:* 1905–1909.

CRISTOFALO, V. (1990). Biological mechanisms of aging: An overview. In: W. Hazzard, R. Andres, E. Bierman, & J. Blass (Eds.), *Principles of Geriatric Medicine and Gerontology.* New York: McGraw-Hill.

DEAN, E. (1994). Cardiopulmonary development. In: B. Bonder & M. Wagner (Eds.), *Functional Performance in Older Adults.* Philadelphia: F.A. Davis.

DESPOPOULOS, A., & SILBERNAGL, S. (1991). *Color Atlas of Physiology,* 4th ed. New York: Thieme Medical Publishers.

EVANS, J. (1994). Aging and disease. In: D. Evered & J. Whalen (Eds.), *Research and the Aging Population.* Chichester: John Wiley and Sons.

FALVO, D. (1991). *Medical and Psychosocial Aspects of Chronic Disease and Disability.* Gaithersburg, MD: Aspen Publishers.

FIFE, R. (1994). Osteoarthritis. In: W. Hazzard, E. Bierman, J. Blass, W. Ettinger, & J. Halter (Eds.), *Principles of Geriatric Medicine and Gerontology.* 3rd ed. New York: McGraw-Hill.

FLETCHER, D. (1994). Low vision: The physician's role in rehabilitation and referral. *Geriatrics, 49:* 50–56.

FRICK, H., LEONHARDT, H., & STARCK, D. (1991). *Human Anatomy 1.* New York: Thieme Medical Publishers.

———. (1991). *Human Anatomy 2.* New York: Thieme Medical Publishers.

HARMAN, D. (1998). Aging phenomena and theories. *Annals of the New York Academy of Sciences, 854:* 1–7.

HAYFLICK, L. (1994). *How and Why We Age.* New York: Ballantine Books.

HOLLWICH, F. (1985). *Opthalmology.* 2d rev. ed. New York: Thieme-Stratton.

KAHANE, J., & BECKFORD, N. (1991). The aging larynx and voice. In: D. Ripich (Ed.), *Geriatric Communication Disorders.* Austin: Pro-Ed.

KAMINER, M., & GILCHREST, B. (1994). Aging of the skin. In: W. Hazzard, E. Bierman, J. Blass, W. Ettinger, J. Halter (Eds.), *Principles of Geriatric Medicine and Gerontology.* 3d ed. New York: McGraw-Hill.

KANE, R., OUSLANDER, J., & ABRASS, I. (1994). *Essentials of Clinical Geriatrics.* 3d ed. New York: McGraw-Hill.

KENNEY, R. (1988). Physiology of aging. In: B. Shadden (Ed.), *Communication Behavior and Aging.* Baltimore: Williams & Wilkins.

KOHN, R. (1978). *Principles of Mammalian Aging.* 2d ed. New Jersey: Prentice Hall.

LAKATT, E. (1990). Heart and circulation. In: E. Schneider & J. Rowe (Eds.), *Handbook of the Biology of Aging.* 3d ed. San Diego: Academic Press.

LEWIS, C. (1990). *Aging: The Health Care Challenge.* 2d ed. Philadelphia: F.A. Davis.

LEWIS, C., & BOTTOMLEY, J. (1990). Musculoskeletal changes with age: Clinical implications. In: *Aging: The Health Care Challenge.* 2d ed. Philadelphia: F.A. Davis.

LIGHTHOUSE, INC. (1995). *The Lighthouse National Survey of Vision Loss: The Experience, Attitudes, and Knowledge of Middle Aged and Older Americans.* New York: The Lighthouse, Inc.

MARTIN, G. (1992). Biological mechanisms of aging. In: J. Evans & T.F. Williams (Eds.), *Oxford Textbook of Aging.* Oxford: Oxford University Press.

MILLER, R. (1990). Aging and the immune response. In: E. Schneider & J. Rowe (Eds.), *Handbook of the Biology of Aging.* 3d ed. San Diego: Academic Press.

MORLEY, J. (1990). Nutrition and aging. In: W. Hazzard, R. Andres, E. Bierman, & J. Blass (Eds.), *Principles of Geriatric Medicine and Gerontology.* New York: McGraw-Hill.

MRAK, R., GRIFFIN, S., & GRAHAM, D. (1997). Aging associated changes in human brain. *Journal of Neuropathologic Experimental Neurology,* 56: 1269–1275.

ORGEL, L. (1963). The maintenance of the accuracy of protein synthesis and its relevance to aging. *Proceedings of the National Academy of Sciences USA,* 49: 517.

PETERSON, M. (1994). Physical aspects of aging: Is there such a thing as "normal"? *Geriatrics,* 49: 2, 45–50.

POIRIER, J., & FINCH, C. (1994). Neurochemistry of the aging human brain. In: W. Hazzard, E. Bierman, J. Blass, W. Ettinger, & J. Halter (Eds.), *Principles of Geriatric Medicine and Gerontology.* 3d ed. New York: McGraw-Hill.

ROCHET, A. (1991). Aging and the respiratory system. In: D. Ripich (Ed.), *Geriatric Communication Disorders.* Austin: Pro-Ed.

ROTH, E. (1991). The aging process. In: R. Hartke (Ed.), *Psychological Aspects of Geriatric Rehabilitation.* Gaithersburg, MD: Aspen Publishers.

ROWE, J., & KAHN, R. (1998). *Successful Aging.* New York: Random House.

RUMNEY, N. (1998). The aging eye and vision appliances. *Ophthalmic Physiol-Opt,* 18: 191–196.

SALTZMAN, A. (1992). Pulmonary disorders. In: E. Clakins, A. Ford, & R. Katz (Eds.), *Practice of Geriatrics.* 2d Ed. Philadelphia: W.B. Saunders.

STREHLER, B. (1977). *Time, Cells, and Aging.* 2d ed. New York: Academic Press.

TABBARA, K. (1989). Anatomy and embryology of the eye. In: D. Vaughan, T. Asbury, & K. Tabarra (Eds.), *General Ophthalmology.* 12th ed. Norwalk: Appleton & Lange.

TIDEIKSAAR, R., & SILVERTON, R. (1989). *Falling in Old Age: Its Prevention and Treatment.* New York: Springer Publishing.

TIMIRIS, P.S. (1988). *Physiological Basis of Geriatrics.* New York: Macmillan.

WAINAPEL, S. (1994). Visual Impairments. In: G. Felsenthal, S. Garrison, & F. Steinberg (Eds.), *Rehabilitation of the Aging and Elderly Patient.* Baltimore: Williams & Wilkins.

WALFORD, R. (1969). The immunologic theory of aging. Munksgaard, Copenhagen. From: G. Martin, Biological mechanisms of aging. In: J. Evans & T.F. Williams (Eds.), (1992), *Oxford Textbook of Aging.* Oxford: Oxford University Press.

WILLIAMS, M. (1994). Clinical management of the elderly patient. In: W. Hazzard, E. Bierman, J. Blass, W. Ettinger, & J. Halter (Eds.), *Principles of Geriatric Medicine and Gerontology.* 3d ed. New York: McGraw-Hill.

YORKSTON, K., & GARRETT, K. (1997). Assistive communication with technology of elders with motor speech disability. In: R. Lubinski & D. Higginbotham (Eds.), *Communication Technologies.* San Diego: Singular Publishing Group.

Chapter 3

Psychosocial Changes with Aging

Society in general and health care professionals in particular should be more sensitive to our plight . . . they too will one day confront the challenge of old age.

—M.L.S. (78-year-old psychiatrist)

Lifestyle choices more than genes determine how well we age.

—Rowe and Kahn, 1998

LEARNING OBJECTIVES

After reading this chapter, you should be able to:

- Explain the social aspects of aging.
- State the psychological changes associated with normal aging.
- Relate psychosocial aspects of aging to evaluative and management strategies for older hearing-impaired adults.

OVERVIEW

Human beings are biological, social, and psychological systems that are in a constant stage of development (Verwoerdt, 1976). Over the life cycle, we are in a continuous state of flux, changing our interests and goals as we mature and pass through various stages of human development (Verwoerdt, 1976). Table 3–1 displays the broad areas in which change occurs. The changes in each of these domains will be discussed along with the implications of these changes for audiologic practice.

TABLE 3–1 Domains of Change

1. The Social Domain
2. The Psychologic Domain
a. personality
b. cognitive

THE SOCIAL DOMAIN

In general, late life is a period of transition and adjustment to loss. Transitions include retirement and relocation. Bereavement is a complex phenomenon associated with loss of companionship primarily because of death of a spouse (Abrams, Beers, & Berkow, 1995). Loss triggers a decline in social interaction and often a change in social status. As would be expected, the social context of aging influences the risk of disease and the experience of illness.

PEARL

The health care professional's ability to deliver timely and appropriate care depends in large part on an understanding of the social context in which illness takes place and on the care ultimately provided.

Social theories have been advanced to explain and account for the behavior of older adults relative to their social context. In particular, four theories of aging have been espoused and in some cases tested by different sociologists. The four theories and the researchers responsible for each are listed in Table 3–2. For the most part there have been few shifts in social–gerontological theory during the past decade (Bengtson, Parrott, & Burgess, 1996).

TABLE 3–2 Sociological Theories of Normal Aging

Theory	Proponent
Disengagement Theory	Cumming and Henry (1961)
Activity Theory	Havighurst (1963)
Continuity Theory	Neugarten (1966)
The Subculture Theory	—

The Disengagement Theory

The disengagement theory is the earliest, most famous, and most controversial theory of American gerontology. The disengagement theory was first described by Cumming and Henry (1961). It posits that normal aging is an inevitable mutual withdrawal or disengagement by the aging individual and the society to which he or she belongs. Cumming and Henry (1961) reasoned that this voluntary curtailment of involvement in social relationships arises from inner psychological changes wherein the individual comes to prefer less input and interactions with the outside world. Based on their interviews of over 200 older adults Cumming and Henry concluded that once the disengagement process is complete, the morale of the individual will be high and the person will be satisfied with his or her niche in life and will no longer have to compete with younger rivals. For society, the withdrawal of older persons allows younger, more energetic persons to assume the functional roles necessary for society to thrive (Cox, 1988). The validity of the contention that disengagement is a voluntary, self-imposed correlate of old age, plus Cumming and Henry's prescription of "withdrawal for happiness," has been challenged due to methodological shortcomings and because of the accumulation of empirical data that fails to support their postulates (Botwinick, 1973; Maddox, 1965). Recently, Cummings and Henry publicly disagreed with their own theory when they concluded that in fact people do not normally disengage. Disengagement can be viewed as adaptive from the perspective of the individual and society. Further, disengagement if and when it occurs is dependent on the lifelong personality of the individual. In addition, disengagement behavior can be viewed as a symptom or consequence of one or more disorders requiring professional attention (Davis, 1990).

Internal factors including physical and mental health status and external variables such as social structure, socioeconomic status, or educational level have been implicated as contributing to disengagement. With regard to health, the insults of old age (e.g., physical incapacity, mental status) preclude the maintenance of social involvement that characterizes one's earlier years. In short, the quality and quantity of interpersonal contacts as well as participation in various activities bears a positive relationship to physical functional status (Maddox, 1965; Tallmer & Kutner, 1969).

Weinstein (1980) reviewed the disengagement literature and found that none of the investigations designed to examine the contribution of physical health to social isolation considered hearing status as a possible determinant of the social withdrawal that characterizes many elderly individuals. As part of her doctoral dissertation, she chose to explore the relation between hearing loss, hearing handicap, and social isolation in a sample of older male veterans. Weinstein (1980) administered a subjective and an objective isolation scale to 80 male veterans ranging in age from 65 to 88 years. The majority (71%) of subjects had mild to moderate, bilaterally symmetrical, sensorineural hearing loss. There was a wide range in the perception of hearing handicap that was based on scores on the Hearing Measurement Scale (Noble & Atherly, 1970). Subjects were in good physical health and had negative histories of psychological problems. The sub-

jective social isolation scale yielded information on the desire to interact with others, interest in engaging in various activities, feelings of loneliness, and satisfaction with the quality of interactions. The objective isolation scale quantified contacts with significant others, participation in leisure/recreational activities, and living arrangements. Scores on the isolation scales were comparable to scores obtained in a Cross-National Study of the physical, social, and mental problems confronting community-based older adults. In the latter study, hearing loss was not considered as an important variable potentially contributing to social isolation.

Weinstein (1980) found that self-perceived hearing handicap, and to a lesser extent the severity of the hearing impairment, was positively associated with the magnitude of subjective social isolation reported by her sample of older adults. Interestingly, self-perceived hearing handicap accounted for more of the variability among subjects in their feelings of subjective social isolation than did the index of physical health. In contrast, objective social isolation did not bear a strong relationship to audiologic measures. More in-depth analysis of responses to the objective social isolation scale revealed that participation in leisure activities, pursuit of solitary activities such as television viewing, telephone usage, etc. were strongly associated with hearing loss severity. A greater proportion of individuals with moderately severe to severe hearing loss withdrew socially than did persons with lesser impairments. Further, it was possible to rank subjects as to their isolation status according to performance on audiologic tasks. In general, persons categorized as being subjectively and objectively isolated had greater hearing handicaps and hearing impairments than did nonisolates or individuals who were not classified as subjectively or objectively isolated. Further, subjective isolates were more impaired and handicapped than objective isolates.

The *Lighthouse National Survey of Vision Loss* (Lighthouse, Inc., 1995), a nationwide study of older adults' experiences with vision impairment revealed that vision loss also impacts on the quantity and quality of social interactions. The overriding complaint was that vision loss makes it difficult to get to places outside the home and interferes with leisure activities. Taken together, the latter study and prior studies challenging the disengagement theory lend support to the notion that disengagement is not universally natural, and very often is imposed from outside (Botwinick, 1973).

PEARL

Age-related chronic conditions, such as hearing and visual loss, are variables that may contribute to inactivity in later life.

The Activity Theory

The activity theory was proposed as an alternative to the disengagement theory, yet maintained some of its philosophy (Havighurst, 1963). The activity theory poses a view of successful aging which is exactly opposite that presented by the disengagement theory. It emphasizes the importance of maintaining an active lifestyle such that for every role that an individual gives up, there should be a suitable replacement. It posits that older people must stay active and involved to continue to maintain their own integrity. Further, as individuals age, the nature of the activities most important to life satisfaction may change (Botwinick, 1973). Whereas, formal activities (e.g., participation in voluntary activities) or solitary activities (e.g., household activities) were a priority early in life, more informal activities (e.g., interaction with friends, relatives, or neighbors) take on greater importance. In general, contact with friends and relatives appears not to decline until the eighties as maintenance of social relationships is critical to life satisfaction. It is of interest that 40 to 50% of older adults with mild to moderate sensorineural hearing loss perceive that hearing impairment interferes with interactions with friends, relatives, and neighbors leading to psychosocial handicap. The extent to which hearing loss that is handicapping in the domain of informal activities interferes with life satisfaction remains a question in need of investigation.

The Continuity Theory

The continuity theory evolved as a bridge between the disengagement and activity theories. Recall that the proponents of the disengagement theory argue that disengagement is a normal, healthy, "functional" adjustment to old age. In contrast, advocates of the activity theory contend that social activity is predictive of better physical function and higher happiness/life satisfaction ratings. Sociologists disenchanted with each of these theories have proposed an alternative view of the aging process, namely the continuity theory (Neugarten, 1966). The latter theory holds that in the course of the aging process, the individual tends to maintain stability in the areas established throughout life. Thus, a person's habits, associations, and lifestyle early on will predispose the person to maintain these preferences in later years. Whereas, proponents of the disengagement and activity theories hold that successful adaptation to the aging process is defined by inactivity or activity, the continuity theory posits that past history and preferred lifestyle mediate the individual's adaptation (Cox, 1988). Thus, the continuity theory allows for a multiplicity of adjustment patterns. Rowe and Kahn (1998) underline the importance of engagements with family and friends as critical to successful aging.

PEARL
From the rehabilitative standpoint, a major implication of the continuity theory is that clinicians must appreciate the life activities that are important to the individual, determine the extent to which hearing loss interferes with pursuing these activities, and design an intervention program that addresses the limitations.

The Subculture Theory

The subculture theory of aging holds that older adults form a subculture unto themselves, with their own values, mores, feelings, and norms. Thus older adults find great comfort in being amongst their own age cohorts. This theory is evidenced in the formation of such groups as the Gray Panthers and the American Association of Retired Persons (AARP) (Hayflick, 1994). This theory that older adults prefer to be part of their own subculture has not yet been substantiated, as in fact older adults do not appear to share similar attitudes or values by dint of age (Hayflick, 1994). However, it stands to reason that older adults would prefer to be part of support groups (e.g., Self Help for Hard of Hearing Persons [SHHH]) or rehabilitation groups comprising individuals of their cohort.

PEARL
The components of successful aging include low risk of disease, high physical and mental function, and active engagement with family and friends (Rowe & Kahn, 1998).

THE PSYCHOLOGIC DOMAIN
Personality

Having overviewed the sociologic theories that seek to explain adjustment to old age, the next step is to establish an understanding of the natural growth process of the personality from birth to late life in order to set the stage for understanding psychologic changes with age. Human development has been described in terms of life cycle phases. The premise of Erikson's model of development is that an individual successfully overcomes or meets the challenges of each stage and emerges as a healthy, mature personality (Table 3–3). Erikson (1968) theorized that if one does not successfully complete a prior phase it will be difficult to meet the demands of a subsequent phase. In fact, failure in one phase can result in psychological problems related to that phase and may predispose the individual to failure in later phases. According to Erikson (1968), there are increasingly more chances to fail at each subsequent phase, making the final phase of life the most challenging and difficult to attain (Verwoerdt, 1976). Erikson's stages of personality and ego development help us to understand the emotional reactions to some of the physical and social changes that older adults undergo as well as the enormous individual variability so characteristic of older adults. His formulations can also be invaluable as a guide to intervening with older adults who may or may not have successfully mastered each of the stages of development (Erikson, 1968; Davis, 1990).

Erikson (1968) also acknowledged that family, the environment, and society influence to a large extent the ability to master the crises associated with each stage, and the ultimate move and mastery of succeeding stages. He hypothe-

TABLE 3–3   Erikson's Stages of Development

Period in life	Erikson's stage	Description
0–12 months	Trust versus Mistrust	Hopeful, self-confident versus mistrustful
1–3 years	Autonomy versus Shame and Doubt	Autonomous, proud versus self-doubt, self-conscious
3–6 years (pre-school)	Initiative versus Guilt	Creative, independent versus guilt and inhibition
6–12 years (school age)	Industry versus Inferiority	Productive, positive learning versus inadequacy, self-doubt, and inhibited
12–18 years (adolescence)	Identity versus Role/ Identity Confusion	Inner solidarity, knowledge of oneself versus role confusion
18–35 years (young adulthood)	Intimacy versus Isolation	Trust, sharing versus distancing from others
35–60 years (middle age)	Generativity versus Stagnation	Mentoring, guiding new generations, nurturance versus self-absorption, preoccupation
Over 60 years (later life)	Integrity versus Despair	Sense of satisfaction, acceptance with oneself and station in life versus despair, anger

Source: Erikson, 1968; Corey, 1991.

sized that psychopathology may develop when the challenges of a stage are not met or resolved. The outcome of the final stage strongly influences the older adult's ability to cope with the losses and stresses of late adulthood. The challenge for older adults is to respond to and be aggressive about positive and negative social and physical forces that arise, with the goal being to maintain and increase self-esteem and to take responsibility for one's life (Davis, 1990). Decline in physical function and vulnerability to illness can lead to depression and psychosomatic illness, thereby interfering with the attainment of integrity (Verwoerdt, 1976; Kaplan, Sadock, & Grubb, 1994). Similarly, loss of independence and the need for physical and economic assistance can have devastating effects. The environment, including shrinkage of one's peer group, retirement, and decline of the nuclear family, can also interfere with resolution of the latter phase of the life cycle. Thus, biological and environmental hazards are likely to interfere with successful completion of the ultimate stage of life. Kaplan and his colleagues underline the importance of active preparation for old age as a way of offsetting some of the negative consequences that arise because of the difficulty in successfully passing through the psychosocial crisis of integrity versus despair.

Personality traits tend to remain the same throughout life, unless of course the social or physical stresses of old age interfere. Costa and McCrae (1994) described the five-factor model of personality (Table 3–4). Each of these domains of personality helps to explain the four basic elements of personality that include motivation, emotion, and interpersonal or experiential style. Cross-sectional and longitudinal studies have been conducted in an effort to measure changes across each of these personality traits. In general, personality traits do not appear to change in individuals over 30 years of age (Costa & McCrae, 1994). It appears that all five of the major dimensions of personality are highly stable in adulthood, the latter defined as after age 30. In short, adult personality is attained by age 30 and barring outside events, personality profiles are maintained throughout life. The extent to which apparent changes in personality can be attributed to physical, cognitive, or social factors is constantly under investigation. Finally, it is important to point out that personality style, such as level of neuroticism or conscientiousness, may provide insight into health behavior and may influence management decisions. For example, an individual who scores high on a neuroticism scale may self-rate a mild hearing impairment as more handicapping than an individual who scores low. Similarly, an individual who scores high on the conscientiousness factor may be motivated to purchase a hearing aid and undergo audiologic rehabilitation whereas an individual who scores low on this factor may require counseling to motivate him or her to seek intervention. Hearing impairment and personality traits influence adjustment to hearing aid use, as will be discussed in later sections of the text.

TABLE 3–4   Traits from the Five Personality Factors

Factor	Characteristics
Neuroticism	Calm, comfortable, unemotional versus worrisome, self-conscious, emotional
Extraversion	Reserved, quiet, passive versus affectionate, talkative, active
Openness	Conventional, conservative, uncreative versus original, liberal, creative
Agreeableness	Ruthless, suspicious, critical versus soft-hearted, trusting, lenient
Conscientiousness	Negligent, lazy, disorganized versus conscientious, hard-working, well-organized

Source: Costa & McCrae, 1994.

Cognitive Function

Cognition is defined as the process of obtaining, organizing, and using intellectual knowledge (Kaplan, Sadock, & Grubb, 1994). Cognition implies an understanding of the connection between cause and effect, between an action and the consequences of that action (Kaplan, Sadock, & Grubb, 1994). It also implies calling up and processing relevant information from stored memory. Cognitive strategies are mental plans used by individuals to understand themselves and the environment in which they function. Cognitive function, in selected domains, tends to decline somewhat with age. It is imperative that audiologists are aware of the magnitude and rate of change in cognitive function because the changes impact on every aspect of the evaluation and management process. For the purposes of the discussion that follows, the four aspects of cognitive function to be discussed will include learning capacity, memory, intelligence, and motivation (Table 3–5). These are the dimensions of information processing that are integral to the diagnostic and rehabilitative process. Further, changes in any of these domains can act as a diagnostic window into some form of medical, neurologic, or psychiatric problem requiring immediate referral.

Learning Capacity

Learning is defined as the change in behavior in a given situation brought about by repeated experiences in that particular situation, provided that the new behavior cannot be explained by the individual's native response tendencies, maturation, or some temporary state of being (Kaplan, Sadock, & Grubb, 1994). Learning can be viewed as the acquisition of connections or associations between stimulus and response through practice and rehearsal. It is the practicing and rehearsing of information to be retained (Kausler, 1988). The neurobiological basis of learning is located in the structures of the brain responsible for forming and storing

TABLE 3–5   Dimensions of Information Processing

Dimension	Definition
Learning	The process of acquisition of skills and information
Memory	The process of storing and retrieval of information
Intelligence	The capacity to manipulate and apply new and old information
Motivation	Having the impetus to seek out opportunities

Source: Bienfeld, 1990.

information, namely the hippocampus, the cortex, and the cerebellum (Kaplan, Sadock, & Grubb, 1994).

SPECIAL CONSIDERATION

Learning capacity does not decline as one ages.

Contrary to common belief, in fact, older adults can learn as much as younger adults. Further, the rate of forgetting what has been learned appears to be independent of age, as well (Kausler, 1988). While the capacity to learn does not change, the amount of effort to learn does. Specifically, the ability to perform new tasks and flexibility of learning style do undergo some decline.

PEARL

Older people learn more slowly than do their younger counterparts, thus it takes more trials for a particular skill to be acquired (Bienfeld, 1990).

The latter is most pronounced in verbal skills. With regard to verbal skills, persons over 60 years of age make more errors on verbal learning tasks than do young adults. In addition to requiring more time to learn new tasks, older adults require more time to integrate new learning and to practice it before it is incorporated into their daily routine (Davis, 1990). Older adults tend to be vulnerable to distracting events that can interfere with their level of concentration. Finally, ability to learn orally presented material (as opposed to written material) declines in persons over 70 years of age (Hayflick, 1994). As is shown in Table 3–6, a number of noncognitive factors will influence an older adult's learning capacity. Table 3–7 lists tips for overcoming learning barriers in older adults

Memory

Learning and memory are related cognitive processes that must be differentiated to understand each (Melton, 1963). Both involve a modification of behavior as a function of

TABLE 3–6 Strategies for Overcoming Barriers to Learning in Older Adults

Factors that affect learning:	Strategies for overcoming learning deficits:
1. Hearing or visual deficits	Make sure that the hearing or visual deficit is compensated for, otherwise it may take longer to learn and/or persons may misunderstand what has been said. Present material orally and in writing, especially to individuals over 70 years of age.
2. Poor physical health or chronic pain can interfere with concentration, stamina, and strength	Make inquiries about health status and physical comfort prior to beginning a new learning task.
3. Reluctance to learn new information	Build on former knowledge, present new information on a continuum with what the older adult already knows.
4. Need more time to integrate new learning	Provide ample opportunity to integrate new learning, separate new learning experiences.
5. Easily distracted by the physical environment.	Minimize auditory and visual distractions.
6. Perform better when self-pace new learning, as they have a slowed rate of information processing	Allow adequate time for responses and for completion of forms. Do not give too much information at one sitting.
7. Experience anxiety in new learning situations	Provide an overview or summary of activities to be covered in each session so that the individual can anticipate the sequence.
8. Motivation influences learning efficiency	Information should be relevant and meaningful to maximize motivation to learn.

Source: Davis, 1990.

TABLE 3–7 Tips for Overcoming Learning Barriers

- Older adults benefit when new material is presented along a continuum with what they already know. Proceed in a slow and careful manner when resistance to new information is expected.
- Older adults need more time to integrate new learning and to rehearse it before it settles into new memory.
- Concentrate on one task at a time.
- Space new learning experiences well enough apart.
- Reduce the potential for distraction whenever possible as this interferes with concentration. Observe the person for signs of interference with concentration.
- Allow the client to set the learning pace.
- Provide an overview of the entire learning session so that the person can organize the sequence of the session.
- Learning is facilitated when the patient can hear and see the same material presented at the same time.

Source: Lewis, 1990.

experience. Whereas learning is measured in relation to a change from one trial to another, memory is measured in terms of the temporal interval between trials (Melton, 1963). Each process is dependent on the other. For example, if one does not learn well, then there is little to recall. Similarly, if memory is poor there is little evidence that one has learned very much (Melton, 1963). Storage is key to a good memory.

Memory has been defined as the product of operations that individuals perform on incoming information regardless of intent to remember or the extent to which practice and rehearsal determine its memorability (Kausler, 1988). Memory has been likened to computer science. Common to both areas are the following processes: input, throughput, and output (Bienfeld, 1990). *Input* refers to the data entry stage, *throughput* to the data manipulation and processing, and *output* to retrieval of meaningful information or data.

Memory can be divided into several categories, depending on the length of time for which information can be stored. Sensory memory or the sensory store refers to the initial, momentary registration of information at the input stage. It is the earliest stage of information processing and

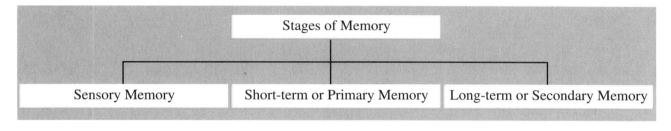

Figure 3–1 Stages of Memory.

relies on perceiving and attending to information (Albert, 1994). Data that are input to the system can be held there for a short period of time (0.25 to 0.5 seconds) so they can be encoded and turned into a format to be relayed to the next compartment for storage. Following this encoding, the next repository is primary or short-term memory. This compartment has a slightly longer, albeit a limited, capacity. It pertains to the ability of individuals to retain a small amount of information over a brief time period (Albert, 1994). Operationally, the capacity of primary memory is defined by the number of items an individual can remember for a few seconds. For example, short-term memory is the compartment used to remember a phone number that is immediately dialed and subsequently forgotten. Information must be rehearsed to be retained in primary memory. Secondary or long-term memory has a large capacity for information storage. It provides for long-term retention of unlimited amounts of information requiring analysis and organization for future storage and retrieval (Hartke, 1991). It can be thought of as a file cabinet filled with a number of folders that hold newly learned material for retrieval or output at a later date. The manner in which information is "filed away" will influence information storage capacity. Figure 3–1 depicts the stages of memory. Examples of each form of information processing are shown in Table 3–8.

As is evident from Table 3–9, the aging process has a differential effect on each of the stages of memory. Few age-related differences have been documented at the sensory phase. Storage capacity is unchanged at this stage of input however, perceptual changes in hearing, vision, or touch can alter input into the sensory store. It is, therefore, imperative that clinicians verify that input into memory (i.e., information has been seen and/or heard) to insure that the individual can later retrieve the information in question. Older adults have minimal difficulty at the next memory repository (i.e., primary memory). For example, absolute digit or word span is relatively unaffected by age. It is important to note that encoding at this stage is highly dependent on attention. With increasing age, encoding becomes more and more susceptible to distracting events that tend to compromise attentional capacity (Hartke, 1991).

When the number of items older adults are asked to recall exceeds the primary memory span, the effects of age become apparent (Robertson-Tchabo & Arenberg, 1988). In general, older adults are less proficient than young adults at tasks that test secondary memory. To facilitate the study of long-term memory, researchers have categorized it into three stages, namely recall, recognition, and retrieval. Figure 3–2 depicts each of these categories within long-term memory. It appears that defects in retrieval appear to be most susceptible to aging effects. Bienfeld (1990) hypothesized that the deficits arise because of a less efficient means of classifying and placing information into long-term storage. That is, older adults use less effective strategies for organizing material. This compromises the ability to retrieve information.

With regard to age decrements on recall tasks, memory for recent events can be viewed as a free recall task. For example, "what did you have for lunch yesterday?" In contrast, cued recall implies that the examiner provides cues for recall (e.g., the first thing you ate was orange juice). The method and timing of the assessment appears to influence performance on tests of memory. Age decrements are greatest on free recall rather than on cued recall tasks and are most evident after age 40. Further, age decrements in delayed recall tasks have been reported in older adults, as well (Albert, 1994). It appears that declines in recall memory can

TABLE 3–8 Examples of Stages of Information Processing

Stage	Examples
Sensory Memory	Time necessary to identify a single letter
Primary Memory	Digit span forward, word span, letter span
Secondary Memory	Who was the third president of the U.S.A., among these five individuals who was the third president?

TABLE 3–9 Memory and Aging

Stage of memory	Effect of aging on storage capacity
Sensory Memory	Unchanged by aging
Primary Memory	Unchanged by aging
Secondary Memory	Age-related differences

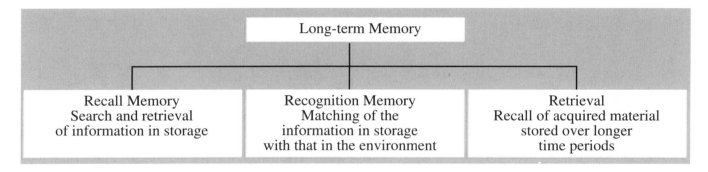

Figure 3–2 Categories of Long-term Memory.

be attributed to age-related deficits in search, retrieval, and storage.

Recognition memory does not depend on retrieval and older adults appear to be as successful as younger adults when asked to match or recognize a stimulus that has been stored away. At all ages recognition memory outperforms recall memory (Bienfeld, 1990). When tests of recognition memory involve storage of information over a brief time interval, there is an age effect. That is, performance on recognition tests administered one month after information has been learned declines with age (Botwinick, 1973). Memory for remote events in part reflects recognition memory, especially when an event or some experience triggers a memory of something similar that happened a long time ago. For example, if an older adult attends grandparents' day at their grandchild's kindergarten class, this may trigger their memory of events that took place when he or she was in kindergarten. According to Bienfeld (1990) stability of recognition memory over free recall memory most likely occurs over the entire life span. It may be more evident in the elderly because they tend to engage in active reminiscence.

In sum, memory is a very intricate form of information processing that must be understood prior to understanding the implications of age-related deficits. The memory task, age, and assessment approach interact to determine decrements due to age. To minimize the effects of age on audiologic tasks that are dependent on memory status, the audiologist should follow the steps listed in Table 3–10. These tips will be quite pertinent during all aspects of the audiologic assessment ranging from diagnostic testing to audiologic rehabilitation.

Intelligence

Intelligence is a multifaceted and complex construct that can be defined as the ability to accumulate, assimilate, process, store, and retrieve information (Bienfeld, 1990). Most studies of intelligence utilize tests designed to predict how individuals would function in an academic environment and thus they do not assess all aspects of cognitive ability (Albert, 1994). Performance on intelligence tests varies as a function of the design (e.g., longitudinal versus cross-sectional), presentation mode and rate, measuring instrument, and form of

TABLE 3–10 Approaches to Minimizing the Influence of Age-Related Memory Defects of Audiologic Tasks

Cognitive Process	Strategy
Sensory Memory	Insure that the new information is acquired. That is, did the individual hear, see, and/or feel the input?
Primary Memory	Allow adequate time for storage of new information.
	Provide opportunity for practicing new information.
	Have individual demonstrate his/her understanding of the instructions or new information.
	Write information or instructions down.
	Provide reinforcement as a way of motivating the individual to store and later retrieve the new information.
Secondary Memory	Provide cues that will help the individual to remember what he/she has learned.
	Provide choices rather than rely on free recall.
	Provide suggestions for storage of new information into memory to facilitate later retrieval.
	Activities must be relevant and meaningful so that it can be integrated into one's knowledge base.

TABLE 3–11 Scales and Corresponding Subtests on the Wechsler Adult Intelligence Scale (WAIS)

Scale	Subtest
Verbal	Information
	Comprehension
	Arithmetic
	Similarities
	Digit Span
	Vocabulary
Performance	Digit Symbol
	Picture Completion
	Block Design
	Picture Arrangement
	Object Assembly

intelligence being assessed. The most popular instrument used to measure intellectual functioning in research and clinical environments is the Weschler Adult Intelligence Scale (WAIS). The WAIS is a battery of tests containing two scales and 11 subtests that assess a wide range of verbal and nonverbal abilities, yielding an index of overall cognitive ability. The verbal scale contains 6 subtests that measure the capacity to retrieve information along each of these dimensions. The performance scale assesses the ability to manipulate data independent of existing knowledge. The scales and corresponding subtests on the WAIS are shown in Table 3–11.

There is widespread agreement that performance on the WAIS is age dependent. The point at which decrements in performance occur varies with age, experimental design, educational level, and cultural variables. Further, decrements vary as a function of the aspect of intellectual life addressed by a particular subtest. In general, it appears that subtests that measure verbal ability are less vulnerable to the effects of age than are tests that quantify psychomotor ability. Further, irrespective of the methodology, performance on the WAIS is stable in adults up to 50 years of age. After this age, conclusions depend on whether a longitudinal or cross-sectional design was employed. It appears that decrements in performance on intelligence tests occur slightly later in the life span when the design is longitudinal (late 60s) rather than cross-sectional (early 60s). Both methodologies demonstrate substantial declines in performance on intelligence tests when individuals are in their mid-70s (Albert, 1994).

Some psychologists have suggested that intelligence should not be divided according to performance on the verbal and performance scales. Rather, intelligence should be viewed as having two rather different components, namely crystallized or fluid intelligence. The former involves experience, meaning, knowledge, wisdom, and professional expertise whereas the latter involves tests of memory and abstract problem solving. Bienfeld (1990) suggested that crystallized intelligence is measured by performance on the

vocabulary and general information subtest of the WAIS. Crystallized intelligence involves experience and consists of a knowledge base acquired early in life. In contrast, fluid intelligence assesses abstract problem-solving ability and is tapped by performance on the block design and the digit symbol subtests. Fluid intelligence can be viewed as a measure of the brain's ability to reorganize data into new pathways and is thought to be dependent on the integrity of the central nervous system (Hartke, 1991). When intelligence is measured according to this categorization scheme, profound age differences are noted, favoring younger adults.

SPECIAL CONSIDERATION

Crystallized intelligence appears to remain stable or increase throughout adulthood whereas fluid intelligence tends to decline with the insults of old age (Horn & Cattell, 1967; Friedan, 1993).

It is critical to emphasize that there is considerable variability in performance on tests of intellectual function. The variability is most likely due to internal factors (e.g., age-related alterations in brain function) and external factors (e.g., environmental variables).

Motivation

Motivation is one of the most important cognitive factors that affects adaptation to chronic disease and resultant disability (Kemp, 1990). As such it has a great impact on the well-being of older disabled adults including those with hearing impairment (Kemp, 1990). The term *motivation* refers to self-directed behavior. It is a state of being that produces a tendency toward some type of action (Kaplan, Sadock, & Grubb, 1994). Motivational theorists including Freud and Lewin have stressed that motivation is a multivariate process comprising four primary variables (Kemp, 1986). Three of the variables encourage or support behavior. These include wants, expectations, and reinforcement. The final variable, cost of the behavior, discourages or prevents behavior. In general, motivation is optimal when: (1) the person knows what he or she wants (W); (2) the person expects or believes it can be obtained (B); (3) the rewards associated with it are meaningful (R); and (4) the costs associated with it are minimal (C) (Kemp, 1990). The motive system can be expressed as the following equation:

$$\text{Motivation} = W \times B \times R/C$$

It is important to emphasize that each of these components of the motivational formula are based on the individual's perceptions rather than on what the clinician might perceive as the facts. The likelihood of success plays a critical role in motivating behavior, as does the expectancy factor, which refers to the subjective probability that, with enough effort, one's goal may be achieved (Kaplan, Sadock, & Grubb, 1994).

In the audiologic domain a person's wants might include desires, wishes, needs, and goals relative to hearing status and audiologic interventions (Kemp, 1990). Goals initiate behavior and are strongly related to behavior and outcomes.

SPECIAL CONSIDERATION

An individual who wants something is more likely to succeed than one who does not.

For example, a person who wants to overcome the handicapping effects of hearing loss and is self-referred for a hearing aid, is more likely to do so than an individual who is brought in reluctantly by a family member. For audiologic treatment to be successful, the clinician must identify: (1) what the person wants from the intervention; (2) why the person wants the treatment; (3) how life might change if the individual receives the treatment; and (4) how the individual's goals were established.

Beliefs, expectations, assumptions, or attitudes all relate back to what the client wants. Beliefs are the cognitive component of motivation and are what the person acts upon. Three areas of belief are important to fully comprehend a person's motivation. These include the situation and/or task the person is facing, the future as the person sees it, and the person himself or herself. In general, the individual must be optimistic about his or her capability to succeed at a task to actually succeed. Belief in one's capabilities will initiate behavior. Behavior that is associated with some form of reward, reinforcement, positive feedback, or benefit will be initiated and maintained. Thus, reward is an important aspect of motivational dynamics. With regard to hearing impairment, the ability to hear birds with a new hearing aid or to finally understand the minister at a church service with an infrared system would be considered rewarding and should be emphasized during a treatment session. It is critical that audiologists relate an intervention to rewards or successes to insure compliance and maintenance of behavior.

Finally, the variables in the numerator of the motivational formula must be weighed against the cost of behavior for it to be initiated and maintained. Costs pertain to effort, physical pain, emotional discomfort, threats to self-esteem, money, and time. Thus, costs can be physical, psychologic, and social. In general, if the denominator or costs are greater than the numerator the person will be unmotivated to pursue a behavior. In contrast, if the benefits of a particular intervention outweigh the costs, the individual will be highly motivated.

Although motivation does not decline with age, there are age-related differences in approaches to motivating older adults. In the latter regard, fulfillment of safety and security

PEARL

Older adults require more and different reinforcement. They respond better to concrete goals that are immediate and affect daily functioning.

needs is a powerful incentive for complying with a particular medical regimen (Kemp, 1986). Older adults often avoid

TABLE 3–12 Tips for Overcoming Motivational Barriers

- Provide a supportive climate for learning.
- Make sure that the patient feels a part of the session.
- Appreciate and value the patient regardless of achievement. This will sustain involvement and progress.
- Materials should be meaningful and instructions clear as this will ensure motivated involvement.

Source: Lewis, 1990.

difficult tasks because of anxiety associated with new or challenging tasks. Accordingly, the older adult should be given every reason to believe that improvement or success is possible prior to attempting a new technique or intervention. Regular corrective feedback presented in a nonthreatening, supportive manner will go a long way toward reducing anxiety about a task, sustaining continued involvement, and promoting motivation and a sense of success (Lewis, 1990). In a later discussion of audiologic rehabilitation, more specific suggestions for assessing and improving motivation will be presented. Table 3–12 lists tips for motivating older adults, especially during rehabilitation sessions.

Miscellaneous Cognitive Variables

In the aging literature a good deal of attention has been focused on the changes in reaction time or speed of response associated with age. The term *reaction time* refers to the time that elapses between a signal being given and a required motor response being undertaken. It appears that portions of peripheral and central nervous systems mediate this cognitive phenomenon, specifically the circuits that lie between the perception of the signal and activation of the intention to respond. The extent to which the aging process is associated with changes in the time required for peripheral and central processing dictates when and if reaction time will be prolonged. In general, one might conclude that as signal pathways deteriorate with age, there is a corresponding decline in reaction time.

SPECIAL CONSIDERATION

To compensate for possible declines in reaction time, the clinician should routinely allow time for the older adult to fully process information prior to demanding a response.

Using the computer analogy put forth earlier, when working with the elderly one should allow sufficent time between data input, data processing, and data output in the event that there is a slowing of reaction time. Clinically, it is a rather simple matter to gain an informal appreciation for a person's reaction time. For example, during the audiological evaluation, upon presentation of the pure-tone stimulus one should monitor the time it takes for the person to respond to the presence of the signal. The stimulus response time should dictate the time interval between stimulus presentations. In a sense, the stimulus response time is an index of reaction time for that particular procedure.

Finally, coping ability is an important cognitive variable in older adults because it influences response to stress, disability, etc. In general, coping is a highly individualized process that appears to evolve with age, rather than changing with increasing years of life. Premorbid personality influences to a great extent an older adult's coping strategies. Further, the type of stressor interacts with lifelong coping ability. For example, as pertains to health stressors, illness severity, and expectations regarding health influence coping ability. Specifically, aging attribution has been shown to undercut the ability to cope with mild as well as severe medical conditions. There is a suggestion in the literature that at any age more effective coping responses are associated with: (1) a higher socioeconomic status; (2) the availability of a wide repertoire of coping strategies; (3) high self-esteem; (4) a good supply of internal resources; (5) assumption of personal responsibility for one's health whenever feasible; and (6) perceptions of disability, health, and aging (Hartke, 1991). Accordingly, clinicians, especially those engaged in audiologic rehabilitation, have a responsibility to understand the older adult's coping ability and introduce strategies for facilitating coping and adaptation to acquired hearing impairment. This is an important aspect of assertiveness and strategies training used during audiologic rehabilitation.

SPECIAL CONSIDERATION

Hartke (1991) suggests that promoting patient involvement in the rehabilitation process, enhancing a sense of realistic mastery or control, and addressing and disspelling age attribution are effective mechanisms for promoting the coping process.

CONCLUDING REMARKS

Psychosocial theories of aging emphasize the individualized nature of the aging process and the complex interaction between internal and external factors as determining the way in which one ages in each domain. The external forces are primarily social and include loss of income, loss of role/status, and bereavement. Along with physical stressors the internal forces are psychological including isolated changes in cognitive status and intellectual functioning. Declines in specific areas of cognition, personality, and coping have been demonstrated in older adults. However, the safest conclusion one can draw from the literature review is that people age in a highly individualized manner and psychological development tends to proceed in such a way as to magnify the diversity of individuals within an aging cohort (Bienfeld, 1990). Life stressors such as illness, loss of job, loss of loved ones, etc. interact with psychological variables to determine age-related declines in the psychologic domain. In general, it appears that the core personality tends to remain stable throughout life as does one's coping mechanisms. Similarly, capacity for new learning remains unaffected by age, as does the capacity for registration and storage of information. In contrast, the speed of learning tends to decline with aging and strategies for retrieval of information tend to become less efficient (Bienfeld, 1990).

Given the multiple stresses associated with aging, the clinician must consider the total person when conducting an evaluation and instituting any form of intervention. Audiologists should operate from the perspective that many older persons have complex problems of a physical, psychological, and social nature that will influence one's diagnostic and treatment approach. We cannot predict what each of these stresses will be because of the individual variability characterizing older adults. Thus, audiologists must have at their disposal a means of assessing and perhaps minimizing the effects of those variables on audiologic management.

REFERENCES

ABRAMS, W., BEERS, M., & BERKOW, R. (1995). *The Merck Manual of Geriatrics.* 2d ed. Whitehouse Station, NJ: Merck & Co., Inc.

ALBERT, M. (1994). Cognition and aging. In: W. Hazzard, E. Bierman, J. Blass, W. Ettinger, & J. Halter (Eds.), *Principles of Geriatric Medicine and Gerontology.* New York: McGraw-Hill.

BENGTSON, V., PARROTT, T., & BURGESS, E. (1996). Progress and pitfalls in gerontological theorizing. *Gerontologist, 36:* 768–772.

BIENFELD, D. (1990). Psychology of aging. In: D. Bienfeld (Ed.), *Clinical Geropsychiatry.* 3d ed. Baltimore: Williams & Wilkins.

BOTWINICK, J. (1973). *Aging and Behavior.* New York: Springer Publishing.

COREY, G. (1991). *Theory and Practice of Counseling and Psychotherapy.* 4th ed. Pacific Grove, CA: Brooks/Cole Publishing.

COSTA, P., & MCCRAE, R. (1994). Personality and aging. In: W. Hazzard, E. Bierman, J. Blass, W. Ettinger, & J. Halter (Eds.), *Principles of Geriatric Medicine and Gerontology.* New York: McGraw-Hill.

COX, H. (1988). Social realities of aging. In: B. Shadden (Ed.), *Communication Behavior and Aging: A Sourcebook for Clinicians.* Baltimore: Williams & Wilkins.

CUMMING, E., & HENRY, W. (1961). *Growing Old: The Process of Disengagement.* New York: Basic Books.

DAVIS, C. (1990). Psychosocial aspects of aging. In: *Aging: The Health Care Challenge.* 2d ed. Philadelphia: F.A. Davis.

ERIKSON, E. (1968). *Identity: Youth and Crisis.* New York: W.W. Norton.

FRIEDAN, B. (1993). *The Fountain of Age.* New York: Simon & Schuster.

HARTKE, R. (1991). The aging process: Cognition, personality, and coping. In: R. Hartke (Ed.), *Psychological Aspects of Geriatric Rehabilitation.* Gaithersburg, MD: Aspen Publishers.

HAVIGHURST, R. (1963). Successful aging. In: R. Williams, C. Tibbit, & W. Donahue (Eds.), *Process of Aging.* New York: Lieber-Atherton.

HAYFLICK, L. (1994). *How and Why We Age.* New York: Ballantine Books.

HORN, J., & CATTELL, R. (1967). Age differences in fluid and crystallized intelligence. *Acta Psychologica,* 26: 107–129.

KAPLAN, H., SADOCK, B., & GRUBB, J. (1994). *Synopsis of Psychiatry.* 7th ed. Baltimore: Williams & Wilkins.

KAUSLER, D. (1988). Cognition and aging. In: B. Shadden (Ed.), *Communication Behavior and Aging: A Sourcebook for Clinicians.* Baltimore: Williams & Wilkins.

KEMP, B. (1986). Psychosocial and mental health issues in rehabilitation of older persons. In: S. Brody & G. Ruff (Eds.), *Aging and Rehabilitation.* New York: Springer Publishing.

———. (1990). Motivational dynamics in geriatric rehabilitation: Toward a therapeutic model. In: B. Kemp, J. Brummel-Smith, & J. Ramsdell (Eds.), *Geriatric Rehabilitation.* Boston: College-Hill Publication.

LEWIS, C. (1990). *Aging: The Health Care Challenge.* 2d ed. Philadelphia: F.A. Davis.

LIGHTHOUSE, INC. (1995). *The Lighthouse National Survey of Vision Loss: The Experience, Attitudes, and Knowledge of Middle Aged and Older Americans.* New York: The Lighthouse, Inc.

MADDOX, G. (1965). Fact and artifact: Evidence bearing on disengagement theory from the Duke geriatrics project. *Human Development,* 1: 117–139.

MELTON, A. (1963). Implications of short-term memory for a general theory of memory. *Journal of Verbal Learning and Verbal Behavior,* 2: 1–21.

NEUGARTEN, B. (1966). Adult personality: A developmental view. *Human Development,* 9: 61–73.

———. (1975). *Middle Age and Aging.* Chicago: University of Chicago Press.

NOBLE W., & ATHERLY, G. (1970). The hearing measurement scale: A questionnaire for the assessment of auditory disability. *Journal of Auditory Research,* 10: 229–250.

ROBERTSON-TCHABO, E., & ARENBERG, D. (1988). Cognitive performance. In: G. Mueller & V. Geoffrey (Eds.), *Communication Disorders in Aging: Assessment and Management.* Washington, DC: Gallaudet University Press.

ROWE, J., & KAHN, R. (1998). *Successful Aging.* New York: Random House.

TALLMER, M., & KUTNER, B. (1969). Disengagement and the stresses of aging. *Journal of Gerontology,* 24: 70–74.

VERWOERDT, A. (1976). *Clinical Geropsychiatry.* Baltimore: Williams & Wilkins.

WEINSTEIN, B. (1980). Hearing impairment and social isolation in the elderly. Doctoral Dissertation. New York: Columbia University.

The Aging Auditory System

Chapter 4

Aging of the Outer, Middle, and Inner Ear, and Neural Pathways

I feel so bad for Uncle Ted,
There's not much hair upon his head,
And what is worse, he barely hears,
There's too much hair in his ears.

—Bruce Lansky, 1996

LEARNING OBJECTIVES

After reading this chapter, you should be able to:

- Explain the age-related changes in the outer ear, middle ear, cochlea, eighth nerve, central auditory pathways, and auditory cortex.
- Understand why the ear is susceptible to age effects.
- Describe the disorders of the outer ear, middle ear, inner ear, eighth nerve, and auditory cortex to which older adults are most susceptible.

The entire auditory system undergoes changes with age. In addition, certain otologic conditions are more prevalent in older than in younger adults. The goal of this chapter is to outline the changes that occur in the peripheral and central auditory systems of the older adult and to describe the ear pathologies prevalent in this population. This chapter will set the stage for Chapters 5 and 6, which discuss the behavioral and electrophysiologic assessment of the ear.

PEARL

Age 65 is an arbitrary cut-off for defining someone as "old."

Sixty-five years of age was adopted by President Franklin D. Roosevelt as the definition of *old* for Social Security purposes. He used Chancellor Otto von Bismarck of Germany's legal criterion for retirement age. Chancellor Bismarck adopted 65 in 1889 because his actuaries advised him that hardly anyone at that time lived to 65 in Germany and thus the plan would rarely have to pay retirement benefits (Nielsen, 1998).

ANATOMICAL AND PHYSIOLOGIC CHANGES IN THE OUTER EAR

The outer ear comprises the auricle (pinna) and the external auditory meatus or external auditory canal. The auricle, which is an irregular ovoid structure, is the external extension of the cartilaginous ear canal and as such is formed of elastic cartilage. Skin covers the auricle, with hairs present primarily in the tragal and anti-tragal regions (Senturia, Marcus, & Lucente, 1980). The external auditory canal is an S-shaped structure approximately 25 mm in length. The anterior wall of the canal is adjacent medially to the temporomandibular joint and laterally to the parotid gland. Also, the inferior wall is closely related to the parotid gland. The external auditory canal is composed of elastic cartilage laterally and bone medially. The cartilage of the outer portion of the canal is continuous with that of the pinna, while the skin of the osseous canal is continuous with the skin covering the lateral surface of the tympanic membrane (Ballachanda, 1995a). Figure 4–1 clearly shows the anatomical distinctions between the cartilaginous and osseous parts of the ear canal and its relation to the middle and inner parts of the ear.

The skin covering the ear canal is thinner in the osseous canal compared to the cartilaginous portion. Specifically, the skin lining the cartilaginous canal consists of epidermis with papillae, a well-developed dermis, and a subcutaneous layer. The epidermis is composed of four layers including basal cell, prickle or squamous cell, granular cell, and cornified layers. As will be shown later, these layers give rise to tumor cells prevalent in older adults. The skin lining the osseous canal is devoid of papillae and has no subcutaneous layer. The osseous canal does not contain glands or hair follicles whereas the skin of the fibrocartilaginous portion of the canal contains hair follicles and apocrine (ceruminous) and sebaceous glands.

The skin of the osseous canal is quite thin (0.2 mm in thickness); it is susceptible to trauma during any type of manipulation including cerumen removal and possibly deep insertion of hearing aids (Ballachanda, 1995a).

55

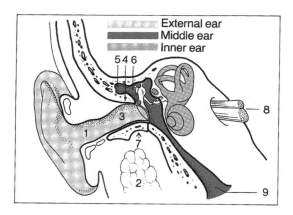

Figure 4–1 Cartilaginous and osseous portions of the external auditory meatus relative to middle and inner portions of the ear. 1, cartilaginous part; 2, parotid gland; 3, bony meatus; 4, lateral attic wall; 5, mastoid antrum; 6, attic; 7, temporomandibular joint; 8, facial vestibular, and auditory nerves; 9, eustachian tube. (From Becker, Naumann, and Pfaltz, 1994, p. 4. Reprinted by permission.)

Cerumen or ear wax is created by secretions from sebaceous and apocrine glands, and from dust particles, desquamated epithelial cells, and dislodged hair follicles (Ballachanda, 1995a). Cerumen, which contains a mixture of lipids, protein free amino acids, and several minerals, serves a protective function for the epithelial lining of the cartilagionus portion of the canal (Ballachanda, 1995a). That is, it lubricates the skin lining the canal, acts as a water repellent, and entraps unwanted material and objects including insects. It is normally cleared by epithelial migration. In some cases, especially in older adults, either excessively large amounts of cerumen are produced or epithelial migration is inadequate, leading to the presence of impacted cerumen (Miyamoto & Miyamoto, 1995).

The outer ear subserves several important functions. In general, the role of the pinna and ear canal is to couple airborne soundwaves to the middle ear. The ear canal, in combination with the concha, alters the spectral content of the signal reaching the tympanic membrane. Specifically, it modifies incoming sound by acting as a resonator or generator of additional sound (Staab, 1995). It is integral to success with hearing aids in that it serves as the location where any type of hearing aid is placed (i.e., in-the-ear, in-the-canal, or behind-the-ear) (Staab, 1995). Finally, the ear canal is an important site for behavioral and electrophysiologic tests and its status often influences the outcomes achieved on these measures as well as the ability to administer selected tests. The audiologist should therefore be familiar with how aging may influence the structure and function of the outer ear.

The primary age-related changes that occur in this structure include degeneration of elastic fibers and decreased collagen, which lead to a loss of elasticity and strength. As such there is a thinning of surface epithelium and atrophy of the subcutaneous tissue. Further, the glandular structure within the ear canal, most notably the sebaceous and cerumen glands, lose some of their secretory ability. There is also a de-

crease in the fat present in the canal and an increase in the thickness and length of hair follicles in the fibrocartilaginous portion. As a result the skin becomes dry and prone to trauma and breakdown, and cerumen becomes more concentrated, hard, and impacted (Ballachanda, 1995a). The bony canal is especially susceptible to trauma that may result from manipulations associated with cerumen removal because the skin covering is so thin. This is also a concern when making ear impressions for completely in-the-canal hearing aids (Ballachanda, 1995a). Associated with the changes in the ear canal is a decrease in tolerance for hard materials, which may impact on hearing aid fittings (Oliveira, 1995). Thus, it is prudent to consider hearing aids made from soft shells that conform to changes in the ear canal during mandibular movements because this will likely promote comfort and long-term use of deep canal hearing aids (Staab, 1995).

Cerumen production and extrusion go uninterrupted in most individuals by virtue of normal epithelial migration from deeper parts of the ear canal. Cerumen impaction can occur for a number of reasons, notably excessive production of cerumen due to increased activity of cerumen glands. Nonphysiological variables accounting for cerumen impaction include physical obstruction due to a hearing aid, frequent use of cotton-tipped swabs, or abnormalities in the shape and size of the ear canal. Older adults are more susceptible to a higher frequency of impaction for still another reason: In older adults there is a reduction in the number of active cerumen glands, which leads to the production of drier and less viscous cerumen. Combined with the presence of thicker and longer hair follicles that are oriented toward the tympanic membrane this leads to a higher frequency of impaction (Ruby, 1986). Gleitman, Ballachanda, and Goldstein (1992) recently completed a study of 892 adults to determine the prevalence of impaction in individuals of varying age groups.

SPECIAL CONSIDERATION

The prevalence of impaction increases with age.

It was notable that the highest prevalence, 34%, was for persons 65 to 75 years, with 22% of adults 75 to 84 years having impacted cerumen. Mahoney (1987) reported the prevalence of cerumen impaction to be as high as 34% in her sample.

COMMON DISORDERS OF THE EXTERNAL EAR

Disorders of the external ear arising in the pinna and external ear, common in older adults, are discussed in the sections to follow.

The Pinna

The most common changes in the pinna associated with the aging process include excessive hair growth on the tragus and on the lower portions of the helix, primarily in males. Enlargement of the pinna has been reported as well as changes in the physical properties of the skin including loss of elasticity, dryness, thinning, and on occasion atrophy (Johnson & Hadley, 1964). For the most part, these changes do not affect hearing; however, they may interfere with hearing aid impressions and hearing aid use.

Chondrodermatitis, a painful or tender pink ulceration, may appear on the helix or antihelix of the ear. It results from degeneration of the epidermis, dermis, and/or cartilage from chronic sun exposure, pressure, or trauma (Young, Newcomer, & Kligman, 1993). If, during audiometry, cerumen management, or the making of an earmold impression, the audiologist notes the presence of a lesion on the ear, referral to a physician, preferably a dermatologist, should be made.

The pinna is a potential site for squamous cell carcinoma, a red-brown appearing nodule associated with chronic sun or radiation exposure (Young, Newcomer, & Kligman, 1993). More than 90% of squamous cell carcinomas in fair-skinned individuals occur on the face or ears, primarily in older adults (Steigleder & Maibach, 1993). The posterosuperior aspect of the pinna is most frequently involved in men whereas these tumors tend to occur closer to the ear canal in women (Abrams, Beers, & Berkow, 1995). Basal cell carcinomas are the second most common malignant tumor of the pinna, occurring more often in males, and like squamous cell carcinomas, occur secondary to sun exposure. Basal cell carcinomas appear as nodules with pearly, heaped-up borders (Abrams, Beers, & Berkow, 1995).

PEARL

If the audiologist notices an unusual-looking growth when examining the pinna, appropriate referral should be made because these tumors have metastatic potential.

The External Auditory Meatus

In light of age-related changes in the structure of the ear canal, which include thinning of the surface epithelium, atrophy of the subcutaneous tissue, and decline in the secretory abilities of the glands, older adults are susceptible to the development of dry skin, which is prone to trauma and breakdown, and to hard and impacted cerumen (Ballachanda, 1995a). Also, older adults are susceptible to selected functional and pathological conditions.

The most commonly reported functional condition of the ear canal is referred to as collapsed canal. In this condition, pressure from earphones applied during audiometric tests may cause the ear canal to collapse. The latter may occur because of atrophy of the supporting cartilage and resulting decreased skin elasticity in the cartilaginous portion of the ear canal. As a result, air conduction threshold shifts may emerge, primarily in the high frequencies leading to the presence of "artificial air-bone gaps." Threshold shifts of 15 dB or more have been reported however, at all frequencies by a number of investigators (Ballachanda, 1995a). The prevalence of collapsed ear canals in older adults varies depending primarily on the population studied but has been reported to be as high as 30 to 40%. While in the past the presence of collapsed canals was a major source of measurement error, the use of insert rather than the traditional supra-aural earphones during testing helps to alleviate the problem.

PEARL

During audiometric testing the presence of a high-frequency air-bone gap, poor test-retest reliability, disagreement between pure-tone and immittance test results should alert the clinician to the potential for collapsed ear canals.

Techniques such as use of sound-field testing, insert earphones, and holding the pinna up and back prior to earphone placement can effectively alleviate the collapsed ear-canal problem (Silman & Silverman, 1991).

Cerumen impaction has been mentioned as a prevalent condition in older adults. Cerumen impaction can have significant medical and audiological consequences, which for the most part are temporary, resolving upon removal of the cerumen. Common medical sequelae of impaction include tinnitus, pain, fullness of the ear, external otitis, and, less frequently, vertigo (Ballachanda, 1995a). An audiologic consequence of gradual cerumen buildup is hearing loss, which is typically high frequency and conductive oftentimes presenting as a conductive component on an already existing sensorineural hearing loss. Hearing loss occurs because the cerumen creates a constriction of the ear canal. The presence of cerumen impaction can restrict audiologists from performing selected diagnostic tests or rehabilitative procedures. For example, blockage can interfere with otoacoustic emissions, immittance measures, electrocochleography, and electronystagmography. Interference with audiological test procedures can create patient inconvenience because of the necessity to postpone testing until the cerumen has been removed. Further, impacted cerumen can preclude real ear hearing-aid measurements, render a hearing aid ineffectual, or cause hearing aids to malfunction. It is incumbent on audiologists to inform professionals working with hearing-aid users to examine the hearing aid or earmold bore in the event of apparent malfunction, as a blocked hearing aid can be a sign of cerumen impaction. In light of the latter considerations, the American Speech-Language-Hearing Association (ASHA), the American Academy of Audiology, the Academy of Dispensing Audiologists, and licensing boards of several states officially recognize cerumen management as within the scope of audiology practice (ASHA, 1992). Audiologists engaged in cerumen management should check state licensure laws, professional insurance policies, and institutional insurance coverage, as well. In addition, universal precautions specified by the Centers for Disease Control and Prevention should be followed. When performing cerumen management in older adults exercise extreme caution in individuals prone to infection such as persons with diabetes mellitus, AIDS infection, auto-immune disease, cancer, or external otitis. With the elderly especially, excessive care should be taken when removing cerumen from the bony portion of the canal to avoid unnecessary abrasion. Finally, if external lesions are present in and around the ear canal, referral to a physician should be made.

SPECIAL CONSIDERATION

Cerumen impaction and collapsed ear canals can jeopardize the validity of pure-tone results.

The external ear canal may be the site of benign, malignant, or premalignant neoplastic changes. These include keratosis obturans, exostosis and osteoma, squamous or basal cell carcinoma, among others. Any unusual appearing outgrowth in the cartilaginous or bony ear canal, bleeding from the earcanal, or otorrhea may signifiy the presence of a neoplasm in the ear indicating the necessity for a medical referral.

Contact dermatitis, an inflammatory process produced by contact of an irritant with the skin, may arise in the ear canal of older adults oftentimes from hearing aids or earmolds. The length of exposure to the agent, combined with individual susceptibility, determines whether skin irritation will arise (Senturia, Marcus, & Lucente, 1980). Symptoms of dermatitis might include itchiness and/or erythema. When dermatitis from hearing-aid use is suspected, the patient should be instructed to remove the etiologic agent and contact the physician for proper treatment.

Pruritis or itching is the most common dermatologic complaint of older adults, and the external auditory meatus is a common site. Dryness of the skin resulting from atrophy of the epithelial sebaceous glands tends to contribute to the development of pruritis. In view of age-related skin atrophy, the skin lining the canal is vulnerable to trauma. Older adults should be advised against using cotton applicators to remove debris because this can induce further itching, trauma, and potential infection (Rees & Duckert, 1995).

Otitis externa is a bacterial infection of the epithelial lining of the ear canal (Miyamoto & Miyamoto, 1995). The symptoms can range from primarily itching to otorrhea, redness, swelling, a blocked feeling within the ear, and tenderness. The severity of the symptoms depends on the duration of the condition and on the pathogen. The most severe form, malignant necrotizing otitis externa, may develop in elderly diabetics and patients whose condition is out of control or in immunocompromised patients (Miyamoto & Miyamoto, 1995). If examination of the ear canal reveals any of the above symptoms, referral to a physician is indicated.

Concluding Remarks

The outer ear has recently become a topic of considerable import to audiologists because of the emergence of interventions and diagnostic procedures that directly involve its visualization and manipulation. In the diagnostic realm, the ear canal is critical to immittance measurements, otoacoustic emissions, electronystagmography, electrocochleography, and auditory brainstem responses. Further, cerumen management is now part of the scope of practice of audiologists, necessitating thorough knowledge of its anatomy and potential disorders. In the rehabilitative arena, the pinna and ear canal serve as the anchor for hearing aids of all shapes and sizes, with the bony portion becoming increasingly important with the advent of completely in-the-canal hearing aids. Precise ear canal impressions are critical for the manufacturing and dispensing of custom-molded products such as hearing aids (Staab, 1995). Finally, the ear canal is critical for performing valid real-ear hearing-aid measurements during hearing-aid fittings. The audiologist working with older adults must be able to identify medical conditions involving the external ear for referral to physicians. At any time during a rehabilitative or diagnostic procedure that any unusual growth or irritation appears, it is incumbent on the audiologist to make the appropriate referral.

ANATOMICAL AND PHYSIOLOGIC CHANGES IN THE MIDDLE EAR

The middle ear consists of the tympanic membrane, an air-filled space containing a chain of three ossicles that mechanically connect the tympanic membrane to the oval window of the cochlea, and the eustachian tube. The tympanic membrane is composed of three layers, an outer epithelial layer that is continuous with the skin of the osseous portion of the ear canal, a fibrous tissue layer, and an inner mucosal layer that is continuous with the lining of the middle ear space, mastoid system, and eustachian tube. The ossicles, within the middle ear cleft, articulate with one another at the incudomalleal (I.M.) and incudostapedial (I.S.) joints, which are lined by articular cartilages. The tensor tympani muscle attaches to the malleus via the tendon of the tensor tympani and the stapedius muscle attaches to the head of the stapes via the stapedial tendon. The ossicles are suspended within the cavity via a system of ligaments and tendons. The eustachian tube connects the middle ear to the nasopharynx, thereby ventilating the middle ear space. A prerequisite for normal transmission of sound to the inner ear is a tympanic membrane of normal position and mobility, a continuous ossicular chain, and adequate ventilation of the middle ear via an intact eustachian tube.

The sound transmission apparatus undergoes changes with the aging process; however, for the most part, the changes do not appear to impact dramatically on hearing sensitivity. The changes are discussed in the following paragraphs. In addition, the diseases prevalent among older adults that affect middle ear status are discussed.

The tympanic membrane, ossicular chain, articular cartilage at the surfaces of the I.M. and I.S. joints, and middle ear muscles and ligaments are susceptible to minor age-related changes. Covell (1952), Rosenwasser (1964), and Etholm and Belal (1974) have performed histological studies of the middle ear structures and have observed a series of age-related changes. The tympanic membrane appears to become stiffer, thinner, and less vascular with increased age. In becoming more translucent with age, selected landmarks appear more visible during the otoscopic examination. Older adults with a history of chronic otitis media (COM) however, may have sclerotic changes on the eardrum. On visual inspection the latter may present as chalky white plaques (White & Regan, 1987). The presence of the white scale-like plaques on the tympanic membrane following COM is a hallmark of tympanosclerosis. This condition typically creates a stiffening effect on the tympanic membrane.

Arthritic changes in the middle ear have been observed in individuals over 30 years of age, increasing in frequency and severity with age. The arthritic changes include thinning and calcification of the cartilaginous I.M. and I.S. joints (Covell, 1952; Rosenwasser, 1964). Etholm and Belal (1974) reported that, according to their histological studies, the arthritic changes were moderate to severe in persons over 70 years of age. Because the I.M. and I.S. joints are synovial in nature, lined by articular cartilage and surrounded by an elastic tissue capsule, these changes are not surprising given the modifications occurring in the articular surfaces of other joints throughout the body. Additional age-related changes include atrophy and degeneration of the fibers of the middle ear muscles and the ossicular ligaments and ossification of the ossicles (Covell, 1952; Rosenwasser, 1964). Finally, calcification of the cartilaginous support of the eustachian tube and atrophy of the musculature has been reported in older adults. The age-related decline in muscle function may interfere with the opening of the eustachian tube especially during swallowing. While these changes do not appear to impact on pure-tone air and bone conduction thresholds, they may account for age effects appearing in selected studies on eustachian tube function, the acoustic reflex, and acoustic immittance results in older adults. These data will be discussed in Chapter 5.

PEARL

The middle ear structures undergo anatomical change with age, though they have little effect on the physiology of the middle ear and on behavioral tests. There is little evidence of substantial stiffening of the middle ear transmission system with age (Wiley, Cruickshanks, Nondahl, & Tweed, 1999).

COMMON DISORDERS OF THE MIDDLE EAR

Older adults are susceptible to developing all of the diseases that arise in the middle ear, yet some are more likely than others to occur early rather than late in adult life. Table 4–1 lists common diseases of the middle ear. Older adults are susceptible to middle ear disease associated with trauma and to neoplastic tumors including squamous cell carcinoma and vascular tumors such as glomus tumors. Otosclerosis, a focal disease of the otic capsule, is generally associated with an early age of onset (e.g., adolescence and young adulthood); however, Farrior (1963) reported that nearly 40% of patients in his sample developed hearing loss from otosclerosis in their fifth, sixth, and seventh decade of life.

TABLE 4–1 Common Diseases of the Middle Ear

Infectious diseases of the middle ear
- Acute or chronic otitis media
- Otitis media with effusion
- Acute mastoiditis
- Tympanosclerosis

Trauma to the middle ear
- Temporal bone injury
- Tympanic membrane or ossicular damage

Neoplastic tumors and diseases of the middle ear
- Polyps
- Cholesteatoma
- Osteomas
- Glomus tumors
- Squamous cell carcinoma

Congenital diseases of the middle ear
- Ossicular anomalies
- Vascular anomalies
- Facial nerve anomalies

Idiopathic diseases of the middle ear
- Otosclerosis

Source: Adapted from Northern, 1996.

When acute otitis media occurs after age 60, the relative incidence of mastoiditis and associated complications is higher in older adults because of the diminished responsiveness of their immune system (White & Regan, 1987). Symptoms include, but are not limited to, facial nerve paralysis, and labrynthitis, while complications may include meningitis and brain abscess. It is noteworthy that otitis media caused by infection with *Mycobacterium tuberculosis* may result from spread associated with pulmonary infection or from an ascending infection through the eustachian tube from the nasopharynx. Tuberculosis otitis media is generally painless, with multiple small perforations that may ultimately lead to total tympanic membrane perforation (Schleuning & Andersen, 1993).

Of all middle ear disorders, persons over 65 years of age are most prone to developing one of the many infectious diseases of the middle ear. Their susceptibility grows out of changes in the musculature of the eustachian tube with age, a less efficient immune system, and tendency toward development of complications from diseases or interventions that may terminate in middle ear infection. Data summarizing the epidemiology of middle ear problems among the elderly are imprecise; however, data from the National Hospital Discharge Survey are somewhat revealing. Among persons over 65 years of age, the most common otolaryngologic diagnoses were as follows: (1) otitis media and upper respiratory infection (URI) with complication or comorbidity, (2) otitis media and URI without complication or comorbidity, (3) dysequilibrium, and (4) ear, nose, and throat (ENT) malignancy. The most common procedures were: sinus and mastoid procedures, major head and neck procedures, and rhinoplasty. The average length of stay for otitis media and URI with or without complications was approximately five days (Korper, 1989). These data suggest that the elderly are at risk for developing such middle ear conditions as otitis media, eustachian tube dysfunction, etc. It is likely that conditions afflicting the elderly such as nasopharyngeal pathology including malignancy and radiation therapy for ENT malignancy also place older adults at risk for otitis media. Similarly, nasotracheal intubation or prolonged nasogastric (NG) tube placement may cause edema of the eustachian tube and nasopharynx, possibly leading to development of otitis media (Kenna, 1993).

SPECIAL CONSIDERATION

Because an older person's immune system may become less effective in its primary function of protecting against infection and neoplastic disease, the case history and audiometric testing should routinely include tests of middle ear status to facilitate early diagnosis and management of middle ear disease.

This is especially true for older adults with URI because the incidence of acute otitis media and otitis media with effusion roughly parallels the incidence of upper respiratory tract infections.

AGING OF THE INNER EAR AND NEURAL PATHWAYS

The inner ear is composed of several functional components that are vulnerable to the effects of aging. These components are sensory, neural, vascular, supporting, synaptic, and/or mechanical (Willott, 1991). The organ of Corti (O of C), which is the site of transduction of mechanical to neural energy, houses the sense organ of hearing. It extends spirally from the basal convolution to the cupula or apex of the cochlea. The O of C rests atop the basilar membrane and is composed of sensory cells (outer and inner hair cells along with their stereocilia), supporting cells, Reissner's membrane, tectorial membrane, and stria vascularis, among other structures. The normal auditory system is tonotopically organized and the tonotopic organization depends on the existence of anatomic connections from the cochlea to regions within the central auditory system (Willott, 1996). This tonotopic organization is the mechanism by which frequencies within the periphery are represented in the central auditory system.

PEARL

The inner ear undergoes dramatic changes with age with corresponding effects on pure-tone threshholds and word recognition tests.

Thus, for example, high-frequency regions within the basal turn of the cochlea connect via a set of neurons within that region, to high-frequency tonotopic regions of the central auditory nervous system (Willott, 1996).

SPECIAL CONSIDERATION

The most critical risk factor for the auditory system is age.

Degeneration of the Organ of Corti

A multivariate study designed to identify risk factors for hearing loss in the elderly revealed that although gender, family history of hearing loss, and noise exposure account for some of the individual variability in hearing loss, the most critical risk factor for the auditory sense organ is age (Moscicki, Elkins, Baum, & McNamara, 1985). The O of C is the structure most susceptible to age-related histopathological changes. Age-related atrophy ultimately interferes with the transduction process integral to the reception of sound. The cells of the inner ear and neural pathways are of the "nonmitotic" variety (Schuknecht, 1993). They are highly differentiated cells such that once their specialized functions have been established, they can no longer reproduce. The length of cell life depends on the ability to maintain their characteristic structural organization while adapting to changes in their fluid environment (Schuknecht, 1993). The changes the aging ear undergoes have been studied most extensively by Schuknecht (1955, 1964) and more recently by Schuknecht and Gacek (1993). Prior to outlining the classic changes extensively studied by Schuknecht and his colleagues, some general age-related histopathological changes within the O of C and spiral ganglion cells will be discussed.

It appears that hair cell loss is the rule rather than the exception among older adults. In general, loss of hair cells is most severe in the basal region of the cochlea. Further, degeneration of the outer row of outer hair cells is often more severe than in the other rows (Willott, 1991).

SPECIAL CONSIDERATION

While both outer and inner hair cells tend to degenerate with age, the outer hair cells are more vulnerable than inner hair cells and most likely account for the typical decline in hearing with age (Willott, 1991).

Both types of hair cells degenerate in the basal turn of the cochlea, with apical and mid-cochlear involvement of the outer hair cells, as well. Figure 4–2 displays outer hair cell versus inner hair cell loss in older relative to younger adults. It is clear that the decrease in hair cell population is greatest in persons over 70 years of age and is most pronounced for outer hair cells. That is, hair cell population is less in older adults, especially for outer hair cells. It is important to note that outer and inner hair cells can degenerate independently.

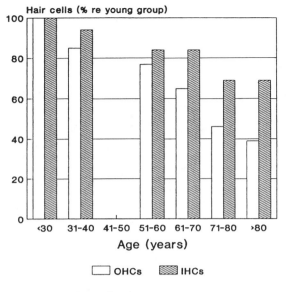

Hair cells (% re young group)

OHCs 100% = 12.4 thousand
IHCs 100% = 3.2 thousand

Figure 4–2 Inner and outer hair cell loss as a function of increasing age. (Adapted from Otte, Schuknecht, and Kerr, 1978. Reprinted by permission.)

PEARL

The substantial loss of outer hair cells in the basal turn of the cochlea affects cochlear mechanics and is responsible for the normal decline in pure-tone hearing with age (Willott, 1991).

In contrast to the effect the loss of hair cells in the basal turn of the cochlea has on cochlear mechanics, hair cell loss in the most apical portions of the cochlea may have little effect on audiometric thresholds. Thus, older adults who experience hair cell damage in selected regions of the cochlea do not necessarily sustain a hearing loss whereas hair cell loss near the cochlea base is associated with hearing loss. According to Willott (1991), a loss of about 20% of hair cells throughout the cochlea may result in minimal sensorineural hearing loss, whereas more severe loss of hair cells extending 10 mm or more from the base of the cochlea is associated with more significant hearing loss in the high frequencies. Bredberg (1968) determined, for example, that a 50 to 75% loss of outer hair cells in the apical region of the cochlea is associated with losses of less than 40 dBHL, whereas a 50% loss of hair cells near the cochlear bases is associated with a hearing loss of approximately 50 to 75 dBHL. The work of Schuknecht and colleagues clearly demonstrates the relation between histopathology and audiometric patterns. Finally, because evoked otoacoustic emissions (OAEs) reflect the active mechanism involving outer hair cell motility, the physiologic vulnerability of these cells to age may influence otoacoustic emission thresholds and amplitude as well as the prevalence

of OAEs. Accordingly, otoacoustic emissions testing has considerable potential for testing older adults and attempting to isolate a site of lesion for presbycusic hearing loss.

PEARL

Hair cell loss near the base of the cochlea produces hearing loss in the high frequencies, which typifies presbycusis.

Degeneration of Spiral Ganglion Cells

Approximately 30,000 neurons join together to form the afferent auditory portion of the eighth nerve. The dendrites of the neurons are located under the hair cells, the cell bodies of the cochlear neurons (spiral ganglion cells) are found in the central core of the cochlea (modiolus), and the axons course centrally to the nuclei in the auditory brainstem. Thus, the auditory nerve comprises first order neurons that link the sensory hair cells of the cochlea to the brainstem. The auditory nerve contains axons from type I and type II spiral ganglion cells. Type I cells are large bipolar neurons composing the vast majority of the spiral ganglion cell population. These myelinated cells synapse with inner hair cells. The remaining 5 to 10% of the spiral ganglion neurons are type II cells (Becker, Naumann, & Pfaltz, 1994). These cells are small and unmyelinated and synapse with outer hair cells. The axons of type I and type II spiral ganglion cells project centrally in the auditory nerve as a spiraling bundle that is tonotopically organized. The center contains axons from spiral ganglion cells innervating the apical part of the cochlea, whereas the periphery of the bundle contains axons from spiral ganglion cells innervating the base (Becker, Naumann, & Pfaltz, 1994). The nerve emerges from the internal auditory meatus and enters the ipsilateral cochlear nucleus where each axon bifurcates to form ascending and descending branches. The centrally directed axons of the ganglion cells transmit sensory information from the periphery, via the eighth nerve, to the central auditory system for processing (Willott, 1991).

The data of Otte, Schuknecht, and Kerr (1978) and Suzuka and Schuknecht (1988) clearly demonstrate a relation between age and loss of ganglion cells. Figure 4–3 depicts total ganglion cell loss as a function of age. The total number of ganglion cells in the cochleas of young adults ranges between 30,000 and 40,000 declining to less than 20,000 for persons between 81 and 90 years of age (Otte, Schuknecht, & Kerr, 1978). Close analysis of the data in Figure 4–3 reveals progressive loss of about 2,000 neurons per decade. As would be expected, neural histopathologic studies suggest that age-related loss in ganglion cells is greatest near the base of the cochlea. The aging process is also associated with a decrease in the average number of fibers in the cochlear nerve. The data of Crowe, Guild, and Polvogt (1934) dramatically demonstrate that nerve fiber loss is greatest within the basal 10 mm of the cochlea. A number of histopathological studies have revealed that neural degeneration can occur before and/or independently of sensory cell loss. That is to say, loss of nerve fibers in one

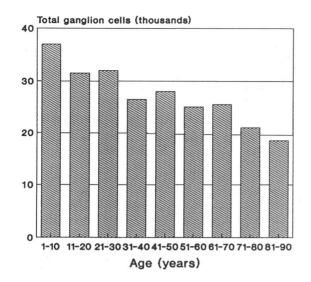

Figure 4–3   Total ganglion cell loss as a function of increasing age. (Adapted from Otte, Schuknecht, and Kerr, 1978. Reprinted by permission.)

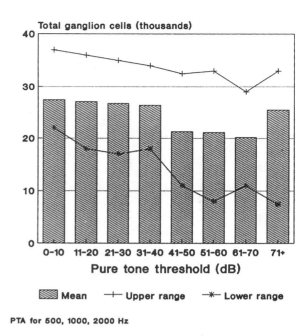

PTA for 500, 1000, 2000 Hz

Figure 4–4   Spiral ganglion cell loss as a function of pure-tone average. (Adapted from Otte, Schuknecht, and Kerr, 1978. Reprinted by permission.)

TABLE 4–2   Criterion for Classification of Types of Presbycusis

Type of presbycusis	Criterion
Sensory	The presence of any total loss of hair cells beginning at the basal end of the cochlea that is at least 10 mm in length so as to involve the region of the speech frequencies on the cochlea.
Neural	Loss of 50% or more of the cochlear neurons as compared to the mean number of cochlear neurons for neonates (i.e., 35, 500).
Strial	Loss of 30% or more of strial tissue.
Cochlear conductive	The criterion set for significant pathologic change in the sensory cells, neurons, or stria vascularis cannot be met and the functional criterion that must be present is a gradual descending audiogram over at least five octaves, no more than a 25 dB difference between any two adjacent frequencies, and a difference of at least 50 dB between the best and the poorest thresholds.
Mixed presbycusis	Presence of significant pathologic change in more than one structure.
Intermediate presbycusis	Cochlear changes do not reach significant levels in any structure, and the audiometric profile of cochlear conductive presbycusis is not met.

Source: Schuknecht & Gacek, 1993.

turn of the cochlea or in all turns has been noted without severe hair cell loss (Willott, 1991). Stated differently, loss of inner or outer hair cells "is not a prerequisite for age-related pathology of ganglion cells" (Willott, 1991, p. 28).

PEARL

Spiral ganglion cell loss in the basal turn of the cochlea is associated with elevated pure-tone thresholds and a decline in word recognition scores. These changes are highly variable.

There appears to be a relation, albeit imperfect, between amount and location of ganglion cell loss and pure-tone thresholds. Suzuka and Schuknecht (1988) reported that hearing status in their subjects was unaffected when ganglion cell loss was less than 20%. Otte, Schuknecht, and Kerr (1978) demonstrated that the most dramatic elevation in pure-tone thresholds occurred when the total ganglion cell population fell below 20,000. Figure 4–4 demonstrates the relation between ganglion cell loss and pure-tone thresholds. Thus, interpolating from Figures 4–3 and 4–4, persons with a ganglion cell population of approximately 25,000 (e.g., 30 to 60 year olds) may be predicted to have mean hearing levels within the mild range. Nadol (1981) demonstrated that ganglion cell loss restricted to the basal 3 to 5 mm of the cochlea is not associated with high-frequency hearing loss, whereas ganglion cell loss in excess of 50% in the basal 10 mm of the cochlea is associated with high-frequency loss. A number of investigators have reported that speech recognition scores are poor in older adults with significant ganglion cell loss. However, cases have been reported where speech recognition performance is good in the face of significant spiral ganglion cell loss (Belal, 1975; Pauler, Schuknecht, & Thornton, 1986; Otte, Schucknecht, & Kerr, 1978).

PEARL

Speech recognition ability also bears a relation to spiral ganglion cell population, although the relation is highly variable.

SCHUKNECHT'S TYPES OF PRESBYCUSIS

Schuknecht and Gacek (1993) examined the temporal bones of approximately 21 cases from the collection at the Massachusetts Eye and Ear Infirmary in an attempt to validate the four pathological types of presbycusis and to determine the extent to which other varieties exist. The value of their temporal bone studies, which describe the various types of presbycusis based on selected atrophy of different morphologic structures in the cochlea, is that they accurately correlated clinical manifestations to pathologic findings. The temporal bones were prepared by a standard method, the cochlea graphically reconstructed, the inner and outer hair cells were plotted separately as being present or absent, and the neuronal population was counted and separated into four segments according to a specific formula. The stria vascularis was plotted in terms of estimated loss of volume of strial tissue. The data on the hair cells, neurons, and the stria vascularis of the 21 cochlea were transferred to histograms in which black filling indicated the percent loss as a function of distance measured from the basal end along the cochlear duct (Schuknecht & Gacek, 1993). The audiogram for each case was placed on a parallel coordinate of equal length to the cytocochleogram with frequency on an anatomic frequency scale. The anatomic frequency scale expresses the spatial distribution of frequency, that is, frequencies of the audiogram are located on the abscissa in accordance with the spatial distribution of their points of maximum excitation along the length of the cochlear duct (Schuknecht, 1993). As is shown in the figures below, the final product for each cochlea contained a cochlear chart consisting of both a matching audiogram and a cytocochleogram.

Schuknecht and Gacek (1993) established a set of criteria connoting significant pathologic change to define the different types of presbycusis. Table 4–2 summarizes the criteria and the six distinct types of presbycusis that emerge according to their classification system.

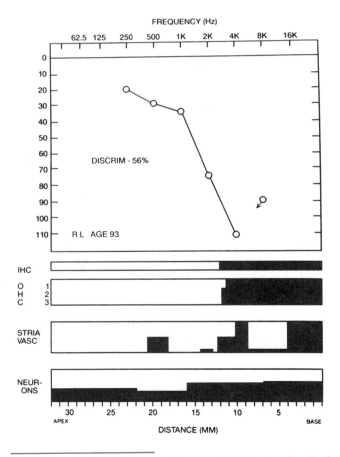

Figure 4–5 Audiogram and cytohistogram for individual with sensory presbycusis. (From Schuknecht, 1993. Reprinted by permission.)

Sensory Presbycusis

Sensory presbycusis appears to be the least important cause of hearing loss in older adults. The sensory cell loss of

SPECIAL CONSIDERATION

With sensory presbycusis it is difficult to distinguish histological and clinical changes due to aging from those associated with acoustic trauma (Schuknecht & Gacek, 1993).

sensory presbycusis is at the extreme basal end of the cochlea (8 to 12 mm region) and the section of involvement rarely includes the speech frequency area of the cochlea. The involved basal end of the cochlea shows a loss of both hair cells and

sustentacular cells (Schuknecht, 1989). As is shown in the audiogram summarized in Figure 4–5, the hearing loss for this 93-year-old male shoemaker is concentrated in the higher frequencies (above 1000 Hz) and is characterized by an abrupt slope (between 1000 and 4000 Hz) and poor word recognition ability. Tonotopically, it is evident that the abrupt high-tone loss is related to a loss of hair cells in the basal 12 mm region of the cochlea. Total neuronal population is 18,315, representing a loss of 49%. This individual likely suffered from acoustic trauma as well. Figure 4–6 shows that in this case, the O of C is totally missing in selected regions (8.25 mm, and 5.25 mm). The neurons supplying this region are diminished in number and those that remain have lost their dendritic fibers. In sensory presbycusis, the loss of speech discrimination is inversely related to the pure-tone loss. It is speculated that the cell death characterizing sensory presbycusis results from the accumulation of lipofuscin granules, a waste

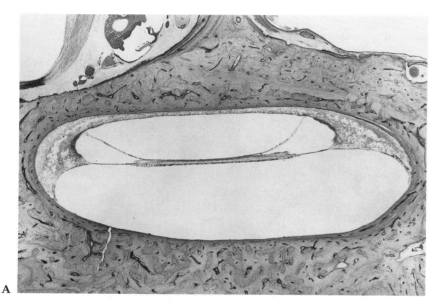

A

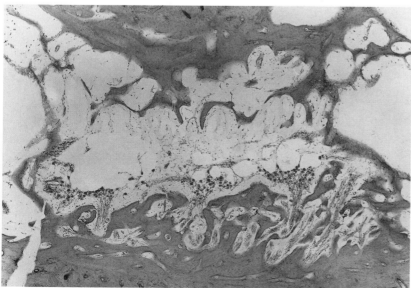

B

Figure 4–6 Views of cochlea in sensory presbycusis for individual in Figure 4–5. Organ of Corti is totally missing in the 5.25 mm and 8.25 mm regions in A. Neurons supplying these regions of the cochlea are reduced in number. (From Schuknecht, 1993. Reprinted by permission.)

product of enzyme activity, in hair and supporting cells of the inner ear (Schuknecht, 1993). Lipofuscin is an indicator of age-associated cell damage. It is present to a greater extent in old rather than young cells (Davies, 1998).

Neural Presbycusis

The most consistent pathologic change in the aging inner ear is the neuronal loss associated with neural presbycusis. Neural presbycusis may begin at any age although hearing loss does not set in until the population of neural units falls below the level required for processing acoustic input (Schuknecht, 1989). Schuknecht and Gacek (1993) reported that, although pure-tone thresholds are variable in persons with neural presbycusis, they are not affected by neuronal loss until about 90% have disappeared. The neuronal loss tends to be diffuse, involving all three turns of the cochlea. Further, the degeneration of the neurons is complete, involving the soma, axon, and dendrites (Schuknecht, 1989). The inner and outer hair cells are rarely involved. Finally, Amesen (1982) reported that the neuronal loss in the periphery is often accompanied by loss of neurons in the ventral and dorsal cochlear nuclei.

According to Otte, Schuknecht, and Kerr (1978), loss of ganglion cell population is much greater in persons with neural presbycusis than in adults over age 80 with no known otologic disease. The relation between ganglion cell loss, otologic disease, and age is depicted in Figure 4–7. Here again, it is clear that the neuronal population is more than 30,000 for younger persons, declining to less than 20,000 in adults over 80 years with no known otologic disease affecting the neurons. Persons diagnosed with neural presbycusis have by far the lowest population of ganglion cells—less than 15,000. The extent of neuronal loss in the 15 to 22 mm region of the

cochlea where the speech frequencies lie is correlated with word recognition ability, whereas loss in the remaining regions of the cochlea is not (Pauler, Schuknecht, & Thornton (1986). Figure 4–8 graphically depicts the relation between loss of cochlear neurons the full length of the cochlea, pure-tone hearing level, and word recognition ability in a case of neural presbycusis based on the cytocochleogram generated by Schuknecht and his colleagues. Note only a slight loss of outer and inner hair cells at the basal 2 mm. In this case the pure-tone hearing loss associated with neural presbycusis was mild to severe involving the entire frequency range, and word recognition ability was severely depressed. In Figure 4–9, the pure-tone hearing loss also involves the entire frequency range; however, the loss is flat in configuration and mild to moderate in degree. Word recognition ability was fair and is consistent with the cytocochleogram, showing partial loss of spiral ganglion cells most pronounced in the basal region of the cochlea.

Strial Presbycusis

Strial presbycusis is characterized by atrophy of the stria vascularis, including loss of strial tissue and loss of strial

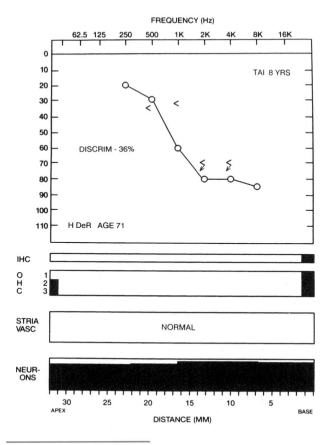

Figure 4–8 Audiogram and cytocochleogram for individual with neural presbycusis. Note, there is no loss of hair cells or stria vascularis, but the total neuronal count is quite low–3924. (From Schuknecht, 1993. Reprinted by permission.)

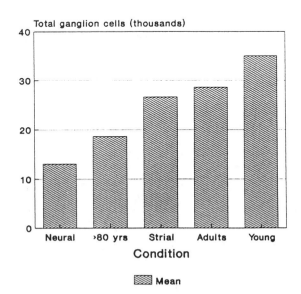

Figure 4–7 Total ganglion cell loss for different conditions within the cochlea. (Adapted from Otte, Schuknecht, and Kerr, 1978. Reprinted by permission.)

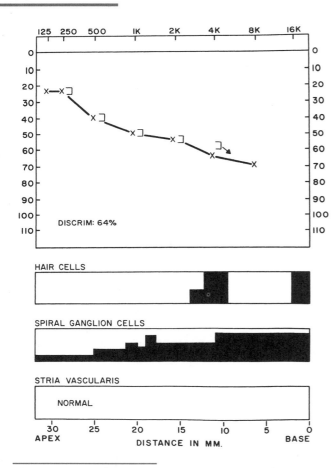

Figure 4–9 Audiogram and cytocochleogram for individual with flat sensorineural hearing loss, associated with neural presbycusis. (From Schuknecht, 1993. Reprinted by permission.)

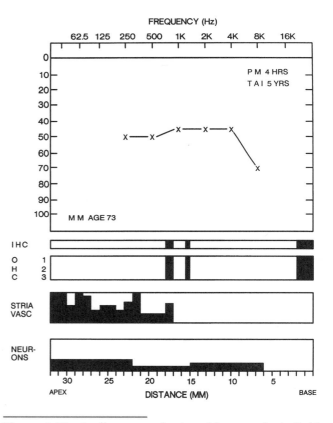

Figure 4–10 Audiogram and cytocochleogram for individual with strial presbycusis. There is a 35% loss of strial vascularis. (From Schuknecht, 1993. Reprinted by permission.)

cells, primarily in the apical and middle turns of the cochlea. Schuknecht (1993) speculated that the loss of strial tissue in aging ears affects some quality of endolymph which in turn has a detrimental effect on the physical and chemical processes by which energy necessary to support cochlear function is made available. The hearing loss that has been found to ensue tends to be flat and mild to moderate in degree as is shown in Figure 4–10. Pauler, Schuknecht, and White (1988) found that severity of the pure-tone hearing loss correlates with the magnitude of strial atrophy and thickness of strial tissue. There is, however, a negligible relationship between strial atrophy and word recognition ability. Figure 4–11 shows a view of the stria vascularis in a 72-year-old male with strial presbycusis. It is evident from Figure 4–11 that strial presbycusis is characterized by a loss of strial tissue, with patchy atrophy of the stria vascularis in the middle and apical turns of the cochlea. Figure 4–12 presents the associated audiogram and cytocochleogram. There is an estimated loss of 44% of the stria vascularis, limited mainly to the apical half of the cochlea. The total neuronal population is 24,903, which represents a 30% loss of neurons. It is evident that in this case strial presbycusis is characterized by a flat threshold pattern and excellent word recognition ability.

Cochlear Conductive Presbycusis

A classification of cochlear conductive presbycusis ensues when the other varieties of presbycusis are histologically excluded and when linear decrements in hearing function appear. There is marked variability in the cytocochleograms. Overall, the cytocochleograms show neuronal loss, degeneration in parts of the stria vascularis, and slight loss of inner and outer hair cells. A decrease in elasticity from the basal to apical end of the basilar membrane has been implicated as a factor in cochlear conductive presbycusis (Schuknecht & Gacek, 1993). Schuknecht (1993) hypothesized that the sharpened thickening of the basilar membrane in cases of cochlear conductive presbycusis is linked to an increase in the number of its fibrillar layers. As is shown in Figures 4–13 and 4–14, the hearing loss tends to be gradually sloping primarily in the high frequencies, with word recognition scores inversely related to the slope of the audiogram. The cytocochleograms are classic showing some neuronal loss, slight loss of hair cells, and degeneration in parts of the stria vascularis.

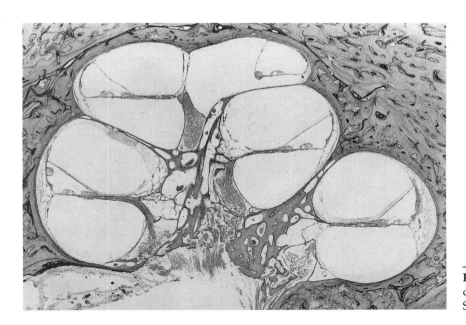

Figure 4–11 View of stria vascularis for individual with strial presbycusis. (From Schuknecht, 1993. Reprinted by permission.)

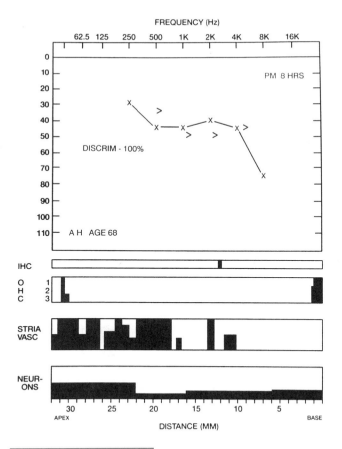

Figure 4–12 Audiogram and cytocochleogram for 68-year-old individual with excellent word recognition scores and strial presbycusis. (From Schuknecht, 1993. Reprinted by permission.)

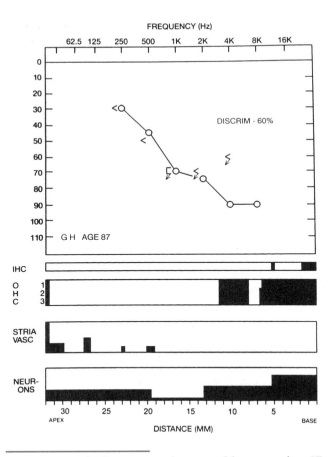

Figure 4–13 Audiogram and cytocochleogram for 87-year-old individual with cochlear conductive presbycusis. (From Schuknecht, 1993. Reprinted by permission.)

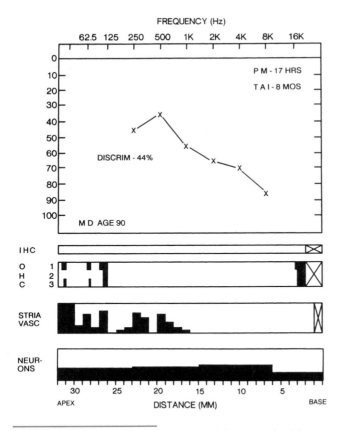

Figure 4–14 Audiogram and cytocochleogram for 90-year-old individual with extremely poor word recognition scores and cochlear conductive presbycusis. (From Schuknecht, 1993. Reprinted by permission.)

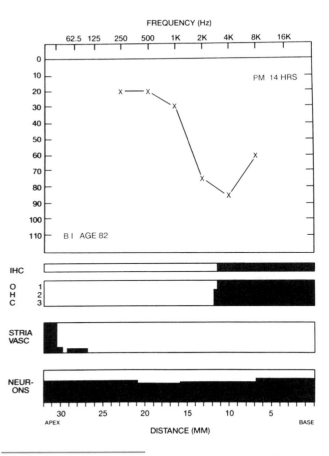

Figure 4–15 Audiogram and cytocochleogram of 82-year-old individual with combined sensory and neural or mixed presbycusis. (From Schuknecht, 1993. Reprinted by permission.)

Mixed Presbycusis

Mixed presbycusis is characterized by the presence of significant pathologic changes in more than one cochlear structure. Stated differently, it is characterized by involvement of two or more of the four classic types of presbycusis. As the types appear to be additive, performance on puretone and word recognition tests is variable. For example, the combination of sensory and strial presbycusis might present as an abrupt high-frequency hearing loss superimposed on a flat audiogram, whereas a sensory and cochlear conductive presbycusis might emerge as an abrupt high-tone loss superimposed on a descending pure-tone audiogram (Schuknecht & Gacek, 1993). The schematic in Figure 4–15, shows how additive effects of different pathologic types of presbycusis might present audiometrically. Figure 4–15 depicts a case of combined sensory and neural presbycusis. Audiometrically, there is an abrupt high-tone hearing loss that correlates tonotopically with a loss of inner and outer hair cells in the basal 12 mm of the cochlea (Schuknecht, 1993). Shown in Figure 4–16 is an audiogram and cytocochleogram of another case of mixed presbycusis of the sensory, strial, neural, and cochlear conductive variety. Here

there is a severe loss of both outer and inner hair cells in the basal 12 mm of the cochlea and an estimated 31% loss of stria vascularis. Total neuronal count was 16,173, representing a loss of approximately 55% relative to normal. The associated audiogram is a steep descending threshold pattern with extremely poor word recognition ability.

Intermediate Presbycusis

Finally, intermediate presbycusis, which has only recently been described by Schuknecht and Gacek (1993), is characterized by the absence of pathologic changes on light microscopy but the presence of submicroscopic alterations in the cochlea. The latter might include alterations in the intracellular organelles that impair cell metabolism, diminished number of synapses on the hair cells, and chemical alterations in the endolymph. The audiograms are primarily flat or mildly descending, without a consistent or distinct pathologic correlate. Figures 4–17 and 4–18 present two cases classified as intermediate presbycusis. Figure 4–17 shows an 89-year-old male factory worker with a flat threshold loss that was slowly progressive in each ear. The cytocochleogram shows a 4 mm sensory lesion at the basal end

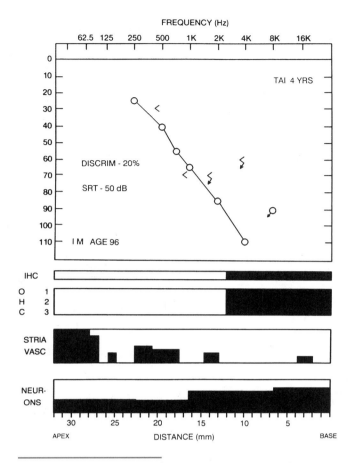

Figure 4–16 Audiogram and cytocochleogram of 96-year-old individual with mixed presbycusis. (From Schuknecht, 1993. Reprinted by permission.)

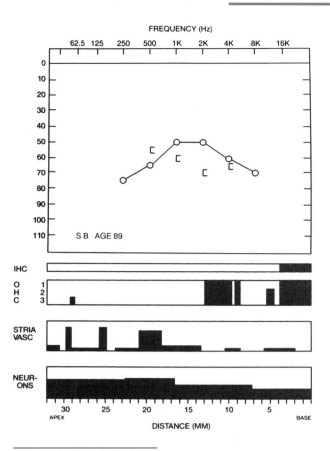

Figure 4–17 Audiogram and cytocochleogram of 89-year-old individual with intermediate presbycusis. (From Schuknecht, 1993. Reprinted by permission.)

and an acoustic trauma lesion in the 9 to 13 mm region. There is patchy atrophy of the stria vascularis for an estimated loss of 22% and a cochlear neuronal count of 18,225 representing a loss of 49% relative to normal (Schuknecht, 1993). Figure 4–18 shows an 85-year-old female with a mildly descending audiogram that was bilateral and symmetrical. Discrimination ability was relatively good considering age and hearing loss. The cytocochleogram showed a sensory lesion in the basal 4.5 mm region and a neuronal count of 19,044. Finally, Figure 4–19 is also a case of intermediate presbycusis that does not appear to fit a particular pathologic schema. This 84-year-old male had extremely poor word recognition scores in the face of a mild (250 to 2000 Hz) sloping from severe to profound hearing loss, thereafter. The cytocochleogram did not support the audiometric findings. Neuronal count was approximately 23,000, reflecting a loss of only 35% of the neuronal population, and the strial loss was only 18%.

In sum, two major age-related structural changes have been observed histologically in the inner ear and auditory nerves of older adults. These include extensive atrophy and degeneration of the hair cells, numerous supporting cells,

and the stria vascularis, as well as a reduction in the number of functional spiral ganglia and nerve fibers that are of the eighth nerve. Further, six different types of presbycusis producing complex pathologic and functional changes have been described by Schuknecht and his colleagues. Figure 4–20 provides a cross-section of the human cochlea that illustrates four of the six types of presbycusis and the locus of pathology. Analysis of the six different types of presbycusis suggests that this clinical entity appears to have variable forms of clinical expression and is not necessarily represented by a single pattern. The evaluation of hearing status in older adults must be comprehensive and individualized to insure that intervention strategies are effective in remediating the functional sequelae of the atrophic changes within the auditory periphery.

SPECIAL CONSIDERATION

The six types of presbycusis described by Schuknecht are associated with specific changes on the audiogram. It is impossible to identify the type of presbycusis from audiometric findings.

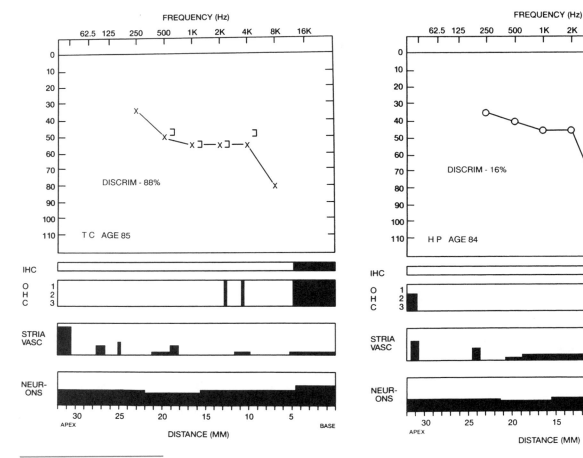

Figure 4–18 Audiogram and cytocochleogram of 85-year-old individual with intermediate presbycusis. (From Schuknecht, 1993. Reprinted by permission.)

Figure 4–19 Audiogram and cytocochleogram of 84-year-old individual with intermediate presbycusis. (From Schuknecht, 1993. Reprinted by permission.)

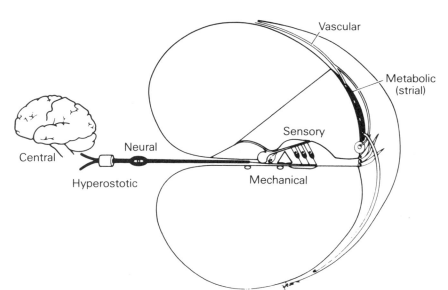

Figure 4–20 Cross-section of the cochlea showing pathological changes associated with various types of presbycusis. (From Johnsson and Hawkins, 1979. Reprinted by permission of the Institute of Gerontology, University of Michigan.)

AGE-RELATED CHANGES IN THE BRAINSTEM AND CORTICAL AREAS

Overview of the Central Auditory Nervous System

Hearing is made possible by the brain's ability to take the electrical impulses from the auditory nerve fibers and transform them into auditory sensations and perceptions (Willott, 1996). Thus, hearing cannot take place without appropriate neural activity within the central auditory system (CAS). The CAS consists of various nuclei that relay information from the cochlea and eighth nerve to other nuclei in the auditory system (Becker, Naumann, & Pfaltz, 1994; Weinstein, 1998). The auditory nerve fiber system projects into centers having progressively larger populations of neurons as it ascends from the cochlea to the cortex. For example, the cell count in the auditory neural system of the monkey is approximately 88,000 at the level of the cochlea nucleus rising to 10,200,000 in the auditory cortex (Schuknecht, 1993). The cochlear nucleus (CN) is the site of an obligatory synapse for all auditory nerve fibers. It is the first location in the central nervous system (CNS) to process and relay acoustic information from the periphery. Upon reaching the CN approximately 75% of the nerve fibers cross over to the contralateral part of the brain, with the remaining 25% traveling along the ipsilateral pathway. There are two principal ascending pathways emanating from the CN. That is, the neurons in the cochlear nuclei send their axons to different targets. These include a bilateral projection from the ventral cochlear nucleus to the nuclei of the superior olivary complex (SOC) and projections from the dorsal (DCN) and ventral cochlear nucleus (VCN) to the contralateral inferior colliculus (IC) and nuclei of the lateral lemniscus (LL). Further, there are different morphological types of neurons within the cochlear nucleus subserving different functions.

The SOC, a major binaural processing, relay, and reflex center, contains three nuclei: the lateral superior olive, the medial superior olive, and the medial nucleus of the trapezoid body. The SOC receives information from both ears through direct and indirect pathways from the respective cochlear nuclei. The SOC and CN are part of the lower brainstem. The LL contains axons from the contralateral CN and ipsilateral SOC. The IC comprises the auditory midbrain and houses the terminal synapse for the vast majority of incoming fibers from the CN, the SOC, and the LL. Virtually all ascending auditory pathways make a synapse in the IC. For example, it receives contralateral input from the DCN and VCN, ipsilateral input from the medial superior olive, and bilateral input ascending from the lateral superior olive. In short, it provides a summation of lower auditory brainstem processing. According to Willott (1996), the brainstem is tonotopically organized such that, for example, neurons in the dorsal portion of the IC respond to low frequencies, and neurons at progressively more ventral locations respond to progressively higher frequencies. The medial geniculate body is the auditory thalamic relay to the auditory cortex. It contains a dorsal, ventral, and medial division. Finally, the auditory cortex is associated with the transverse temporal gyrus and is buried in the sylvian fissure (Becker, Naumann, & Pfaltz, 1994). Figure 4–21 presents a schematic of the central auditory pathways susceptible to age-related degeneration.

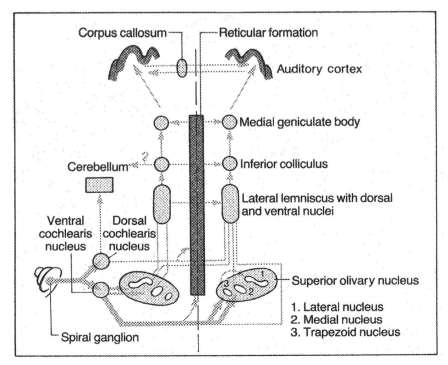

Figure 4–21 Schematic of central auditory pathways susceptible to age-related changes. (From Roeser, 1996, p. 17. Reprinted by permission.)

The aging process impacts on the CNS in general and on the central auditory nervous system (CANS) in particular. Neuronal age-related atrophy is characterized by an overall loss of neurons; a change in neuron size; a decrease in size of the cell body, nucleus or nucleolus; and a decrease in dendritic arborization along with a diminution or disappearance of dendrites (Willott, 1991; Powers, 1994). Another hallmark of the aging CNS is that while neurons do not replicate themselves in the mature brain, they may reorganize synapses and dendritic arborizations. A number of age-related changes have been reported in the CANS from the CN up to and including the auditory cortex. In general, the age-related changes in the nervous system are not uniform across the nuclei within the CANS and vary greatly among individuals.

Kirikae, Sato, and Shitara (1964) and Hansen and Reske-Nielsen (1965) were among the first investigators to perform histological studies of aging brains. While their histopathological descriptions are limited somewhat by the methodology, it seems safe to conclude that the auditory brainstem regions do undergo some age-related changes, which include a decrease in number, size, and density of neurons; reduced cell density in selected nuclei; and an increase in pigmentation. Subsequently Konigsmark and Murphy (1970, 1972), Amesen (1982), and Crace (1970) evaluated portions of the auditory brainstem and expanded upon some of the findings noted above. Konigsmark and Murphy (1970, 1972) found evidence of a decrease in the volume of neurons in the VCN beginning at about 60 years of age; a decrease in the number of well-myelinated fibers in the VCN in older adults; a decrease in the number of small vessels and capillaries per unit area with increasing age; and an increase in lipofuscin accumulation with age. Crace (1970) also noted a slight decrease in neuron size and density with age, as well as a striking increase in the proportion of neurons containing pigment within the CN. Interestingly, Crace as well as Konigsmark and Murphy found that although many neurons within the CN appeared to degenerate, there was no evidence of a decrease in the number of neurons with age. As regards the other brainstem fiber tracts, it appears that there is a slight decrease in the number of nerve fibers within the LL and the IC with age (Willott, 1991).

Brody (1955) conducted an extensive study of the brains of individuals ranging in age from newborn to 95 years. Specifically, he studied age-related changes in the auditory cortex, comparing them to those in the inferior temporal, striate, precentral, and postcentral cortical areas. The magnitude of cell loss was greatest in the superior temporal gyrus (auditory cortex). In fact, there was almost a one-to-one correlation between age and cell loss. Brody also noted a decrease in the thickness of the superior temporal gyrus with increasing age that was not apparent in other cortical regions. Subsequently, Scheibel, Lindsay, Tomiyasu, and Scheibel (1975) also studied the superior temporal cortex, noting a loss of dendrites and cell death in older patients.

In sum, it is evident from histological studies of the CANS that it undergoes some age-related changes. It is also apparent that the changes are not universal across individuals or across the tracts constituting the auditory brainstem. Further, the functional significance of the anatomical and

physiological changes remains the subject of considerable interest among researchers. The speech perception, evoked response, and brain-mapping data presented in Chapters 5, 6, and 7 will hopefully shed light on the functional implications of the age-related changes in the CANS.

PEARL

Age-related changes along the central auditory pathways are highly variable as are the behavioral consequences.

Medical Causes of Hearing Loss Potentially Confused Audiometrically with Presbycusis

Whereas the most fundamental cause of hearing loss among older adults is the biological aging of the cells in the inner ear and auditory pathways, a number of other conditions give rise to the sensorineural hearing loss often exhibited by older adults. These include ototoxicity, noise exposure, metabolic conditions, vascular disease, Ménière's disease, and infections.

Ototoxicity

It is well known that older adults suffer from many chronic illnesses and use more medications than any other age group. In fact, polypharmacy, or the concurrent use of many medications, is the rule rather than the exception among older adults. The average older person uses 4.5 prescription and 2.1 nonprescription drugs and fills approximately 12 to 17 prescriptions a year. Of course, drug use is greater in hospitals and in nursing facilities (Abrams, Beers, & Berkow, 1995). The most commonly used drugs include antiarthritic agents and analgesics, cardiovascular agents and antihypertensives, sedatives, and tranquilizers (Vestal, 1995). Prescription of medications that are ototoxic appears to be somewhat higher in the elderly, predisposing them to drug-induced sensorineural hearing loss.

SPECIAL CONSIDERATION

Physiological changes of aging often alter the drug response of older adults, making them susceptible to potentially dangerous adverse reactions. Specifically, age-related changes in pharmacokinetics account for potential susceptibility to the toxic effects of selected drugs.

The term pharmacokinetics refers to the time course of absorption, distribution, metabolism, and excretion of drugs and their metabolites from the body (Vestal, 1995). The most important pharmacokinetic changes in older adults are: (1) age-related alterations in the physiology of the gastrointestinal system, which produce alterations in drug absorption; (2) age-related changes in body composition coupled with decline in cardiac output, which produce changes in drug distribution; (3) decreased liver mass and decline in regional blood flow to the liver, resulting in decline in hepatic drug metabolism; and (4) diminished glomerular and tubular renal function, resulting in decreased renal elimination of drugs and metabolites. Another variable that influences drug response is pharmacodynamics, which refers to end-organ responsiveness to a given drug concentration. One final factor is homeostasis, or the individual's ability to adapt to drug effects. Adverse reactions from ototoxic agents may result from drug-disease interactions or drug-drug interactions.

Classes of drugs differ in terms of which age-related change in pharmacokinetics will pose the greatest threat to the onset of toxic effects. For example, the main route for elimination of antibiotics including aminoglycosides (e.g., gentamicin, tobramycin), selected cardiovascular drugs, diuretics including furosemide, and psychoactive drugs is the kidney. Renal elimination of these drugs can be reduced in the elderly. In light of this, the standard dosage regimen should be reduced in older adults. Similarly, the hepatic metabolism of cardiovascular drugs such as quinidine, psychoactive drugs such as diazepam, and selected analgesics may be reduced in older adults. There are data to indicate that clearance of analgesics such as salicylates may be reduced in older patients, as well (Abrams, Beers, & Berkow, 1995). Drug toxicity can be associated with some or all of the following: nausea, vomiting, dizziness, fatigue, hearing loss, and tinnitus.

A number of classes of drugs are particularly toxic to the auditory and vestibular systems, the effects of which are exacerbated by the aging process. Table 4–3 displays the drugs reported to produce oto- or vestibulotoxic effects. The site of predilection of the drugs within a particular class differs such that, for example, streptomycin is mainly vestibulo-

toxic; neomycin and kanamycin are particularly toxic to the ear; and gentamicin is both oto- and vestibulotoxic. Neomycin is used topically for some eye, ear, and skin infections or orally before colorectal surgery (Abrams, Beers, & Berkow, 1995). Streptomycin is used to treat tuberculosis and occasionally endocarditis.

The pathogenesis of ototoxicity from aminoglycosides relates to the fact that this class of antibiotics is retained for a longer period and in a higher concentration in the inner ear fluids than in any other body tissue or fluid (Becker, Naumann, & Pfaltz, 1989). This in combination with the potential for reduced renal output may predispose older adults to the development of toxic concentrations of the drug within the inner ear, leading to end-organ damage. Aminoglycosides appear to damage the outer hair cells first and then the inner hair cells if a high enough concentration of the drug is reached. Ototoxicity is related to sustained peak serum levels varying considerably across the family of aminoglycosides. The damage tends to be concentrated in the high-frequency regions, extending into the lower frequencies with prolonged treatment. Audiometrically, the hearing loss manifests itself in the high frequencies and is often occasioned by tinnitus and dizziness. The hearing loss tends to be sensorineural, bilateral, and severe to profound in degree. The severity and time of onset are directly related to the time of onset of drug use, often progressing for several months after cessation of the medication.

PEARL

Older adults are at particular risk for aminoglycoside otoxicity when they have an underlying loss of auditory function associated with the aging process.

The ototoxic effects of aminoglycosides are directly related to serum levels at the end treatment, so that serum concentration monitoring is strongly recommended. The risk of ototoxicity is increased from aminoglycosides in patients receiving cisplatin.

Cisplatin, a chemotherapeutic agent that acts against squamous cell carcinoma of the head, neck, and genitourinary systems, is primarily ototoxic and can lead in some cases to permanent hearing loss. The mechanism of cisplatin ototoxicity has not been elucidated. However, it does appear that the damage associated with cisplatin ingestion is at the level of the hair cell. Initially, it causes damage to outer hair cell stereocilia, followed by hair cell degeneration at the basal turn of the cochlea, progressing apically. Inner hair cells are ultimately affected after all three rows of outer hair cells have degenerated (Boettcher, Gratton, Bancroft, & Spongr, 1992). Of course, loss of inner hair cells may affect survival of ganglion cells. Onset of hearing loss can be detected initially in the ultra-high frequencies soon after the first or second course of chemotherapy (Boettcher et al, 1992). The degree of hearing loss and frequencies affected are directly related to dosing and duration of cisplatin administration (Boettcher et al, 1992). Older adults with

TABLE 4–3 Partial List of Drugs that Produce Toxic Effects on the Auditory and Vestibular Systems

Aminoglycosides
Gentamicin
Streptomycin
Kanamycin
Neomycin
Viomycin
Tobramycin

Analgesics
Salicylates

Diuretics
Furosemide
Ethacrynic acid
Quinine

Cardiovascular Drugs
Quinidine

Chemotherapeutic Agents
Cisplatin
Nitrogen mustard

hearing loss prior to chemotherapy with cisplatin are more likely to experience threshold shift following administration of the drug and thus close monitoring and counseling are recommended for these individuals (Dorr & Dalton, 1993).

PEARL

It is incumbent on audiologists to educate oncologists and the entire chemotherapy team about assistive devices cancer patients can use to facilitate communication should a patient's hearing status deteriorate during and after chemotherapy.

Salicylate ototoxcity is not uncommon given the high prevalence of arthritis and rheumatism and the wide use of this class of drugs in older adults. Salicylate ototoxicity is associated with metabolic damage to the inner ear hair cells. Serum salicylate levels must exceed 12.5 mg% for ototoxic symptoms to present (Myers & Bernstein, 1965). Salicylate otoxicity is associated with tinnitus and mild to moderate sensorineural hearing loss that is gradual in onset. The hearing loss reportedly tends to reverse itself when the drug is discontinued as early as three days following the final administration (Boettcher et al, 1992). It has been postulated that diuretics, such as furosemide and ethacrynic acid, disturb the regulation of ion concentration in the stria vascularis, leading to damage to the outer hair cells primarily (Becker, Naumann, & Pfaltz, 1989). The sensorineural hearing loss resulting from diuretic ototoxicity is potentially reversible, as well.

In sum, it is important to note that the hearing loss associated with ototoxicity from any of the aforementioned ototoxins may interact with that of presbycusis, leading to a more severe hearing loss than that associated with age alone. Audiologists are often called upon to administer pretreatment audiograms to provide baseline information about hearing status prior to the onset of drug use, midtreatment audiograms to monitor hearing status, and posttreatment audiograms to compare hearing status to the baseline information. Audiometric studies are usually conducted in conjunction with laboratory studies of serum levels to assist in maintainance of appropriate dosing and to help monitor potential ototoxic damage. Further, the results of audiometric studies may assist in management of the older adult. With regard to management, for example, older adults sustaining a profound hearing loss from drug ingestion may require hearing aids and/or assistive technology to facilitate the communication process. Given their role in evaluating and managing older adults who develop ototoxic hearing loss, audiologists must have some familiarity with clinical pharmacology including knowledge of pharmacokinetics and the prescribing practices of physicians.

PEARL

In light of polypharmacy, older adults should be questioned extensively about the medications they take to determine if, in fact, hearing loss is due in part to ototoxicity.

Noise-Induced Hearing Loss

Hearing loss in adults can also be attributed to exposure to noise, and the interaction of noise and aging effects. Hearing loss associated with the aging process is often difficult to distinguish audiometrically from hearing loss associated with prolonged noise exposure. The severity and location of the lesion to the inner ear, and corresponding hearing loss, depend on the acoustic characteristics of the sound including its sound pressure level and frequency content, exposure time, and the individual's susceptibility or sensitivity to the effect of the particular type of noise. Noise is associated with irreversible damage to the sensory cells of the inner ear, with outer hair cells degenerating first followed by the inner hair cells. The lesion tends to be concentrated in the region of the cochlea associated with 4000 Hz hearing, namely, the lower basal turn of the cochlea. Unlike presbycusis, there is rarely involvement of the auditory nerve fibers and the brainstem auditory pathways. The audiometric configuration associated with noise exposure is difficult to separate from the patterns typically associated with age (CHABA, 1988). While early on the pure-tone audiogram shows a notch at 3000, 4000, or 6000 Hz, prolonged exposure leads to involvement of higher and lower frequency regions. The loss tends to be bilateral and symmetrical. Tinnitus is a common complaint of persons with a long-term history of noise exposure.

Rosen, Bergman, Plester, El-Mofty, and Sattis (1962) reported that environmental factors such as living in a noise-free versus an industrialized society can influence the extent of the high-frequency hearing loss that emerges in older persons. In fact, individuals living in a noise-free environment reportedly have better hearing in the high frequencies than persons living in industrialized societies (Rosen et al, 1962). The extent to which hearing loss in older persons is attributable to noise rather than age cannot be predicted from the audiogram at this time. There is, however, support for the observation that age and exposure to noise can have a synergistic effect (Moscicki et al, 1985). Gilad and Glorig (1979) speculated that hearing loss among the elderly is a culmination of multiple damaging processes that occur over the life span. In fact, some investigators contend that presbycusis is a multifactorial process in which expression of each factor varies greatly from individual to individual (Gates, Cobb, D'Agostino, & Wolf, 1993). It is the sum of a variety of insults to the auditory system that occur over time, and include age-related degeneration, the effects of environmental noise (sociocusis), and disease of the auditory systems (nosocusis), plus other endogenous factors such as genetics, diet, etc. (Kryter, 1983; Gates et al, 1993).

At the present time isolating the histopathology of presbycusis, nosocusis, and sociocusis and correlating it to audiometric findings is an important research goal yet a challenging one. The difficulty arises because the variables that interact to determine hearing status of older adults are uncontrolled, making it difficult to decide which of the visualized changes on geriatric human temporal bones are solely the result of aging (Gulya, 1991). Despite the difficulties, careful histopathological examination is critical to the practicing clinician. The information can help in test development and the rehabilitation process. Ultimately clinicians may use the data to identify candidates whose word recognition problems are likely to be remedied by a particular treatment such as programmable hearing aids, CIC hearing aids, conventional analog hearing aids, or an assistive listening device such as a behind-the-ear/FM arrangement.

SPECIAL CONSIDERATION

It is clinically impossible to isolate the histopathology of presbycusis, nosocusis, and sociocusis and correlate each to audiometric results.

Acoustic Neuroma

Histologically, cochleovestibular schwannoma, better known as acoustic neuroma, is a benign tumor arising from the Schwann cells of the neurilemma of the vestibular nerve. These are primarily slow growing, well-encapsulated tumors that account for about 8 to 10% of all intracranial tumors. Acoustic tumors occur mainly in mid and later life, with peak incidence at 35 to 40 years of age. The auditory symptoms associated with acoustic neuroma are easily distinguished from those of presbycusis. It is a unilateral disease associated with vestibular symptoms including unsteadiness and occasional frank vertigo and nausea (Schuknecht, 1993). The hearing loss is sensorineural, variable in severity, and often associated with reduced word recognition scores. Individuals often complain of tinnitus in the affected ear. Further, acoustic stapedial reflexes tend to be absent, and brain stem–evoked response audiometry is typically abnormal. An older adult with evidence of acoustic neuroma should be referred to a neuro-otologist for a complete examination.

Cardiovascular Disease

Impaired cardiovascular function is widespread among older adults. By definition, cardiovascular insufficiency compromises the blood supply to organs throughout the body including the cochlea, which is richly supplied with blood vessels. Atherosclerosis, a generic term for thickening or hardening of the arterial wall, plays a major role in cardiovascular disease. A number of investigators have studied the relationship between hearing loss and atherosclerosis. The validity of conclusions is compromised by the high prevalence of each condition in older adults.

SPECIAL CONSIDERATION

There is a substantial amount of support linking cardiovascular disease (CVD) to cochlear pathology in older adults.

Most recently, Gates et al (1993) analyzed data from the Framingham cohort on the relation between CVD and hearing loss in a sample of 1662 subjects. They examined the relation between five risk factors for CVD and hearing loss. The risk factors included: (1) blood pressure and hypertension; (2) serum total cholesterol, triglyceride, and lipoprotein levels; (3) diabetes mellitus; (4) smoking; and (5)

weight. Further, an attempt was made to correlate hearing loss with presence of cardiovascular events including coronary heart disease (CHD), heart attack, and cramping in the leg(s) when walking. In general, it appears that hearing loss is more closely related to coronary vascular disease events including CHD and heart attack than to CVD risk factors. Low-frequency thresholds were more closely correlated to CVD than were high-frequency thresholds, suggesting a possible vascular or metabolic link. The association between CVD and hearing loss was impressive in their sample; however, the authors cautioned that a cause and effect relation cannot be deduced from their findings. It is also important to emphasize that, despite the relationships that emerged, a large number of individuals with cardiovascular disease did not necessarily have hearing loss.

Brant, Gordon-Salant, Pearson, Klein, Morrell, Metter, and Fozard (1996) also examined the relationship among cardiovascular-related risk factors and hearing loss in older adults. Participants in the Baltimore Longitudinal Study of Aging served as subjects in their study. They, too, found a relation between cardiovascular disease and hearing loss in their large sample of older adults who were free of noise-induced hearing loss and other hearing-related disorders. Specifically, their data demonstrated a significant relation between systolic blood pressure and sensorineural hearing impairment. They reported that men who are borderline hypertensive with a systolic pressure of 140 have a 32% greater risk of developing hearing loss than normotensive men. Further, men who are hypertensive with a systolic pressure of 160 have a 74% greater risk of hearing than the borderline hypertensive group. Given the aforementioned association, an additional benefit of controlling blood pressure is the potential for reducing the prevalence of hearing loss (Weinstein, 1998).

PEARL

Audiologists should query their clients regarding cardiovascular disease, and closely monitor audiometrically those who are borderline or definite hypertensives.

Metabolic Disease

A variety of metabolic deficits that develop as individuals age may have a deleterious effect on hearing (Willott, 1991). These include but are not limited to: (1) impaired glucose metabolism, which is a hallmark of diabetes mellitus; (2) selected kidney disorders, which tend to alter fluid and electrolyte metabolism; (3) hyperlipoproteinemia (HLP), a condition that accompanies high serum cholesterol and triglyceride levels and is closely linked to atherosclerosis; or (4) selected thyroid conditions, which may interfere with the production of thyroid hormone. The first two conditions have received the most attention from investigators.

Diabetes Mellitus

Diabetes mellitus is a syndrome characterized by generalized metabolic dysfunction and a variety of clinical disorders. There is an age-related increase in the prevalence of diabetes mellitus, undiagnosed diabetes, and impaired glucose tolerance. Diabetes mellitus is primarily characterized by abnormal glucose metabolism and is associated with abnormal regulation of lipid and protein metabolism. Secondary to diminished insulin secretion and hyperglycemia, persons with diabetes mellitus may undergo vascular changes in small and large vessels. Peripheral neuropathy is not uncommon among diabetic persons. Because diabetes can affect the body's neurochemical balance, fluctuations in communication behavior, including degree of sensorineural hearing loss, have been reported (Groher, 1988). It is noteworthy that in a recent report based on data from the 18th biennial examination of subjects who are part of the Framingham cohort, hearing thresholds and suprathreshold word recognition scores did not appear to vary with the presence or absence of diabetes mellitus or with the presence or absence of glucose intolerance (Gates et al, 1993).

PEARL

Despite these data, clinical experience suggests diabetes that is not properly controlled places older adults at risk for sudden declines in hearing levels that may not be reversible.

I personally witnessed an uncle's hearing decline from a mild to moderate sensorineural hearing loss to the level of a moderately severe to severe loss within one day. The suddenness of the change was devastating and, while the diabetes was brought back into control, hearing levels never returned to their milder levels. Word recognition ability declined as well, to the point that hearing aids became ineffective. Subsequent speech testing revealed the presence of a central auditory processing component superimposed on the peripheral hearing loss.

Kidney Disorders
The kidney undergoes anatomic, histologic, and functional changes as people age. The anatomic changes are primarily vascular, interstitial, and tubular. These changes often leave the older adult vulnerable to a variety of environmental, disease-related, and drug-induced stresses. The major clinical consequences of age-related changes include disorders of salt metabolism, disorders of water metabolism, and disorders of potassium metabolism, etc. The total body content of sodium is the principal determinant of extracellular and intravascular fluid volume. Sodium deficiency results in hypovolemia whereas excess sodium results in edema with or without circulatory congestion (Beck & Burkhart, 1994). Potassium levels may be altered in older adults because of the use of drugs that alter potassium excretion or because of declines in glomular filtration rates. Disturbance in water metabolism is associated with either excess or defects in water conservation. Together the above changes lead to alterations in fluid and electrolyte metabolism. The high level of metabolic activity of the stria vascularis and the high degree of vascularity would make it susceptible to the impairments in sodium, water, and potassium metabolism that attend the age-related decline in

renal function. As such, cochlear pathology and primarily high-frequency sensorineural hearing loss have been reported in older adults with renal disease. Patients with Alport's syndrome (a hereditary nephropathy), chronic renal failure and kidney transplants, or persons undergoing kidney dialysis may have increased susceptibility to hearing impairment. Often, it is difficult to isolate the cause of hearing loss in persons with kidney disease due to the deleterious effects of ototoxic medications conventionally used in the management of individuals with renal disease.

Dementia

Senile dementia is an acquired global impairment involving loss of intellectual function and other cognitive skills that is sufficient to interfere with social or occupational function (Russell & Burns, 1999). It is a slowly progressive, irreversible disorder characterized by impairment in at least one of the four areas listed in Table 4–4. The diagnosis of dementia is based on a thorough history from the patient and an informant, physical examination, brain imaging, laboratory tests, and orally administered neuropsychological tests of cognitive and mental state (Russell & Burns, 1999). Dementia is a common disorder affecting approximately 15% of people over 65 years of age and more than 50% of individuals over 80 years. More than half of nursing home admissions have a diagnosis of senile dementia (Abrams, Beers, & Berkow, 1995).

The known causes of dementia are numerous and quite variable. Structural causes of dementia include Alzheimer's disease and vascular disease; metabolic-toxic causes include anoxia, organ system failure, and hypoglycemia; infectious causes include viral encephalitis, human immunodeficiency virus (HIV), or neurosyphilis; and environmental causes that have been isolated include such contaminants as aluminum. Although the majority of dementias are irreversible, incurable, and progressive, reversible causes of dementia account for some 20 to 30% of all cases. Eye and ear disorders have been isolated as one of eight potential causes of reversible dementia. The latter is not surprising, as significant changes in aging and in dementia occur in the temporal lobe (Grimes, 1995). In particular, neurofibrillary tangles have a propensity for the temporal lobe.

TABLE 4–4 Diagnostic Criteria for Dementia

1. Impairment in abstract thinking, as indicated by difficulty defining words and concepts and difficulty finding similarities and differences between related words, etc.
2. Impaired judgment as indicated by inability to make reasonable plans to deal with interpersonal, family, or job-related issues.
3. Other disturbances of higher cortical function such as aphasia, apraxia, agnosia, or constructional difficulty.
4. Personality change as indicated by alteration or accentuation of premorbid traits.

Source: Modified from Abrams, Beers, & Berkow, 1995.

A definite relation between hearing loss and dementia exists although the nature of the relationship is incomplete. Some investigators have speculated that hearing loss and cognitive decline coexist incidentally as a function of age, others have suggested that the auditory system is preferentially involved in Alzheimer's disease, and a number of investigators have demonstrated a strong positive relationship between hearing impairment and cognitive status (Gates, Cobb, Linn, Rees, Wolf, & D'Agostino, 1996). Further, hearing impairment is reportedly more common and more severe in demented versus nondemented subjects. Specifically, Uhlmann, Larson, Rees, Koepsell, and Duckert (1989); Uhlmann, Rees, Psaty, and Duckert (1989); and Weinstein and Amsel (1986) reported the prevalence of hearing impairment to be higher in a sample of adults with a diagnosis of dementia than in a comparable sample free of the diagnosis. The discrepancy in prevalence is apparent among older adults living in the community and in institutions. They also reported the severity of hearing loss to be greater in subjects with a diagnsois of dementia than in an age-matched group free of cognitive impairment. Uhlmann et al (1989) also noted an increased risk of dementia with increased hearing loss. More recently, Ives, Bonino, and Traven (1995) reported that in their sample of rural older adults, persons with hearing impairment had higher rates of dementia and depression.

More recently, Strouse, Hall, and Burger (1995) performed tests of peripheral and central auditory processing ability on a sample of age-matched older adults with mean hearing levels between 500 and 8000 Hz better than 30 dBHL. One group

was diagnosed with probable senile dementia of the Alzheimer's type while the second group was free of cognitive or neurological deficits. The peripheral test battery consisted of an immittance test battery, pure tone and speech testing, and distortion-product otoacoustic emissions. The central auditory test battery consisted of the synthetic sentence identification test, the dichotic sentence identification test, the dichotic digits test, the pitch pattern sequence, and the duration pattern test. The screening version of the Hearing Handicap Inventory for the Elderly (HHIE-S) was completed by all subjects as well.

Given the subject selection criteria (i.e., hearing levels better than 30 dBHL), it is not surprising that the groups did not differ significantly in their performance on the peripheral auditory measures, with one exception. The Alzheimer's group showed slightly poorer low-frequency pure-tone thresholds than the matched control group. HHIE-S scores were comparable as well. The comparability of HHIE-S scores was to be expected because subjects were selected on the basis of being free of peripheral hearing loss and hearing-

related difficulties (Strouse, Hall, & Burger, 1995). In contrast to performance on peripheral auditory measures, percent correct performance on the majority of tests of central auditory processing was significantly lower in the Alzheimer's group than in the matched controls. Six of 10 subjects scored below normal on all five tests of central auditory function, 3 of 10 were deficient on four measures, and 1 of the subjects failed three of the five tests. On the dichotic digits test and on the dichotic sentence identification test, left ear performance was poorer than right ear performance in more than 50% of subjects with a diagnosis of Alzheimer's disease (AD). In contrast, the majority (70%) of subjects in the control group scored normally on all five central auditory tests. Further, no differences in ear performance was noted among members of the control group. These data attest to the presence of a central auditory processing problem in older adults diagnosed with AD along with the presence of peripheral hearing loss in this population. Weinstein and Amsel (1986) did find that scores on tests of cognitive status improve when people with a diagnosis of dementia can in fact hear the questions on the test of cognitive function. They also reported that the correlation between severity of pure-tone hearing loss and scores on a test of mental status is obliterated when persons with a diagnosis of dementia are able to hear the questions with the assistance of an auditory trainer or hand-held amplifier. As inability to hear questions on orally administered tests of cognitive function can result in lower test scores that confound the interpretation of test results, hand-held amplifiers or desk-top auditory trainers should be used in the diagnostic process to insure reception of the questions. It is incumbent on audiologists to acquaint members of the assessment team with assistive devices that are inexpensive and can be easily incorporated into the diagnostic protocol.

SUMMARY

This chapter has outlined many of the structural and functional changes that occur within the peripheral and central auditory systems as a result of aging and/or disease. It is evident that each part of the ear undergoes changes with age.

As will be discussed in the next chapter, these changes have dramatic effects that are readily tapped using traditional behavioral tests. In light of the high prevalence of hearing loss among older adults and the variety of medical conditions that give rise to hearing loss, audiologists should make every attempt to become part of the extended geriatric health care team. As a member of the team, the role of the audiologist should be to impress upon others the importance of identifying hearing loss and its etiology in older adults undergoing a comprehensive assessment of their health status.

PEARL

Hearing status should be part of the database on each older adult undergoing a routine examination as identification of hearing loss can assist in diagnosing and managing selected conditions (e.g., Alzheimer's disease).

Further, controlling for hearing loss in older adults suffering from a multitude of acute or chronic conditions can promote the quality of life, which may be compromised. Acknowledging that hearing loss among older adults is amenable to medical, surgical, or audiologic intervention, the U.S. Preventive Services Task Force (1989) recommended that elderly persons should be periodically evaluated regarding their hearing, referred for any abnormalities, and counseled regarding the availability of devices to remedy hearing loss. It is incumbent on audiologists to work with physicians to ensure that hearing status is screened as part of an annual check-up. This form of preventive medicine will help reduce the number of older adults who are suffering unnecessarily from the effects of unidentified hearing loss.

PEARL

Audiologists must convince physicians of the importance of including a hearing screen in the routine physical.

REFERENCES

ABRAMS, W., BEERS, M., & BERKOW, R. (1995). *Merck Manual of Geriatrics*, 2d ed. Whitehouse Station, NJ: Merck & Co., Inc.

AMERICAN SPEECH-LANGUAGE-HEARING ASSOCIATION. (1992). External auditory canal examination and cerumen management. *ASHA*, 34: 22–24.

AMESEN, A. (1982). Presbycusis—a loss of neurons in the human cochlear nuclei. *Journal of Laryngology and Otology*, 96: 503–511.

BALLACHANDA, B. (1995a). Cerumen and the ear canal secretory system. In: B. Ballachanda (Ed.), *Introduction to the Human Ear Canal*. San Diego: Singular Publishing Group.

———. (1995b). Ear canal examination. In: B. Ballachanda (Ed.), *Introduction to the Human Ear Canal*. San Diego: Singular Publishing Group.

BECK, L., & BURKART, J. (1994). The renal system and urinary tract. In: W. Hazzard, R. Andres, E. Bierman, & J. Blass (Eds.), *Principles of Geriatric Medicine and Gerontology*, 2d ed. New York: McGraw-Hill.

BECKER, W., NAUMANN, H., & PFALTZ, C. (1989). *Ear, Nose, and Throat Diseases*. New York: Thieme Medical Publishers.

———. (1994). *Ear, Nose, and Throat Diseases*, 2d ed. New York: Thieme Medical Publishers.

BELAL, A. (1975). Presbycusis—physiological or pathological. *Journal of Laryngology and Otology*, 89: 1011–1025.

BESS, F., & STROUSE, A. (1996). Presbycusis. In: J. Northern. (Ed.), *Hearing Disorders*, 3d ed. Boston: Allyn & Bacon.

BOETTCHER, F., GRATTON, M., BANCROFT, B., & SPONGR, V. (1992). Interaction of noise and other agents: Recent advances. In: A. Dancer, D. Henderson, R. Salvi, & R. Hamernik (Eds.), *Noise Induced Hearing Loss*. St. Louis: Mosby.

BRANT, L., GORDON-SALANT, S., PEARSON, J., KLEIN, L., MORRELL, C., METTER, E., & FOZARD, J. (1996). Risk factors related to age-associated hearing loss in the speech frequencies. *Ear and Hearing*, 7: 152–161.

BREDBERG, G. (1968). Cellular pattern and nerve supply of the human organ of Corti. *Acta Oto-Laryngologica Supplement*, 236: 1–135.

BRODY, H. (1955). Organization of the cerebral cortex: III. A study of aging in the human cerebral cortex. *Journal of Comparative Neurology*, 102: 511–556.

COMMITTEE ON HEARING, BIOACOUSTICS AND BIOMECHANICS (CHABA). (1988). CHABA working group on speech understanding and aging. *Journal of the Acoustical Society of America*, 83: 859–895.

COVELL, W. (1952). Histologic changes in the aging cochlea. *Journal of Gerontology*, 7: 173–177.

CRACE, R. (1970). Morphologic alterations with age in the human cochlear nuclear complex. Ph.D. dissertation, Ohio University.

CROWE, S., GUILD, S., & POLVOGT, L. (1934). Observations on the pathology of high-tone deafness. *Johns Hopkins Hospital Bulletin*, 54: 315–380.

DAVIES, J. (1998). Cellular mechanisms of aging. In: R. Tallis, H. Fillit, & J. Brockelhurst (Eds.), *Brockelhurst's Textbook of Geriatric Medicine and Gerontology*. London: Churchill Livingstone.

DORR, R., & DALTON, W. (1993). Cancer chemotherapy. In: R. Bressler & M. Katz (Eds.), *Geriatric Pharmacology*. New York: McGraw-Hill.

ETHOLM, B., & BELAL, A. (1974). Senile changes in the middle ear joints. *Annals of Otology, Rhinology, and Laryngology*, 83: 49–54.

FARRIOR, J. (1963). Stapes surgery in geriatrics: Surgery in the nerve deaf otosclerotic. *Laryngoscope*, 73: 1084–1098.

GATES, G., COBB, J., D'AGOSTINO, R., & WOLF, P. (1993). The relation of hearing in the elderly to the presence of cardiovascular disease and cardiovascular risk factors. *Archives of Otolaryngology, Head and Neck Surgery*, 119: 156–161.

GATES, G., COBB, J., LINN, R., REES, T., WOLF, P., & D'AGOSTINO, R. (1996). Central auditory dysfunction, cognitive dysfunction, and dementia in older people. *Archives of Otolaryngology Head and Neck Surgery*, 122: 161–167.

GILAD, O., & GLORIG, A. (1979). Presbycusis: The aging ear. *Journal of the American Auditory Society*, 4: 195–217.

GLEITMAN, R., BALLACHANDA, B., & GOLDSTEIN, D. (1992). Incidence of cerumen impaction in general adult population. *The Hearing Journal*, 45: 28–32.

GRIMES, A. (1995). Auditory changes. In: R. Lubinski (Ed.), *Dementia and Communication*. San Diego. Singular Publishing Group.

GROHER, M. (1988). Modifications in speech-language assessment procedures for the older adult. In: B. Shadden (Ed.), *Communication Behavior and Aging*. Baltimore: Williams & Wilkins.

GULYA, J. (1991). Structural and physiological changes of the auditory and vestibular mechanisms with aging. In: D. Ripich (Ed.), *Handbook of Geriatric Communication Disorders*. Austin: Pro-Ed.

HANSEN, C., & RESKE-NIELSEN, E. (1965). Pathological studies in presbycusis. *Archives of Otolaryngology*, 82: 115–132.

IVES, D., BONINO, P., & TRAVEN, N. (1995). Characteristics and comorbidities of rural older adults with hearing impairment. *Journal of the American Geriatrics Society*, 43: 803–806.

JOHNSON, J., & HADLEY, R. (1964). The aging pinna. In: J. Converse (Ed.), *Reconstructive and Plastic Surgery*, pp. 1306–1346. Philadelphia: W.B. Saunders.

JOHNSSON, L., & HAWKINS, J. (1979). Age-related degeneration of the inner ear. IN: S. Han & D. Coons (Eds.), *Special Senses in Aging*. Ann Arbor: Institute of Gerontology, University of Michigan.

KENNA, M. (1993). Otitis media with effusion. In: B. Bailey (Ed.), *Head and Neck Surgery-Otolaryngology*. Philadelphia: Lippincott Company.

KIRIKAE, L., SATO, T., & SHITARA, T. (1964). A study of hearing in advanced age. *Laryngoscope*, 74: 205–220.

KONIGSMARK, B., & MURPHY, E. (1970). Neuronal populations in the human brain. *Nature*, 228: 1335–1336.

———. (1972). Volume of the ventral cochlear nucleus in man: Its relationship to neuronal population and age. *Journal of Neuropathology and Experimental Neurology*, 31: 304–316.

KORPER, S. (1989). Epidemiologic and demographic characteristics of the aging population. In: J. Goldstein, H. Kashima, and C. Koopmann (Eds.), *Geriatric Otorhinolaryngology*. Toronto: B.C. Decker.

KRYTER, K. (1983). Presbycusis, sociocusis, and nosocusis. *Journal of the Acoustical Society of America*, 73: 1897–1917.

LANSKY, B. (Ed.) (1996). *Age Happens—The Best Quotes About Growing Older*. New York: Meadowbrook Press.

MAHONEY, D. (1987). One simple solution to hearing impairment. *Geriatric Nursing*, 8: 242–245.

———. (1993). Cerumen impaction: Prevalence and detection in nursing homes. *Journal of Gerontological Nursing*, 19: 23–30.

MIYAMOTO, R., & MIYAMOTO, R. (1995). Anatomy of the ear canal. In: B. Ballachanda (Ed.), *Introduction to the Human Ear Canal*. San Diego: Singular Publishing Group.

MOSCICKI, E., ELKINS, E., BAUM, H., & MCNAMARA, P. (1985). Hearing loss in the elderly: An epidemiologic study of the Framingham Heart study cohort. *Ear and Hearing*, 6: 184–190.

MYERS, E., & BERNSTEIN J. (1965). Salicylate otoxicity. *Archives of Otolaryngology*, 82: 483–493.

NADOL, J. (1981). The aging peripheral hearing mechanism. In: D. Beasley and G. Davis (Eds.), *Aging: Communication Processes and Disorders*. New York: Grune & Stratton.

NATIONAL INSTITUTES OF HEALTH (NIH). (1990). Noise and hearing loss. *NIH Consensus Development Conference Consensus Statement*: 8 (1). Bethesda: Office of Medical Applications of Research.

NIELSEN, N. (1998). Who said 65 was old? *New York Times*, p. 22, 30 June 1998.

NORTHERN, J. (1996). *Hearing Disorders*, 3d ed. Boston: Allyn & Bacon.

OLIVEIRA, R. (1995). The dynamic ear canal. In: B. Ballachanda (Ed.), *Introduction to the Human Ear Canal*. San Diego: Singular Publishing Group.

OTTE, J., SCHUKNECHT, H., & KERR, A. (1978). Ganglion cell populations in normal and pathological human cochleae. Implications for cochlear implantation. *Laryngoscope*, 88: 1231–1246.

PAULER, M., SCHUKNECHT, H., & THORNTON, A. (1986). Correlative studies of cochlear neuronal loss with speech discrimination and pure-tone thresholds. *Archives of Otolaryngology*, 243: 200–206.

PAULER, M., SCHUKNECHT, H., & WHITE, J. (1988). Atrophy of the stria vascularis as a cause of sensorineural hearing loss. *Laryngoscope*, 98: 754–759.

POWERS, R. (1994). Neurobiology of aging. In: *Textbook of Geriatric Neuropsychiatry*. Washington, DC: American Psychiatric Press.

REES, T., & DUCKERT, L. (1995). Auditory and vestibular dysfunction in aging. In: W. Hazzard, R. Andres, E. Bierman, & J. Blass (Eds.), *Principles of Geriatric Medicine and Gerontology*, 2d ed. New York: McGraw-Hill.

ROESER, R. (1996). *Roeser's Audiology Desk Reference*. New York: Thieme-Medical Publishers.

ROSEN S., BERGMAN, M., PLESTER, D., EL-MOFTY, A., & SATTIS, M. (1962). Presbycusis study of a relatively noise free population in the Sudan. *Trans Am. Otol. Soc.*, 50: 135–151.

ROSENWASSER, H. (1964). Otitic problems in the aged. *Geriatrics*, 19: 11–17.

RUBY, R. (1986). Conductive hearing loss in the elderly. *Journal of Otolaryngology*, 15: 245–247.

RUSSELL, E., & BURNS, A. (1999). Presentation and clinical management of dementia. In: R. Tallis, H. Fillitt, & J. Brockelhurst (Eds.), *Brockelhurst's Textbook of Geriatric Medicine and Gerontology.* London: Churchill Livingstone.

SCHEIBEL, M., LINDSAY, R., TOMIYASU, U., & SCHEIBEL, A. (1975). Progressive dendritic changes in aging human cortex. *Experimental Neurology,* 47: 392–403.

SCHLEUNING, A., & ANDERSEN, P. (1993). Otologic manifestations of systemic disease. In: B. Bailey (Ed.), *Head and Neck Surgery-Otolaryngology.* Philadelphia: Lippincott Company.

SCHUKNECHT, H. (1955). Presbycusis. *Laryngoscope,* 65: 402–419.

————. (1964). Further observations on the pathology of presbycusis. *Archives of Otolaryngology,* 80: 369–382.

————. (1989). Pathology of presbycusis. In: J. Goldstein, H. Kashima, & C. Koopman (Eds.), *Geriatric Otorhinolaryngology.* Toronto: B.C. Decker.

————. (1993). *Pathology of the Ear,* 2d ed. Edition. Pennsylvania: Lea & Febiger.

SCHUKNECHT, H., & GACEK, M. (1993). Cochlear pathology in presbycusis. *Annals of Oto-Rhino-Laryngology,* 102: 1–16.

SENTURIA, B., MARCUS, M., & LUCENTE, F. (1980). *Diseases of the External Ear.* New York: Grune & Stratton.

SILMAN, S., & SILVERMAN, C. (1991). *Auditory Diagnosis—Principles and Applications.* San Diego: Academic Press.

STAAB, W. (1995). Deep canal hearing aids. In: B. Ballachanda (Ed.), *Introduction to the Human Ear Canal.* San Diego: Singular Publishing Group.

STEIGLEDER, G., & MAIBACH, H. (1993). *Pocket Atlas of Dermatology.* New York: Thieme Medical Publishers.

STROUSE, A., HALL, J., & BURGER, M. (1995). Central auditory processing in Alzheimer's disease. *Ear and Hearing,* 16: 230–238.

SUZUKA, Y., & SCHUKNECHT, H. (1988). Retrograde cochlear neuronal degeneration in human subjects. *Acta Oto-Laryngologica Supplement,* 450: 1–20.

UHLMANN, R., LARSON, E., REES, T., KOEPSELL, T., & DUCKERT, L. (1989). Relationship of hearing impairment to dementia and cognitive dysfunction in older adults. *Journal of the American Medical Association,* 261: 1916–1919.

UHLMANN, R., REES, T., PSATY, B., & DUCKERT, L. (1989). Validity and reliability of auditory screening tests in demented and nondemented older adults. *Journal of General Internal Medicine,* 4: 90–96.

U.S. PREVENTIVE SERVICES TASK FORCE. (1989). Screening for hearing impairment. In: *Guide to Clinical Preventive Services,* chap. 33. Baltimore: Williams & Wilkins.

VESTAL, R. (1995). Clinical pharmacology. In: W. Hazzard, R. Andres, E. Bierman, & J. Blass (Eds.), *Principles of Geriatric Medicine and Gerontology,* 2d ed. New York: McGraw-Hill.

WEINSTEIN, B. (1998). Disorders of hearing. In: R. Tallis, H. Fillitt, & J. Brockelhurst (Eds.), *Brockelhurst's Textbook of Geriatric Medicine.* London: Churchill Livingstone.

WEINSTEIN, B., & AMSEL, L. (1986). Hearing loss and senile dementia in the institutionalized elderly. *Clinical Gerontologist,* 4: 3–15.

WHITE, J., & REGAN M. (1987). Otologic considerations. In: G. Mueller & V. Geoffrey (Eds.), *Communication Disorders in Aging: Assessment and Management.* Washington, DC: Gallaudet University Press.

WILEY, T., CRUICKSHANKS, K., NONDAHL, D., & TWEED, T. (1999). Aging and middle ear resonance. *Ear and Hearing,* 10: 173–179.

WILLOTT, J. (1991). *Aging and the Auditory System.* San Diego: Singular Publishing Group.

————. (1996). Anatomic and physiologic aging: A behavioral neuroscience perspective. *Journal of the American Academy of Audiology,* 7: 141–151.

YOUNG, E., NEWCOMER, V., & KLIGMAN, A. (1993). *Geriatric Dermatology.* Philadelphia: Lea & Febiger.

Chapter 5

Behavioral Manifestations of Age-Related Changes within the Ear

They say that I am legally deaf, and all I can hear is some background noise, such as the refrigerator humming. I can still hear a whole life time of sounds, people and places—all the details, even if the audiometer says I can't hear anything now.

—N.B., born 1897

LEARNING OBJECTIVES

After reading this chapter, you should be able to:

• Explain the behavioral correlates of the anatomical and physiological age-related changes within the auditory system.
• Identify the elements accounting for variability in speech understanding characteristic of older adults.
• Conduct a behavioral test battery for assessing the hearing problems experienced by older adults.

Presbycusis, the hearing loss associated with aging, implies both decreased hearing sensitivity for tonal stimuli caused by changes in the peripheral auditory system and decrements in speech understanding associated with changes in the peripheral and central auditory nervous systems. Knowledge of the behavioral consequences of the physiologic effects of aging on the ear can guide the audiologist in selecting the most appropriate test protocols. The goal of this chapter is to highlight results of recent studies that describe the audiologic characteristics associated with aging.

PREVALENCE DATA

Approximately 28 million people suffer from some degree of hearing impairment. The majority of these people are over 65 years. Specifically, approximately 10 million people over 65 years of age suffer from hearing impairment. Hearing impairment in individuals over 65 years is considered a significant chronic condition as it has disabling functional consequences.

SPECIAL CONSIDERATION

Of persons 65 and over, nearly one-third report having hearing impairment or heart disease making it the third most prevalent chronic condition in this age group (Adams & Benson, 1992).

The prevalence of hearing loss increases dramatically with age such that while only 5.4% of adults between 18 and 44 years of age report having a hearing impairment, nearly 30% of persons over 65 years of age report a self-reported hearing impairment (Schoenborn & Marano, 1988). Further, hearing impairment among older adults increases with increasing age. Overall 295.2 per 1000 persons over 65 years report a hearing loss, with the prevalence rising from 256.4 per 1000 for persons 65 to 74 years to 354.3 per 1000 for persons over 75 years. If current hearing loss rates are applied to the 2030 population estimates, the number of individuals with hearing loss will be 7 million in the 65 to 75 year age category and 13.3 million for persons in the 75 and older category. Since women represent nearly 60% of the

---

PEARL

It is conceivable that by the year 2030 nearly 21 million Americans 65 years of age and older will have a hearing loss (Garstecki & Erler, 1995).

---

population of individuals over 65, by 2030 nearly 13 million women may present with hearing loss.

The increased prevalence of hearing loss among individuals as they age and live longer explains in part why among nursing home residents the prevalence of hearing loss is quite high, rising to nearly 70 to 80% in the majority of facilities (Schow & Nerbonne, 1980). In fact, some investigators have reported that approximately 92% of persons residing in health care facilities suffer hearing impairment of sufficient degree to interfere with the communication process (Chafee, 1967; Hull, 1995). It will become evident from the

81

discussion below that prevalence estimates vary according to methodology such that audiometric-based studies reveal prevalence to be much higher than health interview surveys. This is not surprising given the incomplete relation between severity of hearing impairment and severity of self-reported hearing handicap.

Audiometric Studies: Cross-Sectional Data

Within the past two decades several large-scale studies have been conducted using an epidemiologic approach to gathering and analyzing data on hearing status of a large, essentially unscreened sample of older adults. These include studies by Moscicki, Elkins, Baum, McNamara (1985) and Gates, Cooper, Kannel, and Miller (1990), both using the Framingham cohort, and most recently the report by Cooper (1994) from the Health and Nutrition Examination Survey. The first of these large-scale studies on the nature of hearing loss in the elderly was conducted by Moscicki et al (1985), using data from the Framingham Heart Study, a prospective investigation of risk factors leading to the development of cardiovascular disease. The study was initiated in 1950 and included biennial physical examinations and histories of all subjects. During the fifteenth cycle of examinations (1977–1979), a hearing study was conducted under the auspices of the National Institute of Neurological and Communicative Disorders and Stroke. Of the 2634 individuals undergoing complete physical examinations, 2293 community-based individuals (87%) received a hearing examination. The age range of subjects was comparable for the men and women, as were the mean ages (i.e., men = 68, women = 69 years). Participants included 935 men and 1358 women. All subjects underwent pure-tone air and bone conduction testing in a sound-treated booth. Sensorineural hearing loss was defined as a hearing level greater/poorer than 20 dBHl at any one frequency from 500 to 4000 Hz and no air bone gap.

Overall, 83% of subjects presented with a hearing loss in the better ear in at least one frequency when hearing loss was defined as pure-tone average (PTA) > 20 dBHL. The prevalence of hearing loss was greater in men (94%) than in women (76%). Using a more traditional definition of hearing loss (PTA > 25 dBHL), 31% of subjects presented with hearing impairment. According to subjective reports, many of the subjects did not feel they had a problem at the time of the study, despite the presence of decrements in pure-tone thresholds. Further, many subjects did not have "purepresbycusic" hearing loss. A significant proportion of subjects attributed their hearing loss to noise exposure and illness among other potential etiologies. Overall, 59% of the cohort had sensorineural hearing loss, 24% had a mixed loss, and the remainder had a conductive loss.

The authors generated threshold values as a function of frequency for men and women and for those with "purepresbycusic" loss and those with a history of noise exposure, illness, etc. Interestingly, the audiometric configuration for the entire cohort was comparable to that obtained for the "purepresbycusics," confirming that it is difficult to conclude from the audiogram whether a hearing loss is due to age or exogenous factors such as noise or illness. Figures 5–1 and 5–2 summarize data on the overall sample for males and females, respectively. Several trends are apparent. First, it is evident that

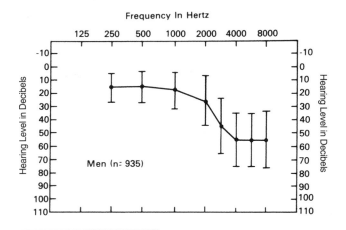

Figure 5–1 Mean pure-tone air-conduction threshold values and standard deviations in the better ear for males. (From Moscicki et al, 1985.)

the configuration differs for men and women. The audiogram for women shows a gradually sloping high-frequency configuration; whereas for the men it is abruptly falling and high-frequency, suggesting a possible noise component (Moscicki et al, 1985). Further, mean pure-tone averages in both ears were poorer for men than for women. Pure-tone thresholds for the women suggested average hearing levels to be within normal limits through 2000 Hz, gradually sloping to the level of a mild hearing loss thereafter. In the males, hearing was within normal limits through 1000 Hz, sloping to the level of a mild to moderate hearing loss thereafter. Close examination of Figures 5–3 and 5–4 reveals several trends. First, mean air-conduction thresholds obtained in men and women tend to increase with age most prominently in the frequencies above 1000 Hz. Second, within age groups, mean low-frequency air-conduction thresholds were comparable for the genders. Third, women tended to have better thresholds than men for thresholds above 2000 Hz. Finally, it was of interest that low-frequency thresholds remained within normal limits for

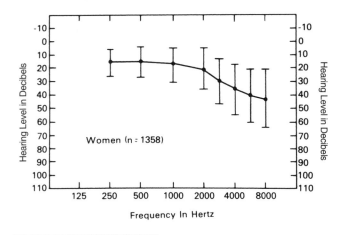

Figure 5–2 Mean pure-tone air-conduction threshold values and standard deviations in the better ear for females (From Moscicki et al, 1985.)

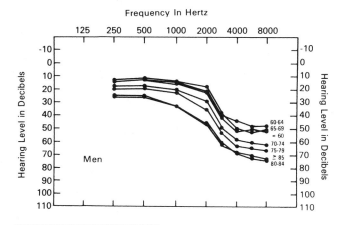

Figure 5–3 Mean air-conduction thresholds in the better ear for men as a function of age. (From Moscicki et al, 1985.)

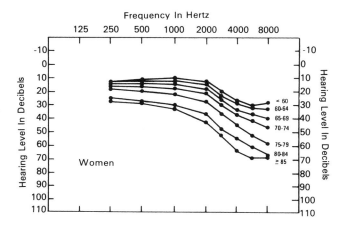

Figure 5–4 Mean air-conduction thresholds in the better ear for women as a function of age. (From Moscicki et al, 1985.)

women of all age groups, and for men up until the oldest age group was reached. The apparent relation between pure-tone threshold and age was borne out upon statistical analysis of the data. According to a logistic regression model used to determine risk factors for hearing loss, age emerged as the most important factor.

SPECIAL CONSIDERATION

Persons 70 years of age and older are more likely than younger persons to have pure-tone hearing loss for the speech frequencies. Additional risk factors for men included history of hearing loss associated with illness and history of noise exposure. Significant risk factors for women included family history of hearing loss, history of Ménière's disease, and illness.

A subsample of subjects underwent repeat testing 6 years later as part of examination cycle 18. In total, 1739 subjects reported for their biennial examination and 1662 persons, or 95% of the cohort, volunteered for follow-up hearing tests, which included pure-tone thresholds, word recognition testing, and immittance measures (Gates et al, 1990). The mean age of subjects was 73 years, 72.7 years for men and 73 years for women. Using a criterion of PTA > 26 dBHL in the better ear, 29% of the cohort had a hearing impairment, with 32.5% of the men and 26.7% of the women having reduced thresholds. On the basis of their self-reports most subjects ascribed their hearing loss to age, noise exposure, infection, injury, or other unknown causes. As is evident from Figures 5–5 and 5–6, which display the mean pure-tone thresholds for the better ear of the men and women by age group, their data corroborate the gender and age effects noted by Moscicki and her colleagues. Mean pure-tone thresholds worsened with age, with the effects being most pronounced in the higher frequencies and for men. Further, among the males, left ear pure-tone thresholds were slightly poorer than right ear thresholds. Finally, the majority of men had

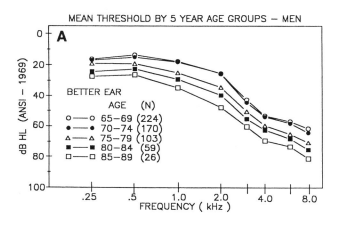

Figure 5–5 Mean air-conduction thresholds for the better ear for men by five-year age group. (From Gates et al, 1990.)

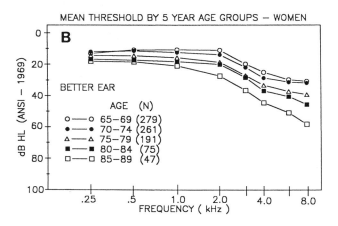

Figure 5–6 Mean air-conduction thresholds for the better ear for women by five-year age group. (From Gates et al, 1990.)

gradually or sharply sloping pure-tone audiograms, whereas the majority of women had flat or gradually sloping configurations.

A recent study, conducted by Cooper (1994), is based on hearing data extracted from the Health and Nutrition Examination Survey of 1971–1975 (HANES). HANES was a multistage, stratified probability sample of 65 geographic areas. As part of the design of the survey, audiograms were obtained from 6913 persons ranging in age from 25 to 74 years. Both air- and bone-conduction thresholds were gathered on the subjects in the sample. The trends emerging from their data corroborate the studies described above. Age and frequency effects emerged such that air-conduction thresholds became poorer as age or frequency increased. Similarly, gender and race effects emerged, as well. Overall, male thresholds were poorer especially in the higher frequencies. At selected frequencies, most notably 500 Hz, females tended to have poorer frequencies than males. There was a trend toward poorer hearing in the black subjects. However, this did not occur in the majority of comparisons. Black females performed more poorly than white females on the majority of comparisons by frequency. Finally, Cruickshanks, Wiley, Tweed, Klein, Mares-Perlman, and Nondahl (1998) conducted a population-based study on the prevalence of hearing loss in older adults residing in Beaver Dam, Wisconsin. In total, 3753 adults with an average age of 65.8 years participated in their study. The prevalence of hearing loss was 45.9%, with the odds of hearing loss increasing with age (odds ratio = 1.88 for every 5 years) and being greater for males than females. They concluded, as did previous investigators, that hearing loss is a very common disorder affecting older adults.

The aforementioned studies have been conducted on essentially the "well-elderly" residing in the community. Thus they did not take into account the approximately 5% of older adults who reside in nursing facilities. The typical nursing home resident is over 85 years of age and presents with a multiplicity of chronic conditions including hearing loss. Further, the majority of residents suffer from intellectual impairments and have a number of functional impairments necessitating assistance in the nursing facility. Specifically, about 63% of elderly nursing home residents exhibit disorientation or memory impairment with nearly half being diagnosed with some form of senile dementia. The potential for hearing loss is great, further complicating the picture of those already-compromised individuals.

SPECIAL CONSIDERATION

The prevalence and severity of hearing loss among nursing home residents is higher than in the community-based population.

Schow and Nerbonne (1980) sampled the hearing levels of residents of five nursing facilities in three cities in Idaho. The mean age of subjects in their sample was 81 years versus 73 years for the Gates et al (1990) sample and approximately 68 years for subjects in the Moscicki et al (1985) study. Approximately 58% of their subjects were 80 years of age and older. Approximately 70 to 80% of subjects sampled

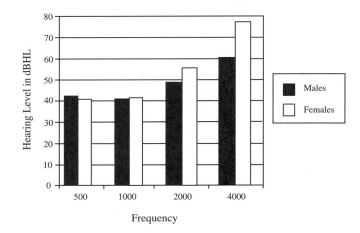

Figure 5–7 Mean hearing levels in dBHL for both ears for nursing home residents. (Modified from Schow and Nerbonne, 1980, p. 128, Table 2.)

had a hearing loss far exceeding prevalence within the noninstitutionalized population of older adults. Figure 5–7 summarizes mean pure-tone thresholds across frequencies averaged across the right and left ears of subjects. The average hearing level ranges from moderate to moderately severe. Figure 5–8 shows the breakdown of hearing levels of nursing home residents by age and severity of loss. It is clear that, as residents age, a greater proportion have more severe hearing loss. Approximately, 50% of subjects in their sample had a mild hearing loss and approximately 50% had a moderate to profound hearing loss, after correcting for contamination attributable to collapsed ear canals. Females had slightly poorer high-frequency thresholds than males. Subsequent studies have verified the finding that nursing home residents have a higher prevalence of hearing loss and more severe hearing loss than older adults residing in the community. This finding has implications for hearing screening protocols and the more widespread use of assistive-listening devices to facilitate communication in this setting.

In sum, the majority of recent cross-sectional studies on hearing loss suggest approximately 30% of individuals over 65 years of age present with a hearing impairment for pure-tones. Available data confirm that hearing loss tends to decline with increasing age in both males and females. Further, the decline in high-frequency sensitivity appears to be greatest in males while low-frequency thresholds are poorer in females of comparable age. The average hearing loss in males can be described as mild to moderately severe, with a sharply sloping configuration, whereas women tend to present with a mild to moderate gradually sloping hearing loss.

SPECIAL CONSIDERATION

Overall nursing home residents have a higher prevalence of hearing loss and more severe hearing loss than the elderly living in the community.

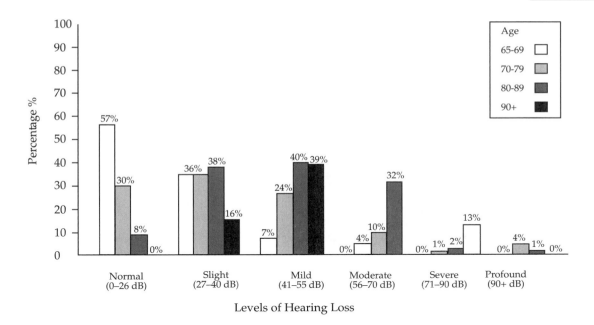

Figure 5–8   Percentage distribution of subjects showing various degrees of hearing loss within various age groups. (Modified from Schow and Nerbonne, 1980, p. 128, Table 3.)

Audiometric Studies: Longitudinal Data

Brant and Fozard (1990) and Pearson, Morrell, Gordon-Salant, Brant, Metter, Klein, and Fozard (1995) have conducted a longitudinal study of changes in hearing thresholds in a sample of adults participating in the Baltimore Longitudinal Study of Aging. This is an ongoing multidisciplinary study of normal human aging that began in 1958. Subjects participating in the study reported on in 1990 were males ($N =$ 813) between the ages of 20 and 95 years. They were generally well educated, white, and financially comfortable, with the majority residing in the Baltimore-Washington metropolitan area. Audiometric tests were performed in an IAC booth at 11 test frequencies using automatic audiometry (i.e., subjects pressed a handheld response to control the loudness of the tonal stimuli). Hearing tests on all participants were gathered on two or more different occasions from 1968 to 1987. Subjects were divided into seven age groups beginning with 20 year olds, and ending with people 95 years. Test results suggested longitudinal and cross-sectional age-related changes in mean hearing thresholds over the range of frequencies tested in all age groups over the 15-year follow-up period. However, the cross-sectional data gathered on a subset of subjects underestimated the rate of hearing loss among the older adults as compared to the longitudinal data. Their data suggest a marked increase in the rate of hearing loss at 500, 1000, 2000, and 3000 Hz starting between 40 and 50 years of age. Further, by 70 years of age, the rate of change in mean hearing thresholds was greater at these frequencies than it was at higher frequencies. Finally, large individual differences in mean pure-tone thresholds emerged across age groups, suggesting that hearing threshold levels cannot accurately be predicted from age data alone. In sum, the data of Brant and Fozard (1990) confirm that hearing threshold

levels at all frequencies change over time, with the rate of change greatest in the high frequencies and for those over 70 years of age.

Pearson et al (1995) recently completed another phase of data analysis using individuals participating in the Baltimore Longitudinal study. This study extends their previous report by incorporating a sample of women to allow for exploration of gender differences in hearing loss as a function of age. Six hundred and eighty-one men and 416 women underwent a series of audiometric tests over a 10-year period of time. Of the women, 48% had 5 or more years of follow-up data whereas in the male data set approximately 60% had 5 or more years of follow-up. Pure-tone threshold data were gathered in a sound-treated IAC booth at nine frequencies using pulsed tones and automatic audiometry. Threshold levels were determined from the audiogram at 1-dB steps from each of the frequencies tested by linear interpolation between the midpoints of the tracking excursions. Several interesting trends emerged from their study and are summarized in Table 5–1. Overall, their data agree with previous studies in that there is an age-associated reduction in hearing sensitivity that is particularly pronounced at higher frequencies. Further, they noted that the rate of decline in hearing sensitivity accelerates with age in both men and women. The change in hearing level with age tended to be gradual and progressive. Gender differences in hearing levels and rates of change in hearing level emerged. Figure 5–9 defines the average 10-year change in hearing level (dB/yr) for men and women at selected frequencies by age group. At most ages and frequencies, the amount of longitudinal change in hearing level over a 10-year period was more than twice as fast in men than in women, with the rate of change converging somewhat after age 60. Among men, decline in hearing sensitivity first became apparent as early as age 30

TABLE 5–1 Gender Differences in Hearing Threshold Level Changes over Time

Men	Women
1. The age-associated longitudinal per decade decline in hearing thresholds is on the order of 2.5 dB to 18 dB.	1. The age-associated longitudinal per decade decline in hearing thresholds is on the order of 2 to 19 dB.
2. Hearing sensitivity declines significantly at age 20 and beyond for 500 Hz and at age 30 and beyond for all other frequencies.	2. Hearing levels worsen at all ages for 500 Hz, after age 50 for 1000 to 3000 Hz, after age 40 for 4000 Hz, and by age 30 for 6000 to 8000 Hz.
3. Decline in hearing sensitivity accelerates at age 20 to 30.	3. Decline in hearing sensitivity accelerates at age 40 to 50.
4. At 3000 to 8000 Hz longitudinal change in rate of hearing loss is 10 dB/decade faster in 50-year olds.	4. At 3000 to 8000 Hz longitudinal change in rate of hearing loss is 10 dB/decade slower in 50 year olds.
5. Longitudinal rate of change in hearing level plateaus after age 60 at 6000 to 8000 Hz.	5. Longitudinal rate of change in hearing level at 6000 to 8000 Hz continues to accelerate even after age 60.
6. At age 30 and above, men have better hearing thresholds than women at 500 Hz and poorer thresholds than women at frequencies above 1000 Hz. Thresholds at 1000 Hz are comparable to those of women.	6. At age 30 and above, women have poorer thresholds than men at 500 Hz, and better thresholds than men at all frequencies above 1000 Hz. Thresholds at 1000 Hz are comparable to those of men.
7. On the average, hearing levels for the left ear are 0.7 dB poorer than right ear thresholds.	7. On the average, hearing levels of the left ear are 0.4 dB poorer than right ear thresholds.

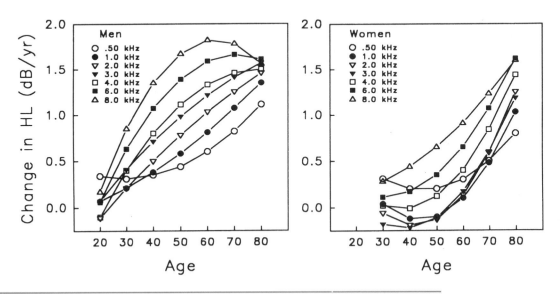

Figure 5–9 Average change over a 10-year period in hearing at selected frequencies for a sample of males and females. (From Pearson et al, 1995.)

whereas in women the age of onset tends to be frequency dependent occurring for the most part when they are somewhat older than males. The largest gender differences in longitudinal rates of hearing loss occurred at the frequencies most affected by noise, namely 3000 to 4000 Hz, with the rate of dB change per decade considerably greater in men than women. Finally, they found that in adults over age 80, the rate of hearing loss was comparable for men and women.

Gates and Cooper (1991) performed a longitudinal study of changes in hearing over a 6-year period in a large cohort of older adults. Pure-tone data were gathered on 1475 individuals as part of the Framingham Heart Study biennial examinations. Pure-tone thresholds at 250 to 8000 Hz obtained in 1978 to 1979 were compared to those obtained in 1983 to 1985. Subjects ranged in age from 58 to 94 years. For the most part, testing was performed by the same individuals, eliminating the examiner as a source of potential variability in thresholds. Mean pure-tone thresholds for men and women at each biennial examination revealed trends similar to those reported by Moscicki and her colleagues using the same cohort. Hearing loss was primarily confined to the high frequencies, men had poorer thresholds than women at frequencies above 2000 Hz and better thresholds at 250 and 500 Hz, and the hearing loss tended to be bilateral and symmetrical. Differences in mean pure-tone thresholds in the right and left ears over the 6-year time interval were rather small for both men and women. In women, the mean difference in PTA was 3.6 ± 0.21 dB and 5.3 ± 0.22 dB for the right and left ears, respectively, whereas in men the mean difference was 2.9 ± 0.25 dB and 4.7 ± 0.26 dB. For men and women, the greatest threshold change occurred at 6000 and 8000 Hz. The magnitude of the change at each of these frequencies was slightly greater in women than men. An interesting finding was the relation between initial age at time of testing and the proportion of subjects whose pure-tone averages changed dramatically over time. Table 5–2 summarizes these data. Overall, only 18% of subjects experienced a significant (> 10 dB) change in the PTA over time while 48% of subjects evidenced a change in the mean high-frequency pure-tone average (PTA$_H$) over time. For both genders, the 6-year rate of hearing loss increased with age in the frequen-

cies below 2 kHz, yet at 4 and 6 kHz men's threshold change slowed with age while the women's increased with age.

Although age had some impact on rate of worsening of hearing thresholds over time, preexisting hearing loss or initial hearing level did not affect the subsequent amount of change in PTA over 6 years. Gates and Cooper (1991) speculated that noise exposure, sociocusis, and other risk factors may interact with age to explain the individual variability in change in hearing level over time. Brant, Gordon-Salant, Pearson, Klein, Morrell, Metter, and Fozard (1996) used information collected from the Baltimore Longitudinal Study of Aging to examine the influence of risk factors other than age on absolute decline in hearing over time. They demonstrated that systolic blood pressure, independent of the effects of age, presents a significant risk for shifts in auditory threshold over time. In short, the risk of developing hearing loss over time appeared to be heightened when systolic blood pressure reached a certain level.

Concluding Remarks—Pure-Tone Data

The data emerging from longitudinal and cross-sectional studies confirm that women and men are at risk for age-associated hearing loss, which begins in men during early adulthood. There is large individual variability in absolute hearing thresholds and in the amount of change with age.

SPECIAL CONSIDERATION

Audiometric thresholds cannot accurately be predicted from age data.

There is a gender reversal in pure-tone thresholds with age. At the lower frequencies, thresholds are better in men whereas, at higher frequencies, thresholds are better in women. Finally, it seems safe to conclude from available longitudinal studies that (1) hearing level declines gradually and progressively with age, (2) the amount of threshold change appears greatest in the highs, (3) there are gender differences in rate of decline in hearing level and in frequencies at which declines take place, and (4) risk factors other than age contribute to the individual variability in decline in hearing level after age 50. Systolic blood pressure and noise exposure appear to be modifiable risk factors for hearing loss.

SPEECH RECOGNITION CORRELATES OF AGING

The majority of audiologists would agree with the statement that older adults frequently report difficulty understanding speech in a variety of situations, most notably in the presence of extraneous noise. Beyond that, there is little agreement regarding the endogenous or exogenous variables underlying their speech understanding difficulties. The literature on aging and performance on speech recognition is formidable, making it impossible to review all of the studies that have attempted to resolve the differences in

TABLE 5–2 Number and Proportion of Subjects in Percent by Age Group Showing Significant (> 10 dB) Change in PTA or PTA$_H$[1] over Time

Age group	Number of subjects	PTA	PTA$_H$
58 to 63	495	13	48
64 to 69	510	17	50
70 to 75	307	20	48
76 to 81	136	33	41
Overall	1448	17.6	48

[1]PTA$_H$ = average thresholds at 4000, 6000, and 8000 Hz.
Source: Modified from Gates and Cooper, 1991.

opinion regarding the source of speech-recognition difficulties among the elderly. The discussion that follows will attempt to provide an overview of the hypothesized factors and mechanisms that may underlie the speech-understanding difficulties experienced by the bulk of our older clients with hearing problems (Humes, 1996).

In general, there is agreement among clinicians and researchers that a pervasive characteristic of aging is an inability to understand speech, particularly in less than optimal circumstances (Crandell, Henoch, & Dunkerson, 1991).

A hallmark of studies on speech understanding in the elderly is the conclusion that there are large individual differences in performance among individuals over 60 years of age. Investigators have attempted to isolate the numerous factors that contribute to the large individual variability. This has led to several hypotheses generated to explain the mechanisms underlying the speech-understanding problems experienced by older adults. The three general hypotheses include the peripheral hypothesis, the central auditory hypothesis, and the cognitive hypothesis (Crandell, Henoch, & Dunkerson, 1991; Humes, Christopherson, & Cokely, 1992; Humes, 1996). In the peripheral hypothesis the auditory periphery is implicated, in the central auditory hypothesis the brainstem pathways and auditory cortex are implicated, and in the cognitive hypothesis the cortex, which is responsible for information processing, labeling, and storage, is implicated (Humes, 1996). The extent to which performance on measures of speech recognition can be accounted for by each of these mechanisms is discussed in the following paragraphs.

The peripheral hypothesis holds that the speech recognition difficulties are attributable to individual differences in the encoding of sound by the outer ear through the inner ear and eighth nerve (Humes, Christopherson, & Cokely, 1992). The peripheral component is reflected in the frequency-specific sensitivity loss revealed by the audiogram, most notable in the high frequencies. The peripheral hypothesis has been further subdivided into two versions. One suggests that simple changes in audibility wherein sound energy falls below an individual's audible region accounts for the speech-understanding problems characterizing older adults. The other suggests that reduced physiological processing associated with age-related changes in the cochlea creates distortions beyond loss-of-hearing sensitivity. Sources of distortion may arise from individual differences in other peripheral encoding mechanisms including loss of spectral and temporal resolution or loss of intensity discrimination.

The second hypothesis, namely the central auditory hypothesis, holds that age-related changes in the central auditory system including the auditory pathways of the brainstem or portions of the auditory cortex degrade the speech signal, leading to central auditory–processing disorders (Humes, 1996). Dysfunction in the auditory pathways within the brainstem or brain tend to impair neural transmission, feature extraction, information processing, labeling, or storage resulting in an impairment commonly referred to as a central auditory processing disorders (CAPD) (Humes, Christopherson, & Cokely, 1992). According to this hypothesis, one is considered to have CAPD when scores on speech audiometric measures of central auditory processing ability are depressed relative to a given norm (Jerger, Oliver, & Pirozzolo, 1990).

The final hypothesis, known as the cognitive hypothesis, implicates higher centers in the auditory pathways as a source of individual variations in cognitive abilities. Cortical functions subsumed under these areas include information processing, storage, and retrieval. These cortical processes underlie performance on speech-understanding tasks and it follows that individual differences in speech-understanding performance may be attributable to deficits in one or more of these areas. It is noteworthy that cognitive deficits are not confined to the auditory modality such that individual differences in short-term memory may emerge on tasks involving auditory or visual presentation of stimuli (Humes, Christopherson, & Cokely, 1992).

Historical Perspective—Studies before 1990

Early studies using elderly subjects revealed that speech recognition scores in the elderly tend to decline with increasing age and that performance on monosyllabic word-recognition tests is poorer than that which can be predicted from the audiogram. The term *phonemic regression* was coined by Gaeth (1948) to describe the latter phenomenon wherein older hearing-impaired adults experience more difficulty understanding speech than one would predict from the pure-tone audiogram. Recently, investigators have challenged Gaeth's hypothesis regarding age-related decrements in speech understanding. Subsequent investigators have speculated that earlier studies were most probably confounded by design problems, leading to erroneous conclusions regarding the contribution of age to decrements in speech understanding. Thus, more recent studies, such as those decribed in the following paragraphs, have attempted to compensate for the threats to the validity of earlier studies by employing better matching techniques and adaptive procedures for estimating word-recognition ability. In general, it appears that auditory processing disorders are not an inevitable concomitant of aging and that, in fact, performance of young adults is comparable to older persons when recognition ability is assessed in quiet and words are presented at sufficient intensity level to overcome the attenuating effects of high-frequency hearing loss (Marshall, 1981).

A comparative study conducted by Townsend and Bess (1980), in which older subjects with high-frequency hearing loss were matched with a young hearing-impaired control group having a similar configuration, revealed that speech-recognition ability in quiet was comparable for the two groups. Their study corroborated an earlier study, contrasting young and elderly subjects with flat audiometric configurations and three-frequency pure-tone averages < 50

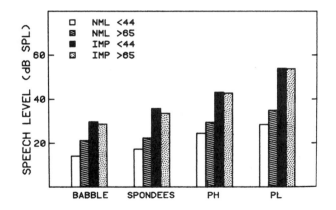

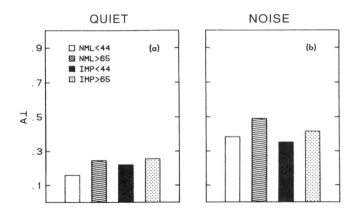

Figure 5–10 Speech level in dBSPL required for 50% recognition of speech materials in young and older subjects with normal and impaired hearing. (From Dubno, Dirks, and Morgan, 1984.)

Figure 5–11 Mean AI for young and older subjects with normal and impaired hearing, for SPIN-LP items in quiet and noise. (From Dubno, Dirks, and Morgan, 1984.)

dBHL. They too found that performance on monosyllabic word-recognition tasks in quiet was comparable. However, word-recognition ability did decline in older subjects with hearing levels exceeding 49 dBHL, implicating audibility as a factor intertwined with age. In the latter study, the differences in word-recognition ability may be due to depressed hearing levels at 3 or 4 kHz, which was not taken into account when the groups were matched. The important contribution of high-frequency hearing to speech understanding is elucidated in the sections to follow.

Dubno, Dirks, and Morgan (1984) employed an adaptive strategy to determine the effects of chronological age on speech-recognition ability in quiet and noise. They noted that mean speech levels required for 50% recognition of spondee words, and of low- and high-predictability items of the speech perception in noise (SPIN) test presented without babble, were comparable for the normals and for the hearing-impaired subjects (Fig. 5–10). That is, within each hearing-loss group, age effects were not observed for speech-recognition levels obtained in quiet at the hearing levels associated with 50% correct performance in quiet. It was of interest that the Articulation Index for 50% performance of low-predictability SPIN sentences in quiet was comparable for the young and old subjects with and without hearing loss. This is illustrated in Figure 5–11. The data

from this classic study support the conclusion that age effects are not observed for speech-recognition procedures conducted in the absence of a background of noise. Frisina and Frisina (1997) also noted that when Northwestern University (NU-6) word lists presented in quiet are used, word-recognition scores do not differ for young and older adults.

Gordon-Salant (1987a) conducted a comparative study of speech-recognition ability of young and older listeners with normal hearing and mild-moderate high-frequency sensorineural hearing loss. She compared open and closed set word-recognition scores for the NU-6 and modified rhyme test (MRT) word lists presented in quiet, at 80 dBSPL and at 90 dBSPL. In general, age effects were usually not observed for recognition of the monosyllabic word lists when presented in a quiet condition. Gordon-Salant and Fitzgibbons (1995a) confirmed these findings when they compared young and elderly listeners with normal hearing, and elderly listeners with mild-moderate sloping sensorineural hearing loss to young listeners with comparable hearing levels in their ability to recognize the low predictability SPIN sentences in quiet at 90 dBSPL. As is evident from Table 5–3, mean percent-correct recognition scores were comparable for the young and old normal hearing individuals and for the young and old hearing-impaired listeners. As would be expected, performance of the hearing impaired was poorer

TABLE 5–3 Mean Percent-Correct Word-Recognition Scores for Young and Elderly Listeners Matched for Hearing Loss

Condition	Young normal	Elderly normal	Young impaired	Elderly impaired
LP-SPIN- Q	98.8% (1.9)	98.8% (1.9)	86.8% (10.5)	88.4% (10.7)

Source: Gordon-Salant and Fitzgibbons, 1995a.

than that of the normal. The latter pattern emerged in the Dubno, Dirks, and Morgan (1984) study, as well.

Jerger and Hayes (1977) analyzed phonetically balanced-maximum (PB-max) scores obtained from PI-functions of 204 subjects with sensorineural hearing loss associated with a cochlear site of lesion. They reported that when monosyllabic speech-recognition ability was assessed at suprathreshold levels (i.e., PB-max), performance was equivalent across hearing-impaired subjects between 35 and 85 years of age. That is, mean percent-correct scores at PB-max were comparable across the age spectrum. Correlational studies using a variety of monosyllabic word-recognition materials confirmed the presence of a weak correlation between age and word-recognition ability, as well.

Finally, the data of Dubno, Lee, Matthews, and Mills (1997) are most compelling. They explored the relationship between gender, age, and word-recognition ability in a large sample of adults with sensorineural hearing loss of cochlear origin. Subjects ranged in age from 55 to 84 years. Mean pure-tone thresholds were indicative of normal hearing in the low frequencies sloping to the level of a mild to moderate hearing loss from 2000 to 8000 Hz. Word-recognition ability was assessed with a variety of materials including the NU-6 monosyllabic word lists, low- and high-predictability word lists from the SPIN test, and the synthetic identification test (SSI) materials. Subjects in three age groups (55 to 64, 65 to 74, 75 to 84) were selected to be closely matched for hearing level. Interestingly, mean scores on the speech-recognition tests were comparable across age groups for each of the six measures of speech recognition. Hence, the authors did not find a significant change in speech recognition with age when average pure-tone thresholds at each frequency were comparable across age groups.

SPECIAL CONSIDERATION

The preponderance of evidence suggests that in good acoustic environments, when speech is presented at high enough levels to receive the weak acoustic cues inherent in the speech signal, age does not influence standard word-recognition ability in quiet for normal or hearing-impaired individuals. However, some researchers have demonstrated age effects with selected materials and procedures. Use of nonsense syllables, an adaptive paradigm, and closed-set materials has been reported to uncover age effects.

Gelfand, Piper, and Silman (1986) found that older adults with minimal hearing loss may experience difficulty understanding nonsense syllables presented in quiet. Gelfand, Piper, and Silman (1986) assigned a sample of 64 adults with normal hearing to one of five age groups ranging from 20 to 69 years. Consonant recognition at MCL in quiet was assessed using the nonsense syllable test (NST). Their data suggest that consonant recognition assessed at MCL tends to decline systematically, albeit slightly with increasing age.

Gordon-Salant (1987a) confirmed some of the findings of Gelfand, Piper, and Silman (1986). She employed an adaptive paradigm to compare speech-recognition performance of young (< 42 years) and elderly (> 65 years) normal-hearing subjects. Open set (NU-6) and closed-set (MRT) monosyllabic word lists were used to gather information about speech-recognition ability. Age-effects emerged and appeared to be task and condition dependent. While mean speech-recognition percent scores of young normal-hearing subjects were comparable in quiet for NU-6 and MRT word lists presented at 80 and 95 dBSPL, age effects did emerge for selected conditions in the hearing impaired subjects. Specifically, in quiet, at 95 dBSPL, mean word-recognition scores on the MRT were better for the young hearing-impaired as compared to the elderly hearing-impaired subjects. Gordon-Salant concluded that while age effects for normal and hearing-impaired individuals did not emerge using the NU-6 word lists, a higher presentation level, coupled with a closed-set response task, helped to produce age effects in hearing-impaired subjects. The latter may be due to the fact that performance on a closed-set response task may be confounded by the cognitive status of subjects making up the sample. It appears from most of the foregoing studies that age effects are not manifest for normal-hearing and elderly subjects with minimal hearing loss when monosyllabic word lists are audible, of good quality, and presented in quiet.

PEARL

There does not appear to be a significant "age effect" for speech understanding when speech-recognition ability is sampled using traditional materials presented at high presentation levels in quiet. However, selected paradigms may be sensitive to uncovering age effects attributable to factors beyond peripheral hearing status.

The data presented in the next section review the endogenous and exogenous variables that may explain the individual differences in performance among older adults on selected speech tasks. The section concludes with a model for evaluating speech understanding in the elderly.

THE PERIPHERAL HYPOTHESIS
Changes in Audibility

In general, the preponderance of recent studies on the relation between hearing level and speech perception in older adults suggests that speech-recognition performance of elderly listeners can be explained in large part by the audibility model (Crandell, Henoch, & Dunkerson, 1991). Studies conducted within the past decade supporting this hypothesis have used better subject-selection criteria and multivariate techniques, thus enabling valid conclusions regarding the role of audibility. For example, Humes and his colleagues have carried out a series of studies designed to identify the correlates of speech-recognition performance among older adults. They used a modeling technique to simulate the perceptual effects of sensorineural hearing loss. Specifically, they introduced a spectrally shaped masking noise into the ear of normal hearing young adults that would induce thresholds shifts identical to the average audiograms of older adults (Humes, 1996). One of the first in the series of studies was a comparative study among three groups of listeners, young normal-hearing adults, elderly hearing-impaired adults (65 to 75 years), and young normal-hearing adults with simulated sensorineural hearing loss comparable to that of the elderly sample (Humes & Roberts, 1990). Both groups had normal hearing out to 1000 Hz, sloping gradually from a mild to severe level. The full 11 subtests of the CUNY NST served as the stimuli in the study. The speech materials were presented in quiet, noise, and in a reverberant environment in an attempt to sample a variety of acoustic conditions. The most striking finding that emerged was that performance of young adults with simulated hearing loss was comparable to that of the older hearing-impaired adults across acoustic conditions. There were, however, large individual differences in performance among the older adults. Pearson product moment correlations between speech recognition performance and average hearing loss revealed that approximately 80% of the variance in speech identification scores could be accounted for by average high-frequency pure-tone hearing loss (1, 2, and 4 kHz), irrespective of the listening condition. Using recordings of the MRT, Humes, Nelson, and Pisoni (1991) confirmed that much of the word-recognition difficulty experienced by older hearing-impaired adults is attributable to their hearing loss. Further, they found that older hearing-impaired adults who had difficulty with natural speech also had difficulty with synthetic speech and that the level of difficulty was similar to a sample of young adults with comparable simulated hearing loss. These data are consistent with the peripheral hypothesis, which ascribes individual differences in speech-recognition ability to the peripheral processing deficits accompanying sensorineural hearing loss.

PEARL

Auditory thresholds are the primary contributor to individual differences in speech-recognition ability (Dubno et al, 1997).

Humes, Watson, Christensen, Cokely, Halling, and Lee (1994) measured speech-recognition performance on a wide range of materials and listening conditions in a sample of 50 older adults from 63 to 83 years. The goal of the study was to attempt to identify the variables that accounted for some of the individual differences in clinical measures of speech recognition. Subjects had normal middle-ear function in the test ear as determined by results of immittance tests. Mean pure-tone thresholds were consistent with a mild to moderate sensorineural hearing loss primarily in the higher frequencies (1000 to 8000 Hz). All subjects underwent a complete battery of speech tests, cognitive tests, and tests of auditory discrimination. Three sets of speech materials were used in this study,

namely, the CUNY NST, the Central Institute for the Deaf (CID) W-22 word lists, and the revised SPIN test. Selected speech tests were presented in quiet and noise, and some of the speech materials were spectrally shaped. Further, the speech tests were presented at two levels, 70 and 90 dBSPL. In total, 20 measures of speech recognition were administered to each of the 50 subjects over four test sessions.

Table 5–4 presents mean performance for the subjects on the five speech tests in quiet and noise at 70 and 90 dBSPL. Several trends emerged. First, performance in quiet was better than performance in noise on all speech tests. Next, subjects clearly performed better at the higher presentation level in quiet. However, this trend was not as clear cut in noise. Finally, in quiet and noise, at 70 and at 90 dBSPL, subjects overwhelmingly performed best on the SPIN-HP. A correlational analysis among the speech-recognition measures revealed a strong correlation among measures, suggesting that subjects who obtained a high score on one of the speech-recognition measures likely scored high on the other tests. Similarly, subjects scoring poorly on one task tended to perform poorly on all of the speech-recognition tasks. Results of the principal components analysis among the 20 speech-recognition measures and hearing loss revealed that 74% of the variance in scores on the speech-recognition measures could be accounted for by the peripheral hearing status. That is to say, among the 50 older adults participating in the study, individual differences in average high-frequency hearing loss accounted for the bulk of the variability in performance on speech-recognition tests, across a variety of materials and conditions (Humes et al, 1994).

The data of van Rooij, Plomp, and Orlebeke (1989) and van Rooij and Plomp (1992) are in agreement with Humes' findings, in that they too found that high-frequency hearing loss was highly predictive of speech-understanding ability. Their data suggest that degree of sensorineural hearing loss is the primary factor, accounting for individual differences in speech recognition among the elderly. Their subjects ranged in age from 60 to 93 years and presented with symmetrical high-frequency hearing loss. Speech materials pri-

TABLE 5–4 Mean Score in Percent on Five Speech Tests (*N* = 50)

Speech materials	70 dBSPL Quiet	Noise	90 dBSPL Quiet	Noise
SPIN-LP[1]	67.1	44.1	82.9	42.5
SPIN-HP[2]	86.6	81.4	95.5	87.4
W-22S[3]	85.5	72.0	90.1	72.1
W-22U[4]	81.5	65.6	86.0	64.3
NST	71.4	55.3	78.9	61.1

Source: Modified from Humes et al, 1994.
[1]LP = low predictability
[2]HP = high predictability
[3]S = spectrally shaped
[4]U = unshaped

marily consisted of tests of phoneme perception and spondee perception in noise. Van Rooij and Plomp (1992) found that speech perception ability correlated with age as well. However, a large component of the latter relation was attributable to the association between progressive high-frequency hearing loss and age. Their conclusion, that hearing loss is the primary determinant of individual differences in speech-recognition ability of older adults, has been echoed by Jerger, Jerger, and Pirozzolo (1991); Helfer and Wilber (1990); Divenyi and Haupt (1997a); Wiley, Cruickshanks, Nondahl, Tweed, Klein, and Klein (1998), and other investigators.

Jerger, Jerger, and Pirozzolo (1991) administered a battery of speech audiometric and neuropsychologic measures to a sample of 200 older adults (mean age = 69.7 years) to determine the contribution of these factors to speech recognition performance. The average high-frequency hearing loss (average of 1, 2, and 4 kHz) of subjects in the sample was 32 dBHL for the right ear and 31 dBHL for the left ear. The speech materials included the phonetically balanced (PB) word test, the SSI test, SPIN test, and the dichotic sentence identification test (DSI). Once again, across all of the test conditions, the most powerful predictor of speech-recognition performance was degree of hearing loss. Age was significantly correlated with speech-recognition performance. However, when hearing loss was controlled, the relation was minimized for most of the comparisons. As will be discussed in a later section, to a much lesser degree, cognitive status affected speech-recognition performance on selected measures, as well.

Dubno and Schaefer (1992) confirmed the primary source for the speech-understanding difficulties of hearing-impaired adults to be reduction in audibility of important portions of the speech signal. They argued that loss of frequency selectivity is not strongly associated with deficits in consonant recognition. Using a paradigm similar to Humes and his colleagues, Dubno and Schaefer (1992) compared frequency selectivity and speech-recognition performance of hearing-impaired listeners to a sample of masked normal-hearing listeners with comparable thresholds. Although frequency selectivity was poorer for the hearing-impaired listeners, their consonant-recognition scores fell within the range of scores for the masked normal-hearing subjects. They concluded that their data support the hypothesis that differences in speech-spectrum audibility accounts for a significant proportion of the variance in speech-recognition scores of the hearing impaired.

Several interesting trends emerged in a study of consonant recognition and confusion patterns among elderly subjects with normal hearing and hearing impairment conducted by Gordon-Salant (1987b). Three groups of subjects ranging in age from 65 to 75 years participated. One group had normal hearing, the second sensorineural hearing loss with gradually-sloping configurations, and the third group had sensorineural hearing loss with sharply sloping configurations. Consonant recognition was assessed at 70 and 90 dBSPL in the presence of a +6 dB signal to babble ratio. Consonant recognition in noise at 75 and 90 dBHL was best among normal-hearing elderly and poorest among those with sharply sloping configurations. Consonants paired

with /u/ were recognized with greater accuracy then those paired with /i/ and /a/. At the higher presentation level, normal-hearing elderly and subjects with gradually sloping loss achieved higher consonant-recognition scores than those with sharply sloping loss. Performance differences emerged as a function of hearing-loss group and presentation level. Finally, differences in consonant-recognition patterns emerged between normal-hearing and hearing-impaired subjects, but few differences emerged between the hearing-impaired subject groups in terms of error patterns. That is, the hearing-loss configuration did not influence the pattern of errors in consonant recognition. Gordon-Salant (1987b) concluded that the attenuation imposed by the hearing loss that could not be compensated by a higher presentation level accounted for decrements in consonant recognition. Further, hearing loss experienced by older adults does not appear to affect the pattern of performance. Her data, once again, lent some support to the audibility model.

Together, the results of these comparative and multivariate studies suggest that much (albeit not all) of the variance in speech-recognition performance of young and older subjects can be explained by differences in speech-signal audibility. Factors other than shifts in hearing sensitivity that

---

SPECIAL CONSIDERATION

Studies conducted by van Rooij, Plomp, and Orlebeke (1989); Helfer and Wilber (1990); Humes and Roberts (1990), among others indicate that roughly 70 to 95% of the variance in speech-recognition performance is associated with individual differences in pure-tone hearing sensitivity. There is, however, increasing evidence that other peripheral deficits, beyond loss of hearing sensitivity, accompany the cochlear pathology of aging and may account for an additional proportion of the individual variation in scores on speech tests.

---

may in fact contribute to deficits in speech-recognition performance experienced by older adults include distortions produced by noise and deficits in auditory temporal processing.

PEARL

The audibility of speech is a primary contributor to variations in word-recognition scores in older adults (Wiley, Cruickshanks, Nondahl, Tweed, Klein, & Klein, 1998).

Other Peripheral Deficits

There is a good deal of support in the literature for the concept that age-related changes in the cochlea lead to reductions in physiological processing of speech information (Crandell, Henoch, & Dunkerson, 1991). Specifically, this theory posits that hearing loss for speech arises because sensorineural hearing impairment attenuates the auditory signal and introduces distortion even when speech is presented within the audible range of the individual (Plomp & Duquesny, 1982). According to Plomp and Duquesny, attenuation that results from the threshold loss causes speech and noise signals to fall below the individual's audible region. Difficulty understanding speech in noise, which is characteristic of the vast majority of elderly listeners, may be due in part to the distortion component, accompanying the sensitivity loss (Crandell, Henoch, & Dunkerson, 1991). The distortion factor results in a reduction in the "functional" signal-to-noise ratio. Further, distortion may be associated with deficits in frequency resolution, or temporal resolution, or frequency or intensity discrimination, etc., even when speech is within the audible range of the individual (Crandell, Henoch, & Dunkerson, 1991).

External distortions such as noise explain in part the speech-recognition deficits experienced by older adults. As discussed in an earlier section, Dubno, Dirks, and Morgan (1984) used an adaptive procedure, spondee words, and the high- and low-predictability items on the SPIN test to assess speech-recognition differences between young (< 44 years of age) and elderly (> 65 years of age) listeners with normal hearing and mild sensorineural hearing loss. Dubno, Dirks, and Morgan (1984) found that elderly listeners with and without hearing loss performed more poorly than younger listeners with matched hearing sensitivity in their recognition of low-predictability items from the SPIN test presented in the presence of multitalker babble. Similarly, irrespective of speech level (i.e., 56, 72, and 88 dBSPL), normal- and hearing-impaired subjects over 65 required more advantageous signal to babble ratios to achieve a 50% criterion score on the low-predictability sentences. The differences are apparent in Figure 5–12. Pure-tone thresholds of subjects could not be used to accurately predict overall performance in quiet and noise underlining the large individual variability inherent in sentence recognition. Their data were noteworthy in that they suggested that even in the presence of normal hearing, older listeners require more advantageous signal to babble ratios for their performance to be equivalent to young normal-hearing subjects. Frisina and Frisina (1997) also

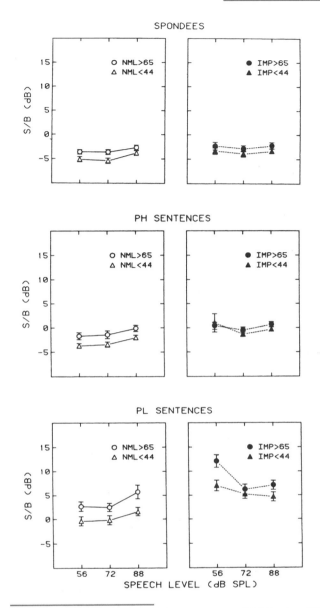

Figure 5–12 Signal-to-babble ratios in dBSPL for 50% recognition of spondees and SPIN sentence material for young and older subjects with normal and impaired hearing. (From Dubno, Dirks, and Morgan, 1984.)

PEARL

Age, independent of hearing loss, is a significant variable influencing speech-recognition ability in noise.

---

found that even after adjusting for audibility, older adults have greater difficulty understanding words in the presence of noise than do young adults. Dubno, Dirks, and Morgan (1984) hypothesized that age effects on speech-recognition in noise may be a result of the peripheral effects of the aging process in combination with central processing dysfunction.

Gordon-Salant (1987a) employed an adaptive paradigm to compare speech-recognition performance of young (< 42 years) and elderly (> 65 years) normal-hearing and hearing-impaired subjects when speech was presented in fixed-noise conditions. Open (NU-6) and closed-set (MRT) monosyllabic word lists presented in the presence of 12-talker babble were used to gather information about speech-recognition ability. In addition to comparing percent-correct word-recognition scores, mean signal to babble ratios required for 50% criterion scores on the word lists were compared. The results were noteworthy, supporting for the most part the conclusions of earlier investigators. Age effects did emerge for selected conditions in the hearing-impaired subjects. Specifically, mean percent-correct recognition scores on the MRT were significantly higher for the younger hearing-impaired subjects than for older hearing-impaired subjects in noise at both presentation levels. Age effects were most apparent when the adaptive strategy was applied to determine mean signal to babble ratios necessary for 50% criterion scores. Age effects emerged for the normal and hearing-impaired subjects and for the young and older subjects, such that older subjects consistently required more favorable signal to babble ratios to achieve 50% criterion scores. The conclusions to be reached from this study are as follows: (1) age effects can emerge independent of hearing loss using an adaptive noise paradigm, (2) testing in noise helps to produce age effects in both normal and hearing-impaired subjects, and (3) fixed-noise paradigms are less effective than an adaptive paradigm in uncovering age effects on speech-recognition tasks.

Notwithstanding the data suggesting that the elderly perform more poorly than younger listeners on speech tasks presented in noise, it is critical to emphasize that there are large individual differences among the elderly in their susceptibility to noise (Crandell, Henoch, & Dunkerson, 1991). Crandell (1991) examined speech-recognition performance of 26 older adults with mild to moderate high-frequency sensorineural hearing loss. Speech-recognition ability was assessed using the high-predictability sentences from the SPIN test, presented in quiet and in the presence of multitalker babble. The most notable finding was the lack of a relation between word-recognition ability in quiet and in noise. That is, speech-recognition ability in noise could not be predicted from that obtained in quiet. Similarly, subjects with comparable speech-recognition scores in quiet differed dramatically in their speech-recognition performance in noise. This apparent individual susceptibility to noise underlies the importance of performing tests of speech understanding in both quiet and in noise to determine the quality of the peripheral deficit and the technology most appropriate for the older adult with hearing impairment.

Gelfand, Piper, and Silman (1986) also found that older adults with minimal hearing loss may experience difficulty understanding nonsense syllables presented in noise background. Gelfand, Piper, and Silman (1986) assigned a sample of 64 adults with normal hearing to one of five age groups ranging from 20 to 69 years. Consonant recognition at most comfortable loudness (MCL) in quiet and at a +5 and +10 dB S/N ratio was assessed using the NST. Their data suggested a systematic and significant decline in consonant recognition in noise with advancing age. There was also a decline in consonant-recognition performance in quiet as a function of age but it was rather small. Gelfand, Piper, and Silman (1986) determined the correlations between audiometric thresholds and performance on the NST and found that consonant recognition decreased as hearing threshold levels became more elevated. Overall, high-frequency thresholds consistently correlated with consonant recognition in quiet and in noise (S/N + 10 and S/N + 5). Partial correlations between thresholds at 8000 Hz and the NST scores were statistically significant when controlling for age but were obliterated

when NST scores were correlated with age and hearing loss was controlled. The latter partial correlations led the authors to conclude that age-associated peripheral-auditory deterioration, even in the presence of normal pure-tone thresholds, accounts in part for deficits in consonant recognition in older adults with minimal hearing loss. Finally, it is noteworthy that the pattern of errors or consonant confusions were comparable across age groups. Stated differently, the age-effect may be one of degree rather than one of kind of confusions. Older adults apparently use the same perceptual cues as younger adults for consonant recognition but they appear to use the cues less efficiently, as evidenced by the poorer consonant-recognition scores.

Gordon-Salant and Fitzgibbons (1995b) assessed the impact of age and hearing loss on recognition of undistorted speech materials (i.e., low-predictability [LP] SPIN sentence-materials) presented at various S/N. Forty subjects were assigned to one of four groups, normal-hearing young and elderly, and hearing-impaired young and elderly. The hearing-impaired subjects presented with essentially mild to moderate sensorineural hearing loss. The LP-SPIN sentences were presented in five noise conditions at 90 dBSPL. S/N were as follows: −8 dB, 0 dB, +8 dB, +16 dB, and +24 dB. As would be expected, hearing level influenced recognition scores. Listeners with hearing loss performed more poorly than listeners with normal hearing at all S/N. The impact of age on speech-recognition ability was highly dependent on the difficulty of the listening condition such that at 0 dB S/N younger listeners scored better than older listeners. However, at more favorable S/N such as +8 dB, +16 dB, and +24 dB age-related differences did not emerge. It was noteworthy that at all signal to noise ratios, performance of the normals was comparable irrespective of condition, whereas at 0 dB S/N mean percent-correct scores were poorer for the elderly hearing impaired even at a relatively high presentation level. Humes et al (1994) also found that even when the presentation level is increased (e.g., 70 to 90 dBSPL), speech-recognition ability in noise remains compromised in older adults with mild to moderate high-frequency sensorineural hearing loss for a range of materials including the revised SPIN test, CUNY NST, and the CID W-22 unshaped or shaped word lists. Wiley et al (1998) tested a large sample of older adults with varying degrees of sensorineural hearing loss and found, as well, that word-recognition ability in the presence of a competing message decreased with increasing age. Hence, decrements in word-recognition ability in the presence of noise are attributable in part to age, even when controlling for audibility.

PEARL

Compensating for audibility (e.g., high-presentation level) may not improve speech-recognition ability in the presence of noise.

Gordon-Salant and Fitzgibbons (1997) have conducted a series of psychoacoustic studies over the past several years on the contribution of auditory temporal processing ability to speech understanding. Gordon-Salant and Fitzgibbons

(1995b) examined the effects of multiple stimulus degradations on speech-recognition performance of young and older listeners with normal hearing and mild to moderate sensorineural hearing loss. Speech-recognition ability was assessed using low-predictability items from the revised speech perception in noise (R-SPIN) test presented in undistorted form, presented in the presence of reverberation, and with the temporal characteristics distorted via time compression, which merely increased the rate of speech without producing spectral distortions. A time compression ratio of 40% and a fixed reverberation time of 0.3 seconds were used. Finally, 12-talker babble presented at a signal to noise ratio of +16 dB was used as a form of degradation as well. In total, seven listening conditions of varying levels of distortion were presented in a randomized fashion to the participants at a fixed level of 90 dBSPL. Their findings support the theory that external distortions such as reverberation, noise, and fast speech may interact with even minor internal distortions (little or no peripheral hearing loss) to disadvantage older listeners (Helfer, 1991). Specifically, they found the following: (1) elderly listeners with normal hearing performed more poorly than younger listeners on time-compressed materials presented in quiet, (2) elderly listeners with normal hearing performed more poorly than young listeners with normal hearing in the time-compressed and reverberant-speech condition and the time-compressed and noise condition, (3) elderly hearing-impaired listeners performed more poorly than young listeners with comparable hearing levels in the time-compressed and noise conditions and in the time-compressed plus reverberant-speech condition, and (4) speech-recognition deficits for the young and older listeners with and without hearing loss were greatest in the condition combining time compression and reverberation. In light of the above findings, the authors concluded that age effects are pronounced even in the presence of minimal hearing loss when speech materials are subjected to multiple external distortions, most notably time compression and noise, or time compression and reverberation.

An earlier study by Gordon-Salant and Fitzgibbons (1993) also revealed age effects independent of hearing loss when speech materials are subjected to varying types of temporal distortion. Four groups of subjects participated in this study, elderly adults with normal hearing and elderly adults with mild to moderate sensorineural hearing loss, young listeners with normal hearing, and young listeners with comparable hearing levels. The low-predictability items of the R-SPIN test were presented in undistorted form and with varying degrees of temporal distortion. The forms of distortion included time compression, reverberation, and interruption. Within each form of distortion were varying degrees or rates of distortion. For example, time compression ratios ranged from 30 to 60%, reverberation time ranged from 0.2 to 0.6 seconds, and the interruption rate ranged from 12.5 to 100 interruptions per second. In the undistorted condition, the young and elderly normal-hearing listeners obtained comparable percent-correct scores, as did the young and older listeners with sensorineural hearing loss. Thus, recognition of the undistorted sentence materials was more affected by hearing loss than age even at a high presentation level, namely 90 dBSPL. For

the most part, hearing loss influenced recognition of the three types of distorted materials at a high presentation level. In the time-compressed condition, an effect of age, hearing level, and time-compression ratio emerged. Older listeners with hearing loss performed more poorly than younger listeners on time-compressed speech tasks such that they might be expected to experience difficulty understanding the speech of fast talkers. Performance scores on the reverberant speech tasks also revealed significant effects for age, reverberation time, and hearing status. The latter finding would suggest that reverberant environments may distort speech in a manner particularly difficult for older listeners. Finally, significant effects of age and hearing status also emerged on the interrupted speech task. The conclusion of Gordon-Salant and Fitzgibbons (1993) that high-frequency hearing sensitivity was the most important variable contributing to understanding of undistorted speech materials, time compressed speech materials (40% time compression [TC]), and reverberant materials (0.2 second reverberation time [RT]) was in agreement with the data of Humes and Christopherson (1991). Further, in light of the decrements in performance for older subjects with and without hearing loss, Gordon-Salant and Fitzgibbons (1993) concluded that there were significant age effects, independent of peripheral hearing loss, in performance on the temporally distorted speech tasks. Specifically, rapid speech appears to be a source of challenge to the slowed processing system of many older adults. However, Wingfield (1996) pointed out that decrements in performance may in fact derive from the speech materials used in their study, which lack the redundancy of normal everyday speech.

Humes and Christopherson (1991) examined the contribution of auditory discrimination to speech understanding as well. They compared the auditory skills of young-old listeners and old-old listeners to those of a sample of young listeners with normal hearing listeners whose hearing loss was simulated via noise masking. Auditory discrimination ability was examined using a battery of discrimination tests known as the Test of Basic Auditory Capabilities (TBAC). This battery of tests makes use of simple tonal stimuli and more complex sequences of tone bursts. Speech materials were nonsense syllables that were spectrally and temporally degraded. Temporal degrading was accomplished using reverberation, and spectral distortion was introduced by band-pass filtering materials from 500 to 4000 Hz. They noted that the primary factor determining performance on the NST was the sensorineural hearing loss of the listener. The greater the hearing loss, the lower the speech-identification scores. Further, simple tonal-frequency discrimination for a 1000 Hz tone accounted for a significant, albeit small, proportion of the individual variability in performance on speech-identification tests. To better isolate the factor(s) that determined scores on the speech-identification tasks, performance of the noise-masked group was compared to that of the young normal-hearing listeners and the elderly hearing-impaired listeners. Decrements in performance emerged for the elderly subjects on auditory discrimination tasks that involved pure-tone frequency discrimination, temporal-order discrimination for sequences of tones or syllables, and intensity discrimination involving complex tonal patterns. The data of

Humes and Christopherson (1991) and Gordon-Salant and Fitzgibbons (1993) suggest that older adults may experience difficulty in the processing of complex signals such as temporal rhythmic structure. These difficulties can be identified using speech materials that have been unnaturally distorted by time compression or interruption.

Jerger and Chmiel (1997) conducted a multivariate analysis of variables contributing to the speech understanding difficulties experienced by older adults. One hundred eighty older adults over 60 years of age participated in their study. The majority of subjects ($n = 100$) were experienced hearing-aid users. The mean pure-tone average was about 45 dBHL in each ear, and the mean score on the Hearing Handicap Inventory for the Elderly (HHIE) was 38%, suggesting significant self-perceived hearing handicap. All subjects underwent a complete audiologic evaluation including comprehensive word-recognition testing. Speech understanding was tested using (1) PB-50 word lists, (2) the SSI test presented dichotically and in the presence of single-talker competition (word materials were presented at several suprathreshold levels to define a performance-intensity function), and (3) conventional immittance testing. The older adult completed the HHIE and their significant other responded to the HHIE-SO (significant other) using a face-face administration. A factor analysis was applied to the data to determine the factor structure of conventional audiometric measures.

Some interesting trends emerged in many respects corroborating some of the findings listed above and on occasion elucidating other facts. Factor one, namely the average of low-frequency thresholds (250, 500, and 1000 Hz) in the right ear and 500 and 1000 Hz in the left ear, accounted for 24% of the variance in the data. In contrast, high-frequency hearing sensitivity, namely the average of 3 and 4 kHz in both ears, accounted for only 16% of the variance in the data (Jerger & Chmiel, 1997). PB scores on both ears that provide an estimate of speech understanding ability accounted for 14% of the variance in the data, and emerged as factor five in the factor analysis. HHIE scores as reported by the client and a significant other accounted for only 8% of the variance in the data. Of interest was the proportion of the variance accounted for by central processing, as quantified using dichotically presented sentences. Specifically, central processing of speech materials presented to the left ear and right ear, respectively, accounted for 20% and 18% of the variance and together accounting for 38% of the variance in the data (Jerger & Chmiel, 1997). As a result of their findings, Jerger and Chmiel (1997) concluded that degree of hearing impairment, which determines speech audibility, is key to the speech-understanding problems characterizing older adults, that central processing of verbal input is a significant factor underlying auditory processing, and that self-perceived hearing handicap emerges as a factor independent of pure-tone and speech audiometric data. Their data lend support to the protocol I will propose toward the end of the chapter for evaluating hearing status of older adults.

In sum, the data reviewed above suggest that sensorineural hearing loss of the listener systematically emerges as the primary variable accounting for performance on measures of speech understanding. The evidence presented in the preceding paragraphs suggests that speech distorted by noise or temporally may be particularly difficult for older adults beyond what one would expect from peripheral hearing level.

Central Auditory Hypothesis

A number of investigators have hypothesized that speech-recognition deficits notable among elderly listeners are attributable to structural or functional changes in the auditory pathways of the brainstem or in the auditory cortex. CAPD

SPECIAL CONSIDERATION

The central auditory hypothesis holds that the existence of a central auditory processing disorder (CAPD) may account for the speech-understanding problems experienced by older adults.

---

refers to functional difficulties revealed through behavioral speech tests that employ degraded or competing acoustic signals (ASHA, 1996). Crandell, Henoch, and Dunkerson (1991) hypothesized that in cases of CAPD, the already degraded signal from the cochlea is being processed through a central auditory system that is unable either to make fine phonemic discriminations or to make use of the redundancy of speech. As a consequence, older adults with presumed CAPD perform poorly on speech-understanding tests that challenge the structural or functional integrity of the central auditory nervous system.

PEARL

The three most widely used tests for detecting the presence of CAPD in the elderly are (1) examining the performance-intensity function (PI) of phonetically balanced word lists for rollover, (2) comparing the SSI test and PI-PB functions or their maxima, or (3) dichotic listening tasks such as the staggered spondaic word (SSW) test, the dichotic digits test (DDT) or the DSI (Bess & Strouse, 1996).

SPECIAL CONSIDERATION

The validity of the central auditory hypothesis has been the subject of debate and controversy among investigators, as demonstrated by disagreement about (1) the prevalence of CAPD in the elderly, (2) the influence of peripheral hearing loss on prevalence of CAPD, (3) the reliability and validity of speech tests used to measure CAPD, and (4) the role other variables may play in influencing auditory processing.

The studies that follow focus on the controversy over the extent to which CAPD is a principal cause of speech perception deficits in the elderly. Studies on prevalence of CAPD in older adults yield estimates ranging from 10 to 90 percent. Stach, Spretnjak, and Jerger (1990) were among the first investigators to report on the prevalence of central presbycusis as a function of age in clinical population. Mean pure-tone averages of their subjects ranged from 15 dBHL in the youngest group (50 to 54) to 40 dBHL in the oldest group (80+). They defined central presbycusis operationally based on the pattern of test scores that emerged when comparing results on the SSI test to those on the PAL PB-50 word lists. According to their definition of CAPD, 17% of persons 50 to 54 years of age, 58% of persons between 65 and 69 years, and 90 to 95% of persons 80 years and older showed evidence of central presbycusis. They concluded that in their sample, 70% of persons over the age of 60 had some degree of speech-understanding deficit that could not be explained on the basis of pure-tone hearing levels.

Jerger, Jerger, Oliver, and Pirozzolo (1989), using a different set of criteria, namely, PB-SSI differences of more than 20%, abnormal SPIN scores, or inter-ear differences on the DSI test that exceeded a criterion level, reported the prevalence of CAPD to be 50% among hearing-impaired adults over 51 years of age. In their sample, cognitive deficits emerged in 54% of subjects with CAPD and in 28% of those without CAPD. Recently, Cooper and Gates (1991), using a stratified random sample of the U.S. population, reported that the prevalence of CAPD may be less than previously believed. They administered a series of central auditory tests to a large sample of adults over 60 years of age. For the most part, mean three-frequency pure-tone averages were within normal limits. Speech-recognition performance was assessed using CID W-22 word lists, the SSI-ICM, and the SSW. Rollover was considered significant and indicative of the presence of CAPD if the rollover index exceeded 0.20 for the CID W-22 word lists. For the synthetic sentences presented with an ipsilateral competing message at a 0 dBMCR, rollover was considered significant and CAPD present if the difference between the minimal and maximal level was more than 20 percentage points. On the SSW test, evidence of CAPD was based on adult norms for the test. The overall prevalence of CAPD in their sample was 22.6% based on abnormal findings on any one of the above speech tests.

Cooper and Gates (1991) attempted to analyze the rate of CAPD as a function of speech test to clarify the relation between CAPD prevalence and test sensitivity. They found that prevalence rates did in fact differ according to the criterion measure. The rate of CAPD was highest, 18%, when comparing PB max to SSI-ICM scores at a 0 dBMCR. The rate was lowest, 1.4%, using the PI-PB rollover index (RO) as the criterion measure. When total corrected SSW error score was the criterion measure for CAPD, the prevalence rate was 10.7%. It was of interest that the prevalence rate declined when the criterion for CAPD was made more stringent, namely abnormal performance on two out of three tests of CAPD, or on all three tests of CAPD. This finding lends support to the theory that loose criterion for CAPD may inflate prevalence estimates (Humes, Christopherson, & Cokely, 1992). Finally, although chronological age had a statistically significant influence on the rate of CAPD, it was of interest that it accounted for no more than 15% of the variability on the three indices of CAPD. Cooper and Gates (1991) concluded that age was not a dominant factor in the etiology of CAPD. However, age may function to increase the likelihood of exposure to events that may produce CAPD.

PEARL

Audiological status is a better predictor of speech understanding than cognitive status or general audiologic performance (Divenyi & Haupt, 1997).

Recently a few investigators have considered the question of whether speech-understanding difficulties experienced by older adults are in fact related to deficits in central auditory processing by studying persons with confirmed Alzheimer's disease. This population lends itself nicely to the question due to focal deficits in temporal areas of the brain in persons with Alzheimer's disease. In addition, early studies have shown a relation between performance on tests of central auditory nervous system, neuroanatomical, physiological, and cognitive function in a sample of patients with Alzheimer's disease. Data from recent studies have revealed a clinically significant relation between central auditory function and tests of cognition in adults with dementia (Grimes, Grady, Foster, Sunderland & Patronas, 1985; Gates, Cobb, Linn, Rees, Wolf, & D'Agostino, 1996). Strouse, Hall, and Burger (1995) compared performance of

SPECIAL CONSIDERATION

Hearing loss lowers performance on the minimental state examination, underlining the important role assistive listening devices can play in the examination of mental status of older adults (Gates et al, 1996).

adults with and without a diagnosis of Alzheimer's disease on a battery of behavioral tests designed to assess central auditory processing ability. Subjects in the Alzheimer's group had a mean age of 72 years, a mean high frequency PTA of 36 dBHL, and mean monosyllabic word-recognition score of 95%. Subjects in the control group had a mean age of 70 years, a mean high frequency PTA of 28.2 dBHL, and a mean monosyllabic word-recognition score of 98%. Statistical analyses revealed that the groups were comparable on the preceding measures. Distortion product otoacoustic emissions revealed that peripheral auditory status was equivalent for both groups. The prevalence of CAPD, defined as an abnormal score on one or more of the five CAPD measures, was 100% for the Alzheimer's group versus 30% for the control group of older adults. On the more widely used scales of central auditory processing ability namely, the SSI and the DSI, scores for all control subjects were within the normal range. The latter finding suggests a lack of support for deficits in central auditory function as a major cause of speech understanding difficulties among older adults with minimal peripheral hearing loss.

PEARL

The high prevalence of central auditory processing disorders in people with a diagnosis of Alzheimer's disease suggests an auditory processing component symptom that could potentially be remedied with assistive listening devices. Central auditory dysfunction may be considered a marker for senile dementia (Gates et al, 1996).

In sum, a number of studies have been conducted to determine the extent to which central auditory processing disorders are a factor contributing to age-related speech-perception difficulties. Some studies have estimated a prevalence rate of 50 to 70%, with prevalence increasing as a function of age. Some of these studies, however, have been criticized because of confounding effects of hearing loss and the questionable reliability and validity of the speech measures. Other studies have reported prevalence rates of 20 to 30% among older adults with minimal peripheral-hearing loss. The more stringent the criterion for CAPD, the less likely the existence of measured CAPD. Together the evidence concerning CAPD as a factor in the speech-perception problems of older adults is incomplete. However, even a prevalence rate as low as 20% would suggest that audiologists must measure central auditory processing ability in older adults to determine which older adults are afflicted and how to manage them. Further, the reasoning of Wiley et al (1998) supports the theory of an underlying central component to the auditory processing abilities of older adults. They found that hearing loss, age, and gender accounted for slightly more than half of the variance in word-recognition scores in noise, and thus central factors must account for some of the individual differences in word-recognition ability so apparent in the elderly.

The choice of test battery to measure CAPD thus becomes an important issue for audiologists. It appears that available tests may not be stable enough to justify their use in validly evaluating CAPD. Dubno and Dirks (1983) reported that interpretation of scores on the SSI is confounded by the large intrasubject variability inherent in scores on this test. Similarly, Cokely and Humes (1992) provided data demonstrating significant test-retest variability in scores on the DSI and SPIN in an elderly population. An additional threat to the validity of the above speech tests as estimates of CAPD is their apparent correlation with peripheral-hearing sensitivity. Cokely and Humes (1992) found that high-frequency pure-tone average had a moderate to high correlation with scores on the SPIN and selected scores on the DSI.

SPECIAL CONSIDERATION

The degree of peripheral hearing loss can confound the interpretation of scores on measures of CAPD.

Absent a reliable and valid test of CAPD, whether an auditory processing disorder exists remains an important question because (1) difficulty understanding speech especially in noise, a hallmark of CAPD, is one of the most frequent complaints of older adults presenting for audiologic assessment and management, (2) the existence of a central auditory processing problem has a significant impact on an older adult's perception of the social and emotional handicap resulting from hearing loss, and (3) of the potential impact of CAPD on successful use of hearing aids. With regard to the second consideration, older adults with minimal, mild, or moderate sensorineural hearing loss and CAPD self-rate their psychosocial handicap to be significantly greater than do those individuals without CAPD. The latter is not the case for older adults with and without cognitive deficits (Jerger, Oliver, & Pirozzolo, 1990). It is noteworthy

---

SPECIAL CONSIDERATION

Older adults with CAPD and with or without peripheral hearing loss who consider themselves handicapped should be considered prime candidates for audiologic intervention in the form of hearing aids and/or assistive-listening devices.

---

that hearing aids are less effective in reducing psychosocial handicap in older adults with CAPD than are frequency

---

PEARL

It is important to determine both the degree of peripheral-hearing sensitivity loss and the possible presence of concomitant CAPD, prior to recommending a particular form of intervention.

---

modulated (FM) systems. An older adult with CAPD who receives a hearing aid must realize that hearing aids may be bothersome to the point that speech understanding in noise is poorer, oftentimes leading to hearing-aid rejection (Jerger, Chmiel, Wilson, & Luchi, 1995).

SPECIAL CONSIDERATION

Remote microphone amplifying systems may be preferable for persons who present with CAPD, because they are more effective than are hearing aids in reducing psychosocial handicaps in these individuals. However, older adults may be reluctant to accept remote microphone amplifying systems because of cosmetic considerations.

Cognitive Factors

The extent to which age-related decline in cognitive abilities is associated with speech-understanding problems has been explored by a number of investigators using global cognitive measures of intelligence and memory span. The theoretical basis for these studies is related in part to two considerations: (1) generalized slowing across a variety of perceptual, cognitive, and motor domains with aging and (2) increased cognitive demands or an increase in the number of mental operations required for selected speech tasks potentially compromising performance of older adults (Gordon-Salant & Fitzgibbons, 1997). Jerger, Jerger, and Pirozzolo (1991) were among the first investigators to explore the relation between speech-recognition ability, age, hearing level, and cognitive abilities. As noted earlier in this chapter, 200 subjects participated in their study. For the most part, subjects presented with mild to moderate sloping sensorineural hearing loss. Speech measures included PB words, the SSI test, the SPIN test, and the DSI test. Several neuropsychologic measures were administered including the WAIS, the Wechsler Memory Scale (WMS), and the Boston Naming Test (BNT). Although their data suggested that degree of hearing loss was the most powerful predictor of speech-recognition performance, they did acknowledge that speed of mental processing as measured by the digit symbol subtest of the WAIS as well as age do account in part for performance on speech tests. Interestingly, the nature of the speech audiometric task determined the extent to which cognitive status or age influenced performance. Whereas hearing loss influenced performance on each of the speech tests, cognitive status and age affected performance on the SSI and DSI. It was of interest that knowledge of the subject's age significantly increased the variance in scores on the SSI test beyond that already accounted for by degree of hearing loss. In contrast, on the DSI, knowledge of speed of mental processing significantly increased the variance in scores beyond that already accounted for by degree of hearing loss. The latter finding is not surprising because the DSI test is a dichotic task that requires the respondent to process two speech targets presented simultaneously and to execute an appropriate response. Interestingly, peripheral-hearing loss accounted for less of the total variance in scores on the DSI than on any of the three other monotic speech-recognition tests (Jerger, Jerger, & Pirozzolo, 1991).

The data of Humes et al (1994) corroborated some of the findings of Jerger and his colleagues (1991). As described in an earlier section, a total of 50 subjects with essentially mild to moderate hearing loss and ages ranging from 63 to 83 years participated in this study. Scores on the CUNY NST, the CID W-22 word lists, and the R-SPIN test presented in quiet and noise were correlated with a variety of measures of cognitive function derived from the Wechsler Adult Intelligence Scale-Revised (WISC-R), the Wechsler Memory Scale Revised (WMS-R), and auditory processing ability. They found that the average hearing loss at 1000, 2000, or 4000 Hz, or the extent of audibility of the speech signal, correlated most strongly with speech-recognition scores, accounting for 70 to 75% of the variability in performance of speech-recognition tests. Cognitive function and auditory processing ability accounted for little of the individual variability in performance on speech tests used in this study.

Finally, van Rooij and Plomp (1992), and van Rooij, Plomp, and Orlebeke (1990) conducted a series of studies exploring the relation among auditive and cognitive factors in speech-understanding abilities of older adults. Their subjects underwent a large battery of tests designed to measure a number of different modalities. Auditory function including sensitivity, frequency selectivity, and temporal resolution was assessed. Cognitive tests that assessed memory, processing speech, and intellectual abilities were administered. Speech understanding in quiet and noise and under varying conditions of reverberation was assessed using phonemes, spondees, and sentence materials. They too found that the extent of high-frequency sensorineural hearing loss was the major factor accounting for individual differences in speech understanding among the elderly and that cognitive status accounted for only a very small portion of additional variability.

Gordon-Salant and Fitzgibbons (1997) explored the role of memory, speech rate, and availability of contextual cues on recognition performance of older as compared to younger adults. They found that older adults with and without hearing loss had more difficulty recalling the low-predictability (LP) sentences of the SPIN than did young listeners but that recall of individual words did not pose as much of a problem for older adults. Understanding of sentence material did not improve for older adults with slowing of the speech-rate. However, Gordon-Salant and Fitzgibbons (1997) did note that availability of contextual cues (e.g., high-predictability sentences on the SPIN) helped older adults with and without hearing loss to achieve excellent word-recognition scores even in the presence of competition.

SPECIAL CONSIDERATION

In general, with the possible exception of memory load, studies on the extent to which age-related cognitive impairments contribute to the speech-recognition difficulties of the elderly have revealed minimal correlations between cognitive changes and speech processing. Some investigators argue that the low correlations are an artifact of the neuropsychological tests used to measure cognitive function and the listening conditions tapped by the speech measures.

Speech-specific cognitive declines using tests of lexical discrimination and tests of language-specific cognitive capacity are presently being explored. The latter tests are designed to assess the use of semantic context as an aid to speech perception. Exploration of the role of semantic context in speech understanding has revealed that older adults derive the greatest benefit from contextual information in the more demanding listening conditions (Pichora-Fuller, Schneider, & Daneman, 1995; Gordon-Salant & Fitzgibbons, 1997). It appears that older listeners may in fact be able to compensate for age-related hearing loss by allowing their increased experience with language to enable them to take full advantage of semantic context (Wingfield, Poon, Lombardi, & Lowe, 1985). Wingfield (1996) reviewed a series of studies used to highlight the role of cognitive factors in auditory performance on selected speech tasks that varied in their linguistic complexity. Wingfield (1996) reported that increasing speech rate beyond the normal 140 to 180 words per minute (wpm) poses a disadvantage to older adults, with the disadvantage influenced by the content and structure of the speech materials. Specifically, he reported that the percent of words correctly identified by older and younger adults tends to be comparable for speech rates ranging from 275 to 425 wpm when normal sentence materials were used. However, older adults are at a significant disadvantage (percent of words correctly identified dramatically less than young adults) at progressively higher speech rates when random strings of words are used. This study highlights the role of linguistic structure as a compensatory agent for understanding speech that has been temporally degraded (i.e., time compression).

The data of Gordon-Salant, LaGuinn, and Sherlock (1992) demonstrate an important clinical implication of the role of linguistic factors, including context, in audiologic rehabilitation in hearing-aid selection. These investigators explored the efficacy of adaptive frequency response hearing aids (AFR) in improving speech perception in noise among a group of older hearing-impaired adults. They found that speech-recognition ability in the presence of noise is improved with AFR circuitry only when contextual cues were provided to aid in recognition. As most listening conditions encountered in daily life are high in contextual cues, and as older adults may be able to compensate for hearing loss by taking greater advantage of the context, use of contextual materials in diagnosis and evaluation should be explored and encouraged. Hence, once again availability and utilization of contextual cues are key to speech understanding.

Gender Differences on Tests of Word Recognition

In an effort to isolate the variables that might account for individual differences in word-recognition ability characterizing older adults, Wiley et al (1998) reported on data evolving from an epidemiologic study of hearing in older adults living in Beaver Dam, Wisconsin. The mean age of the 3753 participants was 65.8 years. Fifty-seven and a half percent of subjects were women and 98.9% were non-Hispanic white. For the most part, subjects presented with high-frequency sensorineural hearing loss, which overall tended to be mild to moderate in degree, with individuals over 80 years of age presenting with poorer hearing levels. Interestingly, a strong gender difference in word-recognition ability emerged in quiet and noise. In general, word-recognition ability using the NU-6 word lists presented in quiet was better for women than men across age groups. When subjects were stratified by gender and hearing-loss category, women tended to have better word-recognition ability than men of comparable age and hearing level. The latter trend emerged when word-recognition ability was assessed in the presence of a competing message (S/N = +8). After adjusting for age, Wiley and his colleagues (1998) found that word-recognition scores in the presence of a competing message were better for women than men overall, and within all hearing-loss categories. As would be expected, word-recognition ability was significantly poorer when assessed in noise than in quiet. Interestingly, results of the analysis of covariance revealed that pure-tone hearing sensitivity accounted for the

greatest proportion of the variance on word-recognition scores in quiet (26%) and competing noise (48%), whereas gender accounted for a small proportion of the variance in word-recognition scores in quiet (4%) and in the presence of competing noise (9%). It is of interest that age, when entered into the equation alone, accounted for a considerable amount of the variance in speech-understanding ability when assessed in the presence of competing noise.

As previously discussed, Dubno et al (1997) were also interested in isolating factors that might account for individual differences in word-recognition ability with age. When Dubno et al (1997) cast the pure-tone data as a function of gender, mean pure-tone thresholds for males were poorer than those for females, an expected finding. PTA accounted for more of the variance in speech-recognition scores for females (0.395 to 0.739) than for males (0.289 to 0.464). Interestingly, when word-recognition score and age were controlled for their mutual relation with PTA, the relation between word-recognition ability and age was reduced dramatically to a statistically insignificant level. Stated differently, in females the correlation between word-recognition ability and age is minimal when controlling for the effect of hearing level ($R^2 = 0.02$) (Dubno et al, 1997). The latter was not the case for males wherein nearly 12% of the variance in scores on word-recognition tests was accounted for by age, after controlling for PTA. Hence, PTA and age account for some of the variance in speech-recognition scores in males. In sum, audibility accounts for the largest proportion of the variance in speech-recognition scores for males and females, "but more for females than males" (Dubno et al, 1997, p. 451).

CONCLUDING REMARKS—SPEECH TESTS

Speech tests are essential to the evaluation of the elderly because they offer the clinician a means of assessing receptive communication function in a quasisystematic manner using materials and procedures that potentially will vary in complexity. They can be used to provide (1) objective quantifiable information about rehabilitative potential, (2) differential diagnostic information relating to site of lesion, and (3) data that can help to identify the etiology of the speech-understanding problems so typical of older adults.

PEARL

Performance on tests of speech understanding can help clinicians unravel the extent to which the difficulties experienced by older adults are attributable to changes in the auditory periphery, changes in the central auditory nervous system, or generalized slowing across the cognitive domain.

Evaluation of empirical and theoretical evidence suggests that peripheral-hearing status emerges as the primary variable accounting for individual variations in speech understanding. Other internal peripheral changes, such as deficits in auditory temporal processing as revealed using reverberant or time-compressed speech, also appear to play a role in explaining the decrements that tend to emerge on selected tests of speech understanding.

This becomes most apparent when controlling for the effects of peripheral hearing loss and test-retest differences on speech measures used to assess CAPD. Similarly, global cognitive function such as memory and overall intelligence does not appear to be a factor contributing to the speech processing problems of older adults. However, speech-specific cognitive declines (e.g., absence of linguistic redundancy) may in fact contribute to the speech-understanding difficulties that emerge when testing older adults (Wingfield, 1996). The role of gender in accounting for some of the individual differences in word-recognition ability that typifies older adults remains to be elucidated. Finally, recent studies have demonstrated that use of contextual information can reduce the difficulty older adults may have processing rapid speech.

OBJECTIVE TESTS: IMMITTANCE AND OTOACOUSTIC EMISSIONS TESTING

Immittance testing is an important part of the routine test battery and it is important for the clinician to be aware of any age effects on test results. While structural changes in the middle ear mechanism due to aging are minimal (e.g., thinning of the tympanic membrane, eardrum becomes less static, increased stiffening of the ossicular chain, atrophy of intra-aural muscles), it is reasonable to suspect that the aging process may impact on acoustic immittance test results. The acoustic immittance test battery, administered to evaluate the status of the middle ear system of older adults, generally includes static admittance, tympanometry, and

acoustic stapedial reflex tests. Table 5–5 summarizes the effects of age on interpretation of immittance test results.

To date, it remains unclear how structural changes in the middle ear affect diagnostic measurements of middle ear function (Holte, 1996). One of the first tests in the battery is static acoustic immittance testing. Static acoustic immittance (a term that encompasses both admittance and impedance) is a test of the immittance of the middle ear at a "rep-

TABLE 5–5 Summary of the Effect of Age on Performance on Immittance Tests

Test	Effect of age on performance
Static admittance values	1. No significant age effect, as static immittance values appear to be within the range considered to be normal for young adults.
Tympanometric pressure peak	1. Majority of ears have peaks between ± 100 daPa.
Middle ear resonant frequency	1. No age effects.
Acoustic reflex thresholds	1. No evidence of a systematic age effect using tonal activators for tonal activators below 2000 Hz. 2. Small age-effect apparent (i.e., elevated reflex levels) when broadband noise is the activator signal. 3. No evidence of an age effect on tests of acoustic-reflex adaptation.

resentative air pressure," be it atmospheric, static or the pressure corresponding to the peak of the tympanogram (Gelfand, 1997). In general, static immittance values, which yield information about the status of the middle ear system in its quiescent state, do not appear to undergo a clinically significant change as a function of the aging process (Holte, 1996). Rather, values change as individuals move through infancy, childhood, and adulthood. While the representative 90% normal range for peak static acoustic admittance in mmhos for children is 0.26 to 0.92, the values are slightly higher for adults, ranging from 0.37 to 1.66 (Gelfand, 1997). Of course, there is some variability depending on methodology. With regard to interpretation, static admittance is considered to be low if it falls below 0.37 mmhos and high if it falls above 1.66 mmhos.

There is a dearth of data on effect of age on the tympanometric pressure peak (TPP), or the value in daPa that corresponds to the ear canal pressure producing the maximum peak. Accordingly, TTP values used for adults (−100 daPa) can be comfortably used with older adults. Holte (1996) reported that median resonant frequency did not change significantly as a function of age, ranging between 800 and 1000 Hz depending on age and where the pressure peak was compensated (e.g., +250 or −300 daPa). Wiley, Cruickshanks, Nondahl, and Tweed (1999) reported that there were no significant age-related trends for middle ear resonant frequency. Their findings support the data of Holte (1996). Holte (1996) did note a statistically significant correlation between age and tympanometric width. However, the correlation was slight, rendering the finding clinically insignificant. Given the above findings, normative values used for adults can be applied to older adults during routine tympanometric testing.

PEARL

A robust age effect on acoustic admittance values, tympanometric peak pressure, middle ear resonance, and tympanometric width has not been documented.

Routine acoustic reflex testing (ART) includes establishing thresholds to tonal stimuli and determining whether a reflex contraction can be maintained during continuous stimulation (i.e, acoustic reflex decay). There is some disagreement among investigators as to the effect of age on acoustic reflex thresholds, depending for the most part on stimulus frequency, hearing level, and the nature of the stimulus. For normal-hearing older adults there appears to be little change in the ART for frequencies between 500 and 2000 Hz (Jepson, 1963; Osterhammel & Osterhammel, 1979; Thompson, Sills, Recke, & Bui, 1979). Jerger, Jerger, and Maudlin (1972) found that for subjects with sensorineural hearing loss, ARTs for high frequencies were slightly higher than those for normals, however this trend was apparent across age groups. In their comprehensive discussion of age and the acoustic reflex, Wilson and Margolis (1991) concluded that the changes in acoustic reflex thresholds to tonal activators ≤2000 Hz are too small to be considered statistically significant. Data on reflex thresholds at 4000 Hz are conflicting, most likely due to the difficulty associated with eliciting reflexes for higher frequency stimuli. For example, Wilson (1981) reported a notable increase in ART with age for an activator signal of 4000 Hz whereas Jerger, Jerger, and Maudlin (1972) reported a decrease in the ART at 4000 Hz for older adults. To further complicate the picture, a number of investigators have reported that the activator signal influences the reflex threshold, such that ARTs for broadband noise stimuli are elevated for normal-hearing older adults (Silman, 1979; Wilson & Margolis, 1991). As would be expected, ARTs are elicited at reduced sensation levels, but normal-hearing levels relative to the 90th percentile values generated by Silman and Gelfand (1981). In sum, for routine tests of the ART, age appears to have a negligible effect on test results. Hence, the values generated by Silman and Gelfand (1981) should be used in interpreting ARTs.

PEARL

ARTs for tonal stimuli (500 to 2000 Hz) are similar across age groups. Age-related increases in thresholds for broadband noise are of statistical and clinical significance and should be considered in drawing conclusions about the status of the auditory system in aged individuals (Wilson & Margolis, 1991).

While otoacoustic emissions (OAEs) may not add relevant information to the routine clinical evaluation of elderly individuals with hearing impairment, the effects of age on emissions should be understood by clinicians, primarily because they have excellent sensitivity to cochlear dysfunction. Evoked otoacoustic emissions are sounds that are produced in the inner ear in response to an evoking stimulus (Prieve & Falter, 1995). They travel through the middle ear and into the external auditory canal where they are detected and measured using an insert microphone. OAEs are generated only when the organ of Corti (O of C) is in near normal condition, and they can be detected only when the middle ear system is operating normally (Kemp, 1997). The sounds produced by the cochlea are small but potentially audible, occasionally amounting to as much as 30 dBSPL (Kemp, 1997). It has been hypothesized that evoked otoacoustic emissions are linked with outer hair cell function and hence may provide insight into the effects of exogenous and endogenous factors on peripheral auditory system function.

OAEs are measured using an instrument that consists of an acoustic ear canal probe assembly containing a loudspeaker to stimulate the ear, a microphone to record all the sounds in the ear canal, and a signal separating process that can discriminate between sounds emerging from the cochlea and other extraneous sound (Kemp, 1997). The probe, which physically seals the ear canal, contains a sensitive microphone and sound delivery transducers. A variety of stimuli can be used to evoke an OAE, including a click (wideband stimulus) and a tone (narrowband stimulus). When a click is used, data are collected from a substantial length of the cochlea, and afterward the response is broken down into separate frequencies. For tonal stimulation, a series of measurements must be made that covers the entire frequency range (Kemp, 1997). Two different classes of OAE instruments are available differing primarily in the manner in which response-signal extraction takes place. In other words, the two different types of OAE technology vary in terms of what the cochlea is doing while one is measuring and which parts of the whole OAE response are captured and which parts are rejected (Kemp, 1997). The two classes of instruments include distortion product otoacoustic emissions (DPOAE) and transient evoked otoacoustic emissions (TEOAE). According to Kemp (1997) TEOAEs are best at detecting threshold elevation below 3000 Hz while DPOAEs are best above 3 kHz. Additionally, TEOAEs provide a view of cochlear activity to soft stimulation, whereas DPOAEs can be obtained at moderate and higher levels of stimulation.

A number of conditions within the peripheral auditory mechanism must be met for OAE generation. These include (Kemp, 1997):

1. Open external auditory meatus
2. A mobile tympanum
3. A well-articulated ossicular chain
4. A mobile and low-loss attachment of the stapes to the oval window
5. A well-formed mobile basilar membrane supporting a normal traveling wave

6. Optimum electrochemical environment of the scala media
7. Optimum condition of the outer hair cells
8. Optimum configuration of the outer hair cells

Interestingly, auditory threshold depends on the sum total of each of the above factors plus (Kemp, 1997):

1. Optimum coupling of motion within the O of C, especially from the basilar membrane to outer and inner hair cells
2. Optimum condition and function of the inner hair cells
3. Optimum synaptic function at the inner hair cell
4. Optimum neural transmission from the inner ear
5. Optimum mapping and processing of the neural signals reaching the cochlear nucleus
6. Optimum function of the entire auditory pathway

As hearing threshold can be computed by adding the above factors, and while OAEs depend on the sum total of the first group of factors, OAE level may not relate directly to audiometric threshold (Kemp, 1997). Hence, while OAEs have excellent sensitivity to cochlear dysfunction at the outer hair cell level, they are only partially correlated with thresholds.

There are two types of OAEs, namely spontaneous (SOAEs) and evoked (EOAEs). SOAEs occur in the absence of any intentional stimulation of the ear. They are low-intensity tonal signals that are typically inaudible to the persons from whose ears they are detected. SOAEs tend to present at stable amplitudes and frequencies (Bright, 1997). The presence of SOAEs suggests that cochlear hearing sensitivity is normal near the frequency of an SOAE (Glattke & Robinette, 1997). It has been suggested that the SOAE may derive from minor irregularities within the cochlea, such as aberrations in outer hair cell arrangement that are typically not significant enough to affect threshold (Bright, 1997). SOAEs are vulnerable to cochlear insults that affect the outer hair cells (e.g., noise, ototoxic medications) and are rarely recorded in the presence of hearing loss greater than or equal to 25 dBHL.

SOAEs are present in approximately 35 to 40% of adult ears. SOAEs can be present in one or both ears, their presence in one ear increases the likelihood that they will be found in the opposite ear (Bilger, Matthies, Hammel, & Demorest, 1990). Women are more likely than men to exhibit SOAEs and interestingly they are more often observed in right ears (Bright, 1997). The majority of adult SOAEs fall within the frequency region of 1000 to 2000 Hz, whereas for infants and newborns they fall in the frequency range between 3000 and 4000 Hz. With regard to amplitude, the majority of SOAEs are measured in adults at mean levels between −3 and 0 dBSPL. In contrast, for infants the mean amplitude is near 10 dBSPL (Bright, 1997).

It appears that the prevalence of SOAEs decreases for subjects over 60 years of age, even when hearing thresholds are within normal limits (Bright, 1997). In addition, the total number of SOAEs observed decreases in aged ears, although other SOAE features (e.g., frequency and amplitude characteristics) remain unchanged and are not affected by age (Bonfils, 1989; Lonsbury-Martin, Cutler, & Martin, 1991). The variability in their appearance and their presence at discrete and unpredictable frequencies, coupled with the fact that SOAEs tend to be present in some but not all persons with normal hearing, limit their validity in the diagnosis of peripheral hearing loss.

SPECIAL CONSIDERATION

SOAEs are not the emission of choice for assessing cochlear functioning (Bright, 1997). However, it is safe to conclude that the presence of an SOAE suggests that hearing is within normal limits within the frequency region of the cochlea tuned to the SOAE frequency (Bright, 1997).

There are three types of EOAEs: (1) TEOAE, (2) stimulus-frequency otoacoustic emissions (SFOAE), and (3) DPOAE. These emissions differ according to when the tonal stimulus is applied. TEOAEs appear after the delivery of a brief stimulus to the ear; SFOAEs appear during the presentation of a tonal stimulus at the frequency of the stimulus; and DPOAEs are produced during stimulation of the ear by tonal stimuli. The discussion below will be limited to TEOAEs and DPOAEs.

TEOAEs can typically be recorded in nearly all persons with normal hearing. TEOAEs have some unique characteristics (Glattke & Robinette, 1997). Responses obtained from stimuli near threshold may reflect energy levels that approach the energy in the applied stimulus. As stimulus intensity increases, response amplitude increases at a slower rate, growing by about 20 to 30 dB for a stimulus increment of 60 to 70 dB. Interestingly, the spectrum of the TEOAE, recorded in response to clicks, contains information that can help determine the spread of the insult along the cochlea, from base to apex. Thus, if the TEOAE spectrum is broadband, it presumably reflects activity from a considerable length of the cochlea whereas if the spectrum is limited to a narrow frequency range, the TEOAE may reflect activity from a narrow cochlear region (Glattke & Robinette, 1997). The presence of TEOAE is integrally related to hearing status such that when a mild hearing loss of 30 to 40 dBHL is present, the TEOAE cannot be measured (Bertoli & Probst, 1997). The latter finding has prompted investigation into the effect of age on the prevalence and characteristics of TEOAE. Bertoli and Probst (1997) gathered click-evoked and otoacoustic emissions (CEOAEs) on a sample of 201 older adults with sensorineural hearing loss. CEOAEs were not detectable in ears with a PTA greater than 30 dBHL and only 60% of ears with PTAs better than 30 dBHL had CEOAEs. As would be expected the prevalence of CEOAEs increased with improved hearing level, rising to 77% for older adults with PTAs better than 15 dBHL. When comparing subjects with and without CEOAEs, age was not a distinguishing variable, but hearing level was. Similarly, amplitude or response level of the OAE did not appear to correlate with age. Bertoli and Probst (1997) concluded that TEOAEs do not substantially contribute to the audiometric test battery for the typical presbycusic who presents with hearing levels in excess of 30 dBHL.

Prieve and Falter (1995) compared the status of CEOAEs in a sample of older adults with normal hearing to that of a group of younger adults. They failed to find a significant difference in CEOAE levels between the two groups, corroborating the results of Robinette (1992) who also sampled adults with normal hearing. While age did not appear to account for a significant proportion of the variance in CEOAE level or threshold, the presence of SFOAEs did. Harris and Probst (1997) also concluded from their literature review that when controlling for the influence of hearing level, age does not have a strong influence on the morphology of the TEOAE. In light of the findings described above, age-adjusted norms may not be necessary for clinical applications. In conclusion, results to date suggest that TEOAEs do not help the audiologist gain specific information about factors in the cochlea that may underlie sensorineural loss (Harris & Probst, 1997). Hence, I do not believe this should be a routine part of the test battery for older adults.

DPOAEs are an intermodulation distortion response produced by the ear in response to primary tones (i.e., two simultaneous pure-tone stimuli) (Lonsbury-Martin, Martin, & Whitehead, 1997). The response is considered distorted because it originates from the cochlea as a tonal signal that was not present in the original pure-tone signal (Lonsbury-Martin, Martin, & Whitehead, 1997). DPOAEs appear to reflect the underlying nonlinear response properties of human cochlea that are associated with the outer hair cell system (Gorga, Neely, Ohlrich, Hoover, Redner, & Peters, 1997). To explain, when outer hair cell damage results from an insult to the cochlea, normal nonlinear processing ability is lost.

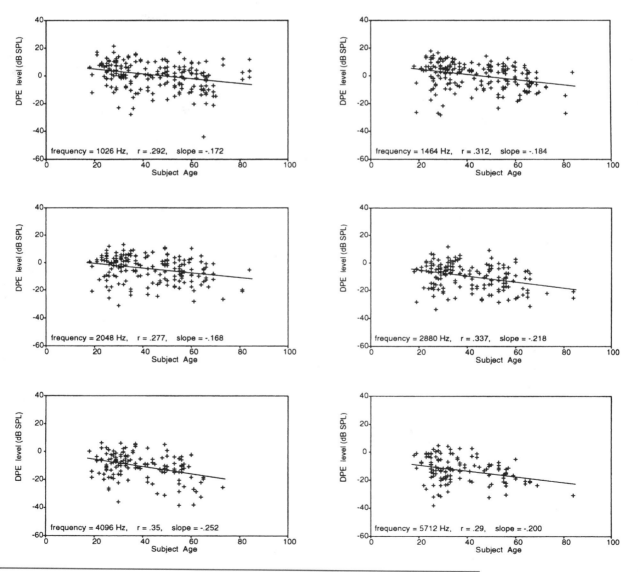

Figure 5–13 Amplitude of DPOAEs by subject age for six different frequencies. (From Glattke and Robinette, 1997, p. 192.)

As otoacoustic emissions are a byproduct of nonlinear processes, otoacoustic emissions are also absent or reduced (Gorga et al, 1997). Outer hair cells, which act over the range of thresholds up to 60 dB, are the source of DPOAE (Gorga et al, 1997). DPOAEs accurately identify hearing status for frequences ranging from 1500 to 6000 Hz, falling off in accuracy for frequencies above and below this range (Gorga et al, 1997). According to Gorga et al (1997) DPOAEs are an inversely graded response of hearing loss over the 50 to 60 dB range especially in the higher frequencies. For hearing levels above 60 dB, ears did not produce measurable emissions minimizing their contribution to the prediction of severe to profound hearing loss (Gorga et al, 1997). In the large-scale study conducted by Gorga et al (1997), these authors did not consider age to be a significant variable when gathering normative data on DPOAE. Their philosophy is in keeping with the conclusions of Karzon, Garcia, Peterein, and Gates (1995) who concluded that when compensating for differences in audiometric threshold, there are no significant changes in DPOAEs that can be attributed to age. Stover and Norton (1993) also examined the effects of age on DPOAE amplitude and concluded that age did not effect the OAE in their sample of normal-hearing individuals.

In contrast, Lonsbury-Martin, Martin, and Whitehead (1997) clearly demonstrated an age effect on the amplitude of the DPOAE. In their sample, older adults clearly had poorer hearing thresholds than did the younger adults. As is evident from Figure 5–13, they found that DPOAE amplitudes decreased with increasing age at most frequencies. These differences were statistically significant. Arnold, Lonsbury-Martin, and Martin (1996) later replicated these findings. Kimberley, Brown, and Allen (1997) also provided evidence of a significant, albeit weak relation between DPOAE level in dBSPL and age. As is evident from Figure 5–14, for individuals with normal hearing, response amplitude appears to decrease with increasing age with the relation varying only slightly with increasing frequency. As researchers do not yet agree on the influence of age on DPOAEs, I would support Kimberley, Brown, and Allen (1997, p. 190) who suggested the use of "age-specific normative DPOAE amplitude data to classify DPOAEs." Given the sensitivity of DPOAEs to

changes in the cochlea due to ingestion of ototoxic drugs, I believe they hold promise as a way to monitor the hearing sensitivity of older adults who are taking ototoxic medications and perhaps cannot be tested behaviorally. Of course, age-adjusted norms should be used.

A TEST BATTERY APPROACH FOR USE WITH THE ELDERLY

Most clinicians and researchers would agree that there is considerable variability among older adults in the pure-tone threshold data, in performance on word-recognition tests, in the reaction to a given hearing impairment, and in their motivation for seeking audiologic assistance at this point in their life. Each area must be explored with the client on a case-by-case basis and the clinician must select from an array of behavioral tests the protocols that best meet the needs of the client. The older adult should be assessed in a comprehensive fashion, with the diagnostic evaluation considered an integral part of the treatment plan. In this era of managed care, the audiologist must take responsibility for the determination and delivery of high-quality care in the most cost-effective way.

Assessment of the older adult should begin with a comprehensive functionally oriented case history. The case history should be administered in a systematic fashion, beginning with exploration of the patient's rationale for purchasing hearing health care services. Further, the clinician should view the case history as an opportunity to learn about the client's attitudes toward hearing loss and hearing aids, and as a chance to gain insight into the communication-specific difficulties attributable to hearing loss. Further, given the link between hearing loss, hearing handicap, and physical functional status, the perceived impact of the hearing loss on physical functional status should be explored.

Every effort should be made to uncover the etiology of hearing loss with a thorough exploration of the auditory and nonauditory symptoms attending the hearing loss. The

SPECIAL CONSIDERATION

A thorough drug history should be taken and a systems analysis should be undertaken to determine whether age-related changes in an organ system or a disease is responsible for the reported hearing impairment.

audiologist should make sure to record the names of all medications, including dosing, should an ototoxic hearing loss be suspected. If the patient's history is incomplete, input from an alternative source (e.g., formal or informal caregiver) should be sought to clarify any confusion that may arise. It is always helpful to have a family member present during the case history.

Audiologists must have a great deal of patience during their interactions with older hearing-impaired patients. They should expect to spend more time interviewing and evaluating the hearing-impaired older adult because a number of

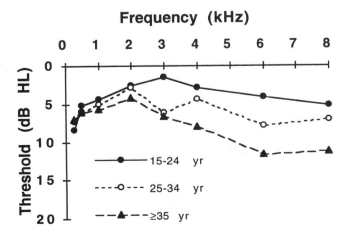

Frequency (kHz)

15–24 yr
25–34 yr
≥35 yr

Figure 5–14 DPOAE amplitude as a function of age. (From Glattke and Robinette, 1997, p. 101.)

conditions can interfere with the interview process including cognitive dysfunction, sensory deficits, etc. A hand-held amplifier, such as a PockeTalker, should be available during the history to assist in taking a valid interview, and in easing the flow of the interview. Audiologists should be sensitive to the nonaudiologic issues raised by their elderly patients. For example, on-going medical, social, or psychologic problems may be more important than a hearing loss.

The medical history should include a psychologic as well as a social history because this information can help guide testing and decisions regarding treatment. Further, every attempt should be made to uncover the perceived communicative and psyschosocial effects of a given hearing impairment on daily function. Self-assessment scales, which quantify the perceived effects of hearing loss on daily life, have emerged as instruments that reliably uncover the functional impact of unremediated and remediated hearing loss. A variety of scales that yield estimates of the degree to which hearing loss is perceived to impact on communication and psychosocial function have evolved for use with older hearing-impaired adults. For the most part scores on these handicap/disability questionnaires bear an imperfect relation to hearing impairment such that each domain must be explored independently. In fact, the data of Jerger and Chmiel (1997) confirmed that perceived auditory handicap emerges as a factor independent of pure-tone and speech data.

In selecting a self-assessment scale, the audiologist must consider its reliability and content validity. Further, the instrument selected by the clinician should fit the purposes and setting for which the instrument was intended. The bulk of audiologists continue to dismiss the contribution of information contained in responses to handicap scales. However, their value in screening, in assessing the functional impact of hearing loss, as a prognostic indicator, in monitoring patient status, and as an outcome measure is undeniable.

> ## PEARL
>
> **The most widely used self-assessment scale is the HHIE, owing in part to its brevity; ease of administration; and scoring, reliability, and validity.**

Since tinnitus is prevalent among older adults, audiologists are encouraged to explore the significance of tinnitus for the individual. Recently, several questionnaires have become available that quantify the individual's perception of the characteristics and physical, emotional, and social response to tinnitus (Newman, Sandridge, & Jacobson, 1998). The Tinnitus Handicap Inventory (THI) which is similar to the HHIE in format and scoring, contains 25 items that explore the functional, emotional, and catastrophic reactions to tinnitus. The THI has high internal-consistency reliability and high test-retest reliability. Individuals can be classified according to the severity of their tinnitus using the THI. Scores ranging from 0 to 16 are indicative of no tinnitus, scores ranging from 18 to 36 suggest mild tinnitus handicap, scores ranging from 38 to 56 suggest moderate tinnitus handicap, and scores 58 and above suggest severe tinnitus handicap. The THI should be administered to clients reporting tinnitus so that audiologists can make the necessary re-

ferral for otological evaluation and/or continued medical management.

Once the history has been completed, the audiologist should discuss the evaluation plan with the patient and move ahead quickly. If cerumen is present, it is within the

> ## PEARL
>
> **It is a good idea to begin the audiological examination with otoscopy to rule out the presence of collapsed canals or impacted cerumen as a source of error in the testing.**

audiologist's scope of practice to undertake cerumen management. If this course is chosen, the necessary precautions listed in Chapter 4 should be taken, including complete documentation of the procedure. If it appears that the external auditory canal walls will collapse under pressure from standard supra-aural earphone cushions, which is often the case in the elderly, especially those residing in nursing facilities, insert earphones should be used to reduce the threat to the validity of air-conduction thresholds posed by collapsed canals.

Pure-tone air and bone-conduction thresholds are at the heart of the audiologic test battery, providing information about hearing status and need for medical and/or rehabilitative intervention. Routine test procedures should be used when the client's mental, cognitive, and physical health status allow. This author recommends routine testing of the interoctave frequencies through 8000 Hz to gain a comprehensive picture of the extent of high-frequency hearing loss and potential impact on speech understanding. It is a good practice to routinely ask about the presence of tinnitus in either ear, given its high prevalence in older adults. Pulsed tones can help minimize the confounding effects of tinnitus on threshold levels. Instructions must be audible, straightforward, and redundant, using examples of sounds they will hear to minimize any confusion. It is a good idea to have one trial run before beginning the testing to insure that the patient understands the response task. Further, the audiologist should emphasize that the patient should respond to the softest tone heard because the goal is to find the patient's best hearing levels. The latter should be reiterated for nursing home residents because clinical experience suggests that often they tend to respond when tones are most comfortable rather than minimally audible. Table 5–6 contains a list of modifications that may be necessary with selected clients. The author has found some of the adjustments invaluable with confused patients and the frail elderly.

> ## PEARL
>
> **When testing nursing home residents, it is often preferable to begin the actual test session with speech testing rather than pure-tone threshold seeking as speech materials have more face validity and enable the respondent to attend to the task more readily.**

Finally, immittance testing should be administered whenever an air/bone gap is present suggesting middle ear involvement. Also, when time or diminished cognitive status precludes masking to obtain valid bone-conduction thresholds, immittance testing is recommended.

Speech testing should include assessment of spondee thresholds or speech awareness thresholds, depending on the patient's cognitive status and word-recognition ability. The purpose of the speech test should dictate the procedure, that is whether you are attempting to gain diagnostic or rehabilitative information. A client-centered speech-understanding profile will help the clinician decide upon the most meaningful intervention strategy for a particular hearing-impaired older adult. It is critical when working with the elderly that the total person be considered and that face valid speech measures be employed to insure that the source(s) of their communication problems can be isolated and remedied. Keep in mind that age-appropriate norms are essential for reaching diagnostic and therapeutic conclusions. Further, when deciding upon a presentation level for word-recognition tests, make every attempt

to compensate for a high-frequency hearing loss to insure audibility of the high-frequency speech spectrum (Gates, Cooper, Kannel, & Miller, 1990). Given the large individual variability in speech-understanding ability among older adults and the importance of quantifying speech-perception abilities, clinicians should thoroughly explore this domain using a variety of speech measures that tap peripheral, central, and cognitive function. Further, speech materials that more accurately reflect everyday communication will provide the clinician with better insight into the problems confronting their clients. As Divenyi and Haupt (1997b) appropriately suggest, speech understanding in less than optimal conditions (e.g., in a babble, in reverberant conditions) should be employed to uncover the problems that may interact with, or be independent from, pure audibility problems. Table 5–7 summarizes the variables the clinician should consider when measuring speech-understanding ability. If, for example, under ideal conditions, the audiologist is interested in using speech testing to identify individuals with the potential for benefiting from hearing aids, the ideal protocol might include a routine test, such as recognition of monosyllabic word lists presented in quiet and noise and at normal and suprathreshold levels; a test of central auditory function (e.g., SSI); a

TABLE 5–6   Modifications to the Standard Test Battery

Behavior	Test modification
Slowed response time	Slow down rate of tonal presentation allowing the patient's pace to dictate the interstimulus interval.
Memory decline	Repeat and simplify instructions.
	Use gestures to supplement voice when instructing.
	Allow an opportunity for practice.
	Provide frequent conditioning/reconditioning trials.
	Provide verbal reinforcement.
Movement deficits	Evaluate different strategies for responding before initiating testing.
	Select response strategy that is the most natural and reflexive.
	Do not change response behavior too often.
Failing attention	Take a break during the session if fatigue begins to set in.
	Sessions should be short, no longer than 45 to 60 minutes.

TABLE 5–7   Factors to Consider When Evaluating Speech-Understanding Abilities of Older Adults

Peripheral status

a. Magnitude of high-frequency hearing loss
b. Temporal acuity—time compression or reverberation task
c. Audibility of signal—suprathreshold, normal conversational level

Cognitive status

a. Performance on a screening test of cognitive status—MMSE
b. Test indicative of speed of mental processing—subtests of WAIS

Central auditory status

a. Performance on a speech in noise test

Environmental factors*

a. Distance between communicators
b. Quiet, noise (e.g., multitalker babble, competing noise)
c. Reverberation
d. Optical conditions (e.g., room illumination)
e. Availability of visible cues

Self-perception of hearing handicap

a. Reliable and valid measure of psychosocial and communicative handicap that bears a minimal relationship to pure-tone data (e.g., HHIE)

Source: Erber, Lamb, and Lind, 1996.

test of cognitive status such as the MMSE; and a self-report test of the extent of perceived psychosocial handicap.

PEARL

If the audiologist is attempting to understand why previously successful hearing aid users are presently dissatisfied with their hearing aid(s), the clinician may wish to assess peripheral and central auditory processing ability and compare it to previous word-recognition scores. Evidence of a disparity between scores on tests of peripheral versus central auditory status or a decline in scores relative to the baseline may implicate a central component.

If an individual is complaining of difficulty understanding speech in particular listening situations, the audiologist should selectively explore factors that may impact on successful communication including use of communication strategies; the acoustic or optical environments in which the individual functions; and the communication partners with which he or she interacts (Erber, Lamb, & Lind, 1996). The data of Jerger and Chmiel (1997) suggesting that central processing of speech is an independent factor underlying auditory processing confirms the importance of assessing central auditory processing ability of older adults being evaluated for diagnostic or rehabilitative reasons.

Following the preliminary test battery the patient should be counseled with a family member present, when possible, regarding the data that were collected during the test session. The test results should be presented in a clear, concise manner, such that the outcome on each of the tests is understood. Assuming further diagnostic testing is not indicated, I find that explaining the audiometric test results relative to the critical frequencies necessary to receive selected speech sounds can facilitate understanding of the test and test results. Thus, using the audiogram, the audiologist should first describe the normal speech spectrum. For example, Figure 5–15 can be used to demonstrate the low-frequency concentration of the vowels and the high-frequency concentration of the consonants, as well as the fact that consonants are weaker in intensity than vowels making them more susceptible to the effects of a high-frequency hearing loss. Next, the audible portion of the speech spectrum (that part which occurs above the patient's threshold) should be clarified as well as the inaudible portion (that part of the speech signal that occurs below the patient's threshold). Figure 5–16 shows the impact of a high-frequency hearing loss on the reception of selected speech sounds, most notably the sibilants, rendering speech difficult to understand especially in the presence of noise. Finally, Figure 5–17 contains aided pure-tone thresholds demonstrating the impact of a hearing aid on speech-reception. It should be pointed out that, theoretically, the goal of a hearing aid is to make speech signals audible to the hearing-impaired individual and in Figure 5–17 it is evident that the previously inaudible high-

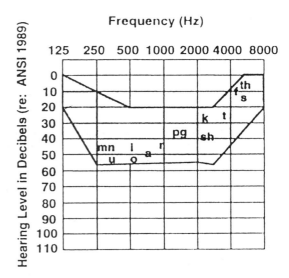

Figure 5–15 Low-frequency concentration of vowels and high-frequency consonants. (From Bess and Humes, 1995.)

frequency consonants have been rendered audible. The concept of the articulation index (AI) can also be invoked to demonstrate the improved audibility of the speech spectrum that results when enough of the speech spectrum is presented above the individual's threshold via amplification. It is often clarifying when a hearing-impaired patient can see that prior to hearing aid use, for example, only 58% of the speech signal was audible whereas following hearing aid use 92% of the speech spectrum, or 34% more of the speech signal, comes in above threshold.

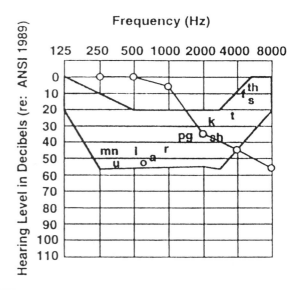

Figure 5–16 Impact of high-frequency hearing loss on reception of selected speech sounds. (From Bess and Humes, 1995.)

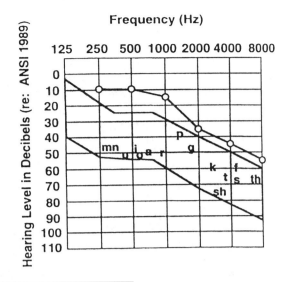

Figure 5–17 Aided pure-tone thresholds relative to hearing level of selected speech sounds. (From Bess and Humes, 1995.)

After explaining the audiometric data, it is important to discuss with the patient and family member their view of the impact of hearing loss on communication in particular and in terms of daily function in general. At this point, it is helpful to review responses to the self-assessment scale, which was completed at the beginning of the test session. If, in fact, it is clear that the patient perceives the hearing impairment to be disabling and/or handicapping, once again it is good to explain the value of hearing aids. In this context, one should explain that in addition to attempting to make speech audible, the goal of hearing aids is to reduce the self-perceived handicapping effects of hearing loss. Thus, if a patient with a moderate sensorineural hearing loss perceives the hearing impairment to be severely handicapping (e.g., score on self-assessment scale of 60%), it is hoped that the hearing aid will reduce the handicap to 30 to 40%, in which case the intervention would be viewed as a success. Conversely, if there is no change in handicap the electroacoustic response of the hearing aid has to be modified or a new hearing aid recommended. Clinical experience suggests that if the patient and/or family member are given well-defined targets, it helps them decide on the next course of action. It goes without saying that the examiner and the patient should decide together on the course of action after the initial examination. The clinician must provide the patient with enough information to make an informed decision. If the patient has an interest in pursuing a hearing aid, he or she should have an opportunity to see the different styles and the advantages and disadvantages of each discussed. On occasion, the opportunity to witness the value of amplified speech by listening through a programmable hearing aid can be instructive. Patients wishing to pursue amplification should be encouraged to return for a complete hearing-aid evaluation and, if necessary, to obtain medical clearance prior to the return visit.

In conclusion, the audiologic evaluation must be comprehensive and the outcomes specified so that patients can make an informed decision about the management of hearing loss, assuming further testing or medical intervention is not indicated. The dimensions of counseling that should be specified and documented should include:

1. Diagnostic results, impressions, and/or recommended diagnostic studies
2. Prognosis
3. Risks and benefits of treatment/management
4. Instructions for treatment/management
5. Importance of compliance with chosen treatment options
6. Patient and family education and responsibilities

Hopefully a comprehensive assessment and counseling will increase the ranks of older adults with hearing loss who pursue hearing aids. Currently only 14 to 15% of older adults with hearing levels exceeding 25 dBHL use hearing aids. (Popelka, Cruickshanks, Wiley, Tweed, Klein, & Klein, 1998). As part of counseling, the audiologist should emphasize that hearing aids can improve the quality of one's retirement years, which are considered by some to be the golden years.

REFERENCES

ABRAMS, W., BEERS, M., & BERKOW, R. (1995). *The Merck Manual of Geriatrics*, 2d ed. Whitehouse Station, NJ: Merck & Co., Inc.

ADAMS, P., & BENSON, V. (1992). Current estimates from the National Health Interview Survey 1991. National Center for Health Statistics. *Vital Health Statistics*, 10: 1–232.

AMERICAN SPEECH-LANGUAGE-HEARING ASSOCIATION. (1996). Central auditory processing: Current status of research and implications for clinical practice. *American Journal of Audiology*, 5: 41–54.

ARNESEN, A. (1982). Presbycusis—a loss of neurons in the human cochlear nuclei. *Journal of Laryngology and Otology*, 96: 503–511.

ARNOLD, D., LONSBURY-MARTIN, B., & MARTIN, G. (1996). Influence of ultra-high-frequency hearing on distortion-product otoacoustic emission levels in humans. Abstracts of the nineteenth midwinter meeting: *Association for Research in Otolaryngology*, 19: 25.

BERTOLI, S., & PROBST, R. (1997). The role of transient-evoked otoacoustic emission testing in the evaluation of elderly persons. *Ear and Hearing*, 18: 286–293.

BESS, F., & HUMES, L. (1995). *Audiology: The Fundamentals,* 2d ed. Baltimore: Williams & Wilkins.

BESS, F., & STROUSE, A. (1996). Presbycusis. In: J. Northern. (Ed.), *Hearing Disorders*, 3d ed. Boston: Allyn & Bacon.

BILGER, R., MATTHIES, M., HAMMEL, D., & DEMOREST, M. (1990). Genetic implications of gender differences in the prevalence of spontaneous otoacoustic emissions. *Journal of Speech and Hearing Research*, 33: 418–432.

BONFILS, P. (1989). Spontaneous otoacoustic emissions: Clinical interest. *Laryngoscope*, 99: 752–756.

BRANT, L., & FOZARD, J. (1990). Age changes in pure-tone hearing thresholds in a longitudinal study of normal human aging. *Journal of the Acoustical Society of America*, 88: 813–820.

BRANT, L., GORDON-SALANT, S., PEARON, J., KLEIN, L., MORRELL, C., METTER, E., & FOZARD, J. (1996). Risk factors related to age-associated hearing loss in the speech frequencies. *Journal of the American Academy of Audiology*, 7: 152–160.

BRIGHT, K. (1997). Spontaneous otoacoustic emissions. In: M. Robinette and T. Glattke (Eds.), *Otoacoustic emissions: Clinical applications.* New York: Thieme Medical Publishers.

CARHART, R. (1965). Problems in the measurement of speech discrimination. *Archives of Otolaryngology*, 82: 253–260.

CHAFEE, C. (1967). Rehabilitation needs of nursing home patients: A report of a survey. *Rehabilitation Literature*, 18: 37–38.

COKELY, C., & HUMES, L. (1992). Reliability of two measures of speech recognition in elderly people. *Journal of Speech and Hearing Research*. 35: 654–660.

COMMITTEE ON HEARING, BIOACOUSTICS, AND BIOMECHANICS. (1988). CHABA Working group on speech understanding and aging. *Journal of the Acoustical Society of America*, 83: 859–895.

COOPER, J. (1994). Health and Nutrition Examination Survey of 1971–75. Part I: Ear and race effects in hearing. *Journal of the American Academy of Audiology*, 5: 30–36.

COOPER, J., & GATES, G. (1991). Hearing in the elderly: The Framingham Cohort 1983–1985. Part II: Prevalence of central auditory processing disorders. *Ear and Hearing*, 12: 304–311.

CRANDELL, C. (1991). Individual differences in speech recognition ability: Implications for hearing aid selection. *Ear and Hearing*, 12: 100S–108S.

CRANDELL, C., HENOCH, M., & DUNKERSON, K. (1991). A review of speech perception and aging: Some implications for aural rehabilitation. *Journal of the Academy of Rehabilitative Audiology*, 24: 121–133.

CRUICKSHANKS, K., WILEY, T., TWEED, T., KLEIN, B., MARES-PERLMAN, J., & NONDAHL, D. (1998). Prevalence of hearing loss in older adults in Beaver Dam, Wisconsin. The Epidemiology of Hearing Loss Study. *American Journal of Epidemiology*, 148: 879–886.

DIVENYI, P., & HAUPT, K. (1997a). Audiological correlates of speech understanding deficits in elderly listeners with mild-to-moderate hearing loss. II. Correlation analysis. *Ear and Hearing*, 18: 100–113.

DIVENYI, P., & HAUPT, K. (1997b). Audiological correlates of speech understanding deficits in elderly listeners with mild to moderate hearing loss. III. Factor representation. *Ear and Hearing*, 18: 189–201.

DODDS, E., & HARFORD, E. (1982). A community hearing conservation program for senior citizens. *Ear and Hearing*, 3: 160–166.

DUBNO, J., & DIRKS, D. (1983). Suggestions for optimizing reliability with the synthetic sentence identification test. *Journal of Speech and Hearing Disorders*, 48: 98–103.

DUBNO, J., DIRKS, D., & MORGAN, D. (1984). Effects of age and mild hearing loss on speech recognition in noise. *Journal of the Acoustical Society of America*, 76: 87–96.

DUBNO, J., LEE, F., MATTHEWS, L., & MILLS, J. (1997). Age-related and gender-related changes in monaural speech recognition. *Journal of Speech and Hearing Research*, 40: 444–452.

DUBNO, J., & SCHAEFER, A. (1992). Comparison of frequency selectivity and consonant recognition among hearing-impaired and masked normal-hearing listeners. *Journal of the Acoustical Society of America*, 91: 2110–2121.

ERBER, N., LAMB, N., & LIND, C. (1996). Factors that affect the use of hearing aids by older people: A new perspective. *American Journal of Audiology*, 5: 11–19.

FITZGIBBONS, P., & GORDON-SALANT, S. (1996). Auditory temporal processing in elderly listeners. *Journal of the American Academy of Audiology*, 7: 183–189.

FRISINA, D., & FRISINA, R. (1997). Speech recognition in noise and presbycusis: Relations to possible neural mechanisms. *Hearing Research*, 106: 95–104.

GAETH, J. (1948). A study of phonemic regression in relation to hearing loss. Ph.D. diss., Northwestern University.

GARSTECKI, D., & ERLER, S. (1995). Older women and hearing. *American Journal of Audiology*, 4: 41–46.

GATES, G., COBB, J., D'AGOSTINO, R., & WOLF, P. (1993). The relation of hearing in the elderly to the presence of cardiovascular disease and cardiovascular risk factors. *Archives of Otolaryngology, Head and Neck Surgery*, 119: 156–161.

GATES, G., COBB, J., LINN, R., REES, T., WOLF, P., & D'AGOSTINO, R. (1996). Central auditory dysfunction, cognitive dysfunction and dementia in older people. *Archives of Otolaryngology Head and Neck Surgery*, 122: 161–167.

GATES, G., & COOPER, J. (1991). Incidence of hearing decline in the elderly. *Acta Otolaryngologica* (Stockholm), 111: 240–248.

GATES, G., COOPER, J., KANNEL, W., & MILLER, N. (1990). Hearing in the elderly: The Framingham Cohort, 1983–1985. Part I: Basic audiometric test results. *Ear and Hearing*, 4: 247–256.

GELFAND, S. (1997). *Essentials of Audiology.* New York: Thieme Medical Publishers.

GELFAND, S., PIPER, N., & SILMAN, S. (1986). Consonant recognition in quiet and in noise with aging among normal hearing listeners. *Journal of the Acoustical Society of America*, 80: 1589–1598.

GENNIS, V., GARRY, P., HAALAND, K., YEO, R., & GOODWIN, J. (1991). Hearing and cognition in the elderly. *Archives of Internal Medicine*, 151: 2259–2264.

GLATTKE, T., & ROBINETTE, M. (1997). Transient evoked otoacoustic emissions. In: M. Robinette & T. Glattke (Eds.),

Otoacoustic Emissions—Clinical Applications. New York: Thieme Medical Publishers.

GORDON-SALANT, S. (1987a). Age-related differences in speech recognition as a function of test format and paradigm. *Ear and Hearing,* 8: 277–282.

GORDON-SALANT, S. (1987b). Consonant recognition and confusion patterns among elderly hearing-impaired subjects. *Ear and Hearing,* 8: 270–276.

GORDON-SALANT, S., & FITZGIBBONS, P. (1993). Temporal factors and speech recognition performance in young and elderly listeners. *Journal of Speech and Hearing Research,* 36: 1276–1285.

GORDON-SALANT, S., & FITZGIBBONS, P. (1995a). Comparing recognition of distorted speech using an equivalent signal-to-noise ratio index. *Journal of Speech and Hearing Research,* 38: 706–713.

GORDON-SALANT, S., & FITZGIBBONS, P. (1995b). Recognition of multiply degraded speech by young and elderly listeners. *Journal of Speech and Hearing Research,* 38: 1150–1156.

GORDON-SALANT, S., & FITZGIBBONS, P. (1997). Selected cognitive factors and speech recognition performance among young and elderly listeners. *Journal of Speech and Hearing Research,* 40: 423–431.

GORDON-SALANT, S., LAGUINN, P., & SHERLOCK, M. (1992). Performance with an adaptive frequency response hearing aid in a sample of elderly hearing-impaired listeners. *Ear and Hearing,* 13: 255–262.

GORDON-SALANT, S., LANTZ, J., & FITZGIBBONS, P. (1994). Age effects on measures of hearing disability. *Ear and Hearing,* 15: 262–265.

GORGA, M., NEELY, S., OHLRICH, B., HOOVER, B., REDNER, J., & PETERS, J. (1997). From laboratory to clinic: A large-scale study of distortion product otoacoustic emissions in ears with normal hearing and ears with hearing loss. *Ear and Hearing,* 18: 440–455.

GRIMES, A., GRADY, C., FOSTER, N., SUNDERLAND, T., & PATRONAS, N. (1985). Central auditory function in Alzheimer's disease. *Neurology,* 35: 352–358.

HANSEN, C., & RESKE-NIELSEN, E. (1965). Pathological studies in presbycusis. *Archives of Otolaryngology,* 82: 115–132.

HARGUS, S., & GORDON-SALANT, S. (1995). Accuracy of speech intelligibility index predictions for noise-masked young listeners with normal hearing and for elderly listeners with hearing impairment. *Journal of Speech and Hearing Research,* 38: 234–243.

HARRIS, F., & PROBST, R. (1997). Otoacoustic emissions and audiometric outcomes. In: M. Robinette & T. Glattke (Eds.), *Otoacoustic Emissions—Clinical Applications.* New York: Thieme Medical Publishers.

HELFER, K. (1991). Everyday speech understanding by older listeners. *Journal of the Academy of Rehabilitative Audiology,* 24: 17–34.

———. (1992). Aging and the binaural advantage in reverberation and noise. *Journal of Speech and Hearing Research,* 35: 1394–1401.

HELFER, K., & WILBER, L. (1990). Hearing loss, aging, and speech perception in reverberation and noise. *Journal of Speech and Hearing Research,* 33: 149–155.

HELFERT, R., SNEAD, C., & ALTSCHULER, R. (1991). The ascending auditory pathways. In: R. Altschuler, R. Bobbin, B. Clopton, & D. Hoffman (Eds.), *Neurobiology of Hearing: The Central Auditory System.* New York: Raven Press.

HOLTE, L. (1996). Aging effects in multifrequency tympanometry. *Ear and Hearing,* 17: 12–27.

HULL, R. (1995). *Hearing in Aging.* San Diego: Singular Publishing Group.

HUMES, L. (1996). Speech understanding in the elderly. *Journal of the American Academy of Audiology,* 7: 161–168.

HUMES, L., & CHRISTOPHERSON, L. (1991). Speech identification difficulties of hearing-impaired elderly persons: The contributions of auditory processing deficits. *Journal of Speech and Hearing Research,* 34: 686–693.

HUMES, L., CHRISTOPHERSON, L., & COKELY, C. (1992). Central auditory processing disorders in the elderly: Fact or fiction? In: J. Katz, N. Stecker, & D. Henderson (Eds.), *Central Auditory Processing: A Transdisciplinary View.* St. Louis: Mosby Year Book.

HUMES, L., NELSON, K., & PISONI, D. (1991). Recognition of synthetic speech by hearing-impaired elderly listeners. *Journal of Speech and Hearing Research,* 34: 1180–1184.

HUMES, L., & ROBERTS, L. (1990). Speech-recognition difficulties of the hearing impaired elderly: The contributions of audibility. *Journal of Speech and Hearing Research,* 33: 726–735.

HUMES, L., WATSON, B., CHRISTENSEN, L., COKELY, C., HALLING, D., & LEE, L. (1994). Factors associated with individual differences in clinical measures of speech recognition among the elderly. *Journal of Speech and Hearing Research,* 37: 465–474.

JEPSON, O. (1963). Middle ear muscle reflexes in man. In: J. Jerger (Ed.), *Modern Developments in Audiology.* New York: Academic Press.

JERGER, J., & CHMIEL, R. (1997). Factor analytic structure of auditory impairment in elderly persons. *Ear and Hearing,* 8: 269–276.

JERGER, J., CHMIEL, R., WILSON, N., & LUCHI, R. (1995). Hearing impairment in older adults: New concepts. *Journal of the American Geriatrics Society,* 43: 928–935.

JERGER, J., & HAYES, D. (1977). Diagnostic speech audiometry. *Archives of Otolaryngology,* 96: 513–523.

JERGER, J., JERGER, S., & MAUDLIN, L. (1972). Studies in impedance audiometry. I. Normal and sensorineural ears. *Archives of Otolaryngology,* 96: 513–523.

JERGER, J., JERGER, S., OLIVER, T., & PIROZZOLO, F. (1989). Speech understanding in the elderly. *Ear and Hearing,* 10: 79–89.

JERGER, J., JERGER, S., & PIROZZOLO, F. (1991). Correlational analysis of speech audiometric scores, hearing loss, age, and cognitive abilities in the elderly. *Ear and Hearing,* 12: 103–109.

JERGER, J., OLIVER, T., & PIROZZOLO, F. (1990). Impact of central auditory processing disorder and cognitive deficit on the self-assessment of hearing handicap in the elderly. *Journal of the American Academy of Audiology,* 1: 75–80.

KEMP, D. (1997). Otoacoustic emissions in perspective. In: M. Robinette & T. Glattke (Eds.), *Otoacoustic Emissions—Clinical Applications.* New York: Thieme Medical Publishers.

KARZON, R., GARCIA, P., PETEREIN, J., & GATES, G. (1995). Distortion product otoacoustic emissions in the elderly. *American Journal of Otology,* 5: 596–605.

KIMBERLEY, B., BROWN, D., & ALLEN, J. (1997). Distortion product emissions and sensorineural hearing loss. In: M. Robinette & T. Glattke (Eds.), *Otoacoustic Emissions—Clinical Applications.* New York: Thieme Medical Publishers.

LONSBURY-MARTIN, B., CUTLER, W., & MARTIN, G. (1991). Evidence for the influence of aging on distortion-product ototacoustic emissions in humans. *Journal of the Acoustical Society of America,* 89: 1749–1759.

LONSBURY-MARTIN, B., MARTIN, G., & WHITEHEAD, M. (1997). Distortion product otoacoustic emissions. In: M. Robinette & T. GLATTKE (Eds.), *Otoacoustic Emissions—Clinical Applications.* New York: Thieme Medical Publishers.

MARSHALL, L. (1981). Auditory processing in aging listeners. *Journal of Speech and Hearing Disorders,* 46: 226–240.

MARSHALL, L., & BACON, S. (1981). Prediction of speech discrimination scores from audiometric data. *Ear and Hearing,* 2: 148–155.

MILLS, J. (1992). Noise-induced hearing loss: Effects of age and existing hearing loss. In: A. Dancer, D. Henderson, R. Salvi, & R. Hamernik (Eds.), *Noise Induced Hearing Loss.* St. Louis: Mosby Year Book.

MOSCICKI, E., ELKINS, E., BAUM, H., & McNAMARA, P. (1985). Hearing loss in the elderly: An epidemiologic study of the Framingham Heart Study Cohort. *Ear and Hearing,* 6: 184–190.

NEWMAN, C., SANDRIDGE, S., & JACOBSON, G. (1998). Psychometric adequacy of the tinnitus handicap inventory (THI) for evaluating treatment outcome. *Journal of the American Academy of Audiology,* 9: 153–160.

OSTERHAMMEL, D., & OSTERHAMMEL, P. (1979). Age and sex variations for the normal stapedial reflex thresholds and tympanometric compliance values. *Scandinavian Audiology,* 8: 153–158.

PEARSON, J., MORRELL, C., GORDON-SALANT, S., BRANT, L., METTER, E., KLEIN, L., & FOZARD, J. (1995). Gender differences in a longitudinal study of age-associated hearing loss. *Journal of the Acoustical Society of America,* 97: 1196–1205.

PICHORA-FULLER, M., SCHNEIDER, B., & DANEMAN, M. (1995). How young and old adults listen to and remember speech in noise. *Journal of the Acoustical Society of America,* 97: 593–608.

PLOMP, R. (1978). Auditory handicap of hearing impairment and the limited benefit of hearing aids. *Journal of the Acoustical Society of America,* 63: 533–549.

PLOMP, R., & DUQUESNY, A. (1982). A model for the speech-reception threshold in noise without and with a hearing aid. In: O. Pedersen & T. Poulsen (Eds.), Binaural Effects in Normal and Impaired Hearing. *Scandivanian Audiology Supplement,* 15: 95–101.

POPELKA, M., CRUIKSHANKS, K., WILEY, T., TWEED, T., KLEIN, B., & KLEIN, R. (1998). Low prevalence of hearing aid use among older adults with hearing loss: The epidemiology of hearing loss study. *Journal of the American Geriatrics Society,* 46: 1075-1078.

POWERS, R. (1994). Neurobiology of aging. In: *Textbook of Geriatric Neuropsychiatry.* Washington, DC: American Psychiatric Press.

PRIEVE, B., & FALTER, S. (1995). COAEs and SOAEs in adults with increased age. *Ear and Hearing,* 16(5): 521–528.

ROBINETTE, M. (1992). Clinical observations with transient evoked otoacoustic emissions with adults. *Seminars in Hearing,* 13: 23–36.

ROSEN S., BERGMAN, M., PLESTER, D., EL-MOFTY, A., & SATTIS, M. (1962). Presbycusis study of a relatively noise free population in the Sudan. *Trans. Am. Otol. Soc.* 50: 135–151.

SCHEIBEL, M., LINDSAY, R., TOMIYASU, U., & SCHEIBEL, A. (1975). Progressive dendritic changes in aging human cortex. *Experimental Neurology,* 47: 392–403.

SCHOENBORN, C., & MARANO, M. (1988). Current estimates from the National Health Interview Survey: United States 1987. *Vital and Health Statistics,* 10, No. 166. Washington, DC: Government Printing Office.

SCHOW, R., & NERBONNE, M. (1980). Hearing levels among nursing home residents. *Journal of Speech and Hearing Disorders,* 45: 124–132.

SCHUKNECHT, H. (1955). Presbycusis. *Laryngoscope,* 65: 402–419.

———. (1964). Further observations on the pathology of presbycusis. *Archives of Otolaryngology,* 80: 369–382.

———. (1989). Pathology of presbycusis. In: J. Goldstein, H. Kashima, & C. Koopman, (Eds.), *Geriatric Otorhinolaryngology.* Toronto: B.C. Decker.

———. (1993). *Pathology of the Ear,* 2d ed. Pennsylvania: Lea & Febiger.

SILMAN, S. (1979). The effects of aging on the stapedius reflex thresholds. *Journal of the Acoustical Society of America,* 66: 735–738.

SILMAN, S., & GELFAND, S. (1981). The relationship between magnitude of hearing loss and acoustic reflex threshold levels. *Journal of Speech and Hearing Disorders,* 46: 312–316.

STACH, B., SPRETNJAK, M., & JERGER, J. (1990). The prevalence of central presbycusis in a clinical population. *Journal of the American Academy of Audiology,* 1: 109–115.

STOVER, L., & NORTON, S. (1993). The effects of aging on otoacoustic emissions. *Journal of the Acoustical Society of America,* 94: 2670–2681.

STROUSE, A., HALL, J., & BURGER, C. (1995). Central auditory processing in Alzheimer's disease. *Ear and Hearing,* 16: 230–238.

SUZUKA, Y., & SCHUKNECHT, H. (1988). Retrograde cochlear neuronal degeneration in human subjects. *Acta Oto-Laryngologica Supplement,* 450: 1–20.

THOMPSON, D., SILLS, J., RECKE, K., & BUI, D. (1979). Acoustic admittance and the aging ear. *Journal of Speech and Hearing Research,* 23: 29–36.

TOWNSEND, T., & BESS, F. (1980). Effects of age and sensorineural hearing loss on word recognition. *Scandinavian Audiology*, 9: 245–248.

UHLMANN, R., LARSON, E., REES, T., KOEPSELL, T., & DUCKERT, L. (1989a). Relationship of hearing impairment to dementia and cognitive dysfunction in older adults. *Journal of the American Medical Association*, 261: 1916–1919.

UHLMANN, R., REES, T., PSATY, B., & DUCKERT, L. (1989b). Validity and reliability of auditory screening tests in demented and non-demented older adults. *Journal of General Internal Medicine*, 4: 90–96.

VAN ROOIJ, J., & PLOMP, R. (1992). Auditive and cognitive factors in speech perception by elderly listeners. III: Additional data and final discussion. *Journal of the Acoustical Society of America*. 91: 1028–1033.

VAN ROOIJ, J., PLOMP, R., & ORLEBEKE, J. (1989). Auditive and cognitive factors in speech perception by elderly listeners. I: Development of test battery. *Journal of the Acoustical Society of America*, 86: 1294–1309.

VAN ROOIJ, J., PLOMP, R., & ORLEBEKE, J. (1990). Auditive and cognitive factors in speech perception by elderly listeners. II: Multivariate analysis. *Journal of the Acoustical Society of America*, 88: 2611–2624.

WEINSTEIN, B., & AMSEL, L. (1986). Hearing loss and senile dementia in the institutionalized elderly. *Clinical Gerontologist*, 4: 3–15.

WILEY, T., CRUICKSHANKS, K., NONDAHL, D., TWEED, T. (1999). Aging and middle ear resonance. *Ear and Hearing*, 10: 173–179.

WILEY, T., CRUICKSHANKS, K., NONDAHL, D., & TWEED, T., KLEIN, R., & KLEIN, B. (1998). Aging and word recognition in competing message. *Journal of the American Academy of Audiology*, 9: 191–198.

WILLOTT, J. (1996). Anatomic and physiologic aging: A behavioral neuroscience perspective. *Journal of the American Academy of Audiology*, 7: 141–151.

WILSON, R. (1981). The effects of aging on the magnitude of the acoustic reflex. *Journal of Speech and Hearing Research*, 24: 406–414.

WILSON, R., & MARGOLIS, R. (1991). Acoustic-Reflex Measurements. In: W. Rintelmann (Ed.), *Hearing Assessment*, 2d ed. Austin: Pro-Ed.

WINGFIELD, A., (1996). Cognitive factors in auditory performance: Context, speed of processing, and constraints of memory. *Journal of the American Academy of Audiology*, 7: 175–182.

WINGFIELD, A., POON, L., LOMBARDI, L., & LOWE, D. (1985). Speed of processing in normal aging: Effects of speech rate, linguistic structure, and processing time. *Journal of Gerontology*, 40: 579–585.

Chapter 6

Performance on Electrophysiologic Tests of Central Auditory Nervous System Function

Craig W. Newman and Sharon A. Sandridge

My grandmother's ninety. She's dating a 92 year old man. It's going great. They never argue. They can't hear each other.

—Cathy Ladman, 1996

LEARNING OBJECTIVES

After reading this chapter, you should be able to:

- Determine whether further clinical investigation is warranted in order to assist in determining abnormal electro-cochleography (ECochG) due to pathologic conditions.
- Use auditory evoked potentials (AEP) to evaluate the temporal processing characteristics of neural activity within the auditory pathway.
- Make appropriate clinical decisions regarding AEP study outcomes in the older adult.
- Determine confounding variables when testing the older adult.

AEPs are represented by a series of positive and negative peaks that can be recorded when the auditory system (peripheral and central) is stimulated by sound (clicks, tones, or speech). These bioelectric potentials, picked up by electrodes placed on the scalp, reflect the contribution of neural events from discrete as well as multiple generator sites along the auditory pathway. Temporal processing information is inferred from the time it takes nerve impulses to travel between each presumed AEP neural generator site. Therefore, AEP techniques offer clinicians a "dynamic" evaluation of the physiology of the auditory system in contrast to a "static" assessment (e.g., magnetic resonance imaging) of anatomy. Accordingly, AEPs provide an electro-physiologic appraisal of auditory function and neural transmission from the cochlea to the cerebral cortex.

Age-related central auditory nervous system (CANS) changes may result in a slowing of neural conduction. This slowing may be attributed to a loss of neurons, dendrite spines, and synaptic contacts, resulting in a reduction of neuronal connectivity in the CANS. Such structural alterations potentially result in reductions in the production of neurotransmitters such as the synthesis of acetylcholine, norepinephrine, dopamine, serotonin, and γ-aminobutyric acid (GABA) (Ritchie, 1982; Toffano, Calderini, Battistella, Scapagnini, Gaitia, Ponzio, Algeri, & Crews, 1982). The rate at which these changes occur varies across the aging population. The resulting heterogeneity of the older population may account for the contradictory AEP findings reported in the literature. It is not surprising then that studies evaluating the impact of age on AEP recordings have been equivocal, leaving many clinical questions unanswered. Knowledge of potential normal age-related changes is critical to clinical decision making. That is, audiologists must be able to differentiate between the effects of normal senescent changes from pathologic conditions requiring further audiologic assessment, neuropsychologic evaluation, or medical/surgical treatment.

This chapter will begin with a brief summary of the various AEP classification schemes. It will be followed by a description of the major AEP components in terms of (1) a description of the response; (2) proposed neural generator sites; and (3) the effects of aging on waveform latency, amplitude and/or morphology, and associated clinical implications. The chapter will conclude with a discussion of confounding variables that may influence the reliability and validity of electrophysiologic tests administered in older adults. Practical considerations for enhancing the clinical utility of the tests will be offered.

115

CLASSIFICATION OF AEPS

Nomenclature

A number of classification schemes have been developed to describe each of the successive levels of electrophysiologic processing within the CANS. The nomenclature for AEP wave components is based on a number of variables including (1) order in sequence (e.g., first, middle, slow, late); (2) latency-polarity combination (e.g., N100, P300); (3) polarity-order (e.g., N1, Pa, Na, P3); (4) latency epoch (e.g., first, last, middle, late); (5) neural generator (e.g., hair cell, auditory nerve, brainstem, cortex); or (6) stimulus-response relationships (e.g., transient, sustained, perceptual). Further, AEPs can be classified as exogenous and endogenous events; that is, exogenous AEPs are determined primarily by the physical characteristics of the eliciting stimulus, such as click intensity or click rate, and endogenous AEPs are relatively unaffected by click intensity but are affected by attention, state of arousal, memory, and cognitive functioning of the individual. For a complete discussion of wave nomenclature and various classifications systems see Davis (1976), Picton and Fitzgerald (1983), Jacobson and Hyde (1985), and Hall (1992).

Measurable Parameters

AEP waveforms consist of a series of peaks and troughs, or wave components. The wave components are described by their amplitude and latency characteristics. These measurable parameters reflect the spatial-temporal organization of the CANS, in addition to reflecting neural synchrony and transmission. AEP absolute latency is determined by the time interval between the stimulus onset and the occurrence of a wave component. Absolute latency coincides temporally with neural activity in peripheral, brainstem, and auditory cortical regions. Interpeak latency is the time between two wave components. Latency is expressed in terms of milliseconds (ms.). Amplitude is measured from peak-to-baseline or peak-to-peak and is notated by microvolts (μV). A wave component's amplitude reflects the collective electrical activity of a large number of cells responding in unison to the syn-

chrony of neural discharge modulations. Figure 6–1 displays a schematic representation of each of the major AEPs. The first 10 ms. represents the early potentials from the cochlea to the brainstem; the segment from 10 to 100 ms. represents the middle potentials arising from the midbrain and cortex; and the remaining represents late cortical potentials.

AUDITORY EVOKED POTENTIALS

Electrocochleography

Description of Response

ECochG is the earliest of the AEPs to be recorded. This response arises from the cochlea and the auditory nerve occurring within the first 2 or 3 ms. following an abrupt stimulus onset, longer if tonal stimuli are used.

The ECochG waveform consists of two cochlear potentials, the cochlear potential (CM) and the summating potential (SP), as well as the compound action potential of the eighth cranial nerve (AP). Figure 6–2 depicts a normal ECochG recording. The CM is an alternating potential characterized by a series of positive and negative peaks that mimics the frequency response of the incoming stimulus. The CM can obscure the SP when using a single polarity stimulus, thus, the use of alternating polarity is desirable to cancel out the CM and maximize the SP. The SP is a baseline shift of the response occurring just prior to the AP. It may appear as a separate peak or a knee on the beginning slope of the AP.

PEARL
The ECochG is primarily used as a tool in the diagnosis of Ménière's disease and to enhance the identification of wave I in order to calculate auditory brainstem response (ABR) interpeak latency values. It can also be used intraoperatively to monitor cochlear and eighth nerve function during surgery that places peripheral auditory structures at risk.

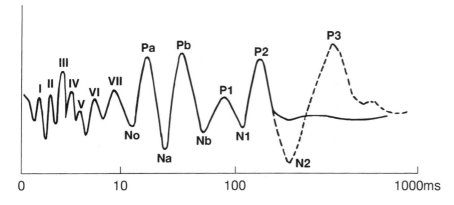

Figure 6–1 A graphic representation of the major auditory evoked potential (AEP) components from early to late. The ABR occurs within the first 10 ms. (labeled I–VII), the MLR occurs within the 10 to 100 ms. time window (labeled No–Nb), and the late components follow the MLR response (labeled P1–P3). Note that the amplitude is not drawn to scale.

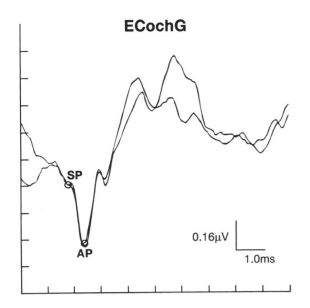

Figure 6–2 ECochG recording from a normal ear. AP is the whole-nerve action potential. SP is the summating potential.

Neural Generators

The CM reflects outer hair cell activity in the basal portion of the basilar membrane. The exact source of the SP is unknown, however, it has been attributed to distortion products associated with irregularities in basilar membrane and hair cell displacement, and to activity of both inner and outer hair cells. The AP is the same as wave I of the ABR, and therefore, arises from the distal portion of the auditory nerve.

Effects of Aging

The effects of aging on the cochlea have been well documented (Schuknecht, 1955, 1964, 1974, 1975) and have been discussed thoroughly in Chapter 4. However, little is known about the effects of aging on the ECochG because few investigations have been conducted. Bergholtz, Hooper, and Mehta (1977) recorded ECochGs in a sample of adults ranging in age from 20 to 78 years (mean age 58 years). The older subjects included individuals with presbycusis, presbycusis with a conductive component, conductive, noise-induced, and sensorineural hearing losses of unknown etiology. The results did not show conclusively that aging was associated with systematic changes of the ECochG. Chatrian, Wirch, Edwards, Lettich, and Snyder (1985) demonstrated some age-related differences in the ECochG, but the differences were not consistent for each response parameter. They did report, however, that the detection level of the SP was positively correlated with age, with a more intense stimulus needed to detect the SP response in older subjects. The SP amplitude was found to be smaller as a function of age, yet only for the left ear. Finally, the amplitude of the AP decreased more than the amplitude of the SP causing an inflated SP:AP ratio.

Summary

While preliminary results suggest that selected ECochG parameters are effected by age, further clinical investigation is warranted in order to assist clinicians in determining abnormal ECochGs due to pathologic conditions. This is especially important given the renewed diagnostic popularity of the ECochG and the clinical utility of the abnormal SP:AP ratio in the diagnosis of Ménière's disease.

Auditory Brainstem Response
Description of Response

During the first 10 ms. following an appropriate acoustic signal, a series of vertex-positive waveforms are recorded, representing the eighth nerve AP and successive generators within the brainstem (see Figure 6–3). These waveforms are generally designated using roman numerals I through VII (Jewett & Williston, 1971). On the basis of several clinico-pathologic studies it appears that waves I, III, and V primarily represent volume-conducted electrical activities from the acoustic nerve and brainstem and that latencies between these three potentials indirectly reflect neural conduction in the corresponding levels of the central auditory pathway. In essence, the auditory brainstem response (ABR) waveform represents the spatial-temporal pattern of brainstem electrical activity.

The presumed association between the various peaks and the ABR waveform and structures within the brainstem has led to clinical applications of the potentials, including auditory sensitivity (Hecox & Galambos, 1974; Picton, Woods, Baribeau-Braun, & Healey, 1977; Galambos & Hecox, 1978), differential assessment of cochlear versus retrocochlear lesions in sensorineural hearing loss (Yamada, Yagi, Yamane, & Suzuki, 1975), neurologic diagnosis of central dysfunction

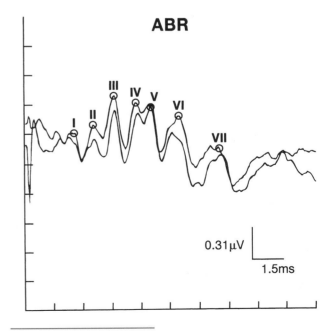

Figure 6–3 An ABR recording from a normal ear.

(Starr & Achor, 1975; Stockard, Stockard, & Sharbrough, 1977), and neurologic maturity (Schulman-Galambos & Galambos, 1975; Salamy & McKean, 1976).

As it pertains to older adults, the ABR is of particular interest because it allows for measurement of central auditory transmission time in an aging system. Central transmission (or conduction) time is inferred from the time required for neural impulses to travel between each presumed ABR wave generator site. Cochlear hearing loss affects basilar

---

SPECIAL CONSIDERATION

It must be kept in mind that age-related changes in ABR latency may be confounded by conductive, cochlear, or retrocochlear impairment. Changes in central transmission time attributable to age alone can be identified only after behavioral testing has ruled out peripheral contamination.

---

membrane travel time, which is the time difference between the arrival of the sound-initiated mechanical motion at the cochlea, and the generation of neural activity. A slowing of basilar membrane travel time due to cochlear impairment has significant effects on ABR latencies and amplitude (Picton et al, 1977).

Neural Generators

Numerous studies (Møller & Jannetta, 1981, 1982a, 1982b, 1983a, 1983b, 1983c; Møller, Jannetta, Bennett, & Møller, 1981) have attempted to locate the neural generator sites responsible for the particular wave components. In general, wave I is attributed to the compound AP in the distal portion of the eighth nerve as the fibers leave the cochlea and enter the internal auditory canal (Hashimoto, Ishiyama, Yoshimoto, & Nemoto, 1981; Møller, 1985; Møller & Jannetta, 1981, 1982b, 1983a, 1983b; Møller, Jannetta, Bennett, & Møller, 1981). Wave II is generated by the proximal eighth nerve as it enters the brainstem (Møller & Jannetta, 1982b; Scherg & von Cramon, 1985). From this point, the auditory system becomes more complex and less well defined. Wave III appears to be the representation of the cochlear nucleus (Møller & Jannetta, 1982a, 1983a, 1983b, 1983c; Grandori, 1986; Møller, Jannetta, & Sekhar, 1988). Wave IV, a component that often appears as a small peak riding on the leading edge of wave V, is attributed to the superior olivary complex with input from cochlear nucleus and lateral lemniscus. Wave V is associated with the termination of fibers from the lateral lemniscus into the inferior colliculus. The precise generator site for waves III, IV, and V are unclear due to conflicting reports from various laboratories. Later waves may come from several structures with ascending and descending input, and ipsilateral, contralateral, or bilateral input. It is best to assume, with the exception of waves I and II, that the later waves have multiple generator sites. The reader is referred to Hall (1992) and Jacobson (1994) for more in-depth information about neural generators of the ABR.

Effects of Aging

Age-related changes in the ABR have been reported for absolute latencies (Maurizi, Altissimi, Ottaviani, Paludetti, & Bambini, 1982; Allison, Hume, Wood, & Goff, 1984; Oku & Hasegewa, 1997), interpeak latencies (Rowe, 1978; Allison et al, 1984; Oku & Hasegewa, 1997), amplitude (Starr & Achor, 1975; Rowe, 1978; Chiappa, Gladstone, & Young, 1979; Psatta & Matei, 1988), morphology (Rosenhammer, Lindstrom, & Lundborg, 1980; Maurizi et al, 1982; Otto & McCandless, 1982), and spectral composition (Spivak & Malinoff, 1990; Ryan & Sandridge, 1993).

SPECIAL CONSIDERATION

In general, it is presumed that with age, absolute latencies increase (Rowe, 1978), amplitudes decrease (Jerger & Hall, 1980; Psatta & Matei, 1988), there is a loss of clarity and organization of waveform morphology (Spivak & Malinoff, 1990), and that the change may be different between females and males (Beagley & Sheldrake, 1978; Rosenhamer, Lindstrom, & Lundborg, 1980).

Rowe (1978) described the ABR response as a technique for documenting age-related slowing of neural transmission time, as well as synchrony of temporally patterned neural activity. In a group of 25 elderly subjects (51 to 74 years old), absolute latencies increased 0.20 to 0.50 ms. compared to a group of 25 young subjects (17 to 33 years old). These findings were supported by a number of other investigations (Rosenhamer, Lindstrom, & Lundborg, 1980; Maurizi et al, 1982; Allison et al, 1984; Rosenhall, Bjorkman, Pedersen, & Kall, 1985; Rosenhall, Pedersen, & Dotevall, 1986; Debruyne, 1986; Trune, Mitchell, & Phillips, 1988; Oku & Hasegewa, 1997). However, Rowe (1978) did not consider the issues of gender and hearing loss as contaminating variables. Rosenhall et al (1986), in a study of 268 subjects with hearing levels no poorer than 35 dBHL at 4000 Hz, noted prolonged absolute latencies of 0.10 to 0.20 ms. for waves I, III, and V when comparing the older adult (55 to 74 years old) group to the young adult (25 to 34 years old) sample. To rule out the influence of even a slight hearing loss at 4000 Hz, a comparison was made in the younger age groups between individuals with normal hearing and individuals with a mild high-frequency hearing loss. The latencies of waves I, III, and V did not show any significant difference between the ears with slight hearing loss and those with normal hearing. However, in a follow-up study, Rosenhall, Pederson, and Dotevall (1986) reported a pronounced age-related delay of wave V for individuals with a slight to moderate hearing loss.

Jerger and Johnson (1988) investigated the effects of gender, hearing loss, and aging on the latency of wave V in 412 subjects. They found a systematic increase in wave V with an increase in high-frequency hearing loss. In addition, results suggested that females showed little wave V latency change with increasing hearing loss, whereas wave V in males lengthened by approximately 0.1 ms. for every 20 dB decrease in effective click level of stimulus. The study by Jerger and Johnson (1988) suggests that ABR latency is affected by the interaction of age, gender, and hearing.

In light of the previously reported findings, Schwartz, Morris, and Jacobson (1994) attempted to clarify the need for separate norms by age and gender group. They plotted data from 240 normal listeners into bivariate scatter plots of ABR latency and amplitude for males and females as a function of age. Note in Figure 6–4 that, although there appear to be more males (indicated by o) in the upper half and more females (indicated by +) in the lower half of each latency distribution, careful examination reveals a relatively inconsequential number of males near the top and females near the bottom. Schwartz, Morris, and Jacobson (1994) also made the point that there was a high degree of overlap between the two gender groups toward the middle of the distribution. They did not see the need for gender specific normative data because, although there may be statistical significance, the gender difference is not clinically significant. In regard to latency and age, there was a slight trend to increasing latency for wave I and V as a function of age, with no relationship evident for interpeak latencies. Conversely, there was a more defined relationship for amplitude and age for wave I only. Schwartz, Morris, and Jacobson (1994, p. 144) concluded from their investigation that "neither age nor gender specific normative data need to be collected."

SPECIAL CONSIDERATION

Although some studies suggest that age and gender influence ABR latency, other studies say the effect is not significant to warrant normative data by age and gender.

Summary

It appears that there is a gender effect and age effect on the ABR but the interaction between age and hearing loss remains controversial. Further, the need to establish separate norms has not been well substantiated because of the lack of convincing evidence that the statistically significant findings are clinically relevant. That is, while the absolute mean latency values for older adults have been shown to be statistically longer than the averages for younger adults, the means tend to fall within the standard deviations established for normative values derived from younger adults.

Middle Latency Response

Description of Response

The middle latency response (MLR) is a series of waveforms that occur within the time epoch of 15 to 50 ms. after the presentation of a high-intensity acoustic stimulus (see Figure 6–5). The response occurs after the ABR and before the auditory late response (ALR). The major sequential peaks are labeled N (negative voltage waves) and P (positive voltage waves). The sequence of waves is denoted as Na, Pa, Nb, and Pb (or P1). The most prominent peak, Pa, normally occurs with a latency of about 25 ms., having an amplitude of, on average, 1.0 μV. The next positive peak, Pb, occurs approximately 25 ms. later. However, this component is highly variable and oftentimes not present even in normal adults (Hall, 1992).

PEARL

At present, the major clinical applications of the MLR include estimation of hearing threshold especially in the low frequencies (Musiek & Geurkink, 1981; Scherg & Volk, 1983), assessment of patients with cochlear implants (Gardi, 1985; Miyamoto, 1986; Kileny, & Kemink, 1987), and neurodiagnostic assessment of auditory pathway disease (Kraus, Ozdamar, Hier, & Stein, 1982; Scherg & von Cramon, 1986; Kileny & Kemink, 1987).

Neural Generators

Both animal and human studies have suggested that the MLR represents complex interactions from multiple generator sites. Using animal models, several investigators (Celesia, Broughton, Rasmussen, & Brach, 1968; Kraus, Smith, & McGee, 1988; McGee, Kraus, Littman, & Nicol, 1992; Amenedo & Diaz, 1998) have suggested that both primary and nonprimary components of the auditory thalamocortical pathway contribute to the MLR. Data discerned from near-field intracranial studies in humans (Celesia et al, 1968; Celesia, 1976; Lee, Lueders, Dinner, Lesser, Hahn, & Klemm, 1984), recordings from patients with computerized tomography (CT) or magnetic resonance imaging (MRI) confirmed brain lesions (Kraus et al, 1982; Scherg & von Cramon, 1986; Kileny, Paccioretti, & Wilson, 1987), and neuromagnetic studies in adults (Makela & Hari, 1987) have indicated that component Pa is generated bilaterally within the primary auditory cortices. Jacobson and his colleagues (Jacobson & Newman, 1990; Jacobson, Newman, Privitera, & Grayson, 1991) manipulated topographic brain maps to examine the physiologic origins of the MLR. Their data supported the hypothesis that Pa is generated by a minimum of two systems, including bilateral sources located in the posterior temporal lobes, and a deeper midline generator system. In addition to neural generators, sonomotor reflexes produced by scalp muscles may also contribute to the response (Kraus, Kileny, & McGee, 1994).

Effects of Aging

The study of aging on the MLR has focused on maturational changes of the Pa component in children (Skinner & Glattke, 1977; Kraus, Smith, Reed, Stein, & Cartee, 1985; Stapells, Galambos, Costello, & Makeig, 1988) with less attention paid to senescent changes on the response. One of the few studies was conducted by Woods and Clayworth (1986).

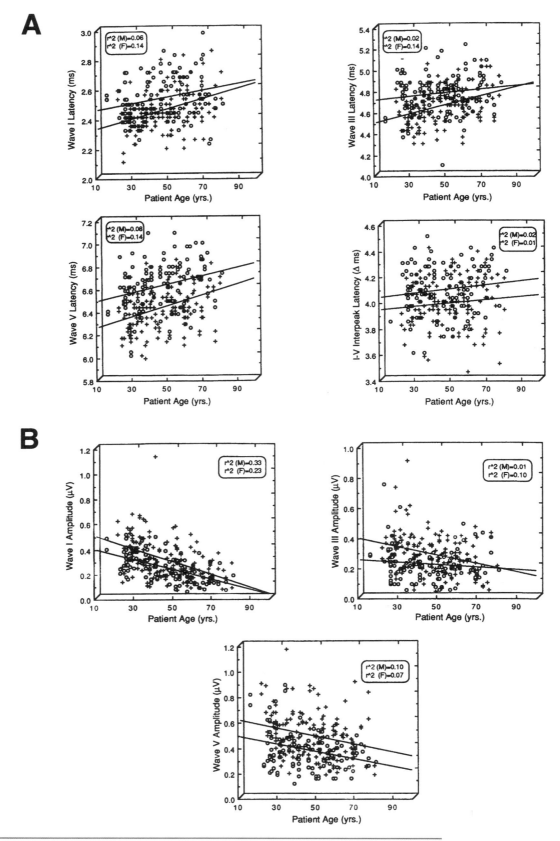

Figure 6–4 (A) Bivariate scatterplots of peak latencies as a function of age and gender (*N* = 240) for ABR waves I, III, V, and I–V interpeak latencies. (B) Bivariate scatterplots of peak amplitude as a function of age and gender (*N* = 240) for ABR waves I, III, and V. Source: The normal auditory brainstem response and its variants. (From Schwartz et al, 1994, pp. 141–142. By permission.)

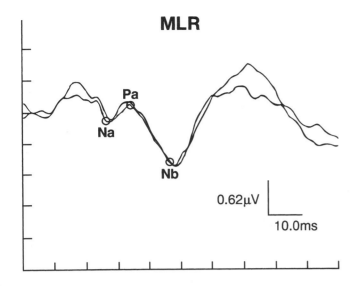

MLR

0.62μV

10.0ms

Figure 6–5 MLR from a normal ear. P indicates positive polarity. N represents negative polarity.

They compared MLRs between 12 young (20 to 35 years) and 12 older (60 to 70 years) adults, with equal number of males and females represented. Pure-tone threshold comparisons between samples showed comparable hearing at 500 Hz and 1000 Hz with the older adults demonstrating high-frequency hearing loss. Stimuli were rarefaction clicks presented at 13 clicks per second at 50 and 60 dB sensation level (SL) in monaural and binaural conditions. Differences in MLR morphology were observed between the two groups. More specifically, in the elderly subjects the Pa component was prolonged in latency, by 2.3 ms. in comparison to the younger adults. Interestingly, there was an enhancement of the Pa amplitude that was consistently observed in each of the conditions. Figure 6–6 displays waveforms generated from individual subjects in the Woods and Clayworth study and shows the striking difference in amplitude between groups. The latter authors argued that differences in amplitude were not attributable to differences in hearing sensitivity. To demonstrate this, they compared six elderly subjects with the lowest click threshold to six younger subjects with the most elevated thresholds, thereby reducing the mean intergroup difference in click threshold to 9.2 dB. Further, responses were then obtained using 50 and 60 dB SL clicks for the elderly and young samples, respectively. Using this paradigm, the enhancement of Pa amplitude was preserved in the older subjects. The authors concluded that age-associated increases in the Pa component may reflect structural or neurochemical production of the inhibitory input of the thalamic reticular nucleus to the medial geniculate nucleus, a proposed neural generator of the MLR. Although the relationship between increased evoked potential amplitudes and deficits in central inhibition is provocative, it has not been documented using independent measures of inhibition (Smith, Michalewski, Brent, & Thompson, 1980).

In a subsequent study, Chambers and Griffiths (1991) evaluated MLRs in a group of normal-hearing, healthy female subjects between the ages of 22 and 68 years. Because older subjects yield a general shift of the response waveform in a positive direction (Pfefferbaum, Ford, Roth, Hopkins, & Kopell, 1979), Chambers and Griffiths evaluated the contribution of such a shift by measuring the area of Pa. Further, the mean deviation from baseline was measured be-

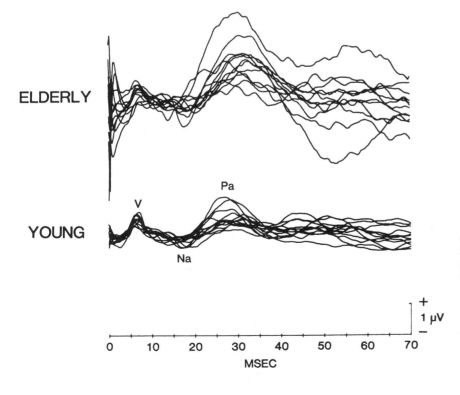

Figure 6–6 MLRs from the Cz electrode averaged over different stimulus conditions and intensities for individual older (top) and younger (bottom) subjects. Each tracing represents the mean MLR from a single subject. (From Woods and Clayworth, 1986, pp. 297–303. Reprinted by permission from Elsevier Science, County Clare, Ireland.)

yond Pa by determining the average amplitude at six different points (at 5 ms. intervals) between 45 and 70 ms. Their findings revealed that the amplitude of Pa increased through middle age, becoming significantly larger in comparison to the younger subjects (22 to 37 years). The larger absolute amplitude observed in the older group (50 to 68 years) resulted from a combination of both an increase in the size of Pa and relatively more positive baseline shift. The area measures of Pa suggested that at least some of the increase in magnitude of Pa is independent of the baseline shift.

Azumi, Nakashima, and Takahashi (1995) demonstrated that aging is not an important factor in latency measures, yet confirmed the observation that amplitude of Na-Pa and Pa-Nb components increased with age. Input levels of the click stimuli did not affect amplitude, further suggesting that the enhanced amplitudes might relate to CANS aging rather than senescent peripheral changes.

Paludetti, Maurizi, D'Alatri, and Galli (1991) evaluated the relationship between Pa and behavioral measures of speech understanding (phonetically balanced bisyllabic word, normal sentences, and compressed sentences) in a sample of 74 subjects (38 males and 36 females) between 60 and 80 years old with varying degrees of hearing loss. Although performance on the speech measures declined with deteriorating listening conditions and hearing loss, the MLRs appeared unaffected by age or hearing sensitivity. No correlations were found between the speech tests and the MLR data. The authors concluded that the generators of MLRs cannot be considered the electrophysiologic substrates for age-related disturbances in speech perception.

Finally, Buchwald, Erwin, Read, Van Lancker, and Cummings (1989) used the MLRs as a probe of brain function in patients with Alzheimer's disease (AD). These investigators compared responses between an age-matched sample of six healthy men and a sample of men with definite (N = 4) or probable (N = 2) AD. Normal findings were observed for the Pa response but a significant decrease in amplitude was seen for component Pb (corresponding to the long-latency response P1 occurring between 50 and 65 ms.). The authors concluded that abnormal responses suggest that the cholinergic cells in the midbrain may be dysfunctional in patients with AD. These conclusions are only hypothetical and the results must be viewed with caution given the small sample size.

Summary

It appears that the primary effect on the MLR is the amplitude of the response. Further clinical studies are needed to investigate the interaction between hearing loss and senescence on latency and amplitude measures of the MLR in normal aging and age-prevalent pathologic conditions.

Auditory Late Responses
Description of Response

The first positive peak following the MLR is the first of four components that constitute the auditory late response

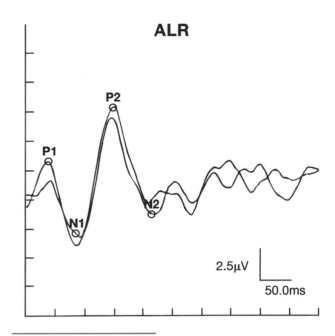

Figure 6–7 ALR from a normal ear. P indicates positive polarity. N represents negative polarity.

(ALR). The ALR (Figure 6–7) comprises P1 (50 to 80 ms.), N1 (100 to 150 ms.), P2 (150 to 200 ms.), and N2 (180 to 250 ms.). The components are labeled according to the polarity and order of occurrence (i.e., P1, P2). The components can also be labeled according to the polarity and latency (P60, N100). The P1, N1, and P2 components are generally considered to be exogenous responses and, hence, are stimulus dependent and relatively psychologically independent. They reflect aspects of acoustic events such as timing, sequencing, and physical dimensions. N2, on the other hand, is considered to be an endogenous response, more dependent upon attentional factors than the other three components of the ALR. N2 may be elicited following a passive task such as acoustic discrimination or a more active task such as semantic discrimination.

The ALR is a highly robust response with latencies ranging from 50 to 250 ms. and amplitudes ranging from 3 to 10 μV. The late response can be elicited with frequency-specific tones presented at a relatively slow rate of one or two stimuli per second. It is recorded from vertex (Cz) to ipsilateral ear. A small number of samples (200 to 250) are averaged because habituation is known to decrease amplitude.

SPECIAL CONSIDERATION

Successful recording of the potential depends on subject state of arousal and rate of stimulus presentation. ALRs cannot be reliably recorded on sedated subjects; subjects must be awake and attend to the stimulus.

Because the ALR has a cortical origin, albeit, specific site unknown, it has been studied in a number of patients with cerebrovascular damage such as temporal lobe infarcts (Rothenberger, Szirtes, & Jurgens, 1982), degenerative disease processes such as dementia (Goodin, 1990), AD (Buchwald et al, 1989), Parkinson's disease (Gil, Neau, Toullat, Rivasseau, & Lefevre, 1989), schizophrenia (Adler, Adler, Schneck, & Armbruster, 1990), and human immunodeficiency virus (HIV) (Ollo, Johnson, & Grafman, 1991). In addition to neurologic applications, ALRs can be used for audiometric testing.

PEARL

The use of frequency-specific tones rather than the broadband click permits a more discrete assessment of hearing sensitivity.

Auditory thresholds may be estimated using the ALR. Similar to the ABR, as stimulus intensity decreases, the latency increases and amplitude decreases. However, the subject must be passively cooperative and the responses must be replicable. Whereas the utility of the ALR is limited for auditory threshold estimation, it may prove useful as a central auditory processing tool in the older adult or as a tool for the investigation of the neurophysiology of speech perception.

Neural Generators

There is little consensus as to the precise generators of the ALRs because of the multiplicity and complexity of the central auditory pathway. Davis (1939) recorded from numerous locations on the scalp and found maximum amplitude from midline over frontal regions suggesting frontal lobe origins. These findings were supported by Picton, Hillyard, Krausz, and Galambos (1974) who purported that the origin of the ALRs was a region in the association cortex of the frontal lobe. Using scalp topography and neuromagnetic correlations in humans, however, a number of researchers proposed the generator or generators in the region of the Sylvian fissure and the superior temporal plane in the temporal lobe (Wood & Wolpaw, 1982; Knight, Scabini, Woods, & Clayworth, 1989; Baumann, Rogers, Papanicolaou, & Saydjari, 1990; Papanicolaou, Baumann, Rogers, Saydjari, Amparo, & Eisenberg, 1990). Intracranial recordings from monkeys (Arezzo, Pickoff, & Vaughan, 1975) and in humans (Chatrian, Petersen, & Lazarte, 1960) supported the temporal lobe origin.

Effects of Aging

The greatest changes seen in the ALR are seen as children develop. ALR latency decreases and amplitude increases from early childhood up to about age 10. Latencies generally increase and amplitude decreases as a function of advancing age in older adults (Callaway & Halliday, 1973; Callaway, 1975; Pfefferbaum, Ford, Roth, & Kopell, 1980), however, this is not without some equivocation (Spink, Johannsen, & Pirsig, 1979).

Summary

ALR is a cortical response that can be used to estimate auditory thresholds as well as a tool for evaluating central auditory processing and/or cortical function. The effects of aging are unknown; however, it is not unreasonable to assume that changes may be observed in latency and amplitude measures reflecting senescent alterations in CNS function.

The P3 Response
Description of Response

The most widely investigated of the endogenous components is the P300 or P3 component. The positive-going P3 component ranges in amplitude between 5 and 30 μV and occurs approximately 300 ms., yet it can occur somewhere between 220 and 900 ms. (Kutas & Hillyard, 1984a, 1984b). Figure 6–8 displays a P3 response from an older adult. It is elicited by task-relevant, "surprising" stimuli presented in an "oddball" paradigm; that is, a series of randomly occurring, infrequent, target (deviant) stimuli are presented within a series of nontarget homogeneous (standard) stimuli. The subject must attend to the stimuli and make a mental count or respond motorically to the target, or deviant stimuli. The P3 component accompanies the occurrence of the rare unexpected or the absence of an expected stimulus.

The P3 component is an endogenous potential, requiring active cognitive participation but relatively independent of stimulus attributes (Duncan-Johnson & Donchin, 1982). It is not modality specific and can be elicited with visual (Kok & Looren de Jong, 1980), auditory (Polich, Howard, & Starr,

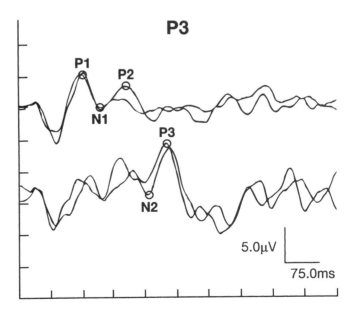

Figure 6–8 An example of the P3 response from an adult with normal hearing. The top tracings are the average of the standard (frequent) stimulus (500 Hz tones). The bottom tracings are the average of the deviant (infrequent) stimulus (2000 Hz tones). P indicates positive polarity. N represents negative polarity.

1985a, 1985b), or somatosensory stimuli (Wood, Allison, Goff, Williamson, & Spencer, 1980). Subject attention, alertness, memory, and cognitive status will influence the P3 response. The P3 component appears to reflect active cognitive processing. Donchin and Coles (1988) suggest that P3 is a by-product of the process, not necessarily an index of the process itself. The theory proposed by Donchin and his coworkers asserts that certain stimulus evaluation activities must be completed prior to the process that is reflected by P3. It does not imply that P3 is an actual measure of stimulus evaluation time; it simply means that if a stimulus is going to be evaluated, it is evaluated before the P3 component occurs.

The P3 component is described by latency, amplitude, and to some degree, topography. While a number of theories have been proposed to account for the latency of the P3 component, the literature most consistently supports the theory that the latency of the P3 component is determined by stimulus evaluation time (Kutas, McCarthy, & Donchin, 1977; Duncan-Johnson, 1981; Duncan-Johnson & Donchin, 1982; Johnson & Donchin, 1985). Manipulation of the discrimination task complexity results in changes in the latency of P3. Research has demonstrated that by increasing the stimulus evaluation process, the P3 latency is increased. For example, latency increased when the frequency difference between target and nontarget stimuli became more narrow (Ritter, Simson, & Vaughan, 1972), hue discrimination decreased (Duncan-Johnson & Kopell, 1981), and the target stimuli was embedded in a noisy background (Polich, Howard, & Starr, 1985a, 1985b). The amplitude of the P3 component has been shown to be a function of the confidence of detection (Squires, Squires, & Hillyard, 1975; Campbell, Courchesne, Picton, & Squires, 1979) and the subjective probability of the target stimuli (Tueting, Sutton, & Zubin, 1970; Squires, Wickens, Squires, & Donchin, 1976; Duncan-Johnson & Donchin, 1977). That is, the more infrequent and unexpected the target, the larger the amplitude (Sutton, Braren, Zubin, & John, 1965; Duncan-Johnson & Donchin, 1977, 1980).

The topography of the P3 has a frontal-parietal distribution. P3 component may consist of a bimodal peak, P3a, and P3b, under certain situations. The "a" component has maximum amplitude over frontocentral regions (Squires, Squires, & Hillyard, 1975) occurring approximately 50 ms. earlier than the P3b, undergoes rapid habituation with repeated trials, is elicited in passive conditions, and represents a central nervous system (CNS) component of the orienting response (Ritter, Vaughan, & Costa, 1968; Knight, 1984). The "b" component occurs later in time, does not habituate, requires active subject participation, and has maximal amplitude over centroparietal scalp regions (Squires, Squires, & Hillyard, 1975).

Neural Origin of P3

The specific neural origin of the P3 remains unknown (McPherson, 1996). Several researchers suggest that the generator site is the hippocampus or surrounding areas such as the parahippocampal gyrus and the amygdala (Begleiter, 1979; Halgren, Squires, Wilson, Rohrbaugh, Babb, & Crandall, 1980; O'Connor & Starr, 1985; Halgren, Stapleton, Smith, & Altafullah, 1986). Others have suggested that the

response has a purely cortical origin (Simson, Vaughan, & Ritter, 1976; Simson, Vaughan, & Ritter, 1977a; Simson, Vaughan, & Ritter, 1977b; Goff, Allison & Vaughan, 1978), or it is from the reticulo-thalamocortical activating system that involves the mesencephalic reticular formation, medial thalamus, and prefrontal cortex (Desmedt & Debecker, 1979; Yingling & Hosobuchi, 1984). Gordon, Rennie, and Collins (1990) proposed that the source of the P3 is either in the hippocampus or temporal lobe. Paller, Zola, Squire, and Hillyard (1988) contradicted Gordon, Rennie, and Collins, (1990) findings by recording, in monkeys, the P3 response following bilateral lesion in the medical temporal lobe. Knight et al (1989), on the other hand, found the P3 was absent in patients with unilateral lesions centered in the posterior superior temporal plane. Pineda, Foote, and Neville (1989) reported a correlation between the extent of damage of locus caeruleus cell bodies and reduction of the P3 response. The literature suggests that the P3 component has several neural generator sites (Wood & Wolpaw, 1982; O'Connor & Starr, 1985; McPherson, 1996) involving the frontal cortex, centroparietal cortex, and hippocampus (McPherson, 1996; Anderer, Pascual-Margui, Semlitsch, & Saletu, 1998).

Effects of Age

Polich, Howard, and Starr (1985a) investigated the changes in latency of the P3 component across age using the classic oddball paradigm in 104 subjects ranging in age from 5 to 86 years. The youngest group (0 to 9 years old) had a mean latency of 355 ms. decreasing to 287 ms. for the 20- to 29-year-old group and then gradually increasing to 387 for the oldest group of 70- to 90-year-old subjects. These findings were consistent with previous investigations (Brown, Marsh, & LaRue, 1983; Pfefferbaum, Wenegrat, Ford, Roth, & Kopell, 1984).

PEARL
There is a clear consensus that peak latency is longer in elderly than younger adults (Goodin, Squires, Henderson, & Starr, 1978; Ford, Hink, Hopkins, Roth, Pfefferbaum, & Kopell, 1979; Pfefferbaum et al, 1980; Barajas, 1991; Schroeder, Lipton, Ritter, Giesser, & Vaughan, 1995).

There is, however, a difference of opinion as to the exact nature of the age/latency function. Most reports have described a linear increase with slopes ranging from 0.91 to 1.85 ms./yr (Goodin et al, 1978; Syndulko et al, 1982; Picton, Stapells, Perrault, Baribeau-Braun, & Stuss, 1984; Polich et al, 1985a; Kraiuhin, Gordon, Stanfield, Meares, & Howson, 1986; Barrett, Neshige, & Shibasaki, 1987; Patterson, Michalewski, & Starr, 1988). In contrast, Brown et al (1983) reported that the relation between the P3 latency and age was curvalinear rather than linear; that is, they observed little change in P3 latencies in individuals younger than 45 years old and then an accelerating positive increase of 3.14 ms./yr thereafter. Barajas (1991), using 103 subjects ranging in age from 6 to 78 years, reported the age/latency slope for subjects 6 to 14 years old was −19 ms./yr, −2.4 ms./yr for subjects 12 to 24 years old, and 1.25 ms./yr for the 18- to 78-year-old group. Iragui, Kutas, Matchiner, and Hillyard (1993) reported similar results with a negative slope for latency for individuals below age 45 years and then changing to a positive slope of 1.09 ms./yr for individuals older than 45 years. Although the addition of a curvalinear factor failed to show significance, the curve did appear to steepen with advancing age.

Age-related findings for amplitude are not as consistent or systematic as the findings for P3 latency. Some authors have not found reductions in amplitude (Ford, Roth, Mohs, Hopkins, & Kopell, 1979; Kraiuhin et al, 1986; Barrett et al, 1987; Amenedo & Diaz, 1998; Friedman, Kazmerski, & Cycowicz, 1998), whereas others have demonstrated a reduction in P3 amplitude with normal aging (Goodin et al, 1978; Syndulko, Hansch, Cohen, Pearce, Goldberg, Monton, Tourtellotte, & Potvin, 1982; Brown et al, 1983; Picton, Stapells, Perrault, Baribeau-Braun, & Stuss, 1984; Pollock & Schneider, 1989; Anderer et al, 1998). Pollock and Schneider (1989) showed maximal P3 amplitude frontally whereas younger subjects showed maximal P3 amplitude in parietal scalp region. Iragui et al (1993) found a gradual decrease of P3 amplitude at central and parietal recording sites and a slight increase in P3 amplitude at frontal sites. Picton et al (1984), recording from the vertex, showed amplitude decreases under one paradigm (counting subvocally) and no change under another paradigm (reaction-time paradigm).

The inconsistent findings of age-related amplitude changes could be due to a number of differences in sampling and recording parameters. For example, both the age range of the sample and the technique employed to measure amplitude (e.g., peak-to-peak, baseline-to-peak, averaged amplitude, or single-trial amplitude) will greatly influence the outcome. In addition, P3a and P3b may show different age-related amplitude changes (Knight, 1987).

The P3a amplitude has been found to remain constant or slightly increase over the frontal regions (Strayer, Wichens, & Braune, 1987; Yamaguchi & Knight, 1991) with age. This increased amplitude may offset any amplitude reduction seen in P3b, obscuring the results. Therefore, age-related decreases in P3 (specifically P3b) may exist.

The changes in P3 with advancing age may be attributed to alterations in the CNS. Shock (1983) reported a decline in the number of functioning neuronal units and decrease in myelin as a function of aging. As a result, there appears to be a decrease in the neural conduction velocity; that is, with age there appears to be a general slowing of the speed at which neural impulses travel. This slowing may result in a longer decision process. In fact, Rabbitt (1965) suggested that the elderly are slower in deciding whether information is relevant.

PEARL

Despite some differences in the degree of age-related changes in the P3, numerous studies have conclusively demonstrated effects of normal aging on P3 latencies and amplitude indicative of a gradual slowing resulting in minor prolongations of stimulus evaluation and slight reductions of selective attention capabilities.

Clinical Applications

Because the P3 component appears to reflect stimulus evaluation time and is influenced by attention, alerting, arousal, and psychological state it has been popular among psychologists, psychiatrists, and neurologists. The P3 has been investigated in conditions associated with memory loss including Huntington's disease (Rosenberg, Nudleman, & Starr, 1985), schizophrenia (Pfefferbaum et al, 1984; Freedman, Waldo, Bickford, & Nagamoto, 1991), Parkinson's disease (Gil et al, 1989; Pang, Borod, Hernandez, Bodis, Raskin, Mylin, Coscia, & Yahr, 1990), dementia (Fein & Turetsky, 1989; Goodin, 1990), and AD (Ball, Marsh, Schubarth, Brown, & Strandburg, 1989; Kuhl, 1990; Marsh, Schubarth, Brown, Riege, Strandburg, Dorsey, Maltese, & Kuhl, 1990; Polich, Ladish, & Bloom, 1990).

Most recently, Attias, Furman, Shemesh, & Bresloff, (1996) reported the use of P3 in the investigation of subjects with noise-induced tinnitus (NIT). They observed significant prolongation of N1, N2, and P3 latencies to both auditory and visual stimuli in NIT subjects compared to hearing-matched control subjects. It appears that event-related potentials may supplement behavioral, audiologic, biochemical, and other physiologic methods for tinnitus assessment (Attias et al, 1996).

Likewise, the P3 may have value as a tool to investigate central auditory aging. Sandridge (1988) investigated the P3 in a group of older adults with some degree of hearing impairment. Twenty-eight healthy males (age 65 to 75 years), with pure-tone thresholds no poorer than 35 dBHL for 500 and 1000 Hz, but with a sloping high-frequency sensorineural hearing loss, underwent both audiometric and electrophysiologic testing. Using a difference score between the PB-max (maximum score for phonetically balanced words) and the SSI-max (maximum score for the Synthetic Sentence Identification; SSI) of 16 or greater, subjects were categorized as having a hearing impairment with a central auditory involvement (centrally impaired, CI), or having a primarily peripheral-hearing impairment (peripherally impaired, PI). Fifteen subjects were considered to be primarily PI while the other thirteen subjects were classified as CI. Both groups were equivalent in all behavioral measurements except the difference score between SSI-max and PB-max. The P3 response was recorded under two conditions: quiet (pure tones of 500 Hz [standard] and 1000 Hz [deviant] presented at 66 dBSPL) and in a medium-band noise (−10 dB signal-to-noise ratio).

The results of this investigation (Figure 6–9) indicated that the latency of the P3 component evoked in quiet was longer for the CI group (Tracing B) when compared to the PI group (Tracing A) and that the introduction of a bandpass noise affected both groups, albeit differently. It was interesting to note that the latency of the P3 component for the PI group, in quiet, was found to be consistent with previously reported age-related norms for auditory stimuli of "easy" discrimination (Goodin et al, 1978; Squires, Chippendale, Wrege, Goodin, & Starr, 1980; Picton et al, 1984; Polich, Howard, & Starr, 1985b). On the other hand, the latency for the CI group was more consistent with Squires et al's (1980) expected latencies for more difficult tasks, suggesting that the CI group had more difficulty and required longer time for stimulus evaluation.

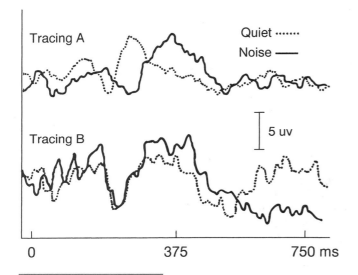

Figure 6–9 Tracing A represents the single recorded responses from a PI subject, demonstrating an obvious shift in the P3 component. Note the earlier occurrence of the P3 component in the quiet condition (the dotted line) when compared to the noise condition (solid line) for the PI subject. Tracing B represents the responses from a CI subject. Note that the P3 component did not shift as a function of the conditions.

The latency of the P3 component evoked in the presence of noise resulted in significantly longer latencies for both the CI and the PI groups when compared to the quiet condition. The introduction of the noise, however, affected each group differently. The PI group shifted from 330 to 393 ms., a 63 ms. shift. The CI group shift was only 36 ms.; from 351 to 387 ms. Whereas the shifts were shown to be significant for each group, the latencies between groups for the noise condition were not significantly different. In effect, the noise served to increase the complexity within bounds. The unequal shift in the P3 component between groups suggests that the noise created more interference for the PI group than the CI group. One explanation is the theory of neural noise. Aging has been associated with an increase in "neural noise" (Talland, 1968; Gregory, 1974) as neurons are lost and the spontaneous activity increases (Brody, 1955, 1985; Shock, 1983; Kenny, 1988). It is possible that the CI group exhibited higher levels of intrinsic neural noise than the PI group. This increased level of internal neural noise may have interfered with the discrimination during the quiet condition, accounting for the prolonged P3 latencies in quiet. When the external noise source was introduced, the overall effect of that noise was diminished because increased level of neural noise was already present.

The P3 component may provide advantages over currently available speech-based tests for investigating cognitive function and speech perception under difficult listening situations. The use of tones over speech stimuli allows the test to be relatively independent of the influence of the peripheral system and/or language biases. Bocca and Calearo (1963) cautioned, however, that tones were not an appropriate stimulus for central auditory processing testing because they do not reduce the extrinsic redundancy sufficiently to tax the intrinsic redundancy of the system. However, because the P3 component is an endogenous potential, it is not influenced by stimulus parameters such as frequency, intensity, rise/fall time, or whether the stimulus is in the auditory, visual, or somatosensory modality. Instead, the P3 component is influenced by motivation, attention, and the cognitive skills of the subject.

Summary

The time needed for stimulus evaluation, as indexed by the P3 component latency, increases as a function of aging. In addition, it appears that the perceptual processes associated with more difficult discrimination tasks are more susceptible to age than easier tasks.

Mismatch Negativity
Description of Response

The mismatch negativity (MMN) is an event-related evoked response to a physically "deviant" (infrequent) stimulus inserted in a train of similar (frequent) stimuli wherein the N1 is elicited but with an additional negativity occurring approximately 100 to 300 ms. post-stimulus onset (Näätänen, Gaillard, & Mäntysalo, 1978). The response is obtained in the absence of attention and reflects a physical mismatch between a memory trace from the frequently occurring stimuli and the incoming features of the infrequently occurring stimuli (Näätänen et al, 1978; Näätänen, 1990). The MMN has been elicited by changes in such parameters as frequency (Sams, Paavilainen, Alho, & Näätänen, 1985), duration (Kaukoranta, Sams, Hari, Hämäläinen, & Näätänen, 1989), intensity (e.g., Näätänen, Paavilainen, Alho, Reinikainen, & Sams, 1987), and location (Paavilainen, Karlsson, Reinikainen, & Näätänen, 1989). A variety of auditory stimuli have been used to evoke the MMN, including simple and complex tones (Schröger, Näätänen, & Paavilainen, 1992), as well as synthesized and natural speech (Kraus, McGee, Sharma, Carrell, & Nicol, 1992; Kraus, McGee, Micco, Sharma, Carrell, & Nicol, 1993; Kraus, McGee, Carrell, & Sharma, 1995; Sandridge & Boothroyd, 1996). The magnitude of the MMN response, quantified by the latency, amplitude, and area of the waveform, is reflective of the degree of difference between the frequently and infrequently occurring stimuli. The greater the difference between the two stimuli, the more pronounced the MMN response (e.g., pairing 1000 and 3000 Hz tones versus pairing 1000 and 1050 Hz tones). The MMN response can be elicited by very fine acoustic differences between auditory signals. Accordingly, the MMN provides the clinical scientist with a method for understanding the central auditory neurophysiology underlying the discrimination of fine acoustic differences. Figure 6–10 displays an example of an MMN response evoked by natural speech (CV) recorded at Cz. The average response to the deviant (/pE/) stimulus is shown as the dotted line; the average response to the standard stimulus (/tE/) is shown as the solid line. The difference wave, obtained by subtracting standard waveforms from deviant waveforms, is shown below the standard and

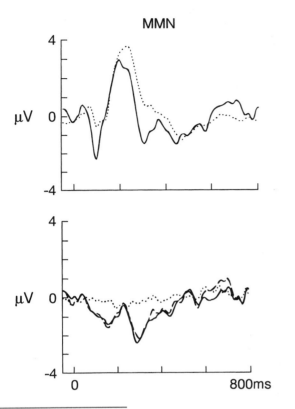

Figure 6–10 An example of the grand average MMN response from a group of young adults (*n* = 10) with normal hearing. The top tracings are the averaged response to the deviant (/pE/) stimulus (dotted line) and the standard (/tE/) stimulus (solid line) recorded at Cz. The bottom tracings are the difference waveforms recorded from Cz, Fz (solid and dashed lines), and A2 (dotted line). The negativity occuring between 200 and 400 ms. represents the MMN.

deviant tracings. For further information regarding the MMN, see the special issue of *Ear and Hearing* (1995) devoted to this topic.

Neural Generators

The neural generators for the MMN response have been studied using magnetoencephalographic (MEG) data, intracranial MMN recordings in animals and humans, scalp distribution recordings, and brain-lesioned recordings. In general, studies have indicated that the major source of the MMN is the auditory cortex, most specifically the supratemporal cortex (Giard, Perrin, Perrier, & Bouchet, 1990; Paavilainen, Alho, Reinikainen, Sams, & Näätänen, 1991; Csépe, Pantev, Hoke, Hampson, & Ross, 1992) with possible contributions from other brain structures such as the medial geniculate body and hippocampus (Csépe, Karmos, & Molnár, 1987). In addition, the exact location of the MMN appears to depend on which feature of a sound, such as frequency, intensity, duration, and interstimulus interval (Deouell, Bentin, & Giard, 1998) is changed. For example, Deouell et al (1998) found that scalp topography varied according to the

type of stimulus change. The dipoles fitting the scalp distribution of MMNs to frequency, intensity, and duration changes were all located along the supratemporal cortex, but were different in their location and/or orientation to each stimulus change. Tiitinen, Alho, Huotilainen, Ilmoniemi, Simola, and Näätänen (1993), using MEG, found that frequency differences corresponded to the tonotopic organization of the supratemporal auditory cortex. That is, the MMNm (MEG) dipole was less vertically oriented on the sagittal plane for higher frequencies and, as frequencies increased, the dipole rotated clockwise (in the right auditory cortex). Also using MEG, Alho, Tervaniemi, Huotilainen, Lavikainen, Tiitinen, Ilmoniemi, Knuutila, and Näätänen (1996) observed that the MMNm dipoles were different for changes in simple and complex sounds, suggesting that these changes are processed in different regions of the auditory cortex. Further, the MMN response appears to be generated in the left and right auditory cortices. Giard et al (1990), using scalp-current density (SCD) maps, recorded greater activity of the auditory cortex in the hemisphere contralateral to the stimulated ear. There is controversy, however, as to the contribution of the primary auditory cortex to the MMN response. Kraus, McGee, Littman, Nicol, and King (1994) recorded MMN responses in guinea pigs in the nonprimary auditory cortex but not in the primary auditory cortex. On the other hand, Javitt, Schroeder, Steinschneider, Arezzo, and Vaughan (1992) observed MMNs to frequency and intensity changes in the primary auditory cortex of the monkey.

Effects of Aging

A number of MMN studies have been conducted with young adult subjects and children (Korpilahti & Lang, 1994; Kraus & McGee, 1994; Kraus et al, 1995; Lang, Eerola, Korpilahti, Holopainen, Salo, Uusipaikka, & Aaltonen, 1995) demonstrating that this is a robust phenomenon. In contrast, little attention has been paid to the impact of advanced aging on the MMN. To our knowledge, one of the few studies on the effects of aging on MMN was conducted by Pekkonen, Jousmäki, Partanen, and Karhu (1993). They evaluated the prevalence of the MMN in 27 subjects between 18 and 85 years of age. All subjects were free from central and peripheral nervous system disease, significant hearing loss (thresholds not specified), and psychiatric disorders, and were not users of drugs that affect the CNS. Sequences of standard (800 Hz) and deviant (552 Hz) tones were presented in four blocks of 300 stimuli. These low-frequency stimuli were selected to help compensate for potential problems associated with high-frequency hearing loss in the older subjects. Interstimulus intervals (ISI) of 1 second and 3 seconds were employed. Because the response partly overlaps other event-related components, amplitude and latency of the MMN are sometimes difficult to specify. To overcome this problem, the authors used the MMN area (area under waveform) as the quantification metric. For the entire sample, when the 3 second ISI was used, the MMN area decreased significantly more in the older subjects than in the young adults. This is shown in Figure 6–11. Representative responses to the standard and deviant tones and the MMN area for a young (38-year-old) and older (65-year-old)

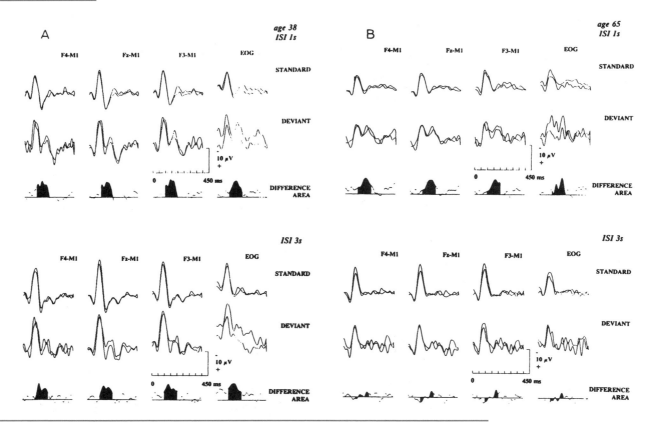

Figure 6–11 Two blocks of averaged responses from three electrode derivations are shown. Note the different ISIs (1 second and 3 seconds). MMN area was obtained from the difference between standard and deviant responses (from 100 to 200 ms., shown in black). The responses from a young subject are shown in A. The responses of older subject are shown in B. EOG is the response from an electrode placed at the eye and referred to the mastoid. (From Pekkonen et al, 1993, pp. 321–325. Reprinted by permission from Elsevier Science, Ireland, County Claire, Ireland.)

adult are displayed. Note that the older subject has smaller MMN areas for the 3 second ISI only. The authors interpreted these findings as a decline in the neuronal representation of the standard stimuli in the older subjects in comparison to the young adults. They concluded that this may provide evidence of shortening of the auditory sensory memory trace with increasing age.

The aforementioned study represents an initial step in the application of the MMN for studying the neurophysiologic mechanism of auditory processing in the older adult. This evoked potential technique is particularly interesting to researchers investigating the effects of aging on the auditory system for several reasons:

1. The MMN is an automatic response; that is, it requires no attention to the task. Thus, it is free from attentional factors that contaminate behavioral and electrophysiologic (e.g., P3) measures of auditory processing. Likewise, auditory function may be studied in individuals who are unable to actively participate, such as patients with AD.
2. The MMN is elicited by any change in a repetitive sound pattern even when the changes are near psychophysical

thresholds. This permits determination of threshold for fine acoustic discrimination for speech or nonspeech auditory signals.
3. The MMN provides a means for studying auditory short-term memory (i.e., echoic memory), which is critical for speech processing and understanding.
4. The MMN provides an objective electrophysiologic index of acoustic discrimination ability for simple (e.g., pure tones) or complex (e.g., speech) signals. Thus, it provides a unique window to view the neurophysiologic processes underlying auditory perception in an aging population.

The future holds much promise for the MMN in studying senescent auditory changes. Gaining a better understanding of the neurophysiologic basis of speech perception using MMN will perhaps enable clinicians to develop more appropriate rehabilitative strategies (e.g., stimulus response training) and technologies (e.g., advanced signal processing in hearing aids) to remediate perceptual problems experienced by older adults with hearing impairment.

Cortical Topography Measures
Electroencephalography (EEG)

Neurophysiologic activity of the brain produces variations in its bioelectric potentials that can be recorded spatially with multiple surface electrodes. These fluctuating potentials range between 50 and 100 μV and consist of continuous rhythmic activity ranging in frequency from approximately 1 to 50 Hz (delta -0.5 to 3.5 Hz; theta -4 to 7.5 Hz; alpha -8 to 11.5 Hz; and beta; < 12 Hz). The brain waves recorded by EEG are basically produced by the electrical activity at the axosomatic synapses, axodendritic synapses, and the all-or-none action potentials in the cerebral cortex. Examination of the EEG has been useful in the identification of brain abnormalities as well as in the identification of brain-behavior relationships (Nobak & Demarest, 1975). In this connection, observations of aberrant EEG recordings in the elderly have been associated with disturbances in auditory temporal processing as well as decreases in response speed.

Over 40 years ago, Busse (1954) and his colleagues were among the first to report a diffuse, slow-wave EEG activity among the elderly. Obrist (1975) reported focal slowing as well as episodic bursts from the left anterior temporal area. The episodic bursts from the temporal region were accompanied by sharp waves and amplitude asymmetries. Earlier, Mundy-Castle (1963) had referred to such episodic bursts as "after-effects," which were noted to occur in subjects beginning at 50 years of age (Obrist & Busse, 1965). Bergman (1980) suggested that time-processing and speech-discrimination difficulties observed among the elderly may be related to "after-effects" seen in EEG recordings.

In a group of 100 subjects between 28 and 99 years of age, Surwillo (1973) found a statistical rank-order correlation between reaction time and alpha period (the time period for completion of one wave, also referred to as alpha slowing). Surwillo hypothesized that the alpha rhythms acted as, or were indicators of, central nervous timing mechanisms, since alpha slowing had been correlated linearly to increases of reaction time across age. Furthermore, he speculated that the frequency of the EEG reflected the operation of a "biological clock" within the central nervous system that determined how rapidly and effectively information could be processed. Surwillo (1963, 1964, 1966, 1973) concluded: (1) that the alpha rhythm reflected the timing or pacing mechanism of the central nervous system and (2) that slowing of alpha was directly correlated with slowing in simple reaction time as well as complex decision-making time.

Duffy, Albert, McAnulty, and Garvey (1984) studied 63 healthy males between 30 and 80 years of age and found that alpha frequency did not decrease with age. However, weak correlations were found between alpha amplitude and age ($r = 1.27; p < 0.05$). A modest relationship ($r = -0.46; p < 0.001$) between alpha reactivity (ratio of eyes-closed alpha amplitude to eyes-open amplitude) and age was observed. It has been suggested that the latter findings are the electrophysiologic correlate of the behavioral effects of declining vigilance and environmental sensitivity (Finitzo, Bartlett, & Pool, 1990).

In general, EEG studies in aging samples have pointed to diffuse increases in delta and theta activity and a slowing of the alpha rhythm. These observations, however, are not universal and have not been consistent across studies.

SPECIAL CONSIDERATION

Two major reasons for the discrepancies in age-related EEG studies include (1) the expertise in visually evaluating EEG records by the electroencephalographer and (2) the inclusion of older subjects with unrecognized disease processes (e.g., hypertension, diabetes, or arteriosclerosis), which could potentially alter EEG findings (Duffy et al, 1984).

Topographic Brain Mapping

Many of the methodologic and technical limitations associated with EEG or evoked potentials (EP) studies (e.g., visual EPs, auditory EPs, and somatosensory EPs) may be overcome through the application of topographic brain mapping. Brain mapping adds the dimension of spatial distribution of the electrical activity. Whereas conventional EP recordings display the temporal components of the response (i.e., changes in voltage as a function of time), topographic maps reveal changes in morphology of the EP as a function of scalp location of the electrodes. Topographic maps are generated using multiple electrode sites and channels. The EP data are converted to colors or shades of gray. Typically, scalp-positive voltages are represented by red colors and scalp-negative voltages are represented by blue colors. Individual maps can be generated to view voltage fields at a given time, or, consecutive maps can be generated in a serial format, called "cartooning." Voltages between electrode sites are interpolated. At present, brain mapping still remains an investigational tool, used primarily to understand the underlying origins of scalp recorded EPs and CNS disease, rather than a proven clinical test. For an excellent overview of brain mapping, the interested reader is directed to Jacobson (1994).

Duffy et al (1984) evaluated the effects of aging on mapped ALRs. Statistically significant differences were found between the 30- to 40- and 50- to 60-year-old groups. The observed differences occurred during the 152 to 172 ms. period in the left frontal polar region and during the 264 to 284 ms. period in the right frontal central- temporal region. Interestingly, these age-associated findings were correlated with alterations in verbal memory ability.

More recently, Marvel, Jerger, and Lew (1992) compared brain maps of the Pa component of the MLRs and the N1 and P2 components of the ALRs in 20 elderly males between 60 and 83 years of age. All subjects demonstrated mild to moderate sloping sensorineural hearing losses with no evidence of cognitive impairment. The group was further divided into two subsamples based on the results of the SSI test scores.

The experimental group was composed of the 10 subjects with the poorest SSI scores whereas the control group contained the 10 subjects with the highest SSI scores. MLRs and ALRs were obtained in response to 1000 Hz signals. The modes of stimulation included left ear only (LE), right ear only (RE), and binaural (BIN). AEPs were converted to gray-scale topographic maps (negative voltages assigned dark shades and positive voltages assigned light shades of gray) using a linear interpolation algorithm. Topographic brain maps for the Pa component of the MLR are displayed in Figure 6–12. As can be seen, for the experimental group an asymmetric distribution of positivity (light gray) with large amplitudes was obtained in the hemisphere contralateral to the stimulated ear. This effect was less apparent in the BIN condition and in any of the three conditions for the control group. No similar hemispheric effects were observed for the N1 or N2 components for the ALR. The authors concluded that the older subjects with reduced speech understanding may have abnormal function of the midline generator sites of the MLR. They hypothesized that perhaps selective attenuation from the midline subcortical neural generator sites of the MLR could have a subsequent effect on the temporal lobe generators, accounting for the asymmetric topographic maps in the experimental group. Further, they presumed that binaural stimulation would reduce or eliminate the asymmetric effect. Moreover, they argued that the observed asymmetry for the MLRs was not due to peripheral sensitivity differences between groups because asymmetries were not found for the ALRs. That is, if the peripheral-hearing loss was the cause of the MLR asymmetry it would also have affected the ALR.

Summary

Topographic brain-mapping techniques allow clinical scientists the potential to evaluate age-related changes in the spatial domain rather than solely in the temporal domain. However, in keeping consistent with the position statement of the American Encephalographic Society (1987), brain mapping must be considered only as an adjunctive method to conventional evoked-potential studies until further results are accumulated.

Concluding Remarks

The exact effects of aging on AEPs remain unclear. Based on the review of literature, a generalization of age-related

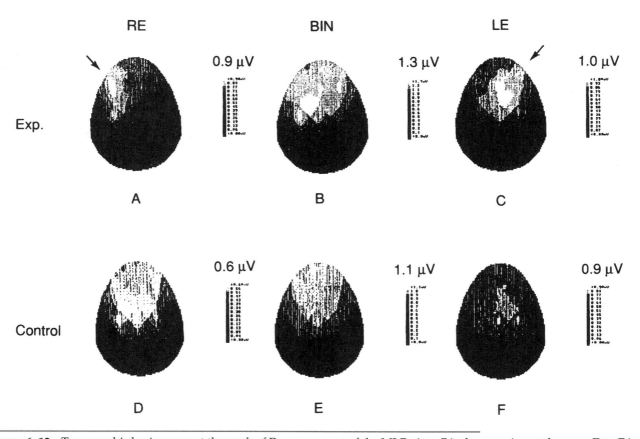

Figure 6–12 Topographic brain maps at the peak of Pa component of the MLR. A to C is the experimental group, D to F is the control group. Note asymmetry of positivity in the experimental group. When sound is presented to the RE or the LE alone, there is a greater response in the contralateral hemisphere. The effect is less evident with BIN or in any of the three modes of stimulation in the control group. (From Marvel et al, 1992, pp. 361–368. Copyright 1992 by Decker Periodicals, Hamilton, Ontario. Reprinted by permission.)

TABLE 6–1 Summary of Age-related Changes on AEPs

AEP	Parameter	Age-related change
ECochG	AP latency	Questionable
	SP/AP ratio	Questionable
ABR	Morphology	Yes
	Absolute latency	Yes
	Interpeak latency	No
	Amplitude	Yes
MLR	Absolute latency	No
	Amplitude	Yes
ALR	Absolute latency	Questionable
	Amplitude	Questionable
P300	Absolute latency	Yes
	Amplitude	Yes

Source: Adapted from Hall, 1992 and Brewer, 1987.

effects on each AEP category is presented in Table 6–1. It is important to note, however, that whereas many studies have shown age-related changes in latency and amplitude measures, the impact on clinical interpretation is equivocal. It would be prudent for the clinician to consider the effects of aging on the various AEPs in their interpretation and the interaction among age and other nonpathologic variables (e.g., hearing loss and gender). These confounding variables are discussed in the next section.

CONFOUNDING VARIABLES WHEN TESTING THE OLDER ADULT

The reliability and validity of AEP data can be compromised by a number of patient characteristics especially when testing the older adult. The clinician needs to keep in mind a few general principles during data acquisition and interpretation of results. A brief summary of these generalizations follows.

Gender

Differences between males and females have been shown to exist for the short latency responses, namely the ABR. Throughout adulthood, females show shorter latency values and larger amplitudes than males for the later ABR waves (III, IV, V, and VI). However, there is disagreement regarding the interaction of age and gender. For example, studies have shown more pronounced age-related increases in ABR latency for females than for males (Rosenhammer, Lindstrom, & Lundborg, 1981) and vice versa (Kjaer, 1980).

SPECIAL CONSIDERATION

Little is known about gender differences for the late potentials, such as auditory late responses (ALR) and the P3.

Body Temperature

Hypo- and hyperthermia exert the greatest effects on short-latency AEPs. Patients at risk for temperature aberrations include those individuals with infection (high temperature), who are comatose, or who are under the effects of alcohol or anesthesia (low temperature).

State of Arousal

The state of arousal is not a factor for the short-latency responses (ECochG or ABR), yet it can have a significant effect on the longer-latency AEPs (e.g., P3). State of arousal can change during the test situation, especially if the test session is lengthy, or if the patient is not feeling well or is medicated. Each of these conditions should be acknowledged by the clinician. For testing requiring an alert state, it may be necessary for repeated breaks or frequent prodding by the examiner.

Drugs

Drugs that influence the CNS (e.g., sedatives, anesthetic agents) have the greatest effect on longer latency, cortically generated AEPs with essentially no effect on ABR. Further,

SPECIAL CONSIDERATION

In light of polypharmacy among older adults, the potential is great that an older adult may be taking medications that can confound the results of AEP testing.

the use of ototoxic drugs (e.g., aminoglycosides, loop diuretics, cisplatin, and salicylates in high doses) places the individual at risk for a drug-induced high-frequency hearing loss, which in turn may have a greater effect on the short latency AEPs. Careful questioning of the patient and examination of the medical record (if available) prior to testing will help reveal any medications that might confound/compromise the interpretation of the obtained data. Further, if the response has greater voltage than "allowable" by the artifact reject setting, averaging of the response will be prevented, thus prolonging the test session.

Muscular Artifact

SPECIAL CONSIDERATION

One of the most prominent problems encountered by clinicians when attempting to collect AEP data in older adults is the high level of muscle artifact. Myogenic potentials are typically larger than neurogenic responses. These larger potentials may distort waveform morphology, making interpretation of the data difficult.

TABLE 6–2 Suggestions for Reducing Myogenic Artifacts from AEP Recordings

AEP	Suggestion
ECochG	1. Attempt to relax patient—explain the purpose of test
	2. Place pillow under neck if patient is lying down
	3. Encourage sleep by turning down lights
ABR	1. Attempt to relax patient—explain purpose of test
	2. Encourage sleep—turn down lights
	3. Sedate the patient
	4. Raise the high-pass filter
AMLR	1. Attempt to relax patient
	2. Encourage sleep if necessary
	3. Raise the high-pass filter cutoff frequency (rarely higher than 10 Hz)
	4. For post auricular muscle (PAM) response decrease intensity, use non-cephalic inverting electrode and reduce neck muscle tension (e.g., use of pillow)
ALR/P300	1. Attempt to relax patient, but do not encourage sleep
	2. Have patient sitting in an upright position but with both neck and head supported.

Source: Adapted from Hall, 1992.

Excessive myogenic potentials can arise from tensing the head, neck, and jaw muscles, possibly from nervousness, and/or possibly from discomfort in the testing situation. Cervical or lumbar arthritic conditions can cause discomfort if the patient needs to assume a certain position for a period of time. For example, patients required to lie in a supine position for ABR testing should be given adequate head elevation in order to reduce neck strain. Tension of the mandibular musculature, resulting from the patient wearing dentures, can be reduced by asking the patient to open his or her jaw slightly or remove the dentures (Brewer, 1987). Involuntary movement tremors (e.g., Parkinson's disease) can be a source of excessive artifact. Muscle artifact appears on the screen as a large, slow artifact. A number of suggestions for reducing myogenic artifact are provided in Table 6–2.

Hearing Loss

Sensorineural hearing loss is another factor that must be taken into account when interpreting all AEPs. The effect of hearing loss on the short latencies (ECochG and ABR) remains under debate. For example, a high-frequency

end-organ hearing loss may result in a shortened wave I–V interpeak latency. This observation stems from the fact that in an intact organ of Corti, wave I originates from the basal portion of the basil membrane and wave V from a broader portion of the basilar membrane. Therefore, if a high-frequency hearing loss exists, activity to generate an AP must originate from more apical parts of the cochlea. The

TABLE 6–3 Suggestions for Minimizing the Effects of Hearing Loss on the Interpretation of AEPs

AEP	Suggestion
ECochG	1. Increase stimulus intensity
	2. Decrease the stimulus rate
	3. Increase the number of sweeps
	4. Use transtympanic (TM) or tymptrode (TT) electrodes
ABR	1. Increase stimulus intensity
	2. Slow stimulus rate
	3. Change stimulus polarity
	4. Increase the number of sweeps
	5. Obtain multiple replicated waveforms
	6. Sum the replicated waveforms
	7. Verify ipsilateral electrode site
	8. Use ear-canal, TM, or TT electrodes
	9. Horizontal electrode array
	10. Lower high-pass filter
MLR	1. Increase stimulus intensity
	2. Use tone-burst (low- versus high-frequency) signals
	3. Slow stimulus rate
	4. Increase number of sweeps
	5. Verify that high-pass filter is less than 30 Hz
	6. Obtain multiple replicated waveforms
ALR/P300	1. Increase stimulus intensity
	2. Verify comparable hearing at rare versus frequent tone-burst stimuli

Source: Adapted from Hall, 1992.

traveling wave transmission time causes wave I to be selectively delayed with reference to wave V. Further, in severe high-frequency hearing loss, there is often a reduction in wave I and wave III amplitude, whereas wave V amplitude remains relatively unaffected. Therefore, the V/I amplitude may be artificially large. In contrast, a P3 response can be obtained at any level as long as the stimulus is 15 dB above the psychophysical threshold at the test frequency.

The challenge faced by audiologists is to distinguish between the age-related hearing loss and any pathologic conditions causing a sensorineural hearing impairment. See Table 6–3 for a few suggestions for minimizing the effects of hearing loss.

Collapsible Canals

Collapsible ear canals when using supra-aural earphones is a well-documented phenomenon associated with audiometric testing. As in behavioral audiometry, collapsing external auditory canals can cause a high-frequency conductive hearing loss, which has the potential to affect the AEP. That is, the collapsing ear canal reduces the overall intensity of the click or tonal stimuli thereby affecting the latency and amplitude of the exogenous AEPs. The most effective

PEARL

As part of the routine otoscopic examination conducted prior to AEP data acquisition, each patient should be checked for collapsed canals.

method for reducing collapsed canal artifact is to use insert tubephones. When using insert tubephones, the clinician must be aware of the associated time delay in latency calculations.

Cognition

Older adults may be at higher risk for disorders (e.g., Alzheimer's disease, dementia) that significantly alter the level of cognitive function. Altered cognitive function will impact greatly on the later responses. Therefore, it is important for the clinician to determine the mental status of the patient through the administration of mental status screenings or surveys such as the Short Portable Mental Status Questionnaire (Pfeiffer, 1975) or the Mini Mental State Examination (Folstein, Folstein, & McHugh, 1975).

CONCLUSION

AEPs provide clinicians an opportunity to evaluate the temporal processing characteristics of neural activity within the auditory pathway. In addition to all of the other stimulus (e.g., click rate, intensity) and subject recording variables (e.g., state of arousal, attention) the influence of aging poses yet another consideration when acquiring and interpreting AEP data. That is, the clinician must account for potential interactions among a variety of factors including, but not limited to, age, gender, and hearing loss. In this way, the responsible audiologist will be able to make appropriate clinical decisions regarding AEP study outcomes in the older adult.

REFERENCES

ADLER, G., ADLER, J., SCHNECK, M., & ARMBRUSTER, B. (1990). Influence of stimulation parameters on auditory stimulus processing in schizophrenia and major depression: An auditory evoked potential study. *Acta Psychiatry Scandinavia*, 85: 453–458.

ALHO, K., TERVANIEMI, M., HUOTILAINEN, M., LAVIKAINEN, J., TIITINEN, H., ILMONIEMI, R.J., KNUUTILA, J., & NÄÄTÄNEN, R. (1996). Processing of complex sounds in the human auditory cortex as revealed by magnetic brain responses. *Psychophysiology,* 33: 369–375.

ALLISON, T., HUME, A.L., WOOD, C.C., & GOFF, W.R. (1984). Developmental and aging changes in somatosensory, auditory, and visual evoked potentials. *Electroencephalography and Clinical Neurophysiology*, 58: 14–24.

AMENEDO, E., & DIAZ, F. (1988). Effects of aging on middle-latency auditory evoked potentials: A cross-sectional study. *Biological Psychiatry*, 43: 210–219.

AMERICAN ENCEPHALOGRAPHIC SOCIETY. (1987). Statement on clinical use of quantitative EEG. *Journal of Clinical Neurophysiology*, 4: 75.

ANDERER, P., PASCUAL-MARGUI, R.D., SEMLITSCH, H.V., & SALETU, B. (1998). Differential effects of normal aging on sources of standard NI, target NI, and target P300 auditory event-related brain potentials revealed by low resolution electromagnetic tomography (LORETA). *Electroencephalography and Clinical Neurophysiology,* 108: 160–174.

AREZZO, J., PICKOFF, A., & VAUGHAN, H.G., JR. (1975). The sources and intracerebral distribution of auditory evoked potentials in the alert rhesus monkey. *Brain Research*, 90: 57–73.

ATTIAS, J., FURMAN, V., SHEMESH, Z., & BRESLOFF, I. (1996). Impaired brain processing in noise-induced tinnitus patients as measured by auditory and visual event-related potentials. *Ear and Hearing*, 17: 327–333.

AZUMI, T., NAKASHIMA, K., & TAKAHASHI, K. (1995). Aging effects on auditory middle latency responses. *Electromyography and Clinical Neurophysiology*, 35: 397–401.

BALL, S.S., MARSH, J.T., SCHUBARTH, G., BROWN, W.S., & STRANDBURG, R. (1989). Longitudinal P300 latency changes in Alzheimer's disease. *Journal of Gerontology*, 44: M195–200.

BARAJAS, J.J. (1991). The effects of age on human P3 latency. *Acta Otolaryngology* 476: 157–160.

BARRETT, G., NESHIGE, R., & SHIBASAKI, H. (1987). Human auditory and somatosensory event-related potentials: Effects of response condition and age. *Electroencephalography and Clinical Neurophysiology*, 66: 409–419.

BAUMANN, S.B., ROGERS, R.L., PAPANICOLAOU, A.C., & SAYDJARI, C.L. (1990). Intersession replicability of dipole parameters from three components of the auditory evoked magnetic field. *Brain Topography*, 3: 311–319.

BEAGLEY, H.A., & SHELDRAKE, J.B. (1978). Differences in brainstem responses latency with age and sex. *British Journal of Audiology*, 12: 69–77.

BEGLEITER, H. (1979). *Evoked Brain Potentials and Behavior*. New York: Plenum Press.

BERGHOLTZ, L., HOOPER, R., & MEHTA, D. (1977). Electrocochleographic response patterns in a group of patients mainly with presbycusis. *Scandinavian Audiology*, 6: 3–11.

BERGMAN, M. (1980). *Aging and the Perception of Speech*. New York: McGraw-Hill.

BOCCA, E., & CALEARO, C. (1963). Central hearing processes. In: J. Jerger (Ed.), *Modern Developments in Audiology*, pp. 337–370. New York: Academic Press.

BREWER, C.C. (1987). Electrophysiologic measures. In: H.G. Mueller, & V.C. Geoffrey (Eds.), *Communication Disorders in Aging: Assessment and Management*, pp. 334–380. Washington, DC: Gallaudet University Press.

BRODY, H. (1955). Organization of the cerebral cortex. Part III: A study of aging in the human cerebral cortex. *Journal of Comparative Neurology*, 102: 511–556.

————. (1985). Neuronal changes with increasing age. In: H.K. Ulatowska (Ed.), *The Aging Brain: Communication in the Elderly*, pp. 23–31. Boston: College-Hill Publication.

BROWN, W., MARSH, J., & LaRUE, A. (1983). Exponential electrophysiological aging: P300 latency. *Electroencephalography and Clinical Neurophysiology*, 55: 277–285.

BUCHWALD, J.S., ERWIN, R.J., READ, S., VAN LANCKER, D., & CUMMINGS, J.L. (1989). Midlatency auditory evoked responses: Differential abnormality of P1 in Alzheimer's disease. *Electroencephalography and Clinical Neurophysiology*, 74: 378–384.

BUSSE, E.W. (1954). Studies of process of aging: VI factors that influence the psyche of elderly persons. *American Journal of Psychiatry*, 110: 897–903.

CALLAWAY, E. (1975). *Brain Electrical Potentials and Individual Psychological Differences*. New York: Grune & Stratton.

CALLAWAY, E., & HALLIDAY, R.A. (1973). Evoked potential variability: Effects of age, amplitude, and methods of measurement. *Electroencephalography and Clinical Neurophysiology*, 34: 125–133.

CAMPBELL, K.B., COURCHESNE, E., PICTON, T.W., & SQUIRES, K.C. (1979). Evoked potential correlates of human information processing. *Biological Psychology*, 8: 45–68.

CELESIA, G.G. (1976). Organization of auditory cortical areas in man. *Brain*, 99: 403–414.

CELESIA, G.G., BROUGHTON, R.J., RASMUSSEN, R., & BRACH, C. (1968). Auditory evoked responses from the exposed human cortex. *Electroencephalography and Clinical Neurophysiology*, 84: 458–466.

CHAMBERS, R.W., & GRIFFITHS, S.K. (1991). Effects of age on the adult auditory middle latency response. *Hearing Research*, 51: 1–10.

CHATRIAN, G.E., PETERSEN, M.C., & LAZARTE, J.A. (1960). Responses to clicks from the human brain: Some depth electrographic observations. *Electroencephalography and Clinical Neurophysiology*, 12: 479–489.

CHATRIAN, G.E., WIRCH, A.L., EDWARDS, K.H., LETTICH, E., & SNYDER, J.M. (1985). Cochlear summating potential to broadband clicks detected from the human external auditory meatus: A study of subjects with normal hearing for age. *Ear and Hearing*, 6: 130–338.

CHIAPPA, K.H., GLADSTONE, K.J., & YOUNG, R.R. (1979). Brainstem auditory evoked responses: Studies of waveform variations in 50 normal human subjects. *Archives of Neurology*, 36: 81–87.

CSÉPE, V., KARMOS, G., & MOLNÁR, M. (1987). Evoked potential correlates of stimulus deviance during wakefulness and sleep in cat—animal model of mismatch negativity. *Electroencephalography and Clinical Neurophysiology*, 66: 571–578.

CSÉPE, V., PANTEV, C., HOKE, M., HAMPSON, S., & ROSS, B. (1992). Evoked magnetic responses of the human auditory cortex to minor pitch changes: Localization of the mismatch field. *Electroencephalography and Clinical Neurophysiology*, 84: 538–548.

DAVIS, H. (1976). Principles of electric response audiometry. *Annals of Otology, Rhinology, and Laryngology*, 85 (Suppl 28): 1–96.

DAVIS, P.A. (1939). Effects of acoustic stimuli on the waking human brain. *Journal of Neurophysiology*, 2: 494–499.

DEBRUYNE, F. (1986). Influence of age and hearing loss on the latency shifts of the auditory brainstem response as a result of increased stimulus rate. *Audiology*, 25: 101–106.

DEOUELL, L.Y., BENTIN, S., & GIARD, M.H. (1998). Mismatch negativity in dichotic listening: evidence for interhemispheric differences and multiple generators, *Psychophysiology*, 35: 335–365.

DESMEDT, J.E., & DEBECKER, J. (1979). Waveform and neural mechanism of the decision P350 elicited without prestimulus CNV or readiness potential in random sequences of near-threshold auditory clicks and finger stimuli. *Electroencephalography and Clinical Neurophysiology*, 47: 648–670.

DONCHIN, E., & COLES, M.G.H. (1988). Is the P300 component a manifestation of context updating? *Behavioral and Brain Sciences*, 11: 357–367.

DUFFY, F., ALBERT, M., McANULTY, G., & GARVEY, A. (1984). Age-related differences in brain electrical activity of healthy subjects. *Annals of Neurology*, 16: 430–438.

DUNCAN-JOHNSON, C.C. (1981). A new metric of information processing. *Psychophysiology*, 18: 207–215.

DUNCAN-JOHNSON, C.C., & DONCHIN, E. (1977). On quantifying surprise: The variation of event-related potentials with subjective probability. *Psychophysiology*, 14: 456–467.

DUNCAN-JOHNSON, C.C., & DONCHIN, E. (1980). The relation of P300 latency to reaction time as a function of expectancy. *Progress in Brain Research*, 54: 717–722.

DUNCAN-JOHNSON, C.C., & DONCHIN, E. (1982). The P300 component of the event-related brain potential as an index of information processing. *Biological Psychology*, 14: 1–52.

DUNCAN-JOHNSON, C.C., & KOPELL, B.S. (1981). The Stroop-effect: Brain potentials localize the source of interference. *Science*, 214: 938–940.

FEIN, G., & TURETSKY, B. (1989). P300 latency variability in normal elderly: Effects of paradigm and measurement technique. *Electroencephalography and Clinical Neurophysiology*, 72: 384–394.

FINITZO, T., BARTLETT, J., & POOL, K.D. (1990). The role of topographic and quantitative electrophysiology in cognitive issues in aging. In: E. Cherow (Ed.), *Proceedings of the Research Symposium on Communication Sciences and Disorders and Aging*, pp. 158–166. ASHA Report 19. Rockville, MD: American Speech-Language-Hearing Association.

FOLSTEIN, M.F., FOLSTEIN, S.E., & MCHUGH, P.R. (1975). Mini-mental state: A practical method for grading the cognitive state of patients for the clinician. *Journal of Psychiatry Research*, 12: 189–198.

FORD, J.M., HINK, R.F., HOPKINS, W.F. III, ROTH, W.T., PFEFFERBAUM, A., & KOPELL, B.S. (1979). Age effects on event-related potentials in a selective attention task. *Journal of Gerontology*, 34: 388–395.

FORD, J., ROTH, W., MOHS, R., HOPKINS, W., & KOPELL, B. (1979). Event-related potentials recorded from young and old adults during a memory retrieval task. *Electroencephalography and Clinical Neurophysiology*, 47: 450–459.

FREEDMAN, R., WALDO, M., BICKFORD-WIMER, P., & NAGAMOTO, H. (1991). Elementary neuronal dysfunctions in schizophrenia. *Schizophrenia Research*, 4: 233–243.

FRIEDMAN, D., KAZMERSKI, V.A., & CYCOWICZ, Y.M. (1998). Effects of aging on the novelty P3 during attend and ignore oddball tasks. *Psychophysiology*, 35: 508–520.

GALAMBOS, R., & HECOX, K.E. (1978). Clinical applications of the auditory brainstem response. *Otolaryngology Clinics of North America*, 11: 709–722.

GARDI, J.N. (1985). Human brainstem and middle latency responses to electrical stimulation: A preliminary observation. In: R. Schindler & M. Merzenich (Eds.), *Cochlear Implants*, pp. 351–363. New York: Raven Press.

GIARD, M.D., PERRIN, F., PERNIER, J., & BOUCHET, P. (1990). Brain generators implicated in the processing of auditory stimulus deviance: A topographic event-related potential study. *Psychophysiology*, 27: 627–640.

GIL, R., NEAU, J.P., TOULLAT, G., RIVASSEAU, J.T., & LEFEVRE, J.P. (1989). Parkinson disease and cognitive evoked potentials. *Annual Review of Neurology* (Paris), 145: 201–207.

GOFF, W.R., ALLISON, T., & VAUGHAN, H.G., JR. (1978). The functional neuroanatomy of event-related potentials. In: E. Callaway, E. Tueting, & S. Koslow (Eds.), *Event-Related Brain Potentials in Man*, pp. 1–79. New York: Academic Press.

GOODIN, D.S. (1990). Clinical utility of long latency "cognitive" event-related potentials (P3): The pros. *Electroencephalography and Clinical Neurophysiology*, 76: 2–5.

GOODIN, D.S., SQUIRES, K.C., HENDERSON, B.H., & STARR, A. (1978). Age-related variation in evoked potentials to auditory stimulus in normal human subjects. *Electroencephalography and Clinical Neurophysiology*, 44: 447–458.

GORDON, E., RENNIE, C., & COLLINS, L. (1990). Magnetoencephalography and late component ERPs. *Clinical and Experimental Neurology*, 27: 113–120.

GRANDORI, F. (1986). Field analysis of auditory evoked brainstem potentials. *Hearing Research*, 21: 51–58.

GREGORY, R.I. (1974). Increase in neurological noise as a factor in aging. In: R.I. Gregory (Ed.), *Concepts and Mechanisms of Perception*. London: Duckworth & Co.

HALGREN, E., SQUIRES, N.K., WILSON, C.L., ROHRBAUGH, J.W., BABB, T.L., & CRANDALL, P.H. (1980). Endogenous potentials generated in the human hippocampal formation and amygdala by infrequent events. *Science*, 210: 803–805.

HALGREN, E., STAPLETON, J.M., SMITH, M., & ALTAFULLAH, I. (1986). Generators of the human scalp P3(s). In: R.Q. Cracco & I. Bodis-Wollner (Eds.), *Evoked Potentials*. New York: Liss.

HALL, J.W., III. (1992). *Handbook of Auditory Evoked Responses*. Boston: Allyn & Bacon.

HASHIMOTO, I., ISHIYAMA, Y., YOSHIMOTO, T., & NEMOTO, S. (1981). Brainstem auditory evoked potentials recorded directly from human brainstem and thalamus. *Brain*, 104: 841–859.

HECOX, K., & GALAMBOS, R. (1974). Brainstem auditory evoked responses in humans and infants and adults. *Archives of Otolaryngology*, 99: 30–33.

IRAGUI, V.J., KUTAS, M., MATCHINER, M.R., & HILLYARD, S.A. (1993). Effects of aging on event-related brain potentials and reaction times in an auditory oddball task. *Psychophysiology*, 30: 10–22.

JACOBSON, G.P. (1994). Brain mapping of auditory evoked potentials. In: J.T. Jacobson (Ed.), *Principles and Applications in Auditory Evoked Potentials*, pp. 517–540. Boston: Allyn & Bacon.

JACOBSON, G.P., & NEWMAN, C.W. (1990). The decomposition of the middle latency auditory evoked potential (MLAEP) Pa component into superficial and deep source contributions. *Brain Topography*, 2: 229–236.

JACOBSON, G.P., NEWMAN, C.W., PRIVITERA, M., & GRAYSON, A.S. (1991). Differences in superficial and deep source contributions to middle latency auditory evoked Pa component in normal subjects and patients with neurologic disease. *Journal of the American Academy of Audiology*, 2: 7–17.

JACOBSON, J.T. (1994). *Principles and Applications in Auditory Evoked Potentials*. Boston: Allyn & Bacon.

JACOBSON, J.T., & HYDE, M.L. (1985). An introduction to auditory evoked potentials. In: J. Katz (Ed.), *Handbook of Clinical Audiology*, pp. 496–533. Baltimore: Williams & Wilkins.

JAVITT, D.C., SCHROEDER, C.E., STEINSCHNEIDER, M., AREZZO, J.C., & VAUGHAN, H.G., JR. (1992). Demonstration of mismatch negativity in the monkey. *Electroencephalography and Clinical Neurophysiology*, 83: 87–90.

JERGER, J., & HALL, J.W., III. (1980). Effects of age and sex on auditory brainstem response (ABR). *Archives of Otolaryngology*, 106: 387–391.

JERGER, J., & JOHNSON, K. (1988). Interactions of age, gender, and sensorineural hearing loss on ABR latency. *Ear and Hearing*, 9: 168–176.

JEWETT, D.L., & WILLISTON, J.S. (1971). Auditory evoked far field potentials averaged from the scalp of humans. *Brain*, 4: 681–696.

JOHNSON, R., JR., & DONCHIN, E. (1985). Second thoughts: Multiple P300s elicited by a single stimulus. *Psychophysiology*, 22: 182–194.

KAUKORANTA, E., SAMS, M., HARI, R., HÄMÄLÄINEN, M., & NÄÄTÄNEN, R. (1989). Reactions of human auditory cortex to a change in tone duration. *Hearing Research*, 41: 15–21.

KENNY, R.A. (1988). Physiology of aging. In: B.B. Shadden (Ed.), *Communication Behavior and Aging: A Sourcebook for Clinicians*, pp. 58–78. Baltimore: Williams & Wilkins.

KILENY, P., PACCIORETTI, D., & WILSON, A.F. (1987). Effects of cortical lesions on middle-latency auditory evoked responses (MLR). *Electroencephalography and Clinical Neurophysiology*, 66: 108–120.

KILENY, P.R., & KEMINK, J.L. (1987). Electrically evoked middle-latency auditory potentials in cochlear implant candidates. *Archives of Otolaryngology, Head and Neck Surgery*, 113: 1072–1077.

KJAER, M. (1980). Variations of brainstem auditory evoked potentials correlated to duration and severity of multiple sclerosis. *Acta Neurologica Scandinavia*, 61: 157–166.

KNIGHT, R.T. (1984). Decreased response to novel stimuli after prefrontal lesions in man. *Electroencephalography and Clinical Neurophysiology*, 59: 9–20.

——. (1987). Aging decreases auditory event-related potentials to unexpected stimuli in humans. *Neurobiology of Aging*, 8: 109–113.

KNIGHT, R.T., SCABINI, D., WOODS, D.L., & CLAYWORTH, C. (1989). Contributions of temporal-parietal junction to the human auditory P3. *Brain Research*, 502: 109–116.

KOK, A., & LOOREN DE JONG, H. (1980). Components of the event-related potential following degraded and undegraded visual stimuli. *Biological Psychology*, 11: 117–133.

KORPILAHTI, P., & LANG, H. (1994). The auditory ERP components in mismatch negativity in dysphasic children. *Electroencephalography and Clinical Neurophysiology*, 91: 256–264.

KRAIUHIN, C., GORDON, E., STANFIELD, P., MEARES, R., & HOWSON, A. (1986). P300 and the effects of aging: Relevance to the diagnosis of dementia. *Experimental Aging Research*, 12: 187–192.

KRAUS, N., KILENY, P., & MCGEE, T. (1994). Middle latency auditory evoked potentials. In: J. Katz (Ed), *Handbook of Clinical Audiology*, pp. 387–405. Baltimore: Williams & Wilkins.

KRAUS, N., & MCGEE, T., (1994). Mismatch negativity in assessment of central auditory function. *American Journal of Audiology*, 3: 139–151.

KRAUS, N., MCGEE, T., CARRELL, T.D., & SHARMA, A. (1995). Neurophysiologic bases of speech discrimination. *Ear and Hearing*, 16: 19–38.

KRAUS, N., MCGEE, T., LITTMAN, T., NICOL, T., & KING, C. (1994). Nonprimary auditory thalamic representation of acoustic change. *Journal of Neurophysiology*, 72: 1270–1277.

KRAUS, N., MCGEE, T., MICCO, A., SHARMA, A., CARRELL, T., & NICOL, T. (1993). Mismatch negativity in school-age children to speech stimuli that are just perceptibly different. *Electroencephalography and Clinical Neurophysiology*, 88: 123–130.

KRAUS, N., MCGEE, T., SHARMA, A., CARRELL, T., & NICOL, T. (1992). Mismatch negativity event-related potential elicited by speech stimuli. *Ear and Hearing*, 13: 158–164.

KRAUS, N., OZDAMAR, O., HIER, D., & STEIN, L. (1982). Auditory middle latency responses in patients with cortical lesions. *Electroencephalography and Clinical Neurophysiology*, 54: 247–287.

KRAUS, N., SMITH, D.I., & MCGEE, T. (1988). Midline and temporal lobe MLRs in the guinea pig originate from different generator systems: A conceptual framework for new and existing data. *Electroencephalography and Clinical Neurophysiology*, 100: 1–18.

KRAUS, N., SMITH, D., REED, N.L., STEIN, L.K., & CARTEE, C. (1985). Auditory middle latency responses in children: Effects of age and diagnostic category. *Electroencephalography and Clinical Neurophysiology*, 62: 343–351.

KUHL, D. (1990). PET and P300 relationships in early Alzheimer's disease. *Neurobiology of Aging*, 11: 471–476.

KUTAS, M., & HILLYARD, S.A. (1984a). Reading senseless sentences: Brain potentials reflect semantic incongruity. *Science*, 207: 203–205.

KUTAS, M., & HILLYARD, S.A. (1984b). Brain potentials during reading reflect word expectancy and semantic association. *Nature*, 307: 161–163.

KUTAS, M., MCCARTHY, G., & DONCHIN, E. (1977). Augmenting mental chronometry: The P300 as a measure of stimulus evaluation time. *Science*, 197: 792–795.

LADMAN, K. (1996). Quotation. In: B. Lansky (Ed.), *Age Happens—The Best Quotes About Growing Older*. New York: Meadowbrook Press.

LANG, A.H., EEROLA, O., KORPILAHTI, P., HOLOPAINEN, I., SALO, S., UUSIPAIKKA, E., & AALTONEN, O. (1995). Clinical applications of the mismatch negativity. *Ear and Hearing*, 16: 117–129.

LEE, Y.S., LUEDERS, H., DINNER, D.S., LESSER, R.P., HAHN, J., & KLEMM, G. (1984). Recording of auditory evoked potentials in man using chronic subdural electrodes. *Brain*, 107: 115–131.

MAKELA, J.P., & HARI, R. (1987). Evidence for cortical origin of the 40 Hz auditory evoked response in man. *Electroencephalography and Clinical Neurophysiology*, 66: 539–546.

MARSH, J.T., SCHUBARTH, G., BROWN, W.S. RIEGE, W., STRANDBURG, R., DORSEY, D., MALTESE, A., & KUHL, D. (1990). PET and P300 relationships in early Alzheimer's disease. *Neurobiology of Aging*, 11: 471–476.

MARVEL, J.B., JERGER, J.F., & LEW H.L. (1992). Asymmetries in topographic brain maps of auditory evoked potentials in the elderly. *Journal of the American Academy of Audiology,* 3: 361–368.

MAURIZI, M., ALTISSIMI, G., OTTAVIANI, F., PALUDETTI, G., & BAMBINI, M. (1982). Auditory brainstem responses (ABR) in the aged. *Scandinavian Audiology,* 11: 213–221.

MCGEE, T., KRAUS, N., LITTMAN, T., & NICOL, T. (1992). Contributions of medial geniculate body subdivisions to the middle latency response. *Hearing Research,* 61: 147–154.

MCPHERSON, D.L. (1996). *Late Potentials of the Auditory System.* San Diego: Singular Publishing Group.

MIYAMOTO, R.T. (1986) Electrically evoked potentials in cochlear implant subjects. *Laryngoscope,* 96: 178–185.

MØLLER, A.R. (1985). Origin of latency shift of cochlear nerve potentials with sound intensity. *Hearing Research,* 17: 177–189.

MØLLER, A.R., & JANNETTA, P.J. (1981). Compound action potentials recorded intracranially from the auditory nerve in man. *Journal of Experimental Neurology,* 74: 862–874.

MØLLER, A.R., & JANNETTA, P.J. (1982a). Evoked potentials from the inferior colliculus in man. *Electroencephalography and Clinical Neurophysiology,* 53: 612–620.

MØLLER, A.R., & JANNETTA, P.J. (1982b). Comparison between intracranially recorded potentials from the human auditory nerve and scalp recorded auditory brainstem responses (ABR). *Scandinavian Audiology,* 11: 33–40.

MØLLER, A.R., & JANNETTA, P.J. (1983a). Auditory evoked potentials recorded from the cochlear nucleus and its vicinity in man. *Journal of Neurosurgery,* 59: 1013–1018.

MØLLER, A.R., & JANNETTA, P.J. (1983b). Interpretation of brainstem auditory evoked potentials: Results from intracranial recordings in humans. *Scandinavian Audiology,* 12: 125–133.

MØLLER, A.R., & JANNETTA, P.J. (1983c). Monitoring auditory functions during cranial microvascular decompression operations by direct recording from the eighth nerve. *Journal of Neurosurgery,* 59: 493–499.

MØLLER, A.R., JANNETTA, P., BENNETT, M., & MØLLER, M.B. (1981). Intracranially recorded responses from the human auditory nerve: New insights into the origin of brainstem evoked potentials. *Electroencephalography and Clinical Neurophysiology,* 52: 18–27.

MØLLER, A.R., JANNETTA, P.J., & SEKHAR, L.N. (1988). Contributions from the auditory nerve to the brainstem auditory evoked potentials (BAEPs): Results of intracranial recording in man. *Electroencephalography and Clinical Neurophysiology,* 71: 198–211.

MUNDY-CASTLE, A.C. (1963). Central excitability in the aged. In: H.T. Blumenthal (Ed.), *Medical and Clinical Aspects of Aging.* New York: Columbia University Press.

MUSIEK, F.E., & GEURKINK, N.A., (1981). Auditory brainstem and middle latency evoked response sensitivity near threshold. *Annals of Otology, Rhinology, and Laryngology,* 90: 236–240.

NÄÄTÄNEN, R. (1990). The role of attention in auditory information processing as revealed by event-related potentials and other brain measure of cognitive function. *Behavioral & Brain Sciences,* 13: 201–288.

NÄÄTÄNEN, R, GAILLARD, A.W.K., & MÄNTYSALO, S. (1978). Early selective-attention effect on evoked potential reinterpreted. *Acta Psychologica,* 42: 313–329.

NÄÄTÄNEN, R., PAAVILAINEN, P., ALHO, K., REINIKAINEN, K., & SAMS, M. (1987). The mismatch negativity to intensity changes in an auditory stimulus sequence. In: R. Johnson, R.W. Rohrbaugh, & R. Parsauraman (Eds.), *Current Trends in Event-Related Potential Research,* pp. 129–130. Amsterdam: Elsevier.

NOBACK, C.R. & DEMAREST, R.J. (1975). *The Human Nervous System.* New York: McGraw-Hill.

OBRIST, W.D. (1975). Cerebral physiology of the aged: Relation of psychological function. In: V.R. Burch, & H. Altshuler (Eds.), *Behavior and Brain Electrical Activity.* New York: Plenum Press.

OBRIST, W.D., & BUSSE, E.W. (1965). The electroencephalogram in old age. In: W.P. Wilson (Ed.), *Application of Electroencephalography in Psychiatry.* Durham: Duke University Press.

O'CONNOR, T.A., & STARR, A. (1985). Intracranial potentials correlated with an event-related potential, P300, in the cat. *Brain Research,* 339: 27–38.

OKU, T., & HASEGEWA, M. (1997). The influence of aging on auditory brainstem response and electrocochleography in the elderly. *Journal of Oto-Rhino-Laryngology & Its Related Specialties,* 59: 141–146.

OLLO, C., JOHNSON, R.J., & GRAFMAN, J. (1991). Signs of cognitive change in HIV disease: An event-related brain potential study. *Neurology,* 41: 209–215.

OTTO, W.C., & MCCANDLESS, G.A. (1982). Aging and the auditory brainstem response. *Audiology,* 21: 466–473.

PAAVILAINEN, P., ALHO, K., REINIKAINEN, K., SAMS, M., & NÄÄTÄNEN, R. (1991). Right hemisphere dominance of different mismatch negativities. *Electroencephalography and Clinical Neurophysiology,* 78: 466–479.

PAAVILAINEN, P., KARLSSON, M.L., REINIKAINEN, K., & NÄÄTÄNEN, R. (1989). Mismatch negativity to changes in spatial location of an auditory stimulus. *Electroencephalography and Clinical Neurophysiology,* 73: 129–141.

PALLER, K.A., ZOLA, M.S., SQUIRE, L.R., & HILLYARD, S.A. (1988). P3-like brain waves in normal monkeys and in monkeys with medial temporal lesions. *Behavioral Neuroscience,* 102: 714–725.

PALUDETTI, G., MAURIZI, M., D'ALATRI, L, & GALLI, J. (1991). Relationships between middle latency auditory responses (MLR) and speech discrimination tests in the elderly. *Acta Otolaryngologica* (Stockholm), 476: 105–109.

PANG, S., BOROD, J.C., HERNANDEZ, A., BODIS, W.I., RASKIN, S., MYLIN, L., COSCIA, L., & YAHR, M.D. (1990). The auditory P300 correlates with specific cognitive deficits in Parkinson's disease. *Journal of Neural Transmission. Parkinson's Disease and Dementia Section,* 2: 249–264.

PAPANICOLAOU, A.C., BAUMANN, S., ROGERS, R.L., SAYDJARI, C., AMPARO, E.G., & EISENBERG, H.M. (1990). Localization of auditory response sources using magnetoencephalography and magnetic resonance imaging. *Archives of Neurology*, 47: 33–37.

PATTERSON, J.V., MICHALEWSKI, H.J., & STARR, A. (1988). Latency variability of the components of auditory event-related potentials to infrequent stimuli in aging, Alzheimer-type dementia, and depression. *Electroencephalography and Clinical Neurophysiology*, 71: 450–460.

PEKKONEN, E.V., JOUSMÄKI, V., PARTANEN, J., & KARHU, J. (1993). Mismatch negativity area and age-related auditory memory. *Electroencephalography and Clinical Neurophysiology*, 87: 321–325.

PFEFFERBAUM, A., FORD, J.M., ROTH, W.T., & KOPELL, B.S. (1980). Age-related changes in auditory event-related potentials. *Electroencephalography and Clinical Neurophysiology*, 49: 266–276.

PFEFFERBAUM, A., FORD, J.M., ROTH, W.T., HOPKINS, W.F., & KOPELL, B.S. (1979). Event-related potential changes in healthy aged females. *Electroencephalography and Clinical Neurophysiology*, 46: 81–86.

PFEFFERBAUM, A., WENEGRAT, B.G., FORD, J.M., ROTH, W.T., & KOPELL, B.S. (1984). Clinical application of the P3 component of event-related potentials: II. Dementia, depression, and schizophrenia. *Electroencephalography and Clinical Neurophysiology*, 59: 104–124.

PFEIFFER, E. (1975). A short portable mental status questionnaire for the assessment of organic brain deficit in elderly patients. *Journal of the American Geriatrics Society*, 23: 433–441.

PICTON, T.W., & FITZGERALD, P.G. (1983). A general description of the human auditory evoked potentials. In: E.J. Moore (Ed.), *Bases of Auditory Brainstem Responses*, pp. 141–156. New York: Grune & Stratton.

PICTON, T.W., HILLYARD, S.A., KRAUSZ, H.I., & GALAMBOS, R. (1974). Human auditory evoked potentials. I: Evaluation of the components. *Electroencephalography and Clinical Neurophysiology*, 36: 179–190.

PICTON, T.W., STAPELLS, D.R., PERRAULT, N., BARIBEAU-BRAUN, J., & STUSS, D.T. (1984). Human event-related potentials: Current perspectives. In: R.H. Nodar & C. Barber (Eds.), *Evoked Potentials II: The Second International Evoked Potentials Symposium*, pp. 3–16. Boston: Butterworth.

PICTON, T.W., WOODS, D.L., BARIBEAU-BRAUN, J., & HEALEY, T.M.G. (1977). Evoked potential audiometry. *The Journal of Otolaryngology* (Toronto), 6: 90–119.

PINEDA, J.A., FOOTE, S.L., & NEVILLE, H.J. (1989). Effects of locus caeruleus lesions on auditory, long-latency, event-related potentials in monkey. *Journal of Neuroscience*, 9: 81–93.

POLICH, J., HOWARD, L., & STARR, A. (1985a). Effects of age on the P300 component of the event-related potentials from auditory stimuli: Peak definition, variation, and measurement. *Journal of Gerontology*, 40: 721–726.

POLICH, J., HOWARD, L., & STARR, A. (1985b). Stimulus frequency and masking as determinants of P300 latency in event-related potentials from auditory stimuli. *Biological Psychology*, 21: 309–318.

POLICH, J., LADISH, C., & BLOOM, F.E. (1990). P300 assessment of early Alzheimer's disease. *Electroencephalography and Clinical Neurophysiology*, 77: 179–189.

POLLOCK, V.E., & SCHNEIDER, L.S. (1989). Effects of tone stimulus frequency on late positive component activity (P3) among normal elderly subjects. *International Journal of Neuroscience*, 45: 127–132.

PSATTA, D.M., & MATEI, M. (1988). Age-dependent amplitude variation of brainstem auditory evoked potentials. *Electroencephalography and Clinical Neurophysiology*, 71: 27–32.

RABBITT, P.M.A. (1965). Age discrimination between complex stimuli. In: A.T. Welford & J.E. Birren (Eds.), *Behavior, Aging, and the Nervous System*, pp. 35–53. Springfield, IL: Charles C. Thomas.

RITCHIE, J.M. (1982). Some pathophysiological aspects of neuronal aging. In: R.D. Terry, C.L. Bolis, G. Toffano (Eds.), *Neural Aging and Its Implications in Human Neurological Pathology, Aging* Vol. 18, pp. 89–98. New York: Raven Press.

RITTER, W., SIMSON, R., & VAUGHAN, H.G., JR. (1972). Association cortex potentials and reaction time in auditory discrimination. *Electroencephalography and Clinical Neurophysiology*, 33: 547–555.

RITTER, W., VAUGHAN, H.G., & COSTA, L.D. (1968). Orienting and habituation to auditory stimuli: A study of short-term changes in average evoked responses. *Electroencephalography and Clinical Neurophysiology*, 25: 550–556.

ROSENBERG, C., NUDLEMAN, K., & STARR, A. (1985). Cognitive evoked potentials in early Huntington's disease. *Archives of Neurology*, 42: 984–987.

ROSENHALL, U., BJORKMAN, G., PEDERSEN, K., & KALL, A. (1985). Brainstem auditory evoked potentials in different age groups. *Electroencephalography and Clinical Neurophysiology*, 62: 426–430.

ROSENHALL, U., PEDERSEN, K., & DOTEVALL, M. (1986). Effects of presbycusis and other types of hearing loss on auditory brainstem responses. *Scandinavian Audiology*, 15: 179–185.

ROSENHAMER, H.J., LINDSTROM, B., & LUNDBORG, T. (1980). On the use of click-evoked electric brainstem responses in audiological diagnosis. II: Influence of sex and age upon normal response. *Scandinavian Audiology*, 9: 93–100.

ROSENHAMER, H., LINDSTROM, B., & LUNDBORG, T. (1981). On the use of click-evoked electric brainstem responses in audiological diagnosis. III: Latencies in cochlear hearing loss. *Scandinavian Audiology*, 10: 3.

ROTHENBERGER, A., SZIRTES, J., & JURGENS, R. (1982). Auditory evoked potentials to verbal stimuli in healthy, aphasic, and right hemisphere damaged subjects. *Archives of Psychiatry and Neurological Sciences*, 231: 155–170.

ROWE, M.J., III. (1978). Normal variability of the brainstem auditory evoked response in young and old adult subjects. *Electroencephalography and Clinical Neurophysiology*, 44: 459–470.

RYAN, J.N., & SANDRIDGE, S.A. (1993). Effects of older age and stimulus rate on ABR spectra. Paper presented at the

American Speech-Language-Hearing Association Convention, Anaheim, CA.

SALAMY, A., & MCKEAN, C.M. (1976). Postnatal development of human brainstem potentials during the first year of life. *Electroencephalography and Clinical Neurophysiology*, 41: 418–426.

SAMS, M., PAAVILAINEN, P., ALHO, K., & NÄÄTÄNEN, R. (1985). Auditory frequency discrimination and event-related potentials. *Electroencephalography and Clinical Neurophysiology*, 62: 437–448.

SANDRIDGE, S.A. (1988). The event-related potential "P3": A central auditory test for older adults? Unpublished Ph.D. diss., University of Florida, Gainesville.

SANDRIDGE, S.A., & BOOTHROYD, A. (1996). Using naturally produced speech to elicit the mismatch negativity. *Journal of the American Academy of Audiology*, 7: 105–112.

SCHERG, M., & VOLK, S.A. (1983). Frequency specificity of simultaneously recorded early and middle latency auditory evoked potentials. *Electroencephalography and Clinical Neurophysiology*, 56: 443–452.

SCHERG, M., & VON CRAMON, D. (1985). Two bilateral sources of late AEP as identified by a spatiotemporal dipole model. *Electroencephalography and Clinical Neurophysiology*, 62: 32–44.

SCHERG, M., & VON CRAMON, D. (1986). Evoked dipole source potentials of the human auditory cortex. *Electroencephalography and Clinical Neurophysiology*, 65: 344–360.

SCHROEDER, M.M., LIPTON, R.B., RITTER, W., GIESSER, B.S., & VAUGHAN, H.G., JR. (1995). Event-related potential correlates of early processing in normal aging. *International Journal of Neuroscience*, 80: 371–382.

SCHROGER, E., NÄÄTÄNEN, R., & PAAVILAINEN, P. (1992). Event-related potentials reveal how nonattended complex sound patterns are represented by the human brain. *Neuroscience Letter*, 146: 183–186.

SCHUCKNECHT, H.F. (1955). Presbycusis. *Laryngoscope*, 65: 402–419.

———. (1964). Further observations on the pathology of presbycusis. *Archives of Otolarynology*, 80: 369–382.

———. (1974). *Pathology of the Ear*. Cambridge, MA: Harvard University Press.

SCHUKNECHT, H.F. (1975). Pathophysiology of Ménière's disease. *Otolaryngologic Clinics of North America*, 8: 507–514.

SCHULMAN-GALAMBOS, C., & GALAMBOS, R. (1975). Brainstem auditory evoked responses in premature infants. *Journal of Speech and Hearing Research*, 18: 456–465.

SCHWARTZ, D.M., MORRIS, M.D., & JACOBSON, J.T. (1994). The normal auditory brainstem response and its variance. In: J.T. Jacobson (Ed.), *Principles and Applications in Auditory Evoked Potentials*, pp. 123–154. Boston: Allyn & Bacon.

SHOCK, N.W. (1983). Aging of regulatory mechanism. In: R.D.T. Cape, R.M. Coe, & I. Rossman (Eds.), *Fundamentals of Geriatric Medicine*, pp. 51–62. New York: Raven Press.

SIMSON, R., VAUGHAN, H.G., & RITTER, W. (1976). The scalp topography of potentials associated with missing visual or auditory stimuli. *Electroencephalography and Clinical Neurophysiology*, 40: 33–42.

SIMSON, R., VAUGHAN, H.G., & RITTER, W. (1977a). The scalp topography of potentials in auditory and visual go/no go tasks. *Electroencephalography and Clinical Neurophysiology*, 43: 864–875.

SIMSON, R., VAUGHAN, H.G., & RITTER, W. (1977b). The scalp topography of potentials in auditory and visual discrimination tasks. *Electroencephalography and Clinical Neurophysiology*, 42: 528–535.

SKINNER, P., & GLATTKE, T.J. (1977). Electrophysiologic responses and audiometry: State of the art. *Journal of Speech and Hearing Disorders*, 42: 179–198.

SMITH, D.B.D., MICHALEWSKI, H.J., BRENT, G.A., & THOMPSON, L.W. (1980). Auditory averaged evoked potentials and aging: Factors of stimulus, task, and topography. *Biological Psychology*, 11: 135–151.

SPINK, U., JOHANNSEN, H.S., & PIRSIG, W. (1979). Acoustically evoked potential: Dependence upon age. *Scandinavian Audiology*, 8: 11–14.

SPIVAK, L.G., & MALINOFF, R. (1990). Spectral differences in the ABRs of old and young subjects. *Ear and Hearing*, 11: 351–358.

SQUIRES, K.C., CHIPPENDALE, T.J., WREGE, K.S., GOODIN, D.S., & STARR, A. (1980). Electrophysiological assessment of mental function in aging and dementia. In: L. Poon (Ed.), *Aging in the 1980s: Psychological Issues*, pp. 125–134. Washington, DC: American Psychological Association.

SQUIRES, K.C., WICKENS, C., SQUIRES, N.K., & DONCHIN, E. (1976). The effects of stimulus sequence on the waveform of the cortical event-related potential. *Science*, 153: 1142–1145.

SQUIRES, N.K., SQUIRES, K.C., & HILLYARD, S.A. (1975). Two varieties of long-latency positive waves evoked by unpredictable auditory stimuli in man. *Electroencephalography and Clinical Neurophysiology*, 38: 387–401.

STAPELLS, D.R., GALAMBOS, R., COSTELLO, J.A., & MAKEIG, S. (1988). Inconsistency of auditory middle latency and steady-state responses in infants. *Electroencephalography and Clinical Neurophysiology*, 71: 289–295.

STARR, A, & ACHOR, L. (1975). Auditory brainstem responses in neurological disease. *Archives of Neurology*, 32: 761–768.

STOCKARD, J.J., & ROSSITER, V. (1977). Clinical and pathologic correlates of brain stem auditory response abnormalities. *Neurology*, 27: 316–325.

STOCKARD, J.J., STOCKARD, J.E., & SHARBROUGH, F.W. (1977). Detection and localization of occult lesions with brainstem auditory responses. *Mayo Clinic Proceedings*, 52: 761–769.

STRAYER, D.L., WICHENS, C.D., & BRAUNE, R. (1987). Adult age differences in the speed and capacity of information processing. 2: An electrophysiological approach. *Psychology of Aging*, 2: 99–110.

SURWILLO, W.W. (1963). The relation of simple response time to brain wave frequency and the effects of age. *Electroencephalography and Clinical Neurophysiology*, 15: 105–114.

———. (1964). The relation of decision time to brain wave frequency and to age. *Electroencephalography and Clinical Neurophysiology*, 16: 510–514.

————. (1966). On the relation of latency of alpha attention to alpha rhythm frequency and the influence of age. *Electroencephalography and Clinical Neurophysiology*, 20: 129–132.

————. (1973). Choice reaction time and speed of information processing in old age. *Perceptual & Motor Skills*, 36: 321–322.

Sutton, S., Braren, M., Zubin, J., & John, E.R. (1965). Evoked potential correlates of stimulus uncertainty. *Science*, 150: 1187–1188.

Syndulko, K., Hansch, E.C., Cohen, S.N., Pearce, J.W., Goldberg, Z., Monton, B., Tourtellotte, W.W., & Potvin, A.R. (1982). Long-latency event-related potentials in normal aging and dementia. In: J. Courjon, F. Mauguiere, and M. Revol (Eds.), *Clinical Applications of Evoked Potentials in Neurology*, pp. 279–285. New York: Raven Press.

Talland, G. A. (1968). *Human Aging and Behavior*. New York: Academic Press.

Tiitinen, H., Alho, K., Huotilainen, M., Ilmoniemi, R.J., Simola, J., & Näätänen, R. (1993). Tonotopic auditory cortex and the magnetoencephalographic (MEG) equivalent of the mismatch negativity. *Psychophysiology*, 30: 537–540.

Toffano, G., Calderini, G., Battistella, A., Scapagnini, U., Gaitia, A., Ponzio, F., Algeri, S., & Crews, F. (1982). Biochemical changes related to neurotransmission in the aging brain. In: R.D. Terry, C.L. Bolis, & G. Toffano (Eds.),

Neural Aging and Its Implications in Human Neurological Pathology, Aging Vol. 18, pp. 119–128. New York: Raven Press.

Trune, D.R., Mitchell, C., & Phillips, D.S. (1988). The relative importance of head size, gender, and age on the auditory brainstem response. *Hearing Research*, 32: 165–174.

Tueting, P., Sutton, S., & Zubin, J. (1970) Quantitative evoked potential correlates of the probability of events. *Psychophysiology*, 7: 385–394.

Wood, C.C., Allison, T., Goff, W., Williamson, P., & Spencer, D. (1980). On the neural origin of P300 in man. *Progress in Brain Research*, 54: 51–56.

Wood, C.C., & Wolpaw, J.R. (1982). Scalp distribution of human evoked potentials. II: Evidence for overlapping sources and involvement of auditory cortex. *Electroencephalography and Clinical Neurophysiology*, 54: 25–38.

Woods, D.L., & Clayworth, C.C. (1986). Age-related changes in human middle latency auditory evoked potentials. *Electroencephalography and Clinical Neurophysiology*, 65: 297–303.

Yamada, O., Yagi, T., Yamane, H., & Suzuki, J.I. (1975). Clinical evaluation of the auditory evoked brainstem response. *Auris-Nasus-Larynz*, 2: 97–105.

Yamaguchi, S., & Knight, R.T. (1991). Age effects on the P300 to novel somatosensory stimuli. *Electroencephalography and Clinical Neurophysiology*, 78: 297–301.

Yingling, C.D., & Hosobuchi, Y. (1984). A subcortical correlate of P300 in man. *Electroencephalography and Clinical Neurophysiology*, 59: 72–76.

Chapter 7

Aging and the Balance Control Systems

Jaynee H. Calder

I am so afraid that I am going to get dizzy and that my husband will not hear me scream if I fall, because he refuses to wear his hearing aids around the house.

—R.D., 78-year-old retired professor

I smoke cigars because at my age if I don't have something to hang on to I might fall down.

—George Burns, 1996

LEARNING OBJECTIVES

After reading this chapter, you should be able to:

- Be more aware of the prevalence of falls and dizziness among older adults.
- Gain an understanding of the age-related changes in the structure and function of the vestibular system.
- Be conversant with the tests used to assess balance function in older adults including electronystagmography, rotational tests, and dynamic posturography.
- Understand how aging impacts on normative values on tests of balance function and on the interpretation of test results.
- Have access to a test protocol for assessing balance function of older adults.

Two problems frequently experienced by aging people are dizziness and falls (Dewane, 1995). The National Safety Council reported that in 1991 falls were the second leading cause of accidental deaths in the United States, and that, among people 75 years and older, falls were the leading cause of accidental death (Kippenbrock & Soja, 1993). Researchers have estimated that between one-third and one-half of older adults experience falls each year, with as many as 15% resulting in serious physical injury (Coogler, 1992; Ginter & Mion, 1992). Interestingly, the incidence of falls increases with age such that 22% of adults between 65 and 69 years, 31% of adults between 75 and 79 years, and 40% of adults between 80 and 84 years report falling. Over one-third of falls in the elderly are caused by dizziness (Cutson, 1994). Sloane, George, and Blazer (1989) reported that approximately one-fifth of community-living elders experience dizziness severe enough to warrant medical attention or to impair daily activities and that dizziness has been reported to be the most common complaint of patients aged 75 years and older in medical practices of internists and family physicians (Sloane, 1989). Boult, Murphy, Sloane, Mor, & Drone (1991) studied the relationship between dizziness, functional disability within two years, and death in a group of 3798 elderly Americans, and found that dizziness is predictive of functional decline, but not mortality. Similarly, gait and balance disturbances are associated with significant psychosocial sequelae, including loss of self-esteem, loss of autonomy, and depression (Tedeiksaar, 1998).

Audiologists are becoming more involved in the management of dizzy patients, both in terms of performing tests of balance function that are used by physicians in making a medical diagnosis, and in terms of providing nonmedical treatments to chronically dizzy or unsteady patients. As the population ages, a higher proportion of the caseload consists of older adults. Audiologists rarely receive extensive training in vestibular system anatomy and physiology in general, and as related to tests designed to evaluate vestibular function in particular. In turn, little emphasis is placed on the effects of normal aging on the status of the vestibular function, or the impact of those normal changes on test performance and function. The purpose of this chapter is to briefly review the normal aging effects on the anatomy and physiology of the systems involved in the maintenance of balance. Further, the goal is to discuss the various clinical tools available to evaluate balance function and the effects of age-related changes on test outcome. Finally, the chapter will conclude with a protocol to be used in evaluating balance function in older adult patients.

Geriatric Audiology. B.E. Weinstein. Thieme Medical Publishers, Inc., New York © 2000

STRUCTURAL CHANGES WITH AGING

The basic task of balance, which involves the condensation of the visual vestibular and proprioceptive systems, is to maintain the body's center of gravity (Tedeiksaar, 1998).

SPECIAL CONSIDERATION

The vestibular system, like the auditory system, undergoes degenerative changes with age.

Similar to the auditory system, the neuronal and sensory cells in the vestibular system are nonmitotic. As such, they are highly differentiated cells that cannot reproduce during adulthood. Their lifespan is determined by the ability to maintain structural organization within the tissue environment in which they reside. Degenerative changes have been demonstrated throughout the entire vestibular system, with the components of the peripheral vestibular system undergoing change to different degrees. Specifically, the utricular maculae are apparently less affected than are the cristae ampullares and the saccular maculae. Within the vestibular system, significant degenerative changes have been demonstrated in the otoconia, the vestibular epithelium, the vestibular nerve, Scarpa's ganglion, and the cerebellum. The specific changes reported to occur within the vestibular system are discussed in the following sections. Figure 7–1 shows the normal vestibular system, including the membranous semicircular canals, endolymphatic sac, utricle, saccule, cochlear duct, heliocotrema, perilymphatic duct, round and oval windows, and ampulla.

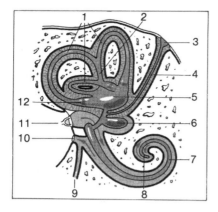

Figure 7–1 Normal vestibular system: 1, membranous semicircular canals (horizontal, superior, and posterior); 2, crus commune of the posterior and superior canal; 3, saccus endolymphaticus on the posterior surface of the pyramid; 4, ductus endolymphaticus; 5, utricle; 6, saccule; 7, cochlear duct; 8, helicotrema; 9, perilymphatic duct; 10, round window; 11, oval window; 12, ampulla of the posterior semicircular canal with a cupula. (Data from Becker, Naumann, and Pfaltz, 1994.)

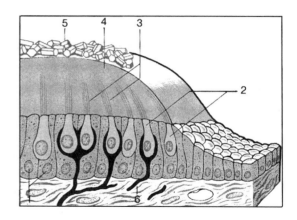

Figure 7–2 Diagram of a static macula: 1, supporting cells; 2, sensory cells; 3, cilia; 4, statolith membrane; 5, statoliths; 6, afferent nerve fibers. (Data from Becker, Naumann, and Pfaltz, 1994.)

Sensory Receptors

Johnsson (1971) reported evidence of age-related degeneration in the sensory cells in the cristae of the semicircular canals and the maculae of the saccule and utricle. Richter (1980) reported decreased cell density in the vestibular receptors after the age of 50, with more noticeable degeneration present in the saccule and cristae than in the utricle. In the cristae, the hair-cell population remains stable until age 40 years (Rosenhall, 1972; Engstrom, Bergstrom, & Rosenhall, 1974), after which there is a significant decrease in the cell population, eventually resulting in an average 40% loss in individuals over 70 years of age (Rosenhall, 1973). Some specimens demonstrated as much as a 60% loss of hair cells. After age 70, there is as much as 40% reduction of hair cells in the semicircular canals (Tedeiksaar, 1998). Further, when comparing the number of macular hair cells of subjects aged 17 to 40 years with those of subjects over 70 years of age, Rosenhall (1973) found a 21% reduction for utricular maculae and a 24% for saccular maculae. Figure 7–2 shows a static macula, the site of age-related degeneration. While the periphery of the cristae is much less affected than the summit, the entire macula appears to be affected.

Ross, Johnsson, Peacor, and Allard (1976) reported that the effects of aging on otoconia include decreased numbers, particularly in the saccule. Moving anteriorly from the posterior part of the macula, otoconia progress from pit formation to the assumption of a fibrous appearance. Subsequently, the mid-portion disappears, and finally the otoconia become fragmented. Migration of fragmented otoconial debris into the ampulla of the posterior semicircular canal has been implicated as a cause of positional balance disturbances in older adults (Schuknecht, 1969).

Using light and electron microscopy, researchers have demonstrated distinct nuclear and cytoplasmic changes in the labyrinths of aging animals and humans. Specifically, these changes include: cell shrinkage, changes in stereocilia and kinocilia including cilia loss, disarrangement, fusion, and formation of giant cilia, formation of inclusion bodies, and vesicle formation. Rosenhall and Rubin (1975) reported that sensory hair loss in elderly human specimens may be related either to chemical changes in the cupula resulting in the cilia becoming tethered in the cupular canals, or to a preparation artifact arising from an increased fragility of the stereociliar attachment on to the cuticular plate. Loss of cilia affects the hair cells of the cristae less than those of the maculae. Apical osmiophilic inclusions of the maculae, especially in the type I hair cells, were noted as well. Because of these inclusions, the striola in the elderly appear as dark stripes.

Engstrom, Ades, Engstrom, Gilchrist, & Bourne (1977) reported on findings observed in the ears of old monkeys, and compared them with what had been described already in older adults. They reported that there is evidence of degeneration in the vestibular sensory epithelia in both older adults and monkeys. There is strong evidence that, in monkeys, type I hair cells may be more vulnerable to senescent changes than type II cells. One constant finding reported is the presence of laminated structures in both the sensory and the supporting cells. Another is the appearance of vesicular structures, especially in the supporting cells. Modifications of sensory hairs such as fusion, appearance of modified kinocilia, and "bleb" formations were also reported. Finally, they reported the occurrence of modifications in synaptic membranes appearing as patchy, dark, irregular areas at the base of type I cells.

Vestibular Nerve

There is lack of agreement regarding changes in the number of nerve fibers with aging. In an often cited study, Bergstrom (1973) counted nerve fibers in 11 individuals ranging in age from birth to 85 years. Her sample population was free of vestibular disorders and had no history of treatment with ototoxic drugs or radiation therapy to the head. The author reported a significant decrease in the number of vestibular nerve fibers with increasing age. Specifically, when comparing the young group (≤ 35 years of age) to those 75 years and older, a 37% reduction was noted. She also reported a selective loss of thick myelinated fibers, particularly in the ampullary nerve branches containing fibers from the semicircular canals. It is logical to assume that this loss may explain in part a decrease in conduction velocity notable with age.

In a more recent study, however, Fujii, Goto, and Kikuchi (1990) used a new technique for studying the human vestibulocochlear nerve in cadaver preparations. Specimens were harvested from one 24-year-old and two individuals from each of the fifth through tenth decades of life. For measuring nerve fibers, three sampling sites on each nerve were selected. In this study, the number of vestibular nerve fibers reported ranged from 13,996 to 20,760. This number is consistent with other investigations. While most of the thick fibers appeared to be myelinated, there were some unmyelinated fibers that were not included in the counts. In this recent study, the number of nerve fibers did not appear to decrease with age, nor did the average size of the axons in the vestibular nerve. When discussing the differences in the age-related findings between their data and those of Bergstrom (1973), Fujii, Goto, and Kikuchi (1990) reported that the discrepancy may be due to differences in sample size and counting techniques.

Fujii, Goto, and Kikuchi (1990) also studied axonal shape and reported that vestibular nerve axons were generally circular or oval, with no club-shaped, crescent-shaped, or asterisk-shaped axons found. However, they reported that amyloid bodies (i.e., abnormal intercellular products) were found in the transverse sections of the vestibulocochlear nerve of every individual except the 24-year-old, and there was a slight increase in the number with age. Richter (1980) reported a decrease in the number of cells in Scarpa's ganglion after age 60 years. He also concluded that hair-cell degeneration precedes neuronal degeneration at Scarpa's ganglion.

Central Vestibular Structures

Generally, studies of human brainstem nuclei have not demonstrated a decrease in numbers of neuronal cells with age, although structural and metabolic variations do develop (Babin & Harker, 1982). Similarly, significant loss of neurons in the flocculonodular lobe of the cerebellum have not been reported, although cell loss in the cerebellar vermis has been demonstrated. Torvik, Torp, Lindboe (1986) studied 67 adult males, and they reported frequent atrophy in the vermis with advancing age, as well as decreased numbers and density of Purkinje cells. Hall, Miller, and Corsellis (1975) reported a 25% reduction in the number of Purkinje cells from birth to the tenth decade, with the most rapid neuronal loss after age 60. Purkinje cell loss is highly variable among individuals, with some retaining normal numbers of cells into their 90s.

In a recent investigation, Lopez, Honrubia, and Baloh (1997) studied age-related effects on the human vestibular nerve complex (VNC). Specifically, the purpose of their investigation was to document quantitative morphometric changes within the VNC in humans as a function of age. To that end, the VNC of normal human subjects was examined using computer-based microscopy. Neuronal counts, neuronal density, and nuclear length of each of the four vestibular nuclei were determined for 15 normal individuals, age 40 to 93 years. Overall, a 3% neuronal loss per decade was documented. Additionally, VNC volume and nuclear density decreased significantly with age, although to a lesser degree than did neuron number. Furthermore, neuronal loss was greatest in the superior vestibular nucleus, and least in the medial vestibular nucleus. Interestingly, despite the overall decrease in neuron number, the number of giant neurons increased in older adults. Overall, the rate of neuronal loss in the VNC is comparable to that previously observed in hair cells, primary vestibular neurons, and cerebellar Purkinje cells, but is in contrast to previous reports of no age-related loss of neurons in other brainstem nuclei.

Examination of vestibular nerve synapses revealed changes in the synaptic bars in humans over age 40 years (Engstrom, Bergstrom, & Rosenhall, 1974). When counting synapses in the molecular layer of the cerebellar vermis of rats, Glick and Bondareff (1979) noted a 24% decrease in the axodendritic synapses with age. This loss appeared to be selective, affecting dendritic spines and sparing synapses involving shafts.

There is a great deal of evidence from animal studies that age-related changes in vestibular nerve electrophysiology do take place. Rogers, Silver, Shoemaker, and Bloom (1980) identified a three- to five-fold decrease in the spontaneous firing rate of parallel fibers with age, with stable activity of climbing fibers across all ages. Additionally, Rogers, Zornetzer, and Bloom (1981) reported changes in electrophysiology including a two-fold increase in the threshold current required to initiate a discharge by Purkinje cells, slower conduction velocities, reduced-response amplitudes, longer refractory periods after discharge, and increased resistance to inhibitory stimuli.

Vascular Supply

Studies of the vasculature of the human inner ear have revealed arteriolar narrowing, loss of capillaries, and thickening of the walls of small arterioles (Jorgensen, 1961; Johnson & Hawkins, 1972; Johnsson, 1973). Interestingly, while the vasculature of the vestibular system does change with aging, the vestibular end organs appear to be less affected than the cochlear end organ. Within the vestibular system, the semicircular canals show the most obvious changes, with atrophy of the capillaries crossing the perilymphatic spaces (Johnsson, 1973). The largest vessels do not exhibit age-related changes.

SPECIAL CONSIDERATION

In addition to considering vascular changes within the vestibular organs themselves, it is important to remember that all three of the sensory systems involved in the maintenance of balance, as well as the central nervous system (CNS) portions, are susceptible to acquired pathologic and pathophysiologic changes in the blood vascular system. It is equally important to consider that it is difficult to discretely separate the effects of vascular insufficiency from those of primary degenerative processes (Babin & Harker, 1982).

In conclusion, progressive deterioration in the structures of the peripheral and central vestibular system as a function of age has been well documented. One might expect that the effect of these changes would be reduced efficiency in performance of motor activities depending on vestibular input (Nadol & Schuknecht, 1989). In an older person, this loss of vestibular function is part of a multisensory deterioration of function. Specifically, in addition to vestibular deficits, there may be reductions in vision, proprioception, muscle strength, joint mobility, and overall CNS function. All of these factors, which have been discussed in Chapter 2, may impact on the sense of stability and equilibrium.

In the following sections, tests of balance function, the impact of age-related changes within the vestibular system on function, and changes in the function of the other systems involved in maintenance of postural control will be discussed.

TESTS OF BALANCE FUNCTION

Maintenance of postural control and balance is affected by input and integration of information from the vestibular, visual, and somesthetic systems. Figure 7–3 shows the oculomotor system. Under normal circumstances, the visual and somesthetic systems interact with the vestibular system and support balance by providing the brain with information about the location of the body in space. Together these systems, with the efferent activity to muscles of the neck, lower limbs, and trunk, enable individuals to remain upright in varying environments. With age, the function of all three systems tends to decline along with the brain's ability to integrate sensory input from these systems.

PEARL

Belal and Glorig (1986) coined the term *presbyastasis*, referring to dysequilibrium associated with aging.

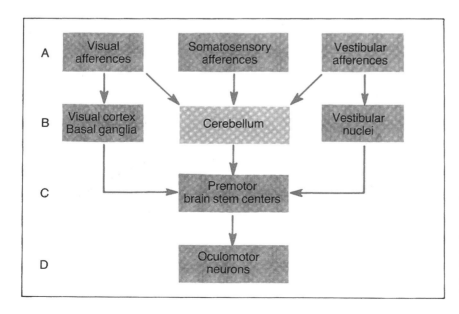

Figure 7–3 Oculomotor system. All three sensory systems **(A)** send their afferences via relay stations **(B)** in premotor centers of the reticular formation of the brain stem **(C)**. The motor neurons **(D)** which innervate the eye muscles begin at that point. (Data from Becker, Naumann, and Pfaltz, 1994.)

Presbyastasis is the diagnosis made when all other specific etiologies have been ruled out. The etiology of presbyastasis is multifactorial, related in large part to the structural and physiologic deterioration of selected components of the vestibular system. In Belal and Glorig's (1986) study of 740 patients over 65 years of age with a presenting complaint of dizziness, only 21% received diagnoses associated with a specific pathologic process. On the other hand, in a review of 116 patients aged 70 years and older, Sloane, Baloh, and Honrubia (1989) were able to identify specific etiologies in 85% of their subjects. The reason for the differences in the outcomes of these studies is unclear. However, inasmuch as older adults may present with a variety of vestibular disorders, completion of a thorough clinical evaluation, including a clear and detailed case history, is essential before assigning a diagnosis of presbyastasis. Some vestibular disorders prevalent among older adults include benign positional vertigo, Ménière's disease, unilateral or bilateral vestibular deficits of various etiologies, defective CNS adaptation to vestibular injury, cervical vertigo, cerebrovascular disease, and vertebrobasilar insufficiency (Maclennan, 1992; Konrad, Girardi, & Helfat, 1999). A brief review of the clinical tools available for evaluating balance function will set the stage for a more detailed discussion of the impact of age on balance function in the elderly.

Balance function laboratory tests can be divided into vestibulo-ocular tests and vestibulospinal tests. Both types rely on a measure of a motor response, either in the form of eye movements or postural sway, resulting from vestibular sensory input. Currently available tests provide only an indirect measure of vestibular system function (Furman & Cass, 1996). The three test batteries typically used clinically in the evaluation of balance system function are electronystagmography (ENG), rotational testing, and dynamic posturography. In the following section, each test battery will be briefly reviewed, including the purpose of each, how performance is measured, and normal data.

ENG

The ENG test battery consists of tests of oculomotor and vestibular function. In ENG testing, the data obtained are recorded eye movements, most commonly using electro-oculography. The physiological basis for electro-oculography is the corneal-retinal dipole potential. Specifically, the eye is similar to a battery, with the cornea having a positive electrical charge, and the retina a negative charge. When electrodes are placed lateral to each eye, voltage changes associated with eye movement are recorded. Similarly, when electrodes are placed above and below the eye, voltage changes associated with vertical eye movements are recorded. Signals recorded from electrodes are typically amplified using a DC-coupled amplifier, the output of which is directed to a strip chart recorder or a digital computer. By convention, for horizontal eye movements, upward deviations represent rightward and downward deviations represent leftward eye movements. Figure 7–4 shows the principle of nystagmography. The direction of eye movements is shown by the negative or positive signs of the corneoretinal potential.

Nystagmus is characterized by two components or phases: a slow deviation in one direction and a rapid return to midline

(Fig. 7–5). In vestibular nystagmus, the vestibular portion is the slow phase, while the return to baseline is associated with CNS function. Nystagmus is described in terms of direction and speed. Direction is described relative to the direction of the fast phase, with nystagmus "beating" in the direction of the fast phase. The slow phase velocity (SPV) is the number of degrees of eye deviation occurring in one second. Right beating nystagmus of 12 degrees per second specifies an eye movement that deviates leftward at a speed of 12 degrees per second with an instantaneous return to midline (rightward).

The dependent variable in vestibular function tests is a particular eye movement (i.e., nystagmus), so it is important to evaluate the neural motor system to insure that disorders affecting that system do not inadvertently affect tests of vestibular function. Oculomotor testing consists of a search for nystagmus with fixation, a search for nystagmus with horizontal and vertical eye deviation, an evaluation of saccadic eye movements by having the patient follow a visual target, a recording of smooth pursuit using a visual target, and a recording of optokinetic nystagmus (OKN). The presence of nystagmus with gaze is an abnormal finding. Saccades are evaluated in terms of accuracy, latency, and peak velocity of the eye movements recorded relative to the target. Smooth pursuit traces are evaluated for the presence of saccadic eye movements, and in terms of tracking gain. OKN gain is evaluated for rightward versus leftward moving targets.

The vestibular function subtests include evaluation of spontaneous and positional nystagmus, with and without fixation, positioning testing (i.e., the Dix-Hallpike maneuver), and caloric testing. Positional testing is performed by placing the patient in a variety of positions while recording eye movements in the dark. The purpose of positional testing is to find nystagmus resulting from gravitational effects. When nystagmus is detected, the examiner must look for the effect of fixation on the nystagmus. Failure of fixation suppression is a strong indication of a CNS disorder.

Positioning testing involves performing the Dix-Hallpike maneuver while observing the eyes and recording eye movements. It is designed to test for the presence of benign paroxysmal positional vertigo (BPPV). The nystagmus associated with BPPV is primarily torsional and must meet the following specific criteria: delay prior to the appearance of nystagmus; duration of 15 to 45 seconds; fatigability; and occurrence in connection with vertigo that subsides when a neutral position is assumed. Nystagmus recorded following the Dix-Hallpike maneuver that does not conform to all of the above criteria is not indicative of BPPV.

Caloric testing involves delivery of a thermal stimulus into the ear canal using either water or air. Figure 7–6 shows a schematic of caloric labyrinthine testing. The basis for caloric testing is establishment of a thermal gradient across the horizontal semicircular canal. Various methods of evaluating the vestibular response to caloric stimulation have been proposed, including the use of monothermal cool or warm irrigations, alternate binaural bithermal irrigations, and simultaneous binaural bithermal irrigations. The water or air stimulus used is presented at a calibrated temperature for a prescribed length of time. Both open and closed loop irrigators are available. Discussion of the relative strengths and weaknesses of each procedure is beyond the scope of this chapter. Suffice it to say, whichever procedure is

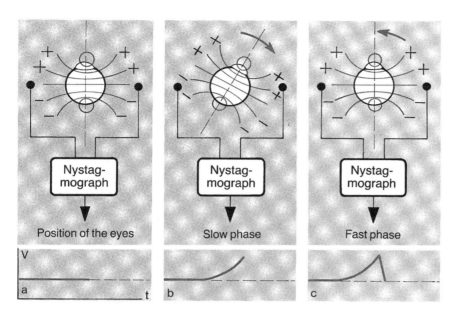

Figure 7–4 Principle of nystagmography. (a) Gaze straight ahead. The nasal and temporal electrodes are positive, and the isoelectric baseline is horizontal. (b) The bulb is turned slowly to the left. The nasal electrode is positive, the temporal electrode negative, and the baseline is displaced superiorly. (c) The bulb returns quickly, the baseline returns to the neutral position, and both electrodes are positive. (Data from Becker, Naumann, and Pfaltz, 1994.)

employed to stimulate the system, eye movements are recorded, nystagmus responses to each irrigation are analyzed by measuring the SPV at its peak, and the responsiveness of one ear is compared to the other. For bithermal irrigations, the formula of Jonkees is typically used to determine the presence of a unilateral weakness (UW) or directional preponderance (DP):

$$UW = \frac{(RC + RW) - (LC + LW)}{RC + RW + LC + LW} \quad DP = \frac{(RC + LW) - (RW + LC)}{RC + RW + LC + LW}$$

Because of differences in instrumentation and test environments, each laboratory should use its own data to determine the limits of normal for each value. In our laboratory, UW $\geq 20\%$ and DP $\geq 27\%$ are considered abnormal.

In ENG testing, nystagmus is expected to occur normally during optokinetic and caloric testing, however, when it occurs during spontaneous, gaze, positional, or positioning testing it is considered abnormal. For a more detailed discussion of ENG procedures, please refer to Jacobson, Newman, and Kartush (1993) or Shepard and Telian (1996).

Older adults may be referred for ENG testing by their primary care physician, an otolaryngologist, or a neurologist. They are typically referred when they report dizziness (e.g., sense of motion) that is sudden in onset (Kerber, Enrietto, Jacobson, & Baloh, 1998). They may also be referred when unsteadiness is reported or demonstrated during routine walking. ENG is useful in determining whether a peripheral vestibular system disorder is causing the symptoms experienced, and is most sensitive when used as part of a balance function test battery.

Rotational Tests

The purpose of rotary chair testing is to evaluate the relationship between a rotational stimulus and the patient's resultant eye movements. The earliest form of velocity-step rotational testing described in literature was the use of the Barany chair, in which a patient was seated with his or her head tilted forward 30 degrees. The patient was manually rotated at a speed of approximately 180 degrees per second until the initial acceleration responses subsided, at which time the patient was abruptly stopped. The clinician was able to observe the patient's eye movements resulting from the rotational stimulus, and record the strength and duration of the resulting nystagmus. The procedure was repeated in both clockwise and counterclockwise directions. Weak or absent responses were generally associated with bilateral vestibular weakness, while asymmetric responses suggested a unilateral vestibular loss. Today, electro-oculography is typically used to record eye movements, with rotational chairs having large motors controlled by computers. As such, the stimuli are precisely controlled. Unlike caloric testing, both ears are stimulated simultaneously during rotational testing. Rotational stimuli may be sinusoidal at various frequencies of rotation, or trapezoidal (rapid acceleration to a constant velocity, followed by an abrupt deceleration to a stop). The most commonly used procedures involve head-on-body, earth-axis rotation, although researchers continue to investigate the use of off-axis rotation. In all cases, the data collected are eye movements.

To analyze the rotationally induced nystagmus, the fast phases are removed by the computer and the slow components are pieced together to generate the slow-component eye position. This derived response is compared with the chair movements to establish the parameters of phase (timing relationship), gain (magnitude ratio), and symmetry (directional preponderance). Rotational testing is a valuable adjunct to the ENG battery in the evaluation of vestibular function. Some of its advantages include precise control of the stimulus and the ability to test at a number of different frequencies and amplitudes. Additionally, rotation is a natural stimulus and is rarely bothersome to the patient. Furthermore, it can be used for serial evaluations to determine changes in the system over time. The primary disadvantage of rotational testing is the fact that it does not permit precise localization or lateralization of a disorder because both ears are stimulated simultaneously. Table 7–1 is a display of the normal ranges for phase, gain, and symmetry for our laboratory.

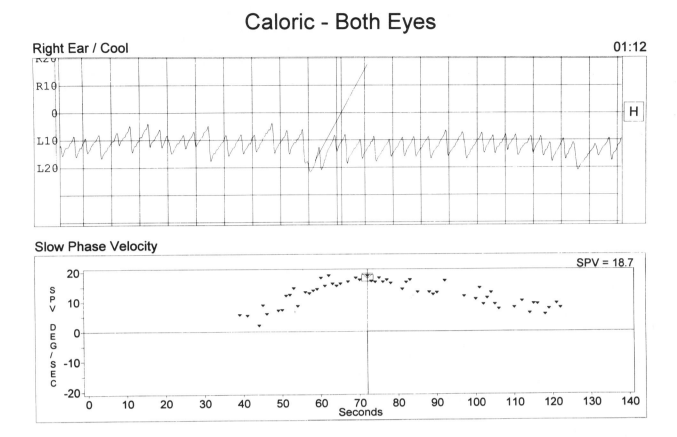

Caloric - Both Eyes

Right Ear / Cool   01:12

Slow Phase Velocity

SPV = 18.7

Figure 7–5   Normal left beating nystagmus in response to cool irrigation of the right ear. Top trace represents a 20-second segment at the peak response. Bottom trace represents the slow-phase velocity for the entire trial, over a period of 40 seconds.

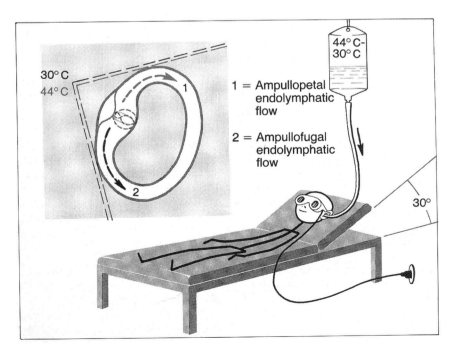

Figure 7–6   Principle of caloric labyrinthine tests. (Data from Becker, Naumann, and Pfaltz, 1994.)

TABLE 7–1 Normal Two-Standard Deviation Ranges for Phase, Gain, and Symmetry Data for Our Laboratory for Chair Frequencies 0.01 to 0.32 Hz

Hz	0.01	0.02	0.04	0.08	0.16	0.32
Phase (deg)	25–52	13–33	5–19	−3–11	−12–7	−12–7
Gain (%)	14–46	23–67	34–100	45–100	45–101	45–101
Asymmetry (%)	−12–22	−8–22	−9–22	−12–19	−12–17	−12–17

Older adults are referred for rotational testing when they experience chronic dizziness or balance disturbances, or when a physician is interested in following the compensation process in an acute peripheral vestibular system disorder. Additionally, because rotational testing evaluates response to a range of stimulus frequencies, it is useful in determining whether there is return to normal function at any frequency in a patient with a bilateral vestibular disorder.

Dynamic Posturography

SPECIAL CONSIDERATION

Whereas ENG and rotational testing are considered objective tests of vestibular and oculomotor function, dynamic posturography is designed to evaluate the ability to utilize sensory input for the maintenance of upright stance.

The test is divided into two portions, namely motor control (MC) and sensory organization (SO). MC testing uses repeated forward and backward translations and up and down rotations of the support surface, and the patient's return to a steady upright stance is quantified. The SO portion of the test battery involves systematic manipulation of the patient's access to vision and somatosensory input across six conditions. Using a technique called "sway referencing," the patient is provided with inaccurate sensory information by rotating the platform and visual surroundings in the same way the patient is swaying. The goal is to determine the patient's ability to use the input from each sensory system for the maintenance of upright stance. The six conditions included are illustrated in Figure 7–7. For each condition, the patient's postural sway is quantified and compared with age-adjusted normative data. Patterns of performance across all six conditions are examined. While dynamic posturography is not considered an objective test of vestibular function, it is useful for evaluation of functional balance. Given the fact that balance problems are

EquiTest™ Conditions

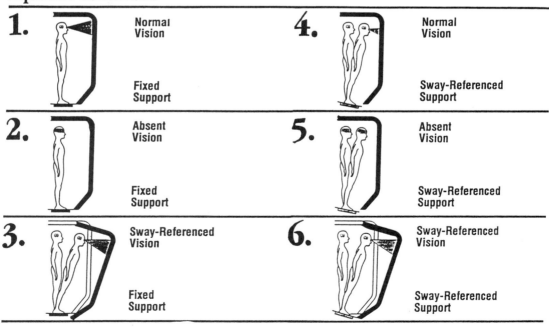

Figure 7–7 The six SO test conditions showing which sensory input cues are available or accurate for each condition. (Data reprinted with permission from NeuroCom International, Inc.)

common in older adults, and that older adults are at increased risk for injury secondary to falls, posturography is an especially valuable evaluation tool. Older adults may be referred for posturography by their primary care physician,

---

PEARL

Posturography is recommended for any patient reporting unsteadiness with standing or walking, as well as patients experiencing chronic dizziness.

---

an otolaryngologist, or a neurologist. Dynamic posturography is especially useful in assessing performance in patients for whom vestibular rehabilitation is a consideration.

AGE EFFECTS ON TESTS OF BALANCE SYSTEM FUNCTION

In examining the literature on the effects of aging on tests of balance system function, it is clear that the effects of age are both widespread across tests, and highly variable across individuals. Specifically, when looking at population trends, small performance declines are seen on every test. However,

within tests, some older adults show large performance decrements while some perform within the range considered normal for younger adults. Age effects on each test in the balance function test battery are discussed in the next sections. It is important to note that performance on each of the balance function tests can be affected by patient state and a variety of medications. For a list of the impact of drugs and toxic agents on oculomotor function, see Tables 7–2 and 7–3. Regarding patient state, oculomotor testing requires a high level of cooperation and attention to the task. For caloric and rotational testing, the patient must be kept alert and quiet, and eye blinking should be minimized. Dynamic posturography requires the patient to stand quietly, which is difficult for most patients for whom this testing is recommended. As such, obtaining valid data requires vigilance on the part of the examiner, and cooperation on the part of the patient.

ENG Test Results: Ocular Motility Testing

Age-related changes in oculomotor control have been reported by numerous investigators (Baloh, Jacobson, & Socotch, 1993; Peterka & Black, 1990b; Mulch & Petermann, 1979). Zackon and Sharpe (1987) studied smooth pursuit responses to sinusoidal and triangular targets in healthy

TABLE 7–2 Toxic Oculomotor Disturbances

Oculomotor sign	Toxic agent
Gaze-evoked nystagmus or saccadic pursuit	Phenytoin, carbamazepine, barbiturates, alcohol, benzodiazepines, methadone, chloral hydrate, marijuana
Slow saccades	Barbiturates, alcohol, benzodiazepines, fentanyl, vestibular sedatives (dimenhydrinate, scopolamine)
Impaired VOR	Vestibular sedatives (dimenhydrinate, scopolamine), barbiturates, alcohol, benzodiazepines
Exaggerated VOR	Industrial solvents (xylene, styrene, trichloroethylene, menthylchloroform)
Internuclear ophthalmoplegia	Phenytoin, barbiturates, tricyclic antidepressants, bromides, hepatic coma
External ophthalmoplegia	Phenytoin, barbiturates, tricyclic antidepressants (imipramine, doxepin, amitriptyline)
Vertical gaze palsy	Barbiturates/primidone
Skew deviation	Lithium, hepatic coma
Downbeat nystagmus/vertigo	Phenytoin, barbiturates, lithium, alcohol, magnesium depletion, vitamin B12 deficiency
Upbeat nystagmus/vertigo	Antiepileptics, tobacco
Periodic alternating nystagmus	Phenytoin
Central positioning nystagmus	Barbiturates, mercury compounds, industrial solvents (xylene, styrene, trichloroethylene, methylchloroform)
Labyrinthine positional nystagmus	Alcohol, glycerol, "heavy" water
Opsoclonus	Amitriptyline, haloperidol, lithium, thallium, chlordecone, DDT

Source: Brandt, T. (1993). Background, technique, interpretation, and usefulness of positional and positioning testing. In: Jacobson, G., Newman, C., and Kartush, J. (Eds.), *Handbook of Balance Function Testing*. St. Louis: Mosby Year Book, Inc. Used by permission.

TABLE 7–3   Oculomotor Abnormalities Caused by Toxic Agents

Drugs and toxic agents	Oculomotor abnormalities
Phenytoin	Gaze-evoked nystagmus, saccadic pursuit, external ophthalmoplegia, internuclear ophthalmoplegia. Rare: periodic alternating nystagmus, downbeat nystagmus/vertigo
Carbamazepine	Gaze-evoked nystagmus, saccadic pursuit, impairment of OKN, external ophthalmoplegia, downbeat nystagmus/vertigo, oculogyric crises
Barbiturates/primidone	Gaze-evoked nystagmus, saccadic pursuit, impairment of OKN, slow saccades, vertical gaze palsy, external ophthalmoplegia, impairment of VOR, internuclear ophthalmoplegia, central positional nystagmus, impaired vergence, decreased accommodative convergence/accommodation ratio
Alcohol	Labyrinthine positional vertigo, saccadic pursuit, slow saccades, downbeat nystagmus/vertigo
Benzodiazepines	Saccadic pursuit, slow saccades, impairment of VOR, impairment of gaze-holding
Tricyclic antidepressants	Internuclear ophthalmoplegia, external ophthalmoplegia, opsoclonus
Tricyclic antidepressants and L-tryptophan	Ocular oscillations and myoclonus
Bromides	Internuclear ophthalmoplegia
Vestibular sedatives	Impairment of VOR, slow saccades
Lithium	Alternating skew deviation, opsoclonus, downbeat nystagmus/vertigo
Thallium	Opsoclonus
Phenothiazines	Internuclear ophthalmoplegia
Methadone	Saccadic pursuit, saccadic hypometria
Haloperidol	Opsoclonus
Marijuana	Gaze-evoked nystagmus, saccadic pursuit
Amphetamine	Increased accommodative convergence/accommodation ratio
Mercury	Spontaneous and/or positional nystagmus, impairment of OKN
Chemotherapeutic anticancer agents	Vestibular/hearing loss
Loop diuretics (ethacrynic acid, furosemide)	Transient vestibular/hearing loss, impaired VOR
Aminoglycoside antibiotics (gentamicin, streptomycin)	Permanent vestibular/hearing loss
Acetylsalicylic acid	Transient vestibulocochlear impairment
Industrial solvents (xylene, trichloroethylene)	Central positional nystagmus, exaggerated VOR, impaired fixation suppression of VOR

Source: Brandt, T. (1993). Background, technique, interpretation, and usefulness of positional and positioning testing. In: Jacobson, G., Newman, C., and Kartush, J. (Eds.), *Handbook of Balance Function Testing.* St. Louis: Mosby Year Book, Inc. Used by permission.

middle-aged (35 to 60 years) and healthy elderly (66 to 87 years) subjects. They found that pursuit gain was significantly lower in elderly than in middle-aged subjects under all target conditions. They reported that the gain reduction seen in older subjects is due to involvement of the steady-state gain element of the pursuit system at slow target accelerations, and to acceleration saturation at higher speeds.

Demer (1994) studied the effects of aging on vertical smooth pursuit, small field OKN, the vestibulo-ocular reflex (VOR), and visual-vestibular interactions. They evaluated eleven normally sighted young subjects (age 30 ± 6 years) and nine normally sighted elderly subjects (age 70 ± 8 years). Eye movements were recorded using a magnetic search coil imbedded in a contact lens affixed to the right eye, and testing was completed in darkness. The authors reported that, in terms of gain for predictable motion, tracking gain was lower in the elderly subjects than it was in younger subjects. Further, they noted that most older subjects were unable to achieve the coherence criteria at the highest frequency tested. Regarding phase for predictable motion, while phase lags were near zero at the lowest test frequencies for both groups of subjects, elderly subjects demonstrated increased phase lags with increasing frequency. At 3.2 Hz, phase errors were quite variable. For poorly predictable targets, both OKN and tracking gains were markedly reduced in both age groups, but phase lag of both pursuit and OKN tended to be greater in elderly subjects than in young subjects. Further, the phase lag seen in the elderly was consistently greater for pursuit than for OKN.

A number of researchers have investigated the effects of aging on saccade performance. Sharpe and Zackon (1987) employed infrared oculography to record saccades in healthy young (19 to 31 years), middle-aged (35 to 63), and older adult (66 to 87) subjects. Saccades were elicited in response to targets with predictable and unpredictable amplitudes and timing. They found that peak velocities were significantly reduced in older adults when the target amplitude and direction were unpredictable. However, saccade latencies were prolonged and saccade accuracy was reduced in all conditions in older subjects. Additionally, hypometric saccades were frequently seen in the elderly. The authors concluded that the use of age-based normative data is essential when evaluating saccade performance clinically.

Sonderegger, Meienberg, and Ehrengruber (1986) published normative data on saccadic eye movements based on examination of 20 healthy adult subjects. They used infrared oculography, and evaluated the parameters of accuracy, peak velocity, and duration of symmetrically midline-crossing 30- and 20-degree saccades. The specific data were reported separately for adducting and abducting eye movements. In addition, they proposed the use of standardized fatigue and Tensilon tests, and provided normative data for those tests. Unfortunately, only four subjects were evaluated per age decade, so the representativeness of the data is questionable.

Pitt and Rawles (1988) studied saccade performance of 85 healthy adult subjects (20 to 68 years) using electro-oculography and horizontal targets moving 20 degrees from midline. Only outgoing saccades were recorded, and the latency and peak velocity of adducting and abducting eye

movements were analyzed separately. As was the case in the other investigations, these authors reported that saccade latency increased with age. However, unlike in the earlier studies, saccade velocity decreased with age. Additionally, saccade latency for adduction was greater than for abduction, while saccade velocity was greater in adduction than abduction.

In a recent study, Shepard (personal communication, 1996) evaluated the effects of aging on smooth pursuit and saccade function. The study was considered normative in that the researchers wanted to establish norms for a variety of age groups for saccades and sinusoidal smooth pursuit. They proposed that some of the reason for variability in the literature regarding aging effects on oculomotor function is lack of consistency regarding stimulating and recording parameters. For that reason, they utilized commercially available clinical hardware and software, and recorded conjugate and individual eye movements using electro-oculography. A total of 82 normal adults served as subjects, ranging in age from 19 to 88 years. Subjects performed saccades that were presented as a randomly located series of abduction and adduction eye movements. Sinusoidal smooth pursuit was also evaluated.

The authors found no differences in the values they obtained for conjugate saccades and smooth pursuit relative to the normal values included in the software from the manufacturer (Shepard, personal communication, 1996). While statistically significant age and gender effects were noted, the authors reported that the differences seen are probably not clinically significant because they accounted for a small proportion of the variance. The findings that were validated in their well-controlled study include age-related decreases in gain and increases in phase lag for smooth pursuit, particularly with increased target speed. Additionally, a clinically significant difference in individual eye saccades was noted based on the direction of eye movement, so that this variable must be considered in interpreting clinical data during ocular motility testing.

ENG Test Results: Caloric Testing

In examining the literature related to the effects of aging on caloric test results, it is clear that conclusions differ across investigations. One possible explanation for some of the

> ### SPECIAL CONSIDERATION
> **Caloric irrigations have resulted in reduced vestibular responses, increased vestibular responses, and normal vestibular responses in older adults.**

response variability has to do with subject selection. While some authors studied adult subjects with no history of dizziness or otologic or neurologic disease, others analyzed data from clinic patients seen for vestibular testing. The clinic patients tested presented with symptoms of dizziness or imbalance, yet had test results within the normal range established for that lab. Including data from symptomatic patients within a "normal" data pool may result in interpretation bias. A second variable worth consideration is methodology, particularly whether subjects were evaluated with eyes open, eyes closed, in darkness or light, and the type and temperature of the irrigations used. A brief review of some of the key studies on this subject follows.

Bruner and Norris (1971) reported on a study of 293 clinic patients with symptoms of dizziness and negative ("normal") findings on vestibular testing. They found that amplitude, slow phase eye velocity (SPEV), and duration increased with age to peak at 60 to 70 years, with a decline noted thereafter. They also reported age-related differences in relative responsiveness to warm and cool irrigations. For older adults, age-dependent changes were most apparent for warm irrigations. A warm irrigation results in increased electrical activity leaving the end organ. Whereas Bruner and Norris (1971) studied clinic patients, Van der Laan and Oosterveld (1974) studied 334 normal adult subjects. They reported that young subjects (through the third decade of life) had lower nystagmus frequency and higher nystagmus amplitude than did older subjects (older than 50 years). They proposed that the obvious age-related changes could be due to decreased blood flow to the vestibular end organ. From their study of 250 subjects divided into seven age groups, Clement, Van der Laan, and Oosterveld (1975) reported a decrease in SPEV with increased age.

Mulch and Petermann (1979) evaluated 102 healthy adult subjects ranging from 11 to 70 years divided into six age groups of 17 subjects each. They reported a clear relationship between age and caloric parameters, but the strength of the response did not simply decrease with increasing age. Rather, the most intense reactions to caloric stimuli occurred in healthy middle-aged and late middle-aged adults, with decrements in function noted only after age 60 years. It was of interest that peak responses were obtained from subjects within the age range where anatomical degeneration had been demonstrated to occur. In light of their findings, the authors emphasized that the degree of alertness warrants consideration when evaluating age effects on caloric response parameters.

Karlsen, Hassanein, and Goetzinger (1981) performed bithermal caloric irrigations on 75 subjects aged 18 to 81 years. Nystagmus amplitude, latency, duration, frequency, and SPEV were quantified. For cool irrigations, the only age-dependent variable was nystagmus duration, with older subjects having shorter nystagmus durations than younger subjects. On the other hand, nystagmus SPEV, duration, amplitude, and frequency all showed significant age effects for warm irrigations, although the effects seen were not always simple. Consistent with the findings of other investigations, this study demonstrated a decline in vestibular system responsiveness beginning at age 65 to 70.

Ghosh (1985) investigated the relationship between age and SPEV for 78 subjects divided into seven age groups from 10 to over 70 years using serial vestibulometry. Overall, a decrease in SPEV as a function of age with greater age-related differences was noted at the temperature extremes. Jacobson and Henry (1989) examined fixation suppression ability as a function of age, and found that fixation suppression becomes significantly poorer with age. These findings may suggest that the neuronal connections between the ves-

tibular nuclei and the midline cerebellar structures become less efficient with age. It is noteworthy that these same pathways facilitate compensation following loss of peripheral vestibular function.

In a recent comprehensive study of vestibular test function, Peterka, Black, and Schoenhoff (1990a) studied the VOR in 216 normal human subjects ranging in age from 7 to 81 years. Unlike the findings of previous investigators, the authors reported no obvious or consistent changes in caloric results as a function of age. There were also no gender differences reported. Examination of the raw data revealed a great deal of variability in the responses, which may have masked any age-related trends.

In summary, then, the literature provides a cloudy picture of the relationship between age and caloric test outcome. Most of the studies reviewed suggested a decline in function when comparing the oldest subjects with young and middle-aged subjects. However, a recent, well-controlled study failed to demonstrate any consistent age-related changes. Rather, the authors reported a high degree of intersubject variability within and across age groups. It is important to note that the high degree of intersubject variability seen in this study may have masked any possible age-related trends.

Rotational Testing

A few studies have been conducted where the effects of age on rotational test results were examined. In one of the largest studies conducted by Van der Laan and Oosterveld (1974), the rotational responses of 779 normal subjects using a torsion swing were calculated. Age-dependent changes in three response parameters were reported. Specifically, they found a slight decline in the average number of nystagmus beats after 80 years of age, a significant decrease in the average SPEV after 70 years of age, and decreased nystagmus amplitude after 40 years of age. Wall and Black (1984) evaluated 50 normal adults aged 20 to 59 years using sinusoidal rotation. They reported diminished gain with increased age for all chair frequencies tested. In contrast to the results obtained in the above studies, Yagi, Sekine, and Shimizu (1983) found that older adults had higher VOR gains when compared with middle-aged subjects.

More recently, Peterka, Black, and Schoenhoff (1990a) measured the VOR resulting from single-frequency sinusoidal stimuli. The authors reported small changes in VOR gain and VOR phase (i.e., measure of the difference between eye position and chair position) associated with age. Specifically, all gains decreased with increasing age, and phase had a tendency to increase with increasing age, with the effect being more consistent at 0.2 and 0.8 Hz than at 0.05 Hz. According to the authors, age-related changes in gain and phase were roughly linear. Rotational test measures of symmetry (i.e., strength of the response for left rotations compared with right rotations) showed no age-dependent effects.

In the same study (Peterka, Black, & Schoenhoff, 1990a), the authors also compared caloric and rotational test findings in the same subjects, and discussed the relationship between their findings and age-related changes in the peripheral vestibular anatomy. Overall, the age-related changes in VOR function identified in their study do not follow the same time course as age-related peripheral vestibular anatomical changes described by others. Specifically, while both VOR gain and the various measures of vestibular anatomic components decline gradually up to about age 50, the rate of decline in anatomy only increases after age 60, resulting in a divergence between anatomical and physiological data. VOR function was shown to be much better in older subjects than would have been predicted based on peripheral vestibular anatomical changes alone.

Having already discussed age-related changes in the VOR in response to caloric and sinusoidal rotational stimulation, it becomes important to know how aging affects the optokinetic and pursuit systems' ability to impact the VOR. Under normal circumstances, the VOR and the optokinetic reflex (OKR) function together to provide clear vision by generating compensatory eye movements that minimize image motion on the fovea of the retina during head movement. Peterka, Black, and Schoenhoff (1990b) studied the dynamic response properties of the VOR and OKR to pseudorandom stimuli in 216 subjects. Subjects demonstrated a wide range of responses on all measures of VOR and OKR function. Age-related changes were identified in most rotation test response measures, however, the magnitude of these changes was small relative to the large individual variability in the data. Despite the variability, the changes were suggestive of a decline in function with age. Stefansson and Imoto (1986) studied OKN and VOR from rotational stimulation in 60 normal subjects aged 13 to 68 years. They found a slight linear correlation with age for both tests. Specifically, while the OKR eye speed increased with increasing age, the rotational SPV decreased with increasing age.

In comparing the VOR measure by single-frequency sinusoidal and pseudorandom rotational stimuli, Peterka, Black, and Schoenhoff (1990b) reported that the results were not significantly different at the lowest frequency (0.05 Hz), but were consistently different at higher frequencies. While the phase findings may represent a small predictive effect, the gain differences may be a procedural artifact. Regarding age-related changes in the VOR and OKR, both the VOR time constant and OKR gain constant increased slightly in subjects up to age 30 years, and then decreased with increasing age. The OKR time-delay parameter demonstrated a clear age-related trend, consistently increasing with increasing age.

Goebel, Hanson, and Fishel (1994b) investigated modulation of the VOR in response to sinusoidal rotation using real and imaginary targets, and the impact of age on modulation effects. Five modulation paradigms were employed including (1) visually enhanced VOR with a real earth-fixed target; (2) mental alerting in darkness with no real or imagined target; (3) mentally enhanced VOR with an imagined earth-fixed target; (4) mentally suppressed VOR with an imagined chair-fixed target; and (5) visually suppressed VOR with a real chair-fixed target. Overall, the results indicated that there was no difference between younger and older subjects in their ability to modulate VOR gain with visual targets. Similarly, both groups were able to suppress VOR gain us-

ing mental imagery. They were not, however, equal in their ability to do so. Neither group of subjects was able to enhance VOR gain with mental imagery. The authors suggested that the ability to modulate the VOR with mental imagery may have important clinical applications. Specifically, the extent to which an individual can mentally suppress the VOR may provide a functional assessment of central adaptive mechanisms. If that is true, it may be used as a predictor of recovery from vestibular ablation. Furthermore, there is

SPECIAL CONSIDERATION

In summary, the literature examining aging effects on the VOR in response to rotational stimulation suggests a decline in function, demonstrated in both gain and phase, with increased age.

evidence to suggest that decrements in function occur at a slower rate than do changes in anatomy, particularly in the highest age groups examined. The OKR, when tested using a sinusoidal stimulus, also declines with age. Finally, no age effects were noted in subjects' ability to modulate VOR gain with real visual targets, although some age-related differences were noted in subjects' ability to suppress the VOR using mental imagery.

Postural Control Testing

The deterioration of postural control in the elderly manifests itself in both static equilibrium problems (falls when standing) and in dynamic equilibrium problems (falls when walking or when moving while standing) (Stelmach & Worringham, 1985). Establishing age-related changes in postural control that are independent of disease is difficult. Data recently emerging suggest age-related changes in the vestibular, visual, and somatosensory systems. In general, when healthy young (20 to 35 years of age) and healthy old (65+ years) are compared in their ability to stand quietly on a firm flat surface with eyes open or eyes closed, differences are minimal. The differences remain minimal when subjects are perturbed slightly (Alexander, 1994). On the other hand, increased severity of the perturbation appears to reveal more substantial age-related differences. Alexander (1994) provided a thorough overview of the literature, and suggested that situations that may bring out age-related differences in postural control include (1) changing the support surface, either in terms of area, compliance, or stability; (2) changing body position prior to the perturbation; (3) changing the accuracy of the visual input provided; and (4) perturbing the support surface or pulling at the waist at a high magnitude. Furthermore, body configuration (e.g., unipedal versus bipedal stance, arms outstretched versus folded on the chest) may influence performance.

Stelmach and Worringham (1985) proposed a scheme of hypothetical processing stages related to protective and/or corrective responses to situations of postural instability. They utilized that scheme to categorize relevant age-related deficits that may affect the prevalence of falls in the elderly. They reported that one of the most convincing findings in the literature on aging is the general slowing of cognitive-motor responses. While the general slowing of responses has been widely observed, the exact causes of the decline are less well understood. For that reason, using a scheme in which response time is partitioned into stages is useful for interpreting a variety of experimental observations.

In the scheme described by Stelmach and Worringham (1985), the first stage is the input, or feedforward stage, which includes "alerting" or "triggering" response-selection centers that a potential fall is imminent. This alerting process may be initiated by one or more of the following sensory inputs: proprioception, vision, vestibular function, or interoception. The second type of alerting input via feedforward mechanisms includes preparatory postural adjustments that precede voluntary motor acts and serve to offset the reaction forces invoked by a motor act. This could include the prediction of an imminent loss of balance. The second stage in fall prevention or amelioration is response selection, including corrective responses that permit a rapid return to a balanced position with minimal interruption of activity, and protective responses that mitigate the effects of an inevitable fall if the delay is too long to prevent a fall. The third stage is response execution, which involves implementing a set of muscle actions that are correctly phased in space and time, and may be characterized as open-loop (without feedback) or closed-loop (with feedback) control.

Using this scheme, it is possible to review what is known about age-related deficits affecting each stage, and the potential effects of each on postural stability in the elderly. Regarding deficits affecting sensory input, decreases in visual acuity, restriction of visual field, susceptibility to glare, and poorer depth perception have all been demonstrated to occur with advancing age (Fozard, Wolf, Bell, McFarland, & Podolsky, 1977). As a result, an older person's ability to utilize visual reference information will be impaired. For example, inasmuch as peripheral vision is most sensitive to movement, a reduction in visual field with age will have a deleterious effect on the elderly person's ability to make use of visual movement cues. In a similar fashion, reduced depth perception will make an older person less sensitive to anterior-posterior sway. These deficits, then, will result in an increase in time taken for the visual system to alert the CNS that a fall is imminent.

Regarding the occurrence of age-related proprioceptive deficits, few data and little agreement are apparent. There is some evidence that proprioceptive deterioration in the elderly is not apparent if the movements in question are preselected by the subject, and that constrained movements are produced less accurately by older adults (Stelmach & Worringham, 1985). Manchester, Woollacott, Zederbaurer-Hylton, and Maria (1989) evaluated age- and pathology-related changes in the relative contributions of visual and somatosensory input to dynamic balance. They studied young adults and older adults by recording electromyographic (EMG) responses to platform perturbations. They manipulated the amounts of visual and somatosensory input while recording muscle response latencies, losses of balance, and muscle sequencing. They found that muscle response latencies did not differ across age groups. However, older adults were less stable than were young adults under conditions in which peripheral vision was occluded and ankle somatosensation was limited. These trends were exaggerated among subjects in whom borderline pathology was diagnosed.

Regarding somatosensory input, Skinner, Barrack, and Cook (1984) reported that both cutaneous vibratory sensation and joint sensation are diminished in older adults. The significance of ankle proprioception for balance retention in the elderly has been demonstrated by Woollacott, Shumway-Cook, and Nasher (1982). In comparing the postural sway of young to elderly subjects, they found that older adults had large increases in postural sway when ankle proprioception was eliminated, and that half of the elderly subjects lost their balance completely when they closed their eyes. These findings suggest that vision takes on a more important role when proprioception is diminished or rendered unreliable. Brocklehurst, Robertson, and James-Groom (1982) reported that vibration sense and proprioception were not correlated, but that impaired vibratory sense and postural sway were highly correlated. He concluded that impaired vibration sense contributes more to postural sway than does any other sensory loss.

Peterka and Black (1990a, 1990b) evaluated postural control in 214 human subjects ranging in age from 7 to 81 years using the sensory organization and motor control portions of dynamic posturography as described earlier. For the sensory organization conditions the dependent variable measured was the magnitude of anterior-posterior body sway (Peterka & Black, 1990a). The authors reported that no age-related changes in postural sway were noted for the conditions in which subjects were standing on a fixed platform with eyes open or eyes closed. However, age-related increases in sway were noted in the sway-referenced conditions, with subjects older than 55 years demonstrating the largest sway increases. Subjects younger than 15 years were also sensitive to alteration of sensory cues. In general, older subjects were affected more by sway-referenced visual input, whereas younger subjects were more adversely affected by sway-referenced support. Peterka and Black (1990a) also discussed that falls which occurred during the sensory organizations testing followed consistent patterns. Specifically, while there are six possible combinations of paired falls within the grouping of the four most difficult conditions, most of the paired falls were limited to two possible combinations (5–6 and 3–6). All of the subjects who fell in three conditions fell in the same set (3–5–6), and most of these subjects were older. Figure 7–7 shows the six conditions of dynamic posturography. Figure 7–8 represents sway as a function of age across the six sensory test conditions.

Similarly, Teasdale, Stelmach, and Breunig (1991) conducted an experiment designed to determine whether a reduction of visual, somatosensory, or both visual and somatosensory inputs were differentially disruptive to postural control of young and older healthy adults. They limited their sample population to individuals having no musculoskeletal defects, taking no medication, not undergoing treatment for neurological disease, and with no history of falling. Their dependent variables were range and variability (standard deviation) of sway on the anterior-posterior and medio-lateral planes; average sway velocity;

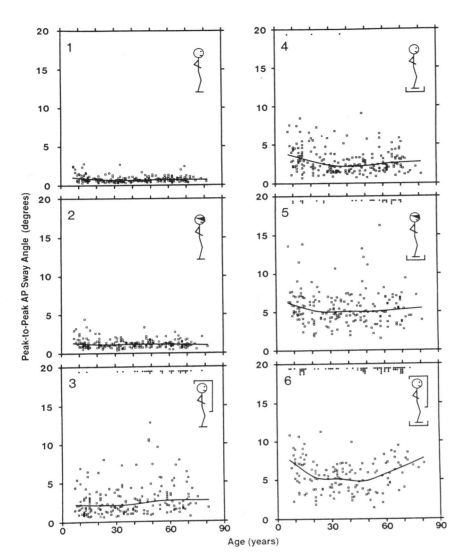

Figure 7–8 Sway as a function of age. (Data from Peterka and Black, 1990a.)

and sway density. Their four test conditions were normal surface with eyes open, altered surface (foam pad added) with eyes open, normal surface with eyes closed, and altered surface with eyes closed. Overall, the older subjects had greater sway range, particularly on the medio-lateral plane, and higher sway velocity than did young subjects. Older subjects also spent more time away from the center of their base of support. Both groups were affected similarly by visual conditions, and the elderly were more affected by the altered surface and the combined altered surface and vision conditions than were young subjects for all measures. For both groups, range, variability, and velocity of sway increased more under the altered vision than that under the altered surface condition, but both groups spent a higher percentage of time in an "at risk" posture-control area, away from center, for the altered surface condition than for the altered vision condition.

Regarding motor control, Peterka and Black (1990b) recorded leg muscle EMG response latencies, body sway, and the amplitude and timing of changes in the center of gravity in response to forward and backward support surface per-turbations. There were very small increases in EMG and center of gravity response latencies as a function of increasing age, and no changes in the amplitude of the center of pressure responses when the amplitude measures were normalized for subject height. The authors reported, further, that a high degree of response variability was noted, irrespective of subject age. Similarly, Lawson, Shephard, Oviatt, & Wang (1994) recorded EMGs from the gastrocnemius and anterior tibialis muscles of 77 adult subjects in response to perturbations of stance by upward toe tilts. They found statistically significant left-right differences in response amplitude, and statistically significant height, gender, and age effects. Specifically, they found significant age differences in onset time and duration of the short latency response (SLR) and for the integrated amplitude and duration of the long latency response (LLR), with onset time, duration, and amplitude increasing with age. Keshner, Allum, and Honegger (1993) also recorded EMG activity in response to support surface rotation, comparing healthy elderly and healthy young subjects. For their study, EMG activity was recorded from the soleus, tibialis anterior, and neck extensor muscles.

They also measured trunk angular acceleration and ankle torque. They observed three group differences. First, EMG response latencies were longer in the elderly subjects. Second, the normal linear correlation between stabilizing ankle muscle activity and ankle torque was disturbed, resulting in decreased ankle torque exerted on the support surface by the elderly. Third, the magnitude of neck muscle activation was increased in the elderly subjects, suggesting an increased compensation at the head for trunk acceleration. The authors reported that their findings suggest that a combination of mechanical and neural changes in the elderly may impact postural corrections, thereby affecting their risk for falling.

Lord, Clark, and Webster (1991) administered a battery of 13 tests including visual, vestibular, sensorimotor, and balance function to 95 residents (mean age of 82.7 years) of an elder hostel in Sydney, Australia. They did not attempt to limit their sample population to those individuals free from illness. Rather, they intended to sample a cross section of elderly people living fairly independently in an attempt to examine the relationship between specific sensorimotor functions and postural instability in that population. The sensory system factors measured included visual acuity, visual contrast sensitivity, touch thresholds, joint position sense, and vibration sense. The motor system factors included quadricep strength and ankle dorsiflexion strength. The authors also measured reaction time and the postural stability variable of sway, measured during a static balance test and a dynamic balance test. Interestingly, while the prevalence of vestibular impairment was high in their study population, vestibular function was not significantly associated with sway under any of the test conditions. Rather, their results suggest that reduced sensation, muscle weakness in the legs, and increased reaction time are all important variables associated with postural instability, with peripheral sensation being the single most important sensory system in the maintenance of static postural stability.

The primary contribution of the vestibular system to posture is in maintaining the reflex associated with keeping the head and neck in a vertical position, and in corrective movements elicited through the vestibulospinal and vestibuloreticulospinal pathways (Stelmach & Worringham, 1985). While we have already discussed the effects of aging on the vestibular system itself, the relationship of vestibular impairment from increased age to balance control has only been studied indirectly, as it is a variable that is less amenable to experimental manipulation than are vision and proprioception. Norre, Forrez, and Beckers (1987) utilized posturography to examine the relationship between unilateral vestibular hypofunction (UVH) and postural stability in the elderly. In humans, postural sway is disturbed when the vestibulospinal reflex is deregulated because of the UVH. The degree of disturbance is dependent upon the effectiveness of the central compensation mechanism. Ocular fixation is also important. Norre, Forrez, and Beckers (1987) studied 117 patients having UVH, divided into four age groups: <30 years, 30 to 49 years, 50 to 59 years, and 60 years or more. Their results indicated that the central compensation mechanism becomes less effective with advancing age. They reported, further, that elderly patients tend to have in-

creased postural instability with their eyes closed. For that reason, they concluded that regarding the problem of falls in the elderly, vestibular function must be assessed, particularly in terms of its influence on postural control.

Apart from the deterioration in the afferent input from the sensory system already discussed is an age-related deficit in the feedforward mechanisms specifically related to postural control. Mankovskii, Mints, and Lysenyuk (1980) demonstrated that old and very old subjects (when compared with young adult subjects) show a low correlation between the latencies of unilateral knee flexion while standing and the postural adjustments that normally precede them, particularly for rapid movements. This led to an increase in the frequency of loss of balance with age, and suggests that there is an age-related breakdown of the postural feedforward mechanism during voluntary movements, particularly when the system is under time stress, as is the case in rapid movements.

In summary, then, deterioration in visual, proprioceptive, somesthetic, or vestibular signals concerning balance as a function of age may produce a central signal detection problem that is common to all of these inputs (Stelmach & Worringham, 1985). In order to accurately detect a peripheral stimulus, a longer sampling period may be necessary, particularly if more noise is contained in the incoming signal. It is evident, then, that any decrease in the time available for response selection will have adverse consequences.

Discussing deficits affecting response selection is somewhat more challenging because response selection is not directly observable. For that reason, Stelmach and Worringham (1985) suggested using the techniques and findings of cognitive motor research to study postural control and falls. Specifically, reaction time (RT) methodology has been used to examine simple and complex tasks. Overall, RT is known to increase with age, and choice RTs increase at a more rapid rate than simple RTs. Furthermore, increasing the complexity of the relationship between the stimulus and the response results in even slower performance associated with age. While older adults are able to make error responses as rapidly as can younger adults, they appear to have particular difficulty in regulating responses that require both accuracy and speed. Since corrective and protective postural actions necessitate both speed and accuracy, Stelmach and Worringham (1985) have suggested that an age-related imprecision in the control of response speed may be a contributory factor in falls.

The third stage of processing proposed by Stelmach and Worringham (1985) is response execution, which includes all processes that follow response selection, including movement planning, motor time, and movement time. Larish and Stelmach (1982) investigated the effect of valid (programming) or invalid (reprogramming) advance information on subjects' movements. They found that older subjects moved more slowly than did younger subjects, but that there was no interaction between age and the three programming conditions studied. There is evidence, however, that the complexity of the required movement affects the age-related slowing that may be seen (Jordon & Rabbitt, 1977). Gottsdanker (1980) demonstrated an impaired ability to prepare responses in elderly subjects, which is presumably independent of selection processes. Motor time has also been demonstrated to increase with age, particularly in physically inactive older adults (Clarkson, 1978; Kroll & Clarkson, 1978). Finally, these same researchers have shown that movement time, or the duration of movement, increases with age.

The relationship between age-related response slowing and falls is somewhat more complicated because it involves the integration of different levels of control, ranging from automatic to volitional. Changes in one part of the system will probably affect the other parts. Salthouse (1985) proposed that slower operations ("hardware" differences) may necessitate different control processes ("software" differences), which in turn may lead to different operations (control and representational differences). If it can be demonstrated that therapy can overcome the age-related deficits discussed, it would imply that deficits exist in the "software" of the system, since sufficient usage would allow optimal availability of relevant operations. If one accepts the relationship between practice and speed of processing, the very caution shown by older people in avoiding unstable positions may inadvertently lead to the production of slower, inadequate responses when these unpracticed, unstable conditions occur (Stelmach & Worringham, 1985). However, the findings of Teasdale, Stelmach, and Breunig (1991) led the authors to conclude that the less stable posture of the older adults was a result of defect, rather than slowing, in the central integrative mechanisms. Inasmuch as both groups showed similar postural adaptation, these findings do not support the hypothesis that a slower reorganizing of the postural control system takes place in the elderly.

Dizziness Handicap Indices

The Dizziness Handicap Index (DHI) was developed in 1990 as a means to assess self-perceived disability/handicap resulting from dizziness and unsteadiness (Jacobson & Newman, 1990). The DHI is a 25-item scale that is intended to evaluate the effects of dizziness and balance problems on the functional, emotional, and physical aspects of daily life. For each item, the patient responds "yes," "sometimes," or "no," and each response is assigned a value of 4, 2, or 0 points, respectively. The highest possible score on the DHI is 100 points. The DHI has been used as an outcome measure to evaluate the effects of nonmedical, medical, and surgical treatments for various balance system disorders. Previously, the relationship between scores on the DHI and performance on vestibulometric and posturographic measures has been evaluated (Jacobson, Hunter, & Balzer, 1991; Robertson & Ireland, 1995). Jacobson, Hunter, and Balzer (1991) reported a statistically significant relationship between scores on the DHI and measures of stability on Condition 5 of the sensory organization subtest of dynamic posturography. No significant relationship was found between the DHI scores and other vestibulometric test results.

More recently, a screening version of the DHI (DHI-S) has been developed and evaluated (Jacobson & Calder, 1998). The DHI-S is a ten-item scale derived from the DHI, including four items from the functional subscale, three items from the emotional subscale, and three items from the

physical subscale. The DHI-S is scored identically to the full DHI. In a recent study, both the DHI and DHI-S were administered to 278 patients seen for balance function testing, with approximately a two-hour interval between administration of the two scales. The results showed that the two scales are highly correlated ($r = 0.86$, $p = 0.001$). Furthermore, abnormal performance on the sensory organization subtest of dynamic posturography was correlated with higher scores on the DHI-S. See Appendix A and Appendix B for copies of the DHI and DHI-S.

Because the DHI and DHI-S are correlated with abnormal postural stability as measured by dynamic posturography, and because older adults are at higher risk for falls than are younger adults, these measures may be useful in screening older patients in order to determine candidacy for further evaluation of balance function. The DHI-S takes less than 5 minutes to administer, and could be given to patients to complete while waiting to be seen by their physician for routine physicals. High scores could signal a need for follow-up questioning, and/or referral for complete balance function testing.

SPECIAL CONSIDERATION

Early identification of balance system disorders, coupled with development of a preventative management strategy, may facilitate a reduction in falls in the older adult population.

EFFECTS OF EXERCISE PROGRAMS ON DIZZINESS AND BALANCE IN THE AGING

PEARL

Vestibular rehabilitation programs generally include exercises designed to address dizziness (vertigo), and/or exercises designed to improve balance function. General conditioning exercise, such as walking, may also be included.

While research has supported the effectiveness of vestibular rehabilitation, relatively few studies have investigated the long-term effects of various exercise programs on older adults. Norre and Beckers (1989) described the use of habituation exercises to reduce motion-provoked vertigo. Subjects were evaluated before therapy using the Vestibular Habituation Training (VHT) test battery, consisting of 19 maneuvers. For each maneuver, the vertigo was described as rotatory or atypical dizziness (A), and the intensity (I) and duration (T) of the symptoms were estimated. A score was computed according to the formula f(A)g(I)log 10(T), and the sum of the scores for the positive maneuvers provided a "total score." When nystagmus was observed, it was also noted.

For this investigation, 40 subjects having rotatory vertigo following at least one of the maneuvers were selected. For each subject, an exercise program was designed consisting of practice of each maneuver that was provocative for the subject. Each maneuver was repeated five times successively, at home, during each of two or three sessions per day. During the study, testing on the VHT test battery was repeated for each subject after one week of treatment and at two months post onset. For subjects who remained symptomatic after one week, testing was repeated at two weeks as well.

The results of the study by Norre and Beckers (1989) revealed that the number of subjects having positive results during testing diminished progressively over time. For the older adults (+ 60 years), progression was slower than it was for the group as a whole (20 to 80 years, mean age = 50.2 years). Additionally, the three subjects for whom at least one maneuver remained provocative at the end of training were all in the + 60 years group. From a clinical perspective, however, the patients with positive findings at the end were very satisfied, as vertigo no longer occurred in their daily life activities. The authors concluded, then, that while some differences were noted in the speed of recovery for the older adult patients treated with VHT, the end results were equally satisfying as in the group as a whole because the goal of the treatment, restoration of normal life activities without vertigo, was reached.

In a relatively large study involving 197 women, Lord, Ward, Williams, & Strudwick (1995) investigated the impact of a 12-month exercise program on postural sway, muscle strength, reaction time, neuromuscular control, and accidental falls. Subjects were divided into two groups, those participating in the exercise program, and a control group. Both groups were tested before, midway through, and at the end of the exercise program. At the initial testing, no between group differences were noted on any of the performance measures.

The exercisers participated in one-hour exercise sessions held twice weekly, with the exception of school holidays. Each class was divided into four sections: a 5-minute warm-up period, a 35-minute conditioning period, a 15-minute stretching period, and a 5- to 10-minute cool-down period. Exercises were done as a group, and the emphasis was on social interaction and enjoyment. The conditioning period contained aerobic exercises, strengthening exercises, activities for balance, flexibility, endurance, and hand-eye and foot-eye coordination. Stretching exercises included all muscle groups, and the muscles were slowly elongated and held for at least 20 seconds.

Of the 100 women originally assigned to the exercise group, 75 completed the program, and the mean number of classes attended throughout the year was 60. At the end of the program, exercise subjects showed improvements in all five strength measures, in reaction time, neuromuscular control, body sway on a firm surface with eyes open, and body sway on a compressible surface with eyes open and eyes closed. On the other hand, no significant improvements were seen in the control subjects. In terms of the program's effect on falling, no significant differences were seen in the proportion of fallers between the exercise and control subjects. However, the exercisers experienced fewer falls due to loss of balance or weak legs than did the control

group, and fewer exercisers experienced multiple falls within the experimental period. Furthermore, fall frequency was correlated with adherence to the exercise program in the experimental group.

These findings are encouraging as they demonstrate that exercise can result in improved lower-limb strength, reaction time, neuromuscular control, and postural sway in older adults. While the exercise program did not provide complete intervention for fall prevention, the significantly improved performance in the physiological tests after the exercise trial demonstrates that exercise can play an important role in improving stability and related factors in older adults. Furthermore, high adherence to an exercise program may reduce fall frequency.

Ledin, Kronhed, Möller, Möller, Ödkvist, and Olsson (1991) investigated the effects of a shorter period of exercise on the balance of older adults. They used dynamic posturography and clinical balance tests to evaluate performance before and after the training sessions. Specifically, the clinical tests were performed 14 days before and 7 days after the training period, and dynamic posturography was performed 7 days before and 5 days after the training sessions were ended. The clinical tests include measurements of the time a subject can stand without losing balance in a variety of conditions, as well as qualitative measurements of the presence or absence of corrective/erroneous steps in various maneuvers. Both the SO and MC tests of dynamic posturography were completed as described earlier in this chapter.

The training program was performed twice weekly over a nine-week period. The training program consisted of 45 minutes of general gymnastic and balance exercises including jogging and jumping; walking straight forward, backward, on toes and heels; walking with sudden turns; walking sideways; rising from sitting; standing on one leg with eyes open and eyes closed; visual fixation during neck flexion, torsion, and lateral flexion; exercise playing with balls; and jumping on a trampoline. Ten to fifteen minutes of muscle relaxation followed the conditioning exercises described.

On the average, the experimental group participated in 16 of a possible 18 sessions. On the clinical tests, significant differences were found for each subject between groups when standing on one leg with eyes open and head shaking, and walking with turning around. Also, a significant difference was found in Condition 4 of dynamic posturography. When comparing within group performance over time (which included training and prior experience effects), the training group showed significant improvements in balance when standing on one leg with eyes closed, standing on one leg while shaking the head, and walking back and forth and turning around. In the SO portion of dynamic posturography, the equilibrium scores in Conditions 4 to 6 improved significantly. In the MC test, the latencies of the training group decreased significantly to large backward perturbations. In the control group, a significant improvement was found in Condition 5 of the SO portion of dynamic posturography only. No other significant changes in clinical test or dynamic posturography performance were seen in the control group.

As was the case with the study by Lord et al (1995), the results of this investigation (Ledin et al, 1991) demonstrate that exercise can have a positive effect on the balance function of older adults. Interestingly, while the exercise program described by Lord, Clarke, and Webster (1991) was not designed specifically as a vestibular rehabilitation program whereas this was, both resulted in improved balance in the older adult subjects studied. Given the difference in time frames and protocols used, making direct comparisons is difficult. Further study to determine the relative impact of various types of exercises, as well as optimal time frame in which the exercises are practiced, may be useful. In any event, it is evident that maintaining an active lifestyle may have the added benefit of improved balance in older adults.

PROPOSED EVALUATION PROTOCOL FOR OLDER ADULT PATIENTS

In determining an appropriate evaluation protocol to be used with older adult patients, the first step is to consider the question being asked. If the intent of the evaluation is to document the presence of a peripheral vestibular disorder, the protocol selected would be the same regardless of the age of the subject, although the use of age-appropriate norms for each of the tests is important.

The first component of any evaluation of balance function is completion of a thorough case history. According to Jacobson (1997) it is the most important part of the test battery. A copy of the case-history form completed in our clinic may be found in Appendix C. It is important to identify the onset of symptoms, specifically whether sudden or gradual, and whether there is any previous history of similar symptoms. Additionally, the characteristics of the symptoms must be identified, including whether the patient experiences vertigo, unsteadiness or lightheadedness, as well as the time course of the symptoms (in spells versus continuous). If the symptoms come in spells, it is important to determine whether they are spontaneous or result from rapid changes in position. Furthermore, the presence of auditory symptoms (e.g., hearing loss, tinnitus, aural fullness) should be considered.

In addition to obtaining information about the dizziness or imbalance itself, it is important to determine whether the patient has any other significant medical history that may be related to the current symptoms, or that may affect testing. For example, eye diseases, such as cataracts and glaucoma, are fairly common in the older adult population, and may impact the patients' feelings of steadiness, as well as their ability to perform on balance function testing. Similarly, orthopedic problems, such as arthritis of the spine, may impact postural stability and the patients' ability to complete positional and positioning subtests of ENG. Diabetes is a disease that may affect each of the sensory systems involved in the maintenance of postural control. Labyrinthitis, Ménière's disease, head trauma, and disorders of the aural spine are associated with vertiginous episodes and should be ruled out as a possible etiology of the dizziness.

It is also critical to determine whether the patient is taking any medications that may either contribute to the symptoms the patient is experiencing, or impact the validity of the test results. Among the medications frequently used by older adults, benzodiazepines (and other anxiolytics/hypnotics), antidepressants, diuretics, and antihypertensives are of particular concern because they have been demonstrated to adversely affect postural control. Additionally, some listed may impact test results. For a thorough discussion of the relationship between medications and falls in older adults, the reader is referred to Thapa and Ray (1996). Tables 7–2 and 7–3 outline the potential impact of various medications on test results.

PEARL

To supplement the completion of a thorough case history, use of the DHI or DHI-S is recommended. As was mentioned earlier, both scales are useful in determining the patient's perception of the handicap caused by his/her symptoms. Additionally, since previous studies have demonstrated a correlation between abnormal performance on dynamic posturography and high self-perceived dizziness handicap, a high score on the DHI may signal the need for assessing postural control.

ENG is recommended for every patient for whom balance function testing is appropriate. Prior to beginning the actual test, it is advisable to informally assess oculomotor function by having the patient follow the examiner's finger while the examiner watches the patient's eyes. In so doing, it is possible to evaluate smooth pursuit and saccadic eye-movement function and to determine whether the patient has gaze-evoked nystagmus. Additionally, disconjugate eye movements will become obvious. Furthermore, the informal evaluation may provide information about the patient's ability to follow instructions, cueing the examiner to the need for modifications in formal test procedures. The informal evaluation may also include assessing fine motor control (e.g., "touch your nose, now touch my finger" while the examiner moves a finger at arm's length to both sides of midline) and balance (e.g., Romberg and sharpened Romberg).

During formal ENG testing, it may be necessary to repeat various subtests to insure that the data obtained reflect the patient's best performance. Additionally, many older adults benefit from continuous feedback from the examiner about performance, particularly during oculomotor testing. For example, during smooth pursuit testing, patients will often get ahead of the target, resulting in saccadic eye movements. Reminding the patient to strive for smooth eye movements and the need to follow, rather than lead, the target frequently results in improved performance. Similarly, reminding the patient to wait for the target to move before moving the eyes, and then moving the eyes quickly to the target, can result in improved performance on saccade testing. The examiner must remember that the goal of testing is to obtain optimal data. Particularly for older adult patients, the instructions and feedback given can make the difference between "normal" and "abnormal" performance.

Rotational testing is a useful addition to the test battery to get a more complete picture of the integrity of the vestibular system. As does the auditory system, the peripheral vestibular system has a range of frequencies over which it is sensitive. Caloric testing assesses only very low frequency function (i.e., 0.003 Hz), most closely related to the frequencies required to sense postural sway while standing. However, the vestibular system is sensitive up to approximately 5 Hz, with the higher frequencies corresponding to head movements while walking and running. Rotational resting generally evaluates function from 0.01 Hz to 0.64 or 1.28 Hz. For patients demonstrating reduced vestibular response to caloric stimulation, it is useful to determine whether there is return to normal function at the higher frequencies, as normal high-frequency function can be a good prognostic indicator for regaining use of vestibular input for maintenance of postural control. Rotational testing is also useful in assessing CNS compensation to peripheral vestibular deficits. Finally, rotational testing provides some measure of internal consistency. Specifically, a vestibular disorder resulting in weak or absent caloric responses bilaterally should be reflected in low-frequency gain reductions in rotational testing.

Dynamic posturography should be added to the balance function evaluation in cases in which the physician is interested in determining whether the patient is able to make normal use of visual, vestibular, and somatosensory input for the maintenance of postural control. Certainly, it should be considered for all patients with a high score on the DHI, or when there are concerns about determining whether the patient is at risk for falling. If equipment limitations preclude inclusion of computerized dynamic posturography, clinical tests designed to evaluate integration of sensory input (i.e., "foam and dome" tests) should be included. Additionally, clinical tests of gait and stance, similar to those described by Ledin et al (1991) are recommended. Again, the use of age-appropriate norms is essential.

The protocols already described are for use with patients presenting with complaints of dizziness and/or imbalance. However, given the high rate of imbalance and falls in the older adult population, and given the fact that exercise has been shown to have a positive impact on both symptoms and function in older adults, it may be appropriate for primary care physicians to perform screening measures on all of their older adult patients. The screening version of the DHI-S may be a useful screening tool. Additionally, a brief clinical evaluation of gait and standing balance could be included without adding much time to a clinic visit. Patients identified as having a high score on the DHI-S, and/or below normal performance on screening tests of standing and walking balance may be referred for complete balance function testing, and vestibular rehabilitation when deemed appropriate. Patients having low DHI-S scores and normal standing and walking balance should be encouraged to maintain an active lifestyle and to participate in some form of exercise on a regular basis. Further study is needed to determine a program that will result in fall prevention in older adults. However, the data presented to date strongly suggest that regular exercise results in improved balance and reduced dizziness in older adults.

In conclusion, as dizziness is a major cause of falls in older adults, and falls are the sixteenth leading cause of accidental death, balance function testing should be an important part of the audiologist's armamentarium. Audiologists who incorporate balance function tests into their scope of practice should make sure to consider age-related changes in their interpretation of the data.

APPENDIX A
Dizziness Handicap Inventory (DHI)

Instructions: The purpose of this questionnaire is to identify difficulties that you may be experiencing because of your dizziness or unsteadiness. Please answer "yes," "no," or "sometimes" to each question. **Answer each question as it pertains to your dizziness problem only.**

	Yes (4)	Sometimes (2)	No (0)
P1. Does looking up increase your problem?			
E2. Because of your problem do you feel frustrated?			
F3. Because of your problem do you restrict your travel for business or recreation ?			
P4. Does walking down the aisle of a supermarket increase your problem?			
F5. Because of your problem do you have difficulty getting into or out of bed.			
F6. Does your problem significantly restrict your participation in social activities such as going out to dinner, going to the movies, dancing, or to parties?			
F7. Because of your problem do you have difficulty reading?			
P8. Does performing more ambitious activities like sports, dancing, household chores, such as sweeping or putting dishes away, increase your problem?			
E9. Because of your problem are you afraid to leave your home without having someone accompany you?			
E10. Because of your problem have you been embarrassed in front of others?			
P11. Do quick movements of your head increase your problem?			
F12. Because of your problem do you avoid heights?			
P13. Does turning over in bed increase your problem?			
F14. Because of your problem is it difficult for you to do strenuous housework or yardwork?			
E15. Because of your problem are you afraid people may think that you are intoxicated?			
P16. Because of your problem is it difficult for you to go for a walk by yourself?			
P17. Does walking down a sidewalk increase your problem?			
E18. Because of your problem is it difficult for you to concentrate?			
F19. Because of your problem is it difficult for you to walk around your house in the dark?			
E20. Because of your problem are you afraid to stay home alone?			
E21. Because of your problem do you feel handicapped?			
E22. Has your problem placed stress on your relationships with members of your family and friends?			
E23. Because of your problem are you depressed?			
F24. Does your problem interfere with your job or household responsibilities?			
P25. Does bending over increase your problem?			

FUNCTIONAL	EMOTIONAL	PHYSICAL	TOTAL SCORE

APPENDIX B
Dizziness Handicap Inventory Screening Version (DHI-S)

Instructions: The purpose of this scale is to identify difficulties that you may be experiencing because of your dizziness or unsteadiness. Please answer "yes," "no," or "sometimes" to each question. **Answer each question as it pertains to your dizziness or unsteadiness problem only.**

	Yes (4)	Sometimes (2)	No (0)
1E. Because of your problem do you feel depressed?			
2P. Does walking down a sidewalk increase your problem?			
3E. Because of your problem, is it difficult to concentrate?			
4F. Because of your problem, is it difficult for you to walk around your house in the dark?			
5P. Does bending over increase your problem?			
6F. Because of your problem do you restrict your travel for business or recreation?			
7F. Does your problem interfere with your job or household responsibilities?			
8E. Because of your problem, are you afraid to leave your home without having someone accompany you?			
9E. Because of your problem, have you ever been embarrassed in front of others?			
10F. Does your problem significantly restrict your participation in social activities such as going out to dinner, going to movies, dancing or to parties?			

FUNCTIONAL	EMOTIONAL	PHYSICAL	TOTAL SCORE

APPENDIX C
Henry Ford Hospital Division of Audiology
Patient History Form

Name: _____   MRN: _____

Date: _____   Age: _____   Sex: M ☐   F ☐

Onset of symptoms:
Date of onset:
Sudden versus gradual:
Past history:
Previous tests to evaluate:

Characteristics:
Vertigo (objective versus subjective):
Direction of rotation:
Continuous or in spells:
Others (e.g., nausea, emesis):

If continuous, is it:
Unsteadiness:
Lightheadedness:
Vertigo:
Other:

If in spells, describe:
Frequency:
Duration:
Symptoms between attacks:
Spontaneous/motion provoked:

Provocative Positions (yes/no):
lie down from sitting: sit from lying:
stand up from sitting: turn head rt or lt:
bending over: straighten from bending:
rolling rt or lt in bed: look up or down:
others:

Auditory Symptoms: (AS AD AU EQ NN)
Tinnitus: If AU, >in:
Aural fullness: If AU, >in:
Perceived hearing loss:

     Sudden: Fluctuant: Gradual:

Ear Surgery (circle one): AS AD AU None Describe:
Procedure: Middle Ear Dx:

Page 1

APPENDIX C *(Continued)*
Henry Ford Hospital Division of Audiology
Patient History Form

Name: _____

Date: _____

MRN: _____

Age: _____   Sex: M ☐   F ☐

Predisposing Factors (yes/no):

Head injury: Neck injury:

Flu/virus: Ototoxic drugs

D.M. self: D.M. family:

Migraine self: Migraine family:

Heart disease: Hypertension:

Eye disease: Orthopedic:

Neuromuscular: Peripheral vascular:

Toxic chemicals: Barotrauma:

Motion Intolerance (yes/no):

Car sickness(now/past):   Sickness on elevators/escalators:

Sickness in store aisles: Sickness from traffic:

Others:

Miscellaneous:

Increase in frequency/duration with exertion:

Oscillopsia:

Falling (or imminent fall and direction):

Numbness/tingling in face or extremities:

Visual symptoms:

Severe memory lapse:

Nervousness Scale: /10

Others:

Current medications (list ALL with dosage):

Disability Scale (Circle One):

  0 No disability, no symptoms

  1 No disability, bothersome symptoms

  2 Mild disability, performs usual duties, but symptoms interfere with social activity

  3 Moderate disability, disrupts usual duties

  4 Recent severe disability, on medical leave or had to change job

  5 Long-term severe disability, unable to work for past year or longer

Comments:

REFERENCES

ALEXANDER, N.B. (1994). Postural control in older adults. *J. Am. Gerontol. Soc.* 2:93–108.

ALEXANDER, N.B., SHEPARD, N., GEE, M.J., & SCHULTZ, A. (1992). Postural control in young and elderly adults when stance is perturbed: kinematics. *J. of Gerontology: Medical Sciences*, 47:79–87.

ANDERSON, R.G., & MEYERHOFF, W.L. (1982). Otologic manifestation of aging. *Otolaryngol. Clin. N. Amer.*, 15:353–370.

BABIN, R.W., & HARKER, L.A. (1982). The vestibular system in the elderly. *Otolaryngol. Clin. N. Amer.*, 15:387–393.

BALOH, R.W., JACOBSON, K.M., & SOCOTCH, T.M. (1993). The effect of aging on visual-vestibulo-ocular responses. *Exp. Brain Res.*, 95:509–516.

BECKER, W., NAUMANN, H.H., & PFALTZ, C.R. (1994). *Ear, Nose, and Throat Diseases: A Pocket Reference*, 2d ed. New York: Thieme Medical Publishers.

BELAL, A., & GLORIG, A. (1986). Disequilibrium of aging (presbyastasis). *J. Laryngol Otol*, 100:1037–1041.

BERGSTROM, B. (1973). Morphology of the vestibular nerve. II. The number of myelinated vestibular nerve fibers in man at various ages. *Acta Otolaryngol*, 76:173–179.

BLOOM, J., & KATSARKAS, A. (1989). Paroxysmal positional vertigo in the elderly. *J. Otolaryngol*, 18:96–98.

BOULT, C., MURPHY, J., SLOANE, P., MOR, V., & DRONE, C. (1991). The relation of dizziness to functional decline. *J. Am Ger Soc*, 39:858–861.

BROCKLEHURST, J.C., ROBERTSON, D., & JAMES-GROOM, P. (1982). Clinical correlates of sway in older age-sensory modalities. *Age Ageing*, 11:1–10.

BRUNER, A., & NORRIS, T.W. (1971). Age-related changes in caloric nystagmus. *Acta Otolaryngol Suppl*, 282:5–24.

BURNS, G. (1996). Quotation. In: B. Lansky (Ed.), *Age Happens—The Best Quotes About Growing Older*. New York: Meadowbrook Press.

CLARKSON, P. (1978). The relationship of age and level of physical activity with the fractionated components of patellar reflex time. *J. Gerontology*, 33:650–656.

CLEMENT, P.A., VAN DER LAAN, F.L., & OOSTERVELD, W.J. (1975). The influence of age on vestibular function. *Acta Otolaryngologica*, 29:163–172.

COOGLER, C.E. (1992). Falls and imbalance. *Rehab Management*, 5:53–117.

CUTSON, T.M. (1994). Falls in the elderly. *Am Fam Physician*, 49:149–156.

DAVIDSON, J., WRIGHT, G., ILMOYL, L., CANTER, R.J., & BARBER, H.O. (1988). The reproducibility of caloric tests of vestibular function in young and old subjects. *Acta Otolaryngologica*, 106:264–268.

DEMER, J.L. (1994). Effect of aging on vertical visual tracking and visual-vestibular interaction. *J. Vestibular Res*, 4:355–370.

DEWANE, J.A. (1995). Dealing with dizziness and disequilibrium in older patients: a clinical approach. *Top Geriatr Rehabil*, 11:30–38.

ENGSTROM, H., BERGSTROM, B., & ROSENHALL, U. (1974). Vestibular sensory epithelia. *Arch Otolaryngol*, 100:411–418.

ENGSTROM, H., ADES, H.W., ENGSTROM, M.B., GILCHRIST, D., & BOURNE, G. (1977). Structural changes in the vestibular epithelia in elderly monkeys and humans. *Adv Oto Rhino Laryngol*, 22:93–110.

ERA, P., & HEIKKINEN, E. (1985). Postural sway during standing and unexpected disturbance of balance in random samples of men of different ages. *J. Gerontol.*, 40:287–295.

FOZARD, J.L., WOLF, E., BELL, B., McFARLAND, R.A., & PODOLSKY, S. (1977). Visual perception and communication. In: J.E. Birrenm, & K.W. Schaie, (Eds.). *Handbook of the Psychology of Aging.* New York: Van Nostrand Reinhold.

FUJII, M., GOTO, N., & KIKUCHI, K. (1990). Nerve fiber analysis and the aging process of the vestibulocochlear nerve. *Ann Otol Rhinol Laryngol*, 99:863–870.

FURMAN, J.M., & CASS, S.P. (1996). *Balance Disorders: A Case Study Approach.* Philadelphia: F.A. Davis.

GACEK, R.R., & HAM, R. (1989). A clinical approach to the management of geriatric dysequilibrium. *Ear Nose Throat J.*, 68:958–960.

GHOSH, P. (1985). Aging and auditory vestibular response. *Ear Nose and Throat Journal*, 64:264–266.

GINTER, S.F., & MION, L.C. (1992). Falls in the nursing home: preventable or inevitable? *J. Gerontol Nurs*, 11:43–48.

GLICK, R., & BONDAREFF, W. (1979). Loss of synapses in the cerebellar cortex of the senescent rat. *J. Gerontology*, 34:818–822.

GOEBEL, J.A., HANSON, J.M., & FISHEL, D.G. (1994a). Interlaboratory variability of rotational chair test results. *Otolaryngol. Head Neck Surg.*, 110:400–405.

GOEBEL, J.A., HANSON, J.M., & FISHEL, D.G. (1994b). Age-related modulation of the vestibulo-ocular reflex using real and imaginary targets. *J. Vestibular Res*, 4:269–275.

GOTTSDANKER, R. (1980). Aging and the maintenance of preparation. *Exp Aging Res*, 6:13–27.

GREER, M. (1981). How serious is dizziness? *Geriatrics*, 36:34–42.

GRYFE, C.I., AMIERS, A., & ASHLEY, M.J. (1977). A longitudinal study of falls in the elderly population. I. Incidence and morbidity. *Age and Aging*, 6:201.

HALE, W.E., PERKINS, L.L., MAY, F.E., MARKS, R.G., & STEWART, R.B. (1986). Symptom prevalence in the elderly. *J. Am. Geriatric Soc.*, 34:333–340.

HALL, T.C., MILLER, A.K.H., & CORSELLIS, J.A.N. (1975). Variations in the human Purkinje cell population according to age and sex. *Neurolpathol App Neurobiol*, 1:267–292.

HORAK, F.B., SHUPERT, C.L., & MIRKA, A. (1989). Components of postural dyscontrol in the elderly. *Neurolbiol Aging*, 10:727–738.

JACOBSON, G. (1997). Ten tips (give or take a couple) for balance function testing. *Hearing Journal*, 50:10–19.

JACOBSON, G.P., & CALDER, J.H. (1998). A screening version of the dizziness handicap inventory (DHI-S). *American Journal of Otology,* 19:804–808.

JACOBSON, G.P., & HENRY, K.G. (1989). Effect of temperature on fixation suppression ability in normal subjects: The need for temperature and age-dependent values. *Ann Otol Rhinol Laryngol,* 98:369–372.

JACOBSON, G.P., & NEWMAN, C.W. (1990). The development of the Dizziness Handicap Inventory (DHI). *Arch Otolaryngol-Head Neck Surgery,* 116:424–427.

JACOBSON, G.P., HUNTER, L., & BALZER, G. (1991). Balance function test correlates of the Dizziness Handicap Inventory (DHI). *JAAA,* 2:253–260.

JACOBSON, G.P., NEWMAN, C.W., & KARTUSH, J.M. (1993). *Handbook of Balance Function Testing.* St. Louis: Mosby.

JENKINS, H.A., FURMAN, J.M., GULYA, A.J., HONRUBIA, V., LINTHICUM, F.H., & MIRKA, A. (1989). Dysequilibrium of aging. *Otolaryngol Head Neck Surg,* 100:272–281.

JOHNSSON, L.G. (1971). Degenerative changes and anomalies of the vestibular system in man. *Laryngoscope,* 81:1682–1694.

JOHNSSON, L.G. (1973). Vascular pathology in the human inner ear. *Adv Oto-Rhino-Laryng,* 20:197–220.

JOHNSSON, L.G., & HAWKINS, J.E. (1972). Sensory and neural degeneration with aging, as seen in microdissections of the inner ear. *Ann Otol Rhinol Laryngol,* 81:179–193.

JORDON, T., & RABBITT, P. (1977). Response times of increasing complexity as a function of ageing. *Br J, Psychology,* 68:189–201.

JORGENSEN, M.B. (1961). Changes of aging in the inner ear. *Archives of Otolaryngology,* 74:164–170.

KARLSEN, E.A., HASSANEIN, R.M., & GOETZINGER, C.P. (1981). The effects of age, sex, hearing loss, and water temperature on caloric nystagmus. *Laryngoscope,* 91:620–627.

KENNEDY, R., & CLEMIS, J.D. (1990). The geriatric auditory and vestibular systems. *Otolaryngol Clin N. Amer.,* 23: 1075–1082.

KERBER, K., ENRIETTO, I., JACOBSON, K., & BALOH, R. (1998). Disequilibrium in older people: a prospective study. *Neurology,* 51:574–580.

KESHNER, E.A., ALLUM, J.H.J., & HONEGGER, F. (1993). Predictors of less stable postural responses to support surface relations in healthy human elderly. *J Vestibular Res,* 3:419–429.

KIPPENBROCK, T., & SOJA, M.E. (1993). Preventing falls in the elderly: interviewing patients who have fallen. *Geriatr Nurs,* 14:205–209.

KONRAD, H., GIRARDI, M., & HELFAT, R. (1999). Balance and aging. *Laryngoscope,* 109:1454–1460.

KROLL, W., & CLARKSON, P.M. (1978). Age, isometric knee-extension strength, and fractionated resisted response time. *Exp Aging Res,* 4:389–409.

LARISH, D., & STELMACH, G. (1982). Preprogramming, programming, and reprogramming of aimed hand movements as a function of age. *J. Mot Behav,* 14:322–340.

LAWSON, G.D., SHEPARD, N.T., OVIATT, D.L., & WANG, Y. (1994). Electromyographic responses of lower leg mus-

cles to upward toe tilts as a function of age. *J Vestibular Res,* 4:203–214.

LEDIN, T., KRONHED, A.C., MÖLLER, C., MÖLLER, M., ÖDKVIST, L.M., & OLSSON, B. (1991). Effects of balance training in elderly evaluated by clinical tests and dynamic posturography. *J. Vestibular Res,* 1:129–138.

LOPEZ, I., HONRUBIA, V., & BALOH, R.W. (1997). Aging and the human vestibular nucleus. *J. Vestibular Res,* 7:77–85.

LORD, S.R., CLARK, R.D., & WEBSTER, I.W. (1991). Postural stability and associated physiological factors in a population of aged persons. *J. Gerontol,* 46:M69–76.

LORD, S.R., WARD, J.A., WILLIAMS, P., & STRUDWICK, M. (1995). The effect of a 12-month exercise trial on balance, strength, and falls in older women: a randomized controlled trial. *J. Amer Geriatrics Soc,* 43:1198–1206.

LUXON, L.M. (1991). Disturbances of balance in the elderly. *Br. J. Hosp. Med.,* 45:22–26.

MACLENNAN, W.J. (1992). Dizziness. In: J.G. Evans, & T.F. Williams (Eds.), *Oxford Textbook of Geriatric Medicine.* Oxford: Oxford University Press.

MANCHESTER, D., WOOLLACOTT, M., ZEDERBAURER-HYLTON, N., & MARIN, O. (1989). Visual, vestibular, and somatosensory contributions to balance control in the older adult. *J. Gerontol,* 44:M118–127.

MANKOVSKII, N., MINTS, Y.A., & LYSENYUK, U.P. (1980). Regulation of the preparatory period for complex voluntary movement in old and extreme old age. *Hum Physiol,* 6:46–50.

MULCH, G., & PETERMANN, W. (1979). Influence of age on results of vestibular function tests. *Ann Otol Rhinol. Laryngol (suppl)* 56:1–17.

NADOL, J.B. JR., & SCHUKNECHT, H.F. (1989). The pathology of peripheral vestibular disorders in the elderly. *Ear Nose Throat,* 68:930–933.

NORRE, M.E., & BECKERS, A. (1989). Vestibular habituation training for positional vertigo in elderly patients. *Arch. Gerontol Geriatr,* 8:117–122.

NORRE, M.E., FORREZ, G., & BECKERS, A. (1987). Vestibular dysfunction causing instability in aged patients. *Acta Otolaryngol* (Stockholm), 104:50–55.

PAIGE, G. (1992). Senescence of human visual-vestibular interactions. I. VOR and adaptive plasticity with aging. *J. Vestibular Res.,* 2:133–155.

PETERKA, R.J., & BLACK, F.O. (1990a). Age-related changes in postural control: sensory organization tests. *J. Vestibular Res,* 1:73–85.

PETERKA, R.J., & BLACK, F.O. (1990b). Age-related changes in postural control: motor coordination tests. *J. Vestibular Res,* 1:87–96.

PETERKA, R.J., BLACK, F.O., & SCHOENHOFF, M.B. (1990a). Age-related changes in human vestibulo-ocular reflexes: sinusoidal rotation and caloric tests. *J. Vestibular Res,* 1:49–59.

PETERKA, R.J., BLACK, F.O., & SCHOENHOFF, M.B. (1990b). Age-related changes in human vestibulo-ocular reflexes: pseudorandom rotation tests. *J. Vestibular Res,* 1:61–71.

PITT, M.C., & RAWLES, J.M. (1988). The effect of age on saccadic latency and velocity. *Neuro-ophthalmology,* 8:123–129.

RICHTER, E. (1980). Quantitative study of human scarpa's ganglion and vestibular sensory epithelia. *Acta Otolaryngol,* 90:199–208.

ROBERTSON, D.D., & IRELAND, D.J. (1995). Dizziness Handicap Inventory correlates of computerized dynamic posturography. *J. Otolaryngol.,* 24:118–124.

ROGERS, J., SILVER, M.A., SHOEMAKER, W.J., & BLOOM, F.E. (1980). Senescent changes in a neurobiological model system: cerebellar Purkinje cell electrophysiology and correlative anatomy. *Neurobiol Aging,* 1:3–11.

ROGERS, J., ZORNETZER, S.F., & BLOOM, F.E. (1981). Senescent pathology of the cerebellum: Purkinje neurons and their parallel fiber afferents. *Neurobiol Aging,* 2:15–25.

ROSENHALL, U. (1972). Vestibular macular mapping in man. *Ann Otol,* 81:339.

ROSENHALL, U. (1973). Degenerative changes in the aging human vestibular geriatric neuroepithelia. *Acta Otolaryngol,* 76:208–220.

ROSENHALL, U., & RUBIN, W. (1975). Degenerative changes in the human vestibular sensory epithelia. *Acta Otolaryngol,* 79:67–80.

ROSS, M.D., JOHNSSON, L.G., PEACOR, D., & ALLARD, L.F. (1976). Observations on normal and degenerating human otoconia. *Ann Otol Rhinol Laryngol,* 85:310–326.

SALTHOUSE, T.A. (1985). Speed of behavior and its implications for cognition. In: J. Birren, & K.W. Schaie (Eds.), *Handbook of the Psychology of Aging,* 2d ed. New York: Van Nostrand Reinhold.

SCHUKNECHT, H.F. (1969). Cupulolithiasis. *Arch Otolaryngol,* 90:765–778.

SHARPE, J.A., & ZACKON, D.H. (1987). Senescent saccades: effects of aging on their accuracy, latency, and velocity. *Acta Otolaryngol* (Stockholm), 104:422–428.

SHEPARD, N.T., & TELIAN, S.A. (1996). *Practical Management of the Balance Disorder Patient.* San Diego: Singular Publishing Group.

SKINNER, H.B., BARRACK, R.L., & COOK, S.D. (1984). Age-related declines in proprioception. *Clin Orthop,* 184:208–211.

SLOANE, P.D., BALOH, R.W., & HONRUBIA, V. (1989). The vestibular system in the elderly: clinical implications. *Amer. J. Olol.,* 10:422–429.

SLOANE, P., GEORGE, L., & BLAZER, D. (1989). Dizziness in a community elderly population. *J. Am. Geriatric Soc.,* 37:101–108.

SONDEREGGER, E.N., MEIENBERG, O., & EHRENGRUBER, H. (1986). Normative data of saccadic eye movements for routine diagnosis of ophthalmoneurological disorders. *Neuro-ophthalmology,* 6:257–269.

STEFANSSON, S., & IMOTO, T. (1986). Age-related changes in optokinetic and rotational tests. *Amer. J. Otol.,* 7:193–196.

STELMACH, G.E., & WORRINGHAM, C. (1985). Sensorimotor deficits related to postural stability: implications for falling in the elderly. *Clinics in Geriatric Medicine,* 1(3):679–691.

TEASDALE, N., STELMACH, G.E., & BREUNIG, A. (1991). Postural sway characteristics of the elderly under normal and altered visual and support surface conditions. *J. Gerontol,* 46:B238–B244.

TEDEIKSAAR, R. (1998). Disturbances of gait, balance, and the vestibular system. In: R. Tallis, H. Fillit, & J. Brocklehurst (Eds.), *Brocklehurst's Textbook of Geriatric Medicine and Gerontology.* England: Churchill Livingstone.

THAPA, P.B., & RAY, W.A. (1996). Medications and falls and fall-related injuries in the elderly. In: A.M. Bronstein, T. Brandt, & M. Woollacott (Eds.). *Clinical Disorders of Balance, Posture and Gait,* pp. 301–325. New York: Oxford University Press.

TINETTI, M.E., SPEECHLEY, M., & GINTER, S.F. (1988). Risk factors for falls among elderly persons living in the community. *N. Eng. J. Med,* 319:1701–1707.

TORVIK, A., TORP, S., & LINDBOE, C.F. (1986). Atrophy of the cerebellar vermis in ageing: a morphometric and histologic study. *J Neurol Sci,* 76:283–294.

URA, M., PFALTZ, R., & ALLUM, J.H.J. (1991). The effect of age on the visuo- and vestibo-ocular reflexes of elderly patients with vertigo. *Acta Otolaryngol* (Stockholm), 481:399–402.

VAN DER LAAN, F.L., & OOSTERVELD, W.J. (1974). Age and vestibular function. *Aerospace Medicine,* 45:540–547.

WALL, C., & BLACK, F.O. (1984). Effects of age, sex, and stimulus parameters on vestibulo-ocular responses to sinusoidal rotation. *Acta Otolaryngol* (Stockholm), 98:270–278.

WARNER, E.A., WALLACH, P.M., ADELMAN, H.M., & SAHLIN-HUGHES, K. (1992). Dizziness in primary care patients. *J. Gen Intern Med,* 7:454–463.

WOOLLACOTT, M., SHUMWAY-COOK, A.T., & NASHER, L.M. (1982). Postural reflexes and aging. In: J.A. Mortimer (Ed.), *The Aging Motor System,* pp. 98–119. New York: Praeger.

YAGI, T., SEKINE, S., SHIMIZU, M. (1983). Age-dependent changes in the gains of the vestibulo-ocular reflex in humans. *Adv Otorhinolaryngol,* 30:9–12.

ZACKON, D.H., & SHARPE, J.A. (1987). Smooth pursuit in senescence: effects of target acceleration and velocity. *Acta Otolaryngol,* 104:290–297.

Rehabilitative Considerations

Chapter 8

Audiologic Rehabilitation: An Integrated Approach

Most people do not realize how depressing this condition can be. . . . People who can hear have no patience for those of us who cannot.

—F.B., 91-year-old woman with hearing loss for 20 years

Compared to all the other health problems I have had to endure, multiple sclerosis, cancer, lupus . . . hearing loss is the most devastating to me. . . . It is isolating, maddening, and it makes me feel so stupid. . . . I hate it!

—C.F., 79-year-old woman

My husband does not even understand the disability he is experiencing. Perhaps if he understood what was happening to him he would do better with his hearing aids.

—B.S., 68-year-old first and only wife of an experienced hearing-aid user

LEARNING OBJECTIVES

After reading this chapter, you should be able to:

- Educate others about the fact that audiologic rehabilitation (AR) will lead to more competent and satisfied hearing-aid users.
- Show that AR is not synonymous with lipreading.
- Better counsel hearing-instrument candidates and users.
- Include AR as part of the evaluation, selection, and dispensing process. Time constraints should not be an excuse for not providing rehabilitation services.
- Integrate AR in your practice as an indispensable component of a treatment program for older adults with hearing impairment. Every new hearing-aid user needs and benefits from some form of AR.
- Apply AR as a cost-effective measure.

AR: AN INTEGRATED APPROACH

AR with older adults requires a perspective different from that adopted for younger individuals, on both a conceptual

and a practical level (Hartke, 1991; Kane, Ouslander, & Abrass, 1994). Rehabilitation of the older adult requires a "biopsychosocial approach" with an emphasis on restoring "functional ability," independence, and the quality of life of the person with a disabling chronic condition (Kane, Ouslander, & Abrass, 1994; Brummel-Smith, 1990; Hartke, 1991; Weinstein, 1991). Stated differently, the process of AR is one that assists persons with hearing impairment to recover lost physical, psychological, or social skills, so that they "may be more independent, live in personally satisfying environments and maintain meaningful social interactions" (Brummel-Smith, 1990, p. 3).

SPECIAL CONSIDERATION

As of this writing it appears that AR in combination with diagnostics is now more often seen as a primary clinical duty than it was in 1980 (Schow, Balsara, Smedley, & Whitcomb, 1993).

According to a survey of 469 clinically active audiologists, 94% report doing some form of AR, ranging from individual hearing-aid orientation to auditory training to counseling with family and friends (Schow, Balsara, Smedley, & Whitcomb, 1993). It is of interest that the proportion of respondents engaged in the more traditional forms of AR has declined from 1980 to 1990. For example, the proportion offering speechreading classes has declined from 38% in 1980 to 19% in 1990 and the proportion engaged in auditory training has declined from 31% to 16%. Conversely, the proportion of clinical audiologists using self-assessment scales has increased from 18% in 1980 to 33% in 1990, as has the proportion counseling the family and friends of the hearing impaired (e.g., 80% in 1980, 86% in 1990) (Schow et al, 1993). Hopefully, this change will continue, with AR becoming a part of the package when a hearing aid is selected and dispensed. Perhaps Carl Binnie (1994, p. 13) was correct when he commented that "the future of audiologic rehabilitation is bright and promising."

The goals of this chapter are: (1) to offer a contemporary view of AR; (2) to present a framework in which audiologists can practice rehabilitation in tune with their

171

understanding of the unique needs of older adults with handicapping hearing impairments; (3) to enable clinicians in rehabilitation to deal more effectively with the special aspects of providing care to older patients with hearing loss by applying more recent information about approaches that are successful; (4) to demonstrate to audiologists that AR is the responsibility of audiologists involved in the diagnosis and management of individuals with hearing impairments, disability, and handicaps (Brummel-Smith, 1990); and (5) to dispel myths about hearing aids and AR.

Myth 1 Hearing aids restore hearing to normal.
Myth 2 Hearing aids eliminate all communication problems.
Myth 3 All hearing-aid users can achieve adequate speech recognition with hearing aids alone.
Myth 4 Most people with hearing aids do not like how they sound.

The organization of the chapter reflects my commitment to dispelling the myths about hearing aids held by patients with hearing impairment using AR as the agent of change. Further, the chapter has been written with deference to the evolving health care system wherein funding is minimal, time is money, and the need for accountability is great. These latter factors convince me more than ever of the importance of an AR program that is brief, efficient, and, above all, comprehensive.

FUNCTIONS OF AUDITION

The older adult's vision and perspective are often clouded by the series of losses attending the aging process that include illness, death of cohorts, retirement, and the possibility of relocation. Hearing loss represents yet another in a series of losses serving to further remind older adults of the necessity of coming to terms with the final life stage. The impact of hearing loss as experienced by older adults is dependent on what the loss does to their lives as well as on what audiologists consider foremost, namely the extent of sound attenuation (Van Hecke, 1994).

SPECIAL CONSIDERATION

As discussed in Chapter 3, the major psychological task facing persons in their last stage of life, late adulthood, and old age, is assigning meaning to their life (Erikson, 1950).

To best understand the impact of hearing loss on older adults the clinician must recall the functions of hearing and the resulting sense of loss. According to Ramsdell (1960), the most fundamental level of hearing is the primitive level, which constitutes "an unconscious link between the individual, and a constantly changing environment." The primitive level of hearing might be conceived of as a basic physiological function." The ability to hear background sounds, such as birds singing and the hum of a car, contributes to our sense of being part of an alive world (Ramsdell, 1960). Persons with severe to profound hearing loss, are often deprived of

the ability to hear background noise, with potentially dramatic psychosocial consequences resulting from such deprivation. Loss at this level may trigger depressive reactions.

PEARL

Presbycusis does not render older adults profoundly deaf and thus the primitive level of hearing remains intact in this population.

Moderately severe, severe, or profound hearing loss can compromise the signal/warning level or the second level of hearing. Ramsdell (1960) postulated that at this level, sound serves as an indicator of an outside stimulus or event and assists in locating the source of sound. In a sense, at this level, hearing serves to inform persons of dangers in the environment including the presence of smoke in the home, an oncoming vehicle, or a knock at the door. The ability to hear warning signals as well as background noise fosters a sense of security and independence. Thus, one's sense of safety and security in the home can be jeopardized when warning signals in the environment are inaudible. The ability to hear signals in the environment is an especially important goal for most hearing-impaired older adults, especially for those who live alone and for those suffering from cognitive problems, including dementia. According to Maslow (1954), older adults are very motivated to pursue intervention when a chronic condition is a threat to safety, either at home or in society at large. People first seek to satisfy their most basic needs, those necessary to survival, after which they will seek to satisfy higher social, self-esteem, and self-actualization needs (Kotler & Clarke, 1987). The availability of assistive-listening devices (ALDs) is an important step toward maintaining a sense of safety and security.

The function subserved by the third level of hearing, namely the symbolic level, is the ability to communicate. When hearing does not function at this level, as is the case with even a mild high-frequency sensorineural hearing loss, older adults may be denied the pleasure of listening to music, of hearing the laughter of children, and of attending cultural events such as films, theater, or lectures. Further, hearing loss may diminish the quantity and quality of social interactions. Hearing-impaired individuals deprived of hearing at the third level may suffer from a loss of social independence. Hence, inability to communicate may interfere with life satisfaction and may impact on one's self-esteem (Kemp, 1990a). According to Kemp (1990a), the latter issues are of greatest concern to persons with disability. Therefore, rehabilitation must be directed toward insuring that life satisfaction and self-esteem are enhanced.

PEARL

Restoration, either in part or in full, of each of these levels of hearing via some form of AR can help promote adjustment to hearing loss contributing to life satisfaction.

CONSEQUENCES OF HEARING LOSS

The sensorineural hearing loss experienced by older adults has dramatic effects on communication and psychosocial function. With regard to communication function the primary deficit is difficulty in understanding speech. As discussed in Chapter 5, an impaired cochlea can lead to hearing impairment for pure-tones, reduced frequency resolution, reduced temporal resolution, and impairment of speech feature detection (Binnie, 1991). Difficulty recognizing and understanding speech in a background of noise typically ensues in a large proportion of adults over 50 with hearing impairment. Communication deficits attributable to the "aging of the sensorineural mechanism" include difficulty at home, difficulty at work, interpersonal difficulties, difficulty understanding speech from a distance, in the context of noise, and on the telephone. Communication disability can place an individual at a disadvantage relative to others leading to a handicap or a "disadvantage experienced through interaction with and adaptation to the environment" (Hyde & Riko, 1994, p. 348).

The goal of most hearing-aid designs is to improve audibility and intelligibility. In turn, most audiologists encourage hearing-impaired persons to wear hearing aids to reduce the extent of the communication deficit. Audiologists spend the majority of time matching the electroacoustic response of the hearing aid to the person's audiometric profile. The goal, namely a well-fit hearing aid wherein real-ear gain is in close agreement with that provided by the National Acoustics Laboratory-Revised (NAL-R), insures that a wide portion of the speech spectrum is inaudible. The latter theoretically leads to significant improvements in speech-recognition performance in quiet and in noise over unaided listening.

It is important to keep in mind that speech-recognition ability bears an imperfect relationship to self-perceived hearing handicap in the psychosocial domain. It is incumbent on

PEARL

Information on receptive ability obtained in the clinic does not assure success in everyday communication exchanges.

the audiologist to gain an understanding of the disabling and handicapping effects of hearing loss and to insure that the audibility and clarity provided by hearing aids facilitate adjustment in the area of psychosocial function. As expressed by Howard "Rocky" Stone (1990), the audiologist must be aware of the psychosocial needs of the whole person and not just focus on the technology.

SPECIAL CONSIDERATION

Psychological and social variables may be more closely linked to hearing-aid success than electroacoustic parameters.

A number of recent studies have demonstrated that hearing loss has an adverse effect on functional status, cognitive function, and emotional, behavioral, and social well-being. Increasing difficulties communicating, combined with the aforementioned changes account for the fact that hearing impairment may inhibit a person's ability to function independently and hence compromise quality of life (Bess, Lichtenstein, Logan, Burger, & Nelson, 1989; Uhlmann, Larson, Rees, Koepsell, & Duckert, 1989; Mulrow, Aguilar, Endicott, & Velez, 1990; Garstecki & Erler, 1996). Garstecki and Erler (1996) examined the behaviors associated with mild to moderate hearing loss in a sample of over 300 older adults. The average age of subjects in their sample was 75. The Communication Profile for the Hearing Impaired (CPHI), which measures self-perceived handicap in four content areas, namely, communication performance, communication environment, communication strategies, and personal adjustment, was completed by the respondents. While subjects did report emotional ramifications of hearing loss, the most problematic situations included work-like or social settings. It was of interest that subjects in this economically advantaged sample judged effective communication in the work setting to be more important than communication in social settings.

SPECIAL CONSIDERATION

Responses of individual subjects in the CPHI indicated a high degree of individual variability in the reactions of older adults to hearing loss, ranging from complete acceptance and positive personal adjustment to feelings of displacement, anger, and withdrawal.

Mulrow, Aguilar, Endicott, and Velez (1990) conducted a cross-sectional study of 204 elderly male veterans selected from a primary care clinic designed to assess the association between hearing impairment and quality of life. Quality of life was defined according to two disease-specific and three generic measures that have been standardized on older adults (Mulrow et al, 1990). The disease specific measures were the Hearing Handicap Inventory for the Elderly (HHIE), which assesses the self-perceived emotional and social effects of hearing loss, and the Quantified Denver Scale of Communication Function (QDS). The QDS quantifies the perceived communication difficulties secondary to hearing impairment (Mulrow et al, 1990). The generic measures included the Short Portable Mental Status Questionnaire (SPMSQ), which yields information about cognitive function; the Geriatric Depression Scale (GDS), which assesses affect; and the Self-Evaluation of Life Function (SELF), which assesses function in several domains including physical disability, social satisfaction, aging, depression, self-esteem, and personal control.

Hearing loss in their sample of older hearing-impaired adults was associated with significant social, emotional, and communication handicaps, as mean scores on the HHIE and QDS were significantly higher for the hearing-impaired group than for the not hearing-impaired group. In contrast, mean scores on the GDS and the SELF did not differ for the groups with and without a hearing impairment. Similarly, mental status was intact for both groups of subjects. As the extent of the perceived social and emotional dysfunction was considerable for their sample (i.e., 66% had HHIE scores > 42 indicative of severe handicap; and 16% had mild to moderate handicaps or HHIE scores between 18 and 40), the authors concluded that hearing loss has an adverse effect on quality of life. A follow-up randomized trial of hearing-aid rehabilitation indicated that hearing-aid intervention was effective at reducing the communication, psychosocial handicaps, as well as depressive and cognitive symptoms experienced by the majority of hearing-impaired older males in their sample (Mulrow, Aguilar, Endicott, & Tuley, 1990). In light of the reduction in depressive symptoms and psychosocial handicap it is tempting to infer a causal relation between hearing loss and these symptoms.

Bess, Lichtenstein, and Logan (1991) reported on the association between hearing loss in older adults and scores on tests of hearing disability and global dysfunction. The Sickness Impact Profile (SIP), a 136-item scale that assesses psychosocial function in a behavioral context, was the index of functional health status, and the screening version of the Hearing Handicap Inventory for the Elderly (HHIE-S) was the hearing specific measure for disability (Bess, Lichtenstein, & Logan, 1991). The authors noted a graded association between measurable hearing impairment and functional health status, such that persons with increasing levels of hearing impairment (speech frequency pure-tone average) demonstrated increased levels of psychosocial and physical dysfunction as measured on the SIP. For example, on the physical scale that assesses ambulation, mobility, and body care/movement, mean SIP scores increased from 3.3 for those with no impairment to 18.9 for those with a loss of 41 dBHL or greater. Thus, on the physical subscale, a SIP score change of 2.8 will occur with each 10 dB increase in hearing loss (Bess et al, 1989). Further, higher HHIE-S scores were associated with higher SIP scores suggesting a relation between hearing disability and global dysfunction (Bess, Lichtenstein, & Logan, 1991). Once again, these findings link hearing loss to functional disability and handicap and demonstrate the importance of including this information in the rehabilitative assessment. Efforts to improve hearing with hearing aids can result in meaningful improvements in quality of life in general and functional status in particular.

SPECIAL CONSIDERATION

Hearing loss is a major determinant of function in older persons. Increasing hearing loss is strongly associated with increased behavioral dysfunction in older adults (Bess, Logan, & Lichtenstein, 1990).

It seems that the effects of hearing loss are first felt in terms of the emotional effects, and as the hearing loss becomes more severe it impacts on social situational function. Weinstein (1980) investigated the relation between audiologic measures and objective and subjective social isolation on a sample of older male veterans with primarily mild to moderately, severe, late-onset sensorineural hearing loss. Objective isolation was quantified using the Objective Present Isolation Scale, which quantifies contacts with significant others, participa-

tion in leisure and recreational activities, and living arrangements. Subjective isolation was quantified using the Subjective Social Isolation Scale, which quantifies interest in engaging in activities, feelings of loneliness, feelings of inferiority, and satisfaction with the quality and quantity of social interactions. The Objective and Subjective Isolation Scales are homogeneous subscales within the Comprehensive Assessment and Referral Evaluation (CARE), a semistructured interview that was developed by Gurland, Kuriansky, Sharpe, Simon, Stiller, and Birkett (1978). The extent of subjective social isolation (e.g., loneliness, withdrawal) was more highly related to severity of hearing impairment and self-perceived hearing handicap than was the extent of objective isolation (e.g., engagement in social activities, visiting friends/family).

Correlations between audiometric measures and feelings of subjective social isolation ranged from 0.40 to 0.52, whereas the correlation between audiometric measures and feelings of objective isolation was approximately 0.25. It was noteworthy that not until the hearing loss became moderately severe did it impact on involvement in social activities such that the majority of persons with moderately severe sensorineural hearing loss lived alone, rarely socialized, kept problems to themselves, rarely visited friends and relatives, rarely engaged in leisure activities, rarely spoke on the telephone, and rarely engaged in volunteer activities. In contrast, even a mild hearing loss left a large proportion of respondents feeling upset, nervous, and handicapped, with the proportion increasing with hearing loss severity. It was of interest that individuals who were considered to be isolated both objectively and subjectively had poorer hearing and were more handicapped than those who were not isolated. Weinstein (1980) concluded that early on, hearing loss is felt in terms of its psychological impact, and as it progresses, it curtails social life.

Data from the nationwide survey of hearing impaired persons over 50 years of age, which was commissioned by the National Council on Aging (NCOA) and funded by the Hearing Instruments Association (HIA), confirmed the detrimental effects on quality of life associated with untreated hearing loss (Kirkwood, 1999). The data from the NCOA study indirectly confirmed that individuals with untreated hearing loss are more likely than hearing aid users to experience depression, anger, and frustration. The former group appears to be less engaged socially than hearing aid users with comparable hearing loss (Kirkwood, 1999).

SPECIAL CONSIDERATION

Hearing aids/AR is critical even for persons with mild hearing loss when its impact on emotional status may be felt at first.

Finally, data are beginning to accumulate documenting a link between hearing loss and cognitive status in persons diagnosed with senile dementia. The major findings of studies on hearing loss in persons with dementia include the following:

1. Hearing loss is more prevalent in older adults with dementia (Weinstein & Amsel, 1986).

2. Older adults with dementia are likely to have more severe hearing loss than those without dementia (Weinstein & Amsel, 1986; Uhlmann et al, 1989).

3. The risk of dementia increases as a function of increasing hearing loss, after adjusting for potentially confounding variables such as depression, number of primary prescriptions, age, etc. (Uhlmann et al, 1989).

4. Unremediated hearing loss lowers performance on aurally administered diagnostic tests used to quantify the severity of senile dementia (Weinstein & Amsel, 1986).

5. Hearing aids lower scores on tests of cognitive function suggesting improved mental status with hearing aid use (Mulrow et al, 1990).

Given the high prevalence of senile dementia among older adults, especially those residing in institutions, and the high prevalence of hearing loss, it is likely that the two disorders will co-occur in a large proportion of older adults. Further unremediated hearing loss can confound the diagnosis of dementia, and oftentimes exacerbates the behavioral manifestations of senile dementia. Similarly, lack of familiarity with the behavioral characteristics of persons with dementia can jeopardize the validity of the audiologic assessment and interfere with the benefits to be derived from audiologic interventions, such as hearing aids and ALDs. Accordingly, audiologists should informally assess mental status in persons being considered for intervention by asking simple questions that yield information regarding memory and orientation, or by administering a validated instrument such as the Short Portable Mental Status Questionnaire (SPMSQ) (Pfeiffer, 1975).

In sum, the behavioral implications of the speech-understanding difficulties characterizing older adults are numerous for the individual, family members, the functioning of nursing facilities, and potentially for society at large.

SPECIAL CONSIDERATION

Hearing loss in older adults restricts one or more dimensions of quality of life including physical functional status and cognitive, emotional, and social function.

Further, the consequences of impaired hearing are highly variable and individualized. The consequences of hearing impairment, some of which are listed in Table 8–1 should be ascertained as part of the routine case history as they should influence decisions regarding the nature and course of AR with hearing aids and ALDs.

WHAT IS THE ROLE OF AR IN THE FITTING AND DISPENSING OF HEARING AIDS AND ALDS?

Once hearing loss is documented, the etiology determined, and the communication disability and handicap quantified, an older adult should undergo some form of AR, assuming medical treatment has been ruled out. Three principles should

TABLE 8–1 Potential Consequences of Hearing Loss Experienced by Older Adults

- Negatively impact on communicative behavior
- Alter psychosocial behavior
- Strain family relations
- Limit the enjoyment of daily activities
- Jeopardize physical well-being
- Interfere with the ability to live independently and safely
- Interfere with long distance contacts on the telephone, potentially jeopardizing safety and security
- Interfere with medical diagnosis, treatment, and management
- Interfere with compliance with pharmacologic regimens
- Interfere with therapeutic interventions across all disciplines including social work, speech-language therapy, physical, or occupational therapy

govern treatment of disabling and handicapping hearing impairment in the older adult: (1) intervention should be aimed at restoring communication function and improving quality of life; (2) the client should be involved in decision making and his/her preferences should guide the goals of treatment; and (3) the approach to treatment should be multifaceted including provision of a hearing instrument in the context of psychological support, social supports, and environmental manipulation. The guiding philosophy underlying AR should be whether the treatment provided actually makes a difference to the patient. That is what has happened to the patient/client as a result or consequence of treatment?

The term AR means different things to different people. It is a highly variable process defined for the most part operationally by the goals set for the remediation process. Most audiologists would agree that provision of custom hearing aids that will make sounds audible, comfortable, tolerable, and comprehensible is an important aspect of audiologic rehabilitation. With regard to the latter, our explicit goal is for the hearing aid to optimize speech comprehension for commonly encountered listening situations (Ross & Levitt, 1997).

PEARL

As of this writing, audiologists readily admit that the hearing-aid fitting should not be the "terminal goal of audiological case management" (Binnie & Hession, 1990, p. 37).

Once the ideal frequency/gain and output characteristics of the hearing aid have been prescribed, AR should be instituted to insure that the patient or client will actually wear the hearing aid (Montgomery, 1991).

SPECIAL CONSIDERATION

While the hearing aid is the focal point of AR, counseling to shape attitudes, increase motivation, modify expectations, and to better understand hearing aids and the communication process should be seen as the cornerstone of any AR effort (Binnie, 1991).

I tend to agree with Trychin (1995) that AR is (1) a process designed to teach older adults who have communication difficulties, and who actually use hearing aids ways to prevent or reduce communication difficulties and (2) a vehicle to help resolve the psychological and social problems resulting from these difficulties. In essence, AR is a comprehensive program of hearing health care for persons with handicapping hearing impairments premised on the assumption that wearing a hearing aid is only a part of the solution to communication problems and their psychosocial manifestations (Trychin, 1995).

Montgomery (1991) outlined five goals of adult AR to which I have added four more. The nine goals are displayed in Table 8–2. Each of these goals dovetails with the components of a comprehensive AR program. The components are displayed in Figure 8–1. In a subsequent section of this chapter I will discuss each of these components in depth. At this point, a description of the purpose of each component with relevance to the goals of AR is in order. The purpose of the hearing-aid fitting is to provide units that will make a wide portion of the speech spectrum audible while at the same time insuring that the SSPL90 of the hearing aid(s) is maintained below the patient's uncomfortable level. An integral part of the hearing-aid fitting is the hearing-aid orientation process wherein the client is counseled regarding the device(s) and given realistic expectations. The purpose of the psychosocial assessment is to gain insight into the client's lifestyle and the extent of self-perceived disability and handicap posed by the hearing loss. This component of AR addresses goals 3 and 4 that are listed in Table 8–2. The purpose of auditory-visual integration (AVI) is to teach the patient how to combine auditory and visual input to maximize receptive communication and promote conversational fluency and spontaneity (Abrahamson, 1995). Goals 4 and 5 are addressed as part of AVI. The purpose of strate-

TABLE 8–2 Goals of Audiologic Rehabilitation

1. Promote an understanding of hearing aids, their care and maintenance and promote realistic expectations regarding their capabilities.
2. Maximize sensory input by providing the best possible visual and auditory signal.
3. Understand the psychological and social problems resulting from hearing impairment.
4. Resolve the psychological and social problems resulting from hearing impairment.
5. Maximize sensory integration by making the best use of the amplified auditory signal and the visible signal.
6. Promote the use of cognitive processes necessary to derive meaning from incomplete sensory messages.
7. Promote an understanding of how to create a positive communication environment.
8. Develop within the individual assertive and interactive ways of communicating and repairing breakdowns.
9. Empower the person with disabling and handicapping hearing impairment.

Source: Modified from Montgomery (1991) and Abrahamson (1995).

gies training is to provide the patient with strategies to reduce communication breakdowns or with strategies to repair them when they occur (Abrahamson, 1995). Promoting assertive behavior helps the hearing-impaired resolve communication problems when they occur or to reduce their occurrence in the first place. Environmental manipulation training entails the provision of strategies necessary for manipulation of the environment to improve communication. In short, the patient is taught to identify barriers to communication that may exist in the environment (e.g., poor lighting, visual distraction, and background noise) and to eliminate or reduce them (Trychin, 1995). Last, but certainly not least, directing patients to consumer organizations is critical as they provide invaluable information about services for the hearing impaired and strategies for coping with hearing loss. The most well known of these organizations being a local Self Help for Hard of Hearing Group (SHHH). In the sec-

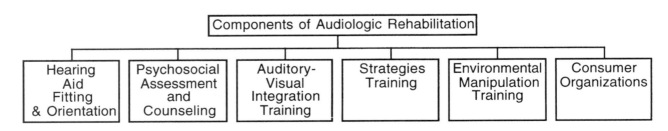

Figure 8–1 Components of audiologic rehabilitation.

tions that follow, I provide a lengthy discussion of each of the components of AR. I have excluded a discussion of the hearing-aid fitting as that information is covered in-depth in Chapter 9.

COMPONENTS OF THE REHABILITATION PROCESS

The Hearing-Aid Fitting and Orientation

Once the hearing aid has been fit it is incumbent on the audiologist to provide an individualized hearing instrument orientation over the 30-day trial period. The components should include an orientation wherein the user is instructed about hearing-aid care and maintenance and is trained in terms of how to manipulate and use all of the options associated with the hearing instrument, and counseling that is designed to insure that realistic expectations regarding hearing-aid function are established (Palmer & Mormer, 1997). The more realistic the expectations, the more satisfied the consumer is likely to be. In fact, Ross and Levitt (1997) suggest that when expectations are reduced to a realistic level, satisfaction with the help provided by hearing aids is likely.

The typical orientation session may last 45 minutes to one hour depending on the hearing aid(s) dispensed and the consumer. Orientation to a programmable hearing aid, for example, may be more time consuming than orientation to a more conventional device, at times requiring 1½ hours for older adults who have never used a hearing aid. Some patients may have to return several times during the 30-day trial period, especially those with physical disabilities or cognitive problems that may limit their ability to concentrate or focus. For those people who have difficulty understanding one-to-one conversation, an ALD should be used while the patient is being familiarized with the components of the unit. Alternatively, one aid of a binaural set can be worn by the patient (Palmer & Mormer, 1997). Before concluding the fitting and orientation session, a return visit should be scheduled and the importance of the follow-up session underscored. The more time spent orienting hearing-aid users, the less likely problems will arise on a regular basis requiring an indefinite number of return visits.

PEARL

It is always helpful to have a family member or caregiver in attendance to facilitate carryover.

Irrespective of the type of unit dispensed, some basic information must be conveyed. The orientation session can be broken into two components, namely, instrument operation and instrument use. The orientation typically begins with a discussion of instrument operation that includes a discussion of care and maintenance. First, the patient should be introduced to the components of the hearing aid, the operation of each of the controls should be demonstrated, and the patient should be given the opportunity to manipulate each of the switches including the volume control, the on/off, and the telephone switch. An overview of the functions of each control should be offered using the instrument owner's manual as a guide to acquaint the patient with the instrument (Palmer & Mormer, 1997).

PEARL

It is helpful to have a magnifier available to enable the patient to see and read the small print as legibility is oftentimes a problem with older adults.

Battery insertion and removal should be demonstrated as well as hearing instrument/earmold insertion and removal. Magnets for inserting and removing batteries should be demonstrated and recommended if it is easier for the patient. The patient should practice adjusting hearing-aid switches when the unit is off the ear and when it is positioned in or behind the ear. The patient should be given the opportunity to demonstrate competency in insertion and removal prior to the completion of the initial orientation session. A checklist such as that displayed in Table 8–3 can insure that basic components of instrument operation have been reviewed and understood (Palmer & Mormer, 1997). Those operations not fully understood should be reviewed at the next orientation session. For patients using multi-memory instruments, the user should be instructed on the use of the memories and how to move from and return to the different channels or memories. This information should be written down to help reduce frustration during the initial stages of use (Palmer & Mormer, 1997).

The discussion of instrument operation is typically followed by a detailed description of care and maintenance of the hearing instrument. As noted in Chapter 9, it is helpful to provide the user with a maintenance kit. This includes a miniature battery tester, a small brush, a packet of extra batteries, a hearing-aid drying kit (especially for persons living in humid climates), a wax pick, and a hot-air blower. Each of these tools should be demonstrated and the patient required to demonstrate his or her ability to clean the instrument independently (Holmes, 1995). These points should be

---

PEARL

The patient should be given a written set of instructions about the care and maintenance of the units.

---

systematically reviewed with the patient, making sure that each is understood. The points to be emphasized are as follows:

- Keep the hearing aid dry.
- Remove the battery when the hearing aid is not in use.
- Test the battery prior to inserting it into the hearing aid.
- Keep a spare battery at all times.

TABLE 8–3 Hearing Instrument Operation and Maintenance Checklist

Name of Unit	Serial Number		R	L

Hearing aid component	Yes	Needs further instruction
Battery Insertion Removal Test Voltage		
Volume Control Adjust to comfortable listening level		
On-Off Function Turn hearing aid on and off		
Hearing Aid / Earmold Removal Insertion		
Telephone Coil Adjust Use with compatible telephone		
Remote Multimemory Control		
Memory 1 2 3		

Source: Modified from Palmer and Mormer (1997).

- Keep spare batteries in a safe place away from children and pets.
- Inform patient of battery life, which ranges from 2 to 3 weeks.
- Lean on a nonslippery table when removing battery to avoid loss of battery.
- Remove hearing aid over a carpeted surface to avoid breakage should it dislodge from the ear or fall out of hands.
- Place hearing aid in dehumidifier to remove moisture and keep hearing aid dry.
- Remove hearing aid when applying hair spray or perfume, or when taking a shower.
- Gently wipe off earmold and aid when removed from the ear. Always check for earwax and gently remove it.
- Check hearing aid opening for wax prior to reinserting it. If necessary, clean opening with a wax pick. If wax buildup constantly occurs, contact a hearing health care professional for possible cerumen management. Also, consider the possibility of a wax guard.
- Check tubing of behind-the-ear hearing aids for debris.
- Clean earmold with mild soap—avoid alcohol. Make sure mold is blown dry prior to reconnecting it to the hearing aid.

- Brush off hearing-aid microphone and receiver with small brush before insertion.

PEARL

Emphasize the following points: patience is important; it will take some time before adjusting to the hearing aid and before feeling completely competent with hearing aid(s); avoid getting frustrated . . . call the audiologist with questions.

Table 8–4 summarizes the dos and don'ts of hearing-aid care and maintenance the patient needs to be made aware of. It is helpful to give the page of dos and don'ts to the patient.

Basic hearing-aid troubleshooting should be considered an integral part of the discussion about hearing-aid care and maintenance. The patient should walk away from the orientation with an understanding of which component to check depending on the symptom (e.g., sound emanating from the hearing aid). For example, if the sound is intermittent, the earmold may be clogged, the tubing may be cracked, the receiver may be damaged, or the batteries may be exhausted

TABLE 8–4   Dos and Don'ts for Hearing Aids

Dos
• Turn on hearing aid
• Adjust volume to a comfortable listening level
• Turn off hearing aid and remove battery at bedtime
• Open battery compartment when hearing aid is not in use
• Check earmold/hearing aid for wax
• Replace batteries routinely every two to three weeks
• Wear hearing aid daily for a couple of hours
• Handle hearing aid with care
• Make sure hearing aid/earmold/battery are inserted correctly
• Check plastic tubing for debris
• Carry spare batteries
• Wash earmold in warm soapy water
• Keep hearing aid dry

Don'ts
• Store battery in a hot/humid space
• Wear someone else's hearing aid
• Use alcohol or cleaning fluid on parts of the hearing aid
• Repair your own hearing aid
• Allow the hearing aid to get wet
• Keep the volume adjusted to a soft level to save battery life
• Expose the hearing aid to radiation from X-rays
HEARING AID NAME: _____
BATTERY TYPE AND NUMBER: _____
_____

Source: Modified from *Audiology and Aural Rehabilitation Resource Guide* (1994). Published by Therapy Management Innovations, Inc., Alta Therapies and Healthcare Rehabilitation.

or corroded. Conversely, if the hearing aid is whistling then the earmold/hearing aid may not be properly positioned, the tubing may be cracked, or the receiver may be worn. If there is no audible sound the earmold may be clogged and need to be cleaned; the volume control may be off; the battery may be exhausted; or the receiver may be defective. The patient should understand when to call the dispensing audiologist because of a potential malfunction of one of the

hearing-aid components. A large-print trouble-shooting guide for the patient to bring home is often helpful. The

---

PEARL

The patient should be encouraged to contact the audiologist if there is any change in how he/she is functioning with the hearing aid.

---

guide should include a listing of the audible symptoms to listen for, the component to check, and the solution to the problem.

Following the above discussion, the dispenser should move into the instrument-use portion of the orientation. This discussion should be conducted with the hearing aid(s) in the ear adjusted (by the patient) to a comfortable listening level. The patient should be given the opportunity to acclimate to the sound of his/her own voice. When people first put hearing aids in the ear, they should understand that their own voice and that of others may sound very strange (Ross, 1996). Their voices may tend to have a hollow booming quality as if talking from the bottom of a barrel. This is often the first hurdle the patient must overcome. The audiologist can make the necessary adjustments to eliminate this sensation. For example, the occlusion effect can be minimized via slight hearing-aid/earmold modifications.

Next, casual conversation between the patient, family member, and dispenser should take place so that the user can experience the sensation of newly amplified sound. It is helpful to introduce some competing background noise to enable the patient to gain insight into the challenges posed by listening through the hearing aid to speech embedded in a background of noise (Palmer & Mormer, 1997). Walking with the patient outside of the sound-treated room to expose the patient to "aided real world sound" is often helpful during the hearing-aid adjustment period. At this point, a brief discussion of strategies for maximizing speech understanding in noise might be initiated, to allay patient anxieties.

A personalized wearing schedule should be developed by the audiologist in consultation with the patient and a family member. Basically, the patient should be encouraged to use the hearing aid(s) for a brief time interval at first, gradually increasing hours of use as the variety of situations in which the patient uses the aid is increased. Palmer and Mormer (1997) recommend that hours of hearing-aid use should be gradually increased during the first week such that on the first day the hearing aid might be worn for an hour a day whereas on the fourth day it might be worn for 4 hours a day and by the end of the first week, perhaps 8 hours a day. The volume control of the hearing aid should be set to a comfortable listening level using the patient's voice as a guide (in the case of a screw-adjust volume control, the patient should understand that this can be changed at any time by the audiologist and in some cases by the patient). It is advisable that hearing-aid users wear their hearing aids in restricted situations at first. Individuals should begin to wear the aid in a quiet place at home, shortly after returning from the clinic (make sure to remind the patient to remove the unit if they are using public transportation such as a train or subway to get home)! Palmer and Mormer (1997) recommend a "listening tour" of household sounds including water from the faucet, toilet flushing, and doorbell ringing. The patient should be encouraged to use the hearing aid in quiet conversation at home, during quiet indoor activities, and when viewing the television or radio. Once the individual feels accustomed to amplified sound at home, he/she should venture into new hearing situations (Ross, 1996). For example, the patient should wear the hearing aid outdoors during quiet activities, and during group conversation when dining or entertaining visitors. Finally, the patient should be encouraged to wear the hearing aid in group situations outside the home, in large listening areas such as a church or synagogue, and at work. Persons with mild hearing loss may find their hearing aids useful in business meetings, but may find them burdensome in noisy situations such as restaurants or parties. If patients complain that some intense sounds produce an uncomfortably loud hearing sensation, they should be told to alert the dispensing audiologist at the follow-up visit so a simple adjustment can be made to the hearing aid. It is helpful for the patient to keep a listening diary and record the situations that are problematic so at the follow-up visit adjustments can be made to the hearing aid and/or strategies can be offered for coping with these situations. Some of these tips are summarized in Table 8–5. These hints can be given to the patient as a large print handout.

The hearing-aid orientation should include a discussion about realistic expectations surrounding hearing aid use. Kricos, Lesner, and Sandridge (1991) contend that the older adult's satisfaction with, use of, and perceived benefits from amplification may be greatly influenced by attitudes and expectations toward hearing aids that exist prior to the actual hearing-aid fitting. In short, "setting realistic expectations is an important component in achieving success with any hearing instrument," be it programmable instruments, true

digital instruments, or conventional analog devices (Stuypulkowski, 1997, p. 57). According to specialists in geriatric rehabilitation, "what a person wants and how specific and realistic their goals are, helps to determine overall perfor-

TABLE 8–5   Helpful Hints for Adjusting to Hearing Aids

- Give time to adjust to the hearing aid.
- Take advantage of the services of the audiologist or hearing-aid specialist.
- Do not get discouraged if the hearing aid does not restore hearing to normal.
- Return to the dispenser for reassurance and counseling regarding realistic expectations. Understand that hearing aids WILL NOT restore hearing capabilities to normal.
- Allow time to adjust as hearing aids do require time to get used to and to attain maximum performance potential.
- At first, wear the hearing aid for as many hours during the day as comfortable—part time use may be preferable for some.
- Gradually adjust to loud incoming signals by first using the hearing aid in quiet and small groups, later moving to larger, less favorable listening situations.
- Maintain a diary of listening experiences—positive and negative—to be reviewed with the audiologist at the return visit.
- Do not hesitate to bring hearing-aid related problems to the attention of the audiologist and work together to resolve them.

mance" (Kemp, 1990b, p. 301), as well as success. Finally, Madell, Pfeffer, Ross, and Chellappa (1991) reported that the major reason for rejection of hearing aids was that performance with hearing aids did not meet expectations.

According to expectations-performance theory, consumer satisfaction is a function of the consumer's product expectations and the product's perceived performance (Kotler & Clarke, 1987). Specifically, if performance with the hearing aid matches expectations, the hearing-impaired consumer will be satisfied, whereas if it falls short he or she will be dissatisfied. In the case of older adult hearing-aid users, personal experience from patients and health care professionals who work with older adults suggests that performance tends to fall short of expectations, hence dissatisfaction, frustration, and disillusionment with the device and hearing health care professionals tend to ensue.

Prior to counseling the patient regarding realistic expectations, it is helpful to listen to the patient's conceptions and misconceptions. They can serve as the foundation on which counseling can be built. The inevitable biological changes

that occur as certain people age make the level of hearing capacity originally enjoyed nearly impossible to attain even with the help of technically advanced instruments. Patients must understand that hearing aids can restore only some degree of hearing and understanding and that the more damage within the auditory system the more difficult it becomes to restore the capabilities that once existed (Stuypulkowski, 1997). Hearing-aid users should not expect to suddenly hear normally. They should, however, expect to have a reduction in the degree of difficulty they have been having, depending on the acoustics of the listening situation.

The audiograms shown in Figures 8–2, 8–3 and 8–4 should be helpful in explaining the hearing loss, its effects on speech understanding, and the value of hearing aids in terms of improving the audibility of speech sounds. My approach is to relate the patient's expressed difficulty to the audiogram. Hence I begin by acknowledging the classic complaint of older adults with presbycusis. I suggest that the comment "I can hear people talking but cannot understand what they are saying especially in noisy situations" very aptly describes the problems that derive from the reduction in transmission, reception, and perception of the speech signal attributable to sensorineuerual hearing loss. I go on to say that these difficulties can easily be predicted from the speech bananna and audiograms depicted in the panel shown in Figure 8–2. The speech bananna shown in Figure 8–2 displays the frequency and intensity levels of typical sounds necessary for speech understanding. I explain that ordinary conversation or the normal speech spectrum is carried out within the range of frequencies from 250 to 6000 Hz and within the range of decibels from 20 to 60 dBHL. Consonant sounds and diphthongs such as "s," "sh," "th," "k," "t," "p," and "g" are relatively high in frequency or pitch and low in intensity or loudness. Conversely, vowel sounds such as "a," "i," "o," "u" are concentrated in the lower frequencies and are somewhat higher in intensity (Bess & Humes, 1995). I proceed to emphasize that

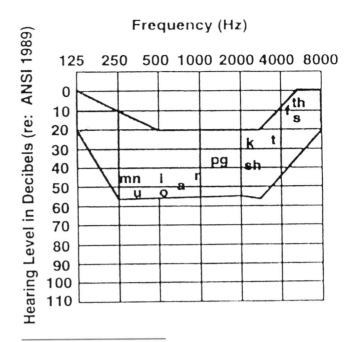

Figure 8–2 Audiogram depicting low-frequency concentration of vowels and high-frequency consonants. (From Bess and Humes, 1995.)

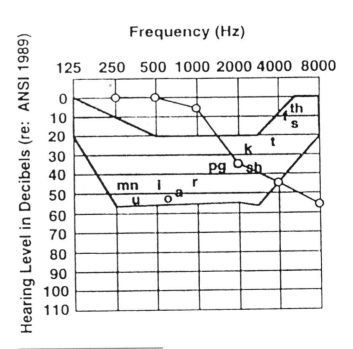

Figure 8–3 Impact of high-frequency hearing loss on reception of selected speech sounds. High frequencies are inaudible. (From Bess and Humes, 1995.)

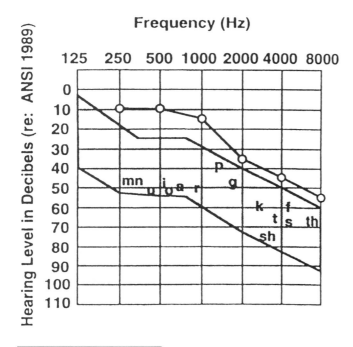

Frequency (Hz)

Figure 8–4 Aided pure-tone thresholds relative to hearing level of selected speech sounds. Aided hearing levels are now audible. (From Bess and Humes, 1995.)

environmental noise is high in intensity and low in frequency, as well. Audibility of the consonant sounds is critical to the understanding of speech. The panel shown in Figure 8–3 depicts a typical hearing loss characterizing older adults suffering from presbycusis (Bess & Humes, 1995). I then show them their audiogram superimposed on a speech bananna that is typically similar to the one I use in counseling. Immediately my patients can relate to what I am saying and gain some confidence in me. This is a key aspect of orientation and counseling sessions.

I proceed to explain that those sounds falling below threshold symbolized by the connected circles are audible (e.g., m, n, e, r, p) whereas those falling above are inaudible (e.g., s, t, th). For most older adults with age-related hearing loss, consonants with energy in the high frequencies are often inaudible, rendering speech-understanding difficult. I emphasize that this difficulty comprehending ordinary conversation is exacerbated in a noisy room, as background noise tends to be audible given good low-frequency hearing, yet consonant sounds important to understanding are inaudible. Further, older adults with good low-frequency hearing can perceive vowels well, even though they may have difficulty with consonant sounds (Bess & Humes, 1995). As a result, older adults claim that they can hear people talking (vowels audible) but they cannot make out the words (consonants inaudible).

I then explain that the goal of hearing aids is to bring consonants into the audible range without amplifying the already audible noise and vowel sounds. This is shown in Figure 8–4. At this point, I call their attention to the fact that the circles in the frequencies above 1000 Hz that represent

aided air-conduction thresholds are now better than (above) the speech sounds depicted in the bananna. The hearing aid has rendered the high-frequency sounds audible. I also explain that if the low-frequency input is too loud relative to the highs the audiologist can make the necessary adjustments to satisfy their "hearing needs." I emphasize that available technology allows the audiologist to "tweek" the audiogram until speech and noise are heard at the intensities that are acceptable to the patient.

Of utmost importance, the hearing-aid user must understand that hearing aids "are not very smart," they do not always do a good job of discriminating between desirable sounds persons want to hear (i.e., speech) and those undesirable sounds they want to ignore (i.e., background noise) (Ross, 1996). However, this situation is changing with the advent of digital hearing aids and the development of more sophisticated electronics. Similarly, hearing-aid users must understand that hearing aids are similar to automobiles in that not all hearing instruments are alike in terms of their performance (Stuypulkowski, 1997). High-end automobiles can make driving a pleasurable experience and high-end hearing instruments may provide improved sound quality, improved speech understanding, and comfortable listening across a variety of environments (Stuypulkowski, 1997).

SPECIAL CONSIDERATION

Hearing-aid users must understand that it takes time to realize the potential benefit from hearing aids, and thus should not become discouraged early on.

Their ears and their brains must become re-educated to hearing selected patterns of sounds that have been made louder by the hearing aid (Ross, 1996). In a sense, new hearing-aid users are suddenly being exposed to or "bombarded with" a world of sounds they have forgotten existed, such as the blare of street noises in the city, and must become re-oriented to or acquainted with the location and source of these "new" sounds.

PEARL

Hearing-aid users should accept their hearing loss and not continue to consider it a disgrace or a stigma. They should not cover their hearing aids as a way of hiding the hearing loss, as hearing aids serve as a signal to others that a hearing loss exists and that they should speak clearly to facilitate speech understanding.

According to Ross, an experienced and successful hearing-aid user and audiologist, the hearing impaired should not worry about people seeing their hearing aids. If hearing-aid users accept hearing loss and hearing aids, so will the people to whom they are speaking. In short, acceptance of hearing loss, and motivation to overcome its consequences, are conditions for hearing-aid satisfaction and success (Ross, 1996). Table 8–6 summarizes the capabilities of hearing instruments that should be communicated to hearing-aid users.

The information presented above should be discussed at the hearing-aid fitting and reviewed at the follow-up session. At the time of the follow-up the disability and handicap questionnaires completed prior to the hearing-aid fitting should be completed and responses compared to determine the extent of improvement associated with hearing aids. Caregivers and family members should complete the questionnaires again as well. If benefit is not achieved, if significant residual disability/handicap remains, or if the patient is not satisfied, additional sessions of AR should be scheduled with the material discussed in the next sections emphasized. Also, at this follow-up visit, the availability of a variety of ALDs should be discussed and consideration should be given to purchase of system(s) to supplement hearing aids.

During the orientation session(s) keep the following points in mind. Older adults require more and different reinforcement, they respond better to concrete goals that are immediate and affect daily functioning. Remember to reassure the patient as often as possible. Be sure to reward

TABLE 8–6 **Realistic Expectations on Capabilities of Hearing Instruments**

Hearing instruments
Should allow you to hear many sounds that you may not be able to hear, or may not hear clearly without amplification
Should allow you to understand speech more clearly and with less effort
Should not amplify normally loud sounds to uncomfortable levels
May enable you to understand speech more clearly in some, but not all, noisy environments
Will require some time for adjustment and maximal performance
WILL NOT restore hearing to normal or to pre-existing levels
WILL be LEAST helpful in the situations YOU MOST NEED THEM
WIL NOT FILTER OUT background noise, rather they will reduce amplification of some types of noise
Will improve sound quality
Will make sounds easier to hear and understand
Will improve the ability to hear environmental sounds including telephone ringing, doorbell, car-horn

Source: Modified from Stypulkowski, P. (1997). Realistic expectations: a key to success. *Supplement to Hearing Review,* 1:56–57.

PEARL

Always keep in mind that in geriatric rehabilitation, even small gains are important and should be communicated to the patient with hearing impairment. Older adults benefit from feedback and reinforcement.

successes and keep reinforcement closely linked to the desired behavior (Kemp, 1990a). Older adults often avoid difficult tasks because of anxiety associated with new or challenging tasks. Accordingly, the older adult should be given every opportunity to experience improvement or success and should be encouraged to move from unaided to aided situations and from quiet to noisy situations gradually. When instructing the patient about use and operation of the hearing aid, regular corrective feedback presented in a nonthreatening, supportive manner will go a long way toward reducing anxiety about a task, sustaining continued involvement and promoting motivation and a sense of success. Instructions should be repeated and the audiologist should verify that the patient has understood the information being conveyed. An older person may have a different

PEARL

It is helpful to employ a variety of modalities to insure that the information has been effectively conveyed to the patient.

learning style. Learn what it is, use it, and respect it. Keep in mind that older adults do not want sympathy from the hearing health care practitioner but do want to work with an empathic professional who understands the problems posed by hearing impairment. Empathy can develop if the clinician remembers that older adults with acquired hearing loss have spent the bulk of their lives with normal hearing. Only recently have they had to live with loss of signal perception at a time when they are experiencing decreased ability to cope successfuly with problems of aging in general and of hearing in particular (Garstecki & Erler, 1996). Above all treat the patient with the respect you expect from health care professionals.

Psychosocial Effects of Hearing Loss: Quantification and Counseling

The rehabilitation process actually begins during the initial encounter with the audiologist. The older adult with hearing impairment typically presents for the audiologic evaluation with a number of questions, one big one being "how can you help me function better in my daily life?" To answer that question the audiologist begins with the routine audiologic evaluation to determine type and severity of hearing loss. Depending on the results and discussions with the patient, a decision is made regarding the appropriate intervention. I find that objective information about the functional impact of hearing loss on daily life is helpful in deciding on candidacy for a hearing aid and AR, and is the basis for personal adjustment counseling, an integral part of rehabilitation. Objective data obtained using a self-report approach is particularly helpful as the psychosocial response to a given hearing loss is quite variable and cannot be predicted from the audiogram. Two individuals with the same level of hearing loss (e.g., mild) will react very differently and will experience different behavioral consequences.

The individual variability in reponse to hearing loss is apparent in the study conducted by Garstecki and Erler (1996) and is apparent from studies on the relation between hearing impairment and self-perceived hearing handicap (Berkowitz & Hochberg, 1971; Swan & Gatehouse, 1990; Weinstein & Ventry, 1983). That is to say, correlations between a number of audiometric variables and varied self-report measures of disability and handicap are moderate at best, albeit statistically significant, varying with the self-report measure, the audiometric variable, and the population. For example, word-recognition ability using monosyllabic word lists bears a weaker relation to self-reported handicap than does the pure-tone average. Similarly, the relation between pure-tone data and scores on disability measures is stronger than the relation between pure-tone data and handicap measures. In recognition of the importance of the above, audiologists

---

PEARL

It is imperative that quantification of the perceived communicative disabilities and handicapping effects of a given hearing loss on communication, social, and emotional function is included in the complete hearing assessment.

---

increasingly are using self-assessment questionnaires to quantify hearing loss (Schow et al, 1993). Table 8–7 includes a description of some of the more popular scales including the domains of function assessed and sample items. As of this writing, the Hearing Handicap Inventory and the Abbreviated Profile of Hearing Aid Benefit (APHAB) (Appendix A) are the most widely used instruments for quantifying handicapping and disabling effects of hearing loss.

In terms of their purpose, several potential uses of self-report measures come to mind. One application is in determining candidacy for and benefit from an amplification system. Another is in counseling both the hearing impaired and family members to alleviate the disabling and handicapping effects of hearing loss and to resolve conflicts between family members that may result from hearing loss. A third application is for purposes of accountability and quality assurance to demonstrate the outcomes achieved with AR and hearing aids dispensed in a particular practice. One final use is in screening to help identify persons who require in-depth audiologic assessments. As a bottom line, whatever questionnaire is selected, for older adults in particular, it is critical that the audiologist attempt to uncover the impact of hearing loss from the perspective of the client to insure that AR is client centered. According to Bicknell (1984, p. 357) we must ascertain the following:

- What does it mean?
- To this person?
- To have this handicap?
- At this time in his/her life?
- With these caretakers?
- In this environment?
- And in this peer group?

In selecting a scale, it is imperative that the questionnaire is appropriate to the population on which it will be used, and appropriate for the desired purpose. For example, with regard to the former, the Hearing Handicap Inventory for Adults was standardized on young adults and would not be appropriate for an elderly person. Similarly, the HHIE was standardized on noninstitutionalized older adults and is not valid for nursing home residents (Appendix B). The Significant Other Assessment of Communication (SOAC) is a companion scale to the Self Assessment of Communication (SAC) and is not appropriate for the person with a hearing impairment. The audiologist must also consider the reason one is utilizing a self-assessment questionnaire. For example, if the audiologist merely wants to quickly screen an older adult to determine need for an audiometric referral, short questionnaires such as the SAC or the HHIE-S (Appendix C) would be appropriate. If however, the clinician wants to design an intervention program, then a more comprehensive questionnaire such as the HHIE or the APHAB might prove more effective. A comprehensive questionnaire would give the clinician a more complete picture of the areas of communication or psychosocial function warranting change so that a client-centered rehabilitation plan can be implemented.

If the audiologist wants to measure the efficacy of treatment, then the scale must be psychometrically robust. If the audiologist needs to identify family counseling needs, then scales with companion versions such as the HHIE, and the SAC might be appropriate because of the availability of spousal versions. In the case of the HHIE, the spousal version is known as the HHIE-SP (Appendix D), whereas the companion version of the SAC is the SOAC. Finally, if the audiologist wants to focus on hearing-aid benefit then perhaps a questionnaire such as the Hearing Aid Performance Inventory (HAPI) developed by Walden, Demorest, and Hepler (1984) or the Shortened Hearing Aid Performance Inventory (SHAPI) described by Schum (1997) may be appropriate. The latter scale provides the hearing-aid user with an opportunity to rate hearing-aid benefit in a variety of situations. The SHAPI was designed to be used with older adults purchasing hearing aids. Subjects in the normative study were older hearing-aid users residing in New Zealand (Schum, 1997).

SPECIAL CONSIDERATION

The handicap and/or disability questionnaire should be administered at several intervals to determine if in fact the AR was successful in reversing the communication deficits and psychosocial handicap associated with hearing loss.

TABLE 8–7   Self-Assessment Scales for Use with Older Adults

Name of scale	Content areas	Number of items	Scoring format
1. CPHI[1]	Communication performance Communication importance Communication environment Communication strategies Personal adjustment	145 questions 25 subscales	Low scores suggest problem areas; high scores indicate more favorable adjustment
2. HHIE/HHIE-S[2]	Social function Emotional function	25/10	Low scores suggest minimal handicap; high scores suggest significant handicap
3. APHAB[3]	Ease of communication Reverberation Background noise Aversiveness	24	The lower the percent score, the fewer problem areas; the higher the percent score the greater the number of problem areas
4. HPI[4] Revised Version	Understanding speech Intensity Response to auditory failure Social problems Personal problems Occupational problems	90	Respondents evaluate the frequency with which they experience a particular degree of difficulty
5. SAC[5]	Communication difficulties Feelings about the handicap Perception about how the loss is perceived by others	10	The higher the score, the greater the difficulty the respondent is experiencing
6. DSCF[6]	Attitudes and feelings of people with hearing impairments and their significant others. Areas covered include family, self, social-vocational, general communication experience.	38	Provides a profile of the areas of strength and weakness for the person with hearing impairment
7. HAPI[7]	Assesses hearing aid benefit in a variety of listening situations including speech in quiet, in noise, nonlive speech or nonspeech, and reduced information in the signal.	64	Provides for direct judgments of the adequacy of hearing aids in given situations
8. SHAPI[8]	Consists of items describing specific listening situations, which includes listening in a background of noise, listening in quiet, and listening with reduced visual cues		Enables the respondent to directly judge the adequacy of the hearing aid. Higher SHAPI ratings suggest lower levels of satisfaction with hearing aids

[1]CPHI: Communication Profile for the Hearing Impaired. (Demorest & Erdman, 1986.)
[2]HHIE/HHIE-S: Hearing Handicap Inventory for the Elderly; Screening version of the Hearing Handicap Inventory for the Elderly. (Ventry & Weinstein, 1982.)
[3]APHAB: Abbreviated Profile of Hearing Aid Benefit. (Cox & Alexander, 1995.)
[4]HPI: Hearing Performance Inventory. (Lamb, Owens, & Shubert, 1983.)
[5]SAC: Self-Assessment of Communication. (Schow & Nerbonne, 1982.)
[6]DSCF: Denver Scale of Communication Function. (J. Alpiner, W. Chevrette, G. Glascoe, M. Metz, & B. Olsen, unpublished studies, 1974.)
[7]HAPI: Hearing Aid Performance Inventory. (Walden, Demorest, & Hepler, 1984.)
[8]SHAPI: Shortened Hearing Aid Performance Inventory. (Schum, 1997.)

As older adults with hearing impairment and their family members often have difficulty communicating with one another, it is often helpful to have a significant other complete a companion questionnaire at the start of rehabilitation and at the same interval as the person with hearing impairment. Typically, a discrepancy exists between ratings of handicap by the significant other and that of the person with hearing impairment. Jerger, Chmiel, Florin, Pirozzolo, and Wilson (1996) reported that at baseline (prior to intervention) significant others tend to judge the handicap as being slightly greater than does the patient. However, interestingly, following intervention with hearing aids or ALDs the perceived residual handicap is judged about the same by both the subject and the significant other. Responses of family members or significant others to a self-report questionnaire can be used during counseling sessions to develop empathy for a communication partner with hearing impairment and to set realistic expectations for hearing aids in difficult listening situations.

Counseling is an important part of the rehabilitation process. Personal-adjustment and informational counseling are

PEARL

Counseling is the cornerstone of AR (Erdman, 1993).

integral to the counseling process. Informational counseling is designed to: (1) instill a basic understanding of the auditory system, normal hearing, and speech perception (e.g., vowel and consonant energy as they relate to audibility and intelligibility); (2) develop an understanding of what a hearing impairment actually is with specific emphasis on the audiogram and how a loss in general and the patient's impairment in particular impacts on audibility and speech understanding. Understanding hearing impairment goes a long way toward helping the patient to accept and adjust to it; and (3) understand the client's motivations for purchasing a hearing aid. This aspect is inextricably intertwined with the hearing-aid orientation designed to instill an appreciation for what the hearing aid can and cannot do, namely hearing aids do not restore hearing to normal, they are merely devices that attempt to maximize residual hearing. Gaining an appreciation for patient motivations will insure that the patient's expectations are fulfilled and motivations satisfied.

PEARL

Personal-adjustment counseling is a facilitative process employed to resolve auditory disabilities and psychosocial handicaps experienced secondary to hearing impairment.

In contrast to informational counseling, personal-adjustment counseling focuses on the adjustment to hearing loss that is, how does a patient cope or adapt to hearing loss. Personal-adjustment counseling addresses the handicap a person attributes to hearing impairment (Schum, 1994). Counseling entails assisting an individual to cope with a particular problem (Schum, 1994). According to Garstecki and Erler (1996), the goal of counseling in association with

hearing-aid use is to bring about changes that will lead to reductions in self-perceived hearing handicap and/or disability as reported on the self-report questionnaires. Hence, counseling theoretically enables individuals to cope effectively with the communicative difficulties (i.e., disability) experienced and helps the patient resolve adjustment problems (i.e., handicaps) (Erdman, 1993). It is well accepted that the effectiveness of counseling determines the extent to which other rehabilitative measures, most notably hearing aids, succeed or fail (Erdman, 1993).

SPECIAL CONSIDERATION

People with hearing loss are persons first who are challenged to cope with a disability using adjustment processes adopted by human beings struggling with other types of chronic conditions (Schum, 1994).

To be successful, counseling should be conducted using a problem-solving approach. The audiologist administering the counseling must view each hearing-impaired patient as a unique individual with his or her own set of idiosyncrasies (Erdman, 1993). They must have an unconditional positive regard, accepting the fact that the patient has a set of inner resources to overcome the handicapping effects of hearing loss (Tye-Murray, 1998). Throughout the counseling process, it is critical that the audiologist remember that improvement in rehabilitation tasks correlates with the patient's own appraisal of his or her potential for recovery. Responses to self-assessment tools can help achieve the

PEARL

It is important to always uncover the subjective viewpoint rather than only relying on your own appraisal of the situation (Kemp, 1990a).

goal of a truly client-centered approach. Thus, information discussed during counseling sessions should evolve from patient responses to one or more of the disability or handicap questionnaires described above. Questionnaires can help the clinician identify the auditory and nonauditory effects of hearing impairment in light of the psychological, interpersonal, environmental, and social variables unique to each individual (Erdman, 1993). The more extensive the questionnaire or the more varied the tools the greater the insight into the individual. Table 8–8 lists the characteristics

SPECIAL CONSIDERATION

The successful counselor should be supportive, facilitative, and at the same time directive.

considered important to successful counseling. Erdman (1993) provides an extensive discussion of practitioner-patient character traits and relationships essential to successful counseling encounters.

TABLE 8–8 Qualities Considered Important to a Successful Counseling Style

- Warm
- Empathic understanding
- Genuine
- Unconditional positive regard
- Good listener
- Good interpersonal skills
- Caring and concerned
- Able to take on another person's point of view
- Able to respond effectively to another person's emotional state
- Understanding

Source: Modified from Erdman (1993).

The goal of personal-adjustment counseling is to help the hearing impaired adapt to a life that has been permanently changed by a chronic condition (Kemp, 1990a). Always keep in mind that chronic disease cannot be cured, yet resulting disabilities and handicaps can. A disability such as hearing loss causes life changes and it is these life changes that are of paramount importance. The changes one encounters after any disabling condition include: (1) a decrease in social independence, (2) compromised life satisfaction, and (3) diminished self-esteem. To the extent that rehabilitation programs help people deal with these changes, they are successful (Kemp, 1990a). It is thus beneficial to focus the hearing impaired on the potential outcomes of AR targeting improvements in these latter domains of function.

Education about the disability and the psychosocial changes that occur as a result of the disability can insure that older persons will lead satisfying lives. Hence, personal-adjustment counseling should help the patient see that the hearing aid has actually been effective in enhancing chances of achieving maximal functioning, life satisfaction, and self-esteem (Kemp, 1990a). Throughout the counseling process, patients should come to understand how hearing loss can impact on aspects of daily life considered important to the older adult and that hearing aids can restore some of the functions lost because of hearing loss.

SPECIAL CONSIDERATION

While from the professional's point of view, psychosocial changes brought on by the disability may not be of clinical relevance, from the older adult's perspective they are a high priority (Kemp, 1990a).

PEARL

Professionals must understand how hearing loss compromises quality of life, and communicate to the hearing impaired how intervention can assist in promoting this quality of life.

Maintenance of independence (i.e., autonomy) is the most desired goal of individuals suffering from a chronic condition such as hearing impairment (Kemp, 1990a). Independence refers to the ability to conduct day-to-day activities without relying on others (Tye-Murray, 1998). Two psychological processes interact to enable a person suffering from a handicapping chronic condition to live independently (Kemp, 1990a). First, the individual must learn the skills necessary to compensate for the effects of hearing loss to enable performance of tasks necessary to daily life. For example, in the case of the hearing impaired, learning to use a hearing aid in the social and communicative situations compromised by the hearing loss is a first step toward restoring independence. Family members or caregivers must be integrated into each phase of the counseling process to facilitate autonomy in each setting the older adult is expected to function in, be it at home, in a nursing facility, or in an acute care setting (Kane, Ouslander, & Abrass, 1994). To this end, we must work with the hearing impaired and family members to structure an environment that is safe and conducive to functional independence (Kane, Ouslander, & Abrass, 1994).

The second psychological process that promotes independence is assertiveness, and development of a positive and realistic attitude regarding hearing loss and hearing aids (Kemp, 1990a). During counseling sessions, especially with the old-old, efforts must be made to facilitate development of these attitudes. Older adults should be encouraged to admit to hearing loss, to offer cues to facilitate communication, and to offer visible reminders to everyone about behaviors that interfere with or facilitate communication (Glass, 1990). This practice will hopefully avoid the tendency for hearing-impaired individuals to be mistakenly labeled "confused" or "forgetful" because of failure to remember what has been spoken. As will be discussed later in the chapter, assertiveness training and participation in self-help groups with other hearing-impaired persons and hearing-aid users can promote the attitudes necessary for independence in the presence of a significant hearing impairment.

Audiologists often pay lip service to the concept of life satisfaction and its importance to older adults. In reality the "topic of life satisfaction after disability is crucial in rehabilitation" (Kemp, 1990a, p. 45). The majority of older adults question the purpose or value of life especially when confronted with a devastating chronic condition such as handicapping hearing impairment (Kemp, 1990a). Rather than confront it and attempt to alleviate it, the older adult will retreat and succumb to depression, declines in physical functional status, and possibly cognitive deficits (Gilhome-Herbst, & Humphrey, 1980; Bess, Lichtenstein, & Logan, 1991).

Pleasurable experiences such as those that derive from our senses (e.g., hearing music), and the experience of success with daily activities are important sources of life-satisfaction (Kemp, 1990a). According to Kemp (1990a), disabling chronic

> ## SPECIAL CONSIDERATION
>
> **Older adults are often unaware of the contribution of hearing loss to life satisfaction, and thus it is incumbent on audiologists to link the benefit of hearing aids to life satisfaction when counseling the elderly.**

conditions are a great source of psychological pain for older adults, and the goal of rehabilitative interventions should be to increase the pleasure-to-pain ratio, to make life satisfying. Audiologists should begin to emphasize life satisfaction as a key outcome of hearing-aid use as a means of promoting this form of intervention. The work of Mulrow, Aguilar, Endicott, and Tuley (1990) demonstrates the contribution of hearing-aid use to life satisfaction.

Experiencing success also contributes to life satisfaction among older adults (Kemp, 1990a). Examples of conditions conducive to feelings of success among the hearing impaired would include restoration of the ability to communicate with family members or caregivers, renewed enjoyment of television and radio, or, at the most basic level, hearing a baby cry or the water run. The ability to successfully engage in communicative behaviors once lost, contributes to feelings of life satisfaction. The final psychological variable contributing to life satisfaction among older adults is "having a sense of meaning or purpose in life" (Kemp, 1990a, p. 44). Similarly, feelings of apathy, loss of self-esteem, and feelings of worthlessness, which are typical signs of depression, also compromise life satisfaction in older adults. Keep in mind that reduction in sensory input deriving from hearing loss is linked to depression and that hearing aids have proven successful in reversing depression in selected older adults (Mulrow, Aguilar, Endicott, & Tuley, 1990; Gilhome-Herbst, & Humphrey, 1980). As hearing loss has been linked to depression, and hearing aids have proven successful at reversing depression in older adults, it is incumbent on audiologists to emphasize to the hearing impaired and their families the potential role hearing aids may play in the management of this prevalent affective disorder. In short, audiologists may have a role to play in the management of depression (Kirkwood, 1999).

> ## PEARL
>
> **Treatment with hearing aids is associated with a number of positive emotional effects, including reduction in depression (Kirkwood, 1999).**

Whereas life satisfaction relates to one's appraisal of their life, self-esteem follows from one's appraisal of themselves (Kemp, 1990a). The onset of a chronic disability, such as impaired hearing, may diminish one's self-esteem because it affects how the individual may be viewed by others (e.g., handicapped, stupid, or dumb), and it may in-

terfere with what a person can do such as engaging successfully in leisure, individual, or group activities (Kemp, 1990a). The latter variables are the ingredients from which self-esteem arises, and the greater the extent to which each is diminished, the greater the probability that the individual will suffer from poor self-esteem (Kemp, 1990a). Once the counseling session(s) is complete it should be clear that the interference with communication, the loss of self-esteem, depression, the loss of independence, and the decrease in functional ability associated with hearing loss are temporary, thanks to the hearing aid delivered in the context of AR.

In sum, audiologists must adopt a rehabilitation approach when managing the elderly person with hearing impairment (Kemp, 1990a). Such an approach implies considering the psychological reaction to a chronic condition such as hearing loss, as these reactions determine how the person copes with disability and the level of motivation for intervention (Kemp, 1990a). Similarly, the audiologist must consider issues and concerns that are of major importance to the patient and that are often at odds with what the clinician views as important (Kemp, 1990a). The latter outcomes are

> ## SPECIAL CONSIDERATION
>
> **Audiologists contend that the primary goal of hearing-aid fittings is enhancing communication, whereas greatest concern to the hearing impaired is that intervention enables them to function independently and safely within their environment (Kemp, 1990a).**

especially relevant to the fastest-growing segment of our population, the old-old, as higher levels of chronic conditions in this population increase the risk of institutionalization and dependence.

Is Counseling-Oriented AR Actually Effective?

A question at this point is whether in fact counseling-oriented AR is actually effective. Abrams, Hnath-Chisolm, Guerreiro, and Ritterman (1992) demonstrated that benefit from hearing aids, namely improvements in emotional and social function, can be enhanced when a hearing aid is dispensed in the context of a counseling-based AR program. Abrams et al (1992) divided their sample of older adults with mild to moderate sensorineural hearing loss into three treatment groups. Treatment group I received a hearing aid and participated in 3 weeks of counseling-based AR. The counseling-based AR included an overview of the anatomy of the ear; an overview of hearing and communication; discussions about speech reading; and an overview of ALDs. Treatment group II received the hearing aid accompanied by a brief counseling session. Treatment group III served as the control group, merely completing the HHIE at baseline and at the 2-month follow-up. Mean HHIE scores for each group were comparable at baseline.

Two months after the hearing-aid fitting, there was a clinically and statistically significant reduction in HHIE scores for treatment groups I and II, but not for the control group. Interestingly, subjects obtaining the hearing aid and counseling-based AR experienced more significant reductions in psychosocial handicap than those who obtained the hearing aid without rehabilitation. Further, self-perceived psychosocial handicap was reduced in 45% of participants in treatment group I versus 18% of subjects in treatment group II. This study demonstrates that the self-perception of hearing handicap can be significantly reduced in persons who have used hearing aids and have participated in a counseling-based AR program. Hence it underlines the value of counseling-based AR in the hearing-aid delivery process. Taylor and Jurma (1999) assessed the relative efficacy of group audiologic rehabilitation programs with adults as well. They concluded that group audiologic rehabilitation as a supplement to initial post-fitting counseling can help to reduce the handicap associated with hearing loss, and help to maintain it at a stable level.

Primeau (1997) found that AR and/or hearing-aid modifications can promote hearing-aid benefit among older adults who initially did not appear to be benefiting from their hearing aids. In his study, 139 older adults were fit with hearing aids. Benefit was assessed in the handicap domain using the HHIE-S. The 95% confidence interval for significant benefit was an improvement of 10 or more points in the score on HHIE-S from the unaided to the aided condition. Primeau's data were impressive in that 81% of subjects fit with hearing aids appeared to be benefiting from their hearing aids in the psychosocial domain. However, some subjects were not in that unaided HHIE-S scores were comparable to aided HHIE-S scores at the 6-week follow-up. The group not benefiting obtained some form of intervention consisting of counseling and/or hearing-aid modifications. Following the additional intervention, benefit in the psychosocial domain was recomputed by combining the hearing aid plus rehabilitation group to the original group, and the percentage benefiting improved to 90%. His data confirm the conclusions of Abrams et al (1992) regarding the contribution of rehabilitation to end-user satisfaction and benefit.

Auditory-Visual Integration Training (AVI)

Auditory-visual speech perception is a natural part of face-to-face communication. From an early age children are encouraged to look at the person to whom they are speaking as it facilitates speech understanding. People differ in their ability to utilize visual cues and as people begin to lose their hearing, the ability to take advantage of visual information takes on greater importance (Garstecki, 1988). Hence AVI training is designed to develop the hearing-impaired individual's potential (Garstecki, 1988). The goal of AVI training or speech reading with auditory cues is to improve speech-recognition ability by training the individual to utilize input from a number of modalities, most notably auditory and visual (Montgomery, 1991). Stated differently, a goal of AVI training is to optimize receptive communication skills during interactive verbal communication by incorporating auditory input, visual sensual information, and nonverbal associational cues into the communication exchange (Gagne, 1994). Nonverbal association cues or relevant talker charac-

teristics include facial expressions, situational cues, contextual cues, and message-related extrafacial gestures. Visual sensual information is available from the speaker's articulatory movements (e.g., lip, tongue, and jaw movements) (Gagne, 1994).

Speechreading with visual cues or AVI training is based on a number of important premises. First, speech understanding is a multisensory event involving the integration of audition, vision, and cognitive processing. Normal-hearing persons and persons with hearing-impaired impairment tend to recognize speech much better when visual cues are available, especially in noisy backgrounds or reverberant conditions (Walden & Grant, 1993). In short, bisensory speech understanding is superior to audition or vision alone (Montgomery, 1993). Second, visual speech cues play a highly significant role in speech perception, acquiring increased significance after hearing becomes impaired (Walden & Grant, 1993). Third, normal-hearing and hearing-impaired persons tend to look at the talker, consciously or unconsciously to maximize input from visual cues. The hearing impaired in particular need to be convinced of the benefit derived from adding visual cues to audition. Fourth, the person with hearing impairment can learn to supplement auditory input with secondary cues (e.g., visual input) to promote speech understanding. Fifth, the auditory-visual communication process requires skills that can be naturally acquired, some that can be slowly acquired, and neurological and cognitive abilities that are not amenable to change (Houston & Montgomery, 1997). Finally, focusing on skills and behaviors that can be changed through a brief period of training is both time and cost efficient.

The typical audiologist does not spend a good deal of time on AVI training yet speechreading is acknowledged by members of Self Help for Hard of Hearing (SHHH) to be the primary way they supplement input from their hearing aids (Sorkin, 1997). Practically speaking, in this era

SPECIAL CONSIDERATION

AVI training is a vital aspect of AR that few audiologists have accepted as their responsibility.

of managed care, if audiologists are to accept responsibility for AVI training, the goals must be modest as the amount of time they have to devote is minimal. Further, to be successful AVI training must target the person with hearing impairment, as well as caregivers and/or family members of persons with hearing impairment.

SPECIAL CONSIDERATION

The goals of AVI training should be to develop the skills that can change including attending behavior, listening abilities, situational control, and the ability to integrate auditory and visual information present in real-life situations (Houston & Montgomery, 1997).

The important points to be emphasized during AVI training vary with the communication partner. The audiologist has responsibility for eliciting the cooperation of both speaking partners after having laid the groundwork. The communication partner must make every effort to apply what he/she has been taught to insure that the appropriate message has been delivered and received. The person with hearing impairment carries the biggest load in AVI training (Trychin, 1997). He/she must: (1) inform others about the existence of hearing loss and speech-understanding difficulties; (2) inform speakers about what to do to be understood; (3) politely remind the speaker how to communicate effectively; and (4) model the desired communication behavior. Modeling the desired behavior or teaching effective communication behaviors serves as encouragement and inducement for others (e.g., people with hearing loss should speak at the rate and loudness level they desire in others).

AVI training should be an integral part of the hearing-aid orientation or the informational counseling session. The variables influencing receptive communication ability are summarized in Table 8–9. Each should be discussed, with the audiologist demonstrating the appropriate behavior to the patient. For example, as regards mouth movements they should be natural, not exaggerated; hands should not cover or obscure the face; and the speaker should always face the listener so that the face is in full view. As regards the rate of speech the speaker should not talk too rapidly—rather at a moderate rate. The speaker should try to speak at a slightly louder than normal level, but not so loud that facial movements are exaggerated. The speaker should avoid dropping his/her voice at the end of sentences. Pitch should be normal, not too high and not too low. The speaker should not speak with food in the mouth nor while chewing gum. Finally, the speaker should be encouraged to use facial expressions to complement and supplement what is being said. For example, a joke might be accompanied by slight laughter, a happy story by a smile. The findings of Helfer (1998) underline the importance of instructing the communication partners that speaking clearly when conversing face-to-face with older adults is in fact a viable aid to communication. She found that the older the listeners the more poorly they recognized conversational speech with auditory and visual speech cues and the greater benefit derived from the talker speaking clearly. Interestingly, Helfer (1998, p. 240) reported that "the difference between A-only perception of conversational speech and AV perception of clear speech was approximately 30 percent, far greater than the benefit obtained from either speaking clearly or using visual speech cues in isolation."

The personal variables listed in Table 8–9 pertain more to the person with hearing loss. With regard to hearing loss,

TABLE 8–9 Factors That Influence Receptive Communication

SPEAKER VARIABLES
Mouth Movements
Rate of Speech
Loudness of Voice
Pitch of Voice
Accent
Dialect
Visibility of Articulators
Objects in the Mouth
Facial Expressions

PERSONAL VARIABLES
Severity of Hearing Loss
Visual Acuity
Mental Status
Physical Functional Status
Listening Skills
Attention Span

ENVIRONMENTAL VARIABLES
Acoustic Factors
Lighting
Visual Distractions

LINGUISTIC VARIABLES
Topic Awareness
Context Awareness
Conversational Context Awareness
Semantic Variables
Syntactic Considerations

Source: Modified from Abrahamson (1995, 1997).

the listener must be instructed to set the stage by admitting to the existence of hearing loss. Acceptance of hearing loss and its impact on communication is the first step to successful communication with or without hearing aids. Trychin (1997) suggested that people often postpone informing others about their hearing loss because they themselves are embarrassed. They prefer to wait until there is an obvious communication problem. This strategy may lead to unnecessary misunderstandings and erroneous assumptions about the listener (Trychin, 1995).

The person with hearing loss may not have good listening habits so that time should be spent developing this aptitude.

The following are some tips that are helpful in promoting listening skills: (1) listen intently yet remain relaxed, (2) show interest and understanding while others are talking by maintaining eye contact and body language, (3) use guessing skills to fill in the blanks for words not heard clearly, (4) disregard noise, (5) maintain good eye-lip contact, (6) sit within 3 to 6 feet from the speaker, and (7) do not give up prematurely (Kricos & Holmes, 1996). Kricos and Holmes (1996) reported that active listening training is an effective treatment for helping individuals with hearing impairment improve their auditory-visual recognition of speech especially in a background of noise.

If the person with hearing impairment has neurological problems such as aphasia, cognitive problems such as Alzheimer's disease, or central auditory processing problems that may compound their communication deficits, communication partners should be taught compensatory communication strategies to facilitate understanding. For example, they should be taught how to break a complex idea into short phrases, to produce clearer speech, to produce more easily understandable messages, or perhaps to try an FM system using proper microphone placement and techniques (Pichora-Fuller, 1997). When communicating with persons with hearing impairment and other physical conditions, the speaking partner should always make sure that the message being discussed has been understood. It is often helpful to repeat what has been agreed upon to keep misunderstandings to a minimum. Message-related gestures are very helpful as well as writing the message down to supplement what is available through audition and speechreading. Of utmost importance, communication partners must try to avoid displaying their feelings of frustration and annoyance with the difficulty associated with getting a message across. Oftentimes, it is the communication partner rather than the person with hearing impairment who needs advice about coping and overcoming the consequences of hearing impairment. Finally, if the person with hearing loss has a visual loss, he/she should be encouraged to wear glasses as this will enable a better view of the speaker's face and gestures and promote better speechreading ability.

Another important component of multimodality speech perception or AVI training is advice about the environment. The focus here is to insure that the patient and communication partner understand that the environment is an information field. It assists individuals in understanding events,

making decisions, and taking appropriate actions (Steinfeld, 1997). Steinfeld (1997) suggests that it is important to emphasize that the ability to detect a signal such as speech depends in large part on the strength of the input relative to the information field in the background, namely noise or visual distractions. One way of increasing signal strength is through hearing aids but this has to be supplemented by reduction or avoidance of noises within the environment such as reverberation from air-conditioning machinery or background music. Additional suggestions include closing the door of a meeting room to eliminate noise from the hallway, turning off the computer in the home or office to eliminate electromagnetic interference, and turning off the television, radio, or computer printer to eliminate background noise.

Of course, lighting is an important environmental variable to be manipulated during any and all discourse. Of utmost importance, the patient should be reminded of the importance of adequate room lighting. Older adults require more light because their pupils are smaller, allowing less light in. Use of natural light should be encouraged, however blinds should be adjusted so that streams of bright, glaring light are kept out. Older adults should avoid talking in an area where there is glare from windows or mirrors. The light should always be focused on the speaker's face for optimal viewing.

Finally, with regard to linguistic variables, the patient must come to understand that communication occurs in an environmental as well as a linguistic context. They must understand that linguistic redundancy can enable the individual to fill in the information not clearly heard or seen. That is it can supplement sensory input. Hence knowledge of language—how sounds and words are strung together, how the context may define the topic of conversation, how world events may define a discussion, and how one's tone of voice can communicate information that is unspoken—is a critical aspect of discourse (Houston & Montgomery, 1997). In short, the "context and general knowledge can disambiguate the sensory stream" (Houston & Montgomery, 1997, p. 148). Hence, the audiologist should encourage the patient to keep abreast of current events as remaining current can aid in the comprehension of compromised auditory and visual input. Interestingly, patients do feel more comfortable entering into or participating in conversation when they have contextual knowledge as a back-up. In sum, AVI training is an integral part of AR in general and of the hearing-aid fitting in particular. Knowledge of realistic strategies for preventing or reducing communication breakdowns and changing communication behaviors should be considered a vehicle that can empower people with hearing impairments, introducing an element of equity into previously threatening situations (Trychin, 1995).

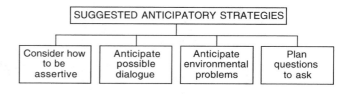

Figure 8–5 Anticipatory strategies.

Conversational Strategies or Assertiveness Training

Throughout the remediation process, the audiologist must strive to establish traits conducive to positive outcomes. Strategies or assertiveness training wherein the patient with hearing impairment is encouraged to manipulate the environment and people in the environment so that communication function is maximized is a relatively recent component of the remediation process. The goal is to use selected strategies to minimize potential communication breakdowns associated with reduced sensory input (Tye-Murray & Witt, 1997). Strategies training has gained some acceptance because of the established link between assertive personality and successful rehabilitation outcomes. Assertiveness in this context implies taking control and influencing outcomes (Kemp, 1990a). Related to this is the fact that when persons are imbued with the ability and power to intervene and make a difference this goes a long way toward setting the stage for success. In general terms, assertiveness training encourages persons with hearing impairment to stick up for their rights, seek answers to questions, and take responsibility for improving communication. It gives people a sense of control in difficult listening situations (Abrahamson, 1995). Key to assertiveness training is willingness on the part of the person with hearing impairment to be open about and willing to admit to hearing loss.

Communication strategies that can be used by the hearing impaired can be classified as anticipatory, repair, or facilitative (Figs. 8–5 to 8–7) (Tye-Murray & Witt, 1997; Tye-Murray, 1998; Abrahamson, 1997). Anticipatory strategies can be used before an event to minimize the number of communication breakdowns that take place. Repair strategies provide directions to the communication partner about how to rectify a breakdown in communication. Facilitative strategies are used to influence speech-recognition performance, the communication environment, the communication partner's presentation of a message, and the message itself. Figures 8–5, 8–6, and 8–7 provide examples of strategies to offer patients with hearing impairment. Facilitative strategies are most effectively employed when the strategies are informa-tive and specific. For example, facilitative strategies wherein the person with hearing impairment informs the communication partner that a hearing loss exists "I have a hearing loss," and then suggests how the message can best be understood, "can you please speak a little louder and slower," are very helpful. Similarly, informing the communication partner of a communication breakdown, "I did not understand your last sentence," and than asking the partner to rephrase, repeat, simplify, or elaborate can be quite effective. Any of the repair strategies listed in Figure 8–6 are very helpful in clarifying misunderstandings. Table 8–10 lists the strategies the communication partner should adopt to facilitate speech understanding (Tye-Murray & Witt, 1997).

Several guided learning activities are available for training patients to use strategies effectively. QUEST?AR, a conversational training technique developed by Erber (1988), provides conversation practice in audition, plus vision- and auditory-only conditions in the presence of noise, or even over the telephone. QUEST?AR is an effective way to teach the hearing impaired how to apply clarification strategies. With QUEST?AR it is helpful if conversational partners first agree on a familiar topic (e.g., grandchildren). Once the topic is selected, the client asks the series of 30 related questions in a conversational order (e.g., do you have any grandchildren?), obtaining an answer prior to proceeding with the next question. If the patient with hearing impairment misses the answer, he/she attempts to identify the sources of difficulty in receiving the message (e.g., too fast, too long) and requests appropriate clarification. The communication partner uses repair or clarification strategies as needed to help the person with hearing impairment retrieve the correct answer. Thus, the communication partner has the opportunity to practice the strategies they have learned for clarification purposes. The QUEST?AR package includes a booklet containing written questions. Clinicians report that this conversational training technique allows for development of natural, interactive conversational skills (Abrahamson, 1995).

TOPICON is another procedure for practice in the use of strategies during conversation (Erber, 1988). It is a conversational sampling, evaluation, and practice procedure for

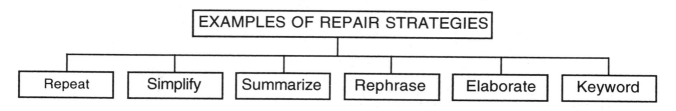

Figure 8–6 Repair strategies.

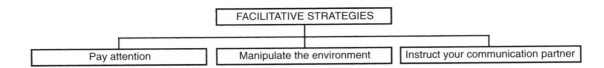

Figure 8–7   Facilitative strategies.

use when the structure provided by the questions in QUEST?AR are no longer needed (Abrahamson, 1995). Tye-Murray and Witt (1997) suggest that continuous discourse tracking can provide practice to clients in using repair and clarification strategies, as well. While QUEST?AR, TOPI-CON, and tracking have many advantages, for the most part older adults may not be able or willing to commit the time or money to intensive long-term communication-strategies training. In my view, communication-strategies training can and should be incorporated into the hearing-aid orientation and/or counseling sessions that take place at the fitting or post-fitting phase. Materials should be client centered and based in the real world. Of course a family member or caregiver should be present.

The WATCH program described by Montgomery (1994) is a simple but effective approach to teaching communication strategies. In this program the acronym WATCH incorporates the strategies people should remember if successful communication exchanges are to take place (Tye-Murray & Witt,

W = Watch the speaker's mouth not his/her eyes
A = Ask specific questions
T = Talk/tell about your hearing loss
C = Change or modify the environment so it is free of distractions
H = Acquire hearing health care knowledge

1997). The W component covers the facilitative strategies used by the patient with hearing impairment to influence speech recognition. Also, the importance of facial expressions, gestures, and intonation to speech recognition can be stressed here. The A component teaches repair strategies to be used with the communication partner. For example, the communication partner should be urged to repeat or rephrase a message when it is unclear; to provide additional information that might help convey the message; or to use gestures. During the T component the patient with hearing impairment is encouraged to inform communication partners that they have a hearing loss and provides instructive strategies for speaking in a more comprehensible fashion. The person with hearing impairment, for example, may be encouraged to say "I have a hearing loss, can you please speak more slowly and face me when you are talking?" During the C component, the client, communication partner, and audiologist discuss the situations that are difficult and how to modify them to one's advantage. For example, the telephone is often a difficult environment for persons with hearing impairment. This conversation should include: (1) repair strategies including verification or confirmation about what has been said, (2) discussions about numbers including asking the speaker to count from zero to the correct number and then stopping; and (3) providing feedback about whether the message was recognized (Abrahamson,

1995). Finally, the H component suggests informing the patient and communication partner about resources available about hearing loss, hearing health care, assistive technology, and consumer organizations.

PEARL

Caregivers or family members need to know how to recognize poor communication environments and create optimal conditions for communicating including rearranging furniture and reducing distractions such as glare and noise. Caregivers or family members should know that it is important to speak slowly and carefully, to make mouth movements visible, to use nonverbal cues, to respond to requests for clarification, and to repeat/clarify when appropriate (Erber & Heine, 1996). Incorporating family members into the rehabilitation process can help to develop communication autonomy (Binnie, 1994).

TABLE 8–10   Improving Communication with Hearing-Impaired Elderly Persons

The following tips should be shared with communication partners:

- Obtain the person's attention before beginning a communication exchange
- Speak face-to-face
- Paraphrase if you have to repeat what has been said
- Speak at a normal level or slightly louder
- Speak slowly but not exaggerated
- Stand within 2 to 3 feet of the listener
- Reduce background noise
- Pause at the end of a sentence
- Avoid appearing frustrated
- If the person can read, write down key words
- Have the person with hearing impairment repeat what you have said to verify that the message was understood

Source: Modified from Walther, A., & Warshaw, G. (1993). Hearing assessment. In: T.T. Yoshikawa, E. Cobbs, & K. Brummel-Smith (Eds.) *Ambulatory Geriatric Care,* p. 158. St. Louis: Mosby.

In sum, assertiveness and strategies training are important components of the rehabilitation process. It tends to come as a sense of relief to people with hearing impairment to learn that they do not have to shoulder all of the responsibility for communication. Providing them with advice on how others should be instructed to modify their behavior to accommodate hearing loss can empower older adults and relieve them somewhat from the worries and anxieties associated with many communication exchanges. The new knowledge that they can use to carry out everyday activities can be easily incorporated and can make a difference in the lives of older persons with hearing impairment.

Environmental Manipulation Training

Many of the important points about the environment were made earlier in the discussion about AVI training. Its importance cannot be underestimated as the environment is a field from which individuals select information on which their attention is focused, for better or for worse (Steinfeld, 1997). For example, information in the environment can be used by persons with hearing impairment to fill in the gaps in a communication exchange, or can detract from communication when too many distractions are present. Older adults must be encouraged to scan the environment around them for information that can supplement conversation. Similarly, they must scan the environment for background elements such as glare from uncontrolled reflections or noise from reverberation that can be detrimental to communication. Older adults have little difficulty identifying distractions. They do, however, find it problematic to manipulate the environment to their advantage. This is where 15 to 20 minutes of training can be essential.

PEARL

The audiologist must emphasize that it is the responsibility of the patient with hearing impairment to ensure that general information can be perceived within the general environment or "information field" in which they are operating.

Environmental manipulation training should include a determination of the need for modifications to facilitate communication and to insure the safety of the hearing-impaired individual. The challenge here is for the audiologist to use technology to help the hearing-impaired obtain information through environmental sound . . . simply restoration of the two most basic levels of hearing (Jensema & Lennox, 1994). The creative use of alerting tehnology can help to inform hearing-impaired people of the presence of environmental sounds that are important to them. In short, the audiologist must work with the patient to determine what he or she needs to hear, and, of course, wants to hear. As part of the environmental assessment, a determination must be made about how to alert the individual to the presence of environmental sound (e.g., enhanced auditory signal, visual signal, and tactile signal). It is especially important to determine whether a hearing-aid user wears the hearing aid at home

because this can influence the necessity for alerting devices in the home. The importance of an environmental assessment cannot be overemphasized especially for older adults with cognitive impairments. In the next section, the technology available to assist the hearing impaired is discussed.

TECHNOLOGY
Signal-Alerting Technology

Signal-alerting technology includes any system that warns, signals, or alerts a person with a hearing impairment, of any degree, to important sounds present in the environment. For the person with hearing impairment, the sound must be enhanced or conveyed through some other sense (Jensema & Lennox, 1994). Devices to alert persons with hearing impairment to conditions in the environment substitute visual signals or tactile signals when warning signals are not audible. Thanks to technological advances and the Americans with Disabilities Act (ADA) of 1992, virtually every sound-producing event used for signaling or warning purposes can be coded into a visual or vibratory stimulus for the benefit of persons with hearing impairment (Ross, 1994). Signal-alerting devices are commercially available and are invaluable to hearing-impaired people who are homebound, for persons with cognitive impairments, and for residents of nursing facilities who cannot hear external events due to hearing loss. They can be used without hearing aids or while wearing amplification.

Independent alerting devices are available for alarm clocks, smoke alarms, doorbells/doorknocks, and the telephone. Devices to indicate that the telephone is ringing are generally visual. They use the telephone ringer as the power source to activate a flash, a strobe, or an incandescent light (Ross, 1994). Remote units can be set up so that the light will flash in an adjacent room, signaling the ring of the telephone. This is very helpful, as most older adults complain of difficulty hearing the telephone ring when they are in an adjoining room (Sandridge, 1995). According to Jensema and Lennox (1994), wired incandescent devices are the most popular visual method of alerting people to a telephone ring signal. The Fone Flasher, available from Radio Shack, is a popular telephone ring signaler that is accessibly priced. Older adults who travel should consider purchasing a portable sound-activated unit while traveling, although hotels should be equipped with signaling and warning devices that can be made available upon request. It is important to note that plug-in devices that provide a loud telephone ring are available for persons with difficulty hearing in noisy environments (Sandridge, 1995). These sound enhancers are relatively inexpensive and easy to set up. The above devices are commercially available through hardware stores, telephone specialty stores, and electronics stores.

The ability to hear the fire alarm, smoke alarm, or carbon monoxide detector is quite important especially in the evening when asleep. People with hearing impairment often are unclear as to whether or not they can hear the alarm with or without the hearing aid. During the initial stage of the rehabilitation assessment, the audiologist should ask the person with hearing loss to test the smoke detector and determine if it is audible even when it is noisy in the room. Some audiologists merely recommend both visual and audio alerts to be safe. Visual alarm systems are required to have certain photometric and location features to insure the safety of persons when they are asleep and awake (Jensema & Lennox, 1994). Powerful white flashing strobe lights have been found to be effective in awakening hard-of-hearing and deaf people from their sleep. Jensema and Lennox (1994) recommend smoke detectors rated at 100 candela or more and audible signals rated at 85 dB or more. Generally speaking, fire/smoke alarms can be plugged into a wall socket and then hung high on a wall close to the ceiling (Jensema & Lennox, 1994). As with telephone devices, remote lights can be set up in various rooms with selected alarms that flash strobe lights when smoke is detected. When purchasing a smoke detector, persons with hearing impairment should be reminded to ask whether the smoke alarm meets the standard set by the National Fire Protection Association. Such standards attempt to insure that the visual light system is bright enough to awaken a sleeping deaf person.

Hearing-impaired persons may not be able to hear an alarm clock with an audio signal. A variety of options are available for home and travel. Most alarm clocks use either light or vibration to wake up the person from sleep. Alarm clocks that chirp loudly can be purchased by persons with milder hearing impairments. Small travel alarms can be purchased which, when placed under the pillow, vibrate to awaken the sleeping traveler. Devices that alert persons with hearing impairment to a door knock or the door bell are available from selected dealers. As with the smoke alarm system, the ability to hear someone at the door generates a sense of security that is so important to older adults. Jensema and Lennox (1994) recommend a doorbell system with visual alerts or audio enhancement over a door-knock system. The simplest solution for the home is installation of a flashing light when the doorbell rings.

If several devices are needed, whole house alerting systems installed centrally may be preferable, albeit more costly (Jensema & Lennox, 1994). Comprehensive alerting systems are equipped with individual sensors for the different systems (e.g., radio alarm, smoke detector, etc.), each with its own response codes (Ross, 1994). Audiologists are well equipped to guide persons and institutions about the system(s) that will best meet their patients' needs and to arrange for the purchase of the necessary ALDs. It is incumbent on audiologists to advise the hearing impaired of the requirements set forth by the ADA to insure that their residence or place of accommodation is in compliance. A simple needs assessment appears in Table 8–11. It should be completed during the audiologic evaluation when decisions are reached about intervention options, or during the hearing-aid evaluation and selection process. It is also helpful to complete the needs assessment at the final rehabilitation session to make sure the device(s) are working to the patient's satisfaction. When reviewing responses to the needs assessment and making recommendations, make sure the patient's visual acuity is adequate enough to detect the visual alerts. If not, consider a tactile signal in combination with an enhanced audio signal. Radio Shack and local

TABLE 8–11   Needs Assessment for Alerting Devices

Without a hearing aid	YES	NO
Do you have difficulty hearing		
a. the telephone ring when in the room with the phone	Y	N
b. the telephone ring when in a room next to the room with the phone	Y	N
c. someone knocking on the door or ringing the doorbell	Y	N
d. the alarm clock at home	Y	N
e. the alarm clock in a hotel	Y	N
f. the smoke detector in your home	Y	N
g. the smoke detector in a hotel	Y	N
With a hearing aid	**YES**	**NO**
Do you have difficulty hearing		
a. the telephone ring when in the room with the phone	Y	N
b. the telephone ring when in a room next to the room with the phone	Y	N
c. someone knocking on the door or ringing the doorbell	Y	N
d. the alarm clock at home	Y	N
e. the alarm clock in a hotel	Y	N
f. the smoke detector in your home	Y	N
g. the smoke detector in a hotel	Y	N

Source: Modified from Sandridge, 1995.

PEARL

Audiologists should consider making available to the consumer brochures that discuss auxiliary aids, the ADA, consumer rights, communication access, etc. SHHH, the Consumer Affairs Division of ASHA, and IBM National Support Center for Persons with Disabilities are examples of organizations that distribute information helpful to persons with hearing impairment.

---

telephone companies make their special needs catalogues available to consumers. The catalogues describe devices available for persons with handicapping conditions. Of course, a number of World Wide Web sites have information available about devices for the hearing impaired. Finally, an ALD center, allowing for hands-on experience with available devices, is an effective way of increasing use of assistive technology by the hearing impaired and their communication partners.

Consumer Organizations

Several consumer organizations have been organized as a resource to older adults with hearing impairments and their families. These groups should be viewed as information-sharing and advocacy groups for persons with hearing impairment. The premise underlying the formation of these organizations is that participation can facilitate the coping and acceptance process. It is a relief to be with others who know how it feels and who routinely experience the frustration and embarrassment of trying to manage when not being able to hear what is being said (Glass, 1990).

PEARL

Learning from others with similar conditions can provide the patient with information beyond what professionals are taught in graduate school.

These organizations make educational materials on a variety of topics available at low cost. Further, a consumer organization such as SHHH publishes a journal for its members providing a good deal of important information about hearing loss, hearing aids, ALDs, legislation, communication skills, technological developments, among other things. SHHH also makes recommendations to professional organizations regarding services that should be offered to patients with hearing impairments. SHHH recently recommended that all hearing-aid dispensers make available and encourage participation in group orientation programs.

Group orientation programs should be short term, 3 to 6 weeks, and should provide sufficient time for an instructional component and for the emergence of group exchanges (SHHH, 1996). Topics for group AR classes should include: (1) discussions about hearing loss and the audiogram; (2) instruction in troubleshooting hearing aids; (3) discussions about the availability of ALDs to supplement hearing aids; (4) an introduction to speechreading/auditory training; (5) overview of coping and conversational repair strategies to facilitate communication; (6) practice in environmental manipulation; and (7) discussions about assertiveness and advocacy. A group environment is a wonderful opportunity for individuals with hearing loss to share experiences and provide each other with support and a sense of belonging. Further, a group environment enables members to learn from each other, and to serve as role models and sources of social and moral support (Abrahamson, 1997). Participants in group intervention programs routinely report that the group experience helps individuals cope with hearing loss. As discussed earlier, Abrams et al (1992) have demonstrated that short-term group programs

do in fact promote hearing-aid benefit among new hearing aid users above that achieved with just a single orientation session.

According to Abrahamson (1997), group rehabilitative sessions are an important supplement to individual sessions as they:

- Provide a support network for the hearing impaired and their family members
- Empower the individual to assume responsibility for the hearing loss
- Confirm some of the negative effects of hearing loss
- Help to set realistic expectations regarding the consequences of hearing loss and the benefits of hearing aids

---

AR WITH HEARING AIDS: AN INTEGRATED APPROACH FOR THE REAL WORLD

Assisting an adult with a bilaterally symmetrical sensorineural hearing loss to accept and use hearing aids is challenging enough. Add to that picture recent retirement, the death of a spouse of 45 years, fixed income, mutiple chronic conditions, and a 78th birthday celebration. This individual may not have a microwave, VCR, computer, or remote control television at home. We do not want this person becoming another statistic . . . hearing aid returned because device

---

PEARL

The challenge for the audiologist is to empower this patient to become a satisfied and successful hearing-aid user in the context of his/her daily life routines and with the cloud of "managed care" hanging over.

---

is too complicated to use . . . hearing aid not being used because it amplifies too much noise . . . situational benefits of hearing aids do not justify the expenditure of $4000 and sacrificing a vacation. How can we "do right by the patient with hearing impairment" and do right by ourselves?

In my view delivering the hearing aid in the context of AR is the best chance we have and is what separates audiologists from other specialists who sell and fit hearing aids. As we move into dispensing more sophisticated and expensive products, managed care organizations will want us to prove that the patient can hear better, can understand better, and, above all, can function better in daily life. Dispensing hearing aids within the context of an integrated rehabilitation program can move us close to our goals. What follows is a suggested protocol for including each of the components of AR into the dispensing process.

PEARL

AR begins at the audiologic evaluation.

The audiologic evaluation provides information used to identify hearing-aid candidates, to select the appropriate amplification system, and serves as a baseline against which to judge the effectiveness of intervention. It should also be considered the first stage of the rehabilitation process as it is at this point that informational and personal-adjustment counseling begins. Audiologists should approach the evaluation as an opportunity to obtain information that will assist in convincing the patient of the need for hearing aids and of their potential value. It should include the following:

- Routine audiometric evaluation including frequency specific UCL's
- Speech-recognition testing with and without visual cues to demonstrate value of speechreading
- Speech-recognition testing at a variety of hearing levels to demonstrate the potential value of amplification
- Speech-recognition testing in the presence of noise to confirm patient complaints of difficulty in noise, and to determine whether there is a central auditory processing component to the hearing loss
- Communication assessment, hearing handicap assessment, and ALD assessment to determine intervention needs and to serve as a baseline against which to judge benefit (Appendices A, B, and C)
- A hearing handicap questionnaire as shown in Appendix D that has been completed by a spouse or caregiver
- Completion of the needs assessment for alerting devices shown in Table 8–11

Following the complete assessment, the patient, caregiver or family member, and audiologist meet to discuss the test results. If the patient has difficulty hearing, an ALD should be used to facilitate communication. The audiologist should discuss the test results and do some informational counseling using Figures 8–2, 8–3, and 8–4 to explain the audiogram in the context of speech sounds, normal conversational speech, and, of course, how hearing aids work to make speech sounds audible. At this point, the audiologist might suggest that, based on the patient's assessment of the situation, the family member's assessment, and outcomes at the evaluation, hearing aids may provide the assistance needed to overcome some of the difficulties expressed or observed during the assessment. If the patient is interested, the audiologist should provide information about hearing aids, available styles, costs, etc. Also, the advantages of binaural over monaural amplification should be discussed, with the patient being encouraged to accept a binaural fitting. If not, always keep in mind that one hearing aid is better than none and the second unit can be purchased later on. Providing the patient with as much information as possible about hearing loss and hearing aids is vital if the patient is to make an informed decision.

At this point during the session, some motivational counseling, as discussed in Chapter 3, may be appropriate. The audiologist must keep in mind that aging affects motivation, that older adults take time to make decisions, and that older adults tend to make choices which tend toward the status quo (Brummel-Smith, 1990). To assist the older

TABLE 8–12 Potential Wants, Needs, and Goals Relative to Hearing Aids

1. Improved television/radio hearing and understanding
2. Improved speech understanding in quiet and noise
3. Maintenance of independence
4. Reduction in emotional and social consequences of hearing loss
5. Restoration of quality of life, self-esteem, and life satisfaction
6. Restoration of a safe environment outside and at home

adult in arriving at a decision to move forward with hearing aids, the audiologist might consider some counseling directed at exploring what the patient might want from hearing aids and then proceed to enumerate some of the benefits and rewards to be garnered from their use. The information in Tables 8–6 and 8–12 could be helpful at this point. The information contained in Table 8–6 is especially important as it is never too early to make sure that the patient's expectations and assumptions regarding hearing aids are realistic. The audiologic evaluation and accompanying counseling session should end with a decision to move forward with the purchase of a particular hearing-aid style and technology. Much of the information discussed at this time can be reviewed at the hearing-aid selection. Further, during the hearing-aid selection the audiologist can begin to discuss hearing-aid use, operation, and maintenance.

Brammer (1982) described the eight stages of a helping relationship that should be kept in mind during the early stages of the clinician's encounter witht the patient. At the initial evaluation or entry point into rehabilitation, the clinician should lay the groundwork for trust and enable the patient and family members to define the problem(s) relating to the hearing impairment. The audiologist should clarify what the patient and/or family member sees as the problem and the effect on daily life. Next, the audiologist should discuss the structure or conditions of the fitting and rehabilitation process. This entails acknowledging the time commitment, fees, restrictions, qualifications, and responsibilities of the audiologist. Exploration of client feelings, client needs, and client expectations should serve as the basis for the planning and execution of the actual rehabilitation. The older adult should be imbued with a sense of power to make a difference. Finally, conditions for terminating rehabilitation based on outcomes data should be established and agreed upon by the patient and audiologist. Each of the points discussed above should be kept in mind throughout.

The Hearing-Aid Fitting

Following the hearing-aid selection, which is discussed in the next chapter, the client returns for the hearing-aid fitting, at which time the electroacoustic response of the hearing aid is verified and aided speech-recognition ability may be assessed. The bulk of this session should be devoted to the hearing-aid orientation that should include discussion of instrument operation, care, and maintenance as well as instrument use. This is a good time to introduce the checklist shown in Table 8–3 and the list of dos and don'ts contained in Table 8–4. A wearing schedule should be mutually decided upon with the patient hopefully agreeing to keep a small diary of situations in which the hearing aid was and was not helpful (Table 8–5). The patient should be reminded to bring the diary to each return visit. Realistic expectations surrounding hearing-aid use should be discussed, with emphasis placed on the fact that hearing aids cannot cure all communication problems and that it could take two to three months before the adjustment or acclimatization process is complete.

Following the hearing-aid orientation, the audiologist should do additional informational counseling and overview some key points about auditory-visual integration, listening strategies, and environmental manipulation training. As time is probably limited from both the audiologist's and the patient's perspectives, some written material about repair strategies and speechreading should be sent home with the patient and caregiver. The patient should be encouraged to call the audiologist if problems arise, and a follow-up visit should be scheduled within 2 to 3 weeks of the fitting. The purpose of the return visit should be discussed, with considerable pressure being applied to keep the appointment. It is helpful to call the patient within 1 week of the fitting to see how things are working out with the hearing aid. Older adults tend to be quite appreciative when a health care professional takes the time to call to see how the hearing aids are working out.

PEARL

I also find it helpful to send the patients a letter reminding them about the "Dos and Don'ts of Hearing Aid Use" and encouraging them to call with questions or concerns.

Finally, all patients leave the clinic with supplies in hand to empower them to care for their hearing aids independently. The "goodies" include a user brochure, daily log, wax pick, dehumidifier or drying kit, miniature battery tester, soft toothbrush, and extra batteries. Upon completion of the session, the audiologist should provide the patient with information regarding hearing-instrument insurance programs and the manufacturer's warranty on the instrument.

The Postfitting or Verification Phase

At the beginning of this visit, the audiologist should ask the patient to remove the hearing aid, insert the battery, reposition the hearing aid, and adjust the hearing aid to make sure that the patient is operating it correctly. The audiologist should make sure that the patient can manipulate the device independently or that the family member understands how to step in when necessary. Next, the audiologist should readminister the communication/disability assessment, the handicap questionnaire, and the ALD needs assessment as a way of monitoring hearing-aid outcomes. If the needs assessment suggests that an additional device is needed to supplement hearing aids, the audiologist should make the appropriate recommendation and referrals.

At the end or termination of the formal rehabilitation process, the outcomes, both subjective and objective, should be discussed, with the professional verifying that the patient and family member understand and are pleased with the progress and behaviors growing out of the remediation process. The audiologist should make sure to demonstrate to the patient the ends achieved via remediation. It is helpful to compare baseline data to that which was gathered over time to demonstrate how successful the intervention has actually been. For example any improvement in scores on tests of speech understanding, or reduction in self-perceived disability or handicap is always impressive to the patient as well as to family members. To this end, the audiologist should compare aided responses obtained on the questionnaires to those obtained at the initial evaluation to determine if in fact the patient is deriving adequate benefit in the disability and handicap domains of function. Results of the comparisons should be shared with the patient and family member. It is reassuring when the older adult learns that some of their functional losses have been restored and that the hearing aid is in fact effective. If the units are not benefiting the patient, then some modifications may be necessary and additional rehabilitation sessions should be scheduled.

The focus of this final session is to promote adaptation of the person to the instrument and to the environment, to adapt the environment to the person using alerting devices when possible, and to promote family adaptation (Brummel-Smith, 1990). The patient and family member should be present once again. At this session, which may be the last, the audiologist should emphasize listening strategies, AVI training, and environmental manipulation. In short, the patient must become conversant with all of the facilitative or repair techniques at his/her disposal to minimize potential communication breakdowns resulting from the communication environment, the communication partner, or the message itself (Tye-Murray & Witt, 1997). On the other hand, the family member must come to understand the speaking behaviors they should adopt. The material contained in Table 8–12 and Figures 8–2, 8–3, and 8–4 should be discussed as it may be valuable throughout this session. Also, material contained in Table 8–10 should be distributed to enable the patient to modify the behaviors of communication partners. Before terminating the session, encourage the patient to contact a local consumer organization, such as SHHH, to meet other people with hearing impairments and to obtain additional information about hearing loss and strategies for coping with hearing loss. Finally, never close the door, take this opportunity to emphasize the importance of periodic follow-ups especially at 3 months, 6 months, 12 months, and 2 years postfitting.

PEARL

Make sure to underline the importance of keeping the follow-up appointments as this is instrumental to sustaining a high level of hearing-aid satisfaction.

PEARL

The patient should be encouraged to return to the audiologist 3 months after the initial fitting and before the end of the first year of hearing-aid use. This time frame will ensure that problems with the hearing aid can be repaired within the 1-year warranty period. The final follow-up sessions also serve as inducements for the patient to continue to use and benefit from hearing aids.

Concluding Remarks

Hopefully my bias has come through in this chapter. I see audiologic rehabilitation as inextricably intertwined with the hearing-aid fitting. In fact, you can't do one without the other. I do not believe hearing aids can cure the hearing impairment. Hearing aids in conjunction with rehabilitation can reduce disability, improve function, and eliminate handicap (Weinstein, 1996). Always keep in mind that a person with hearing impairment does not cause his or her disability or handicap. People with hearing impairment are disabled and/or handicapped to the extent that they have difficulty interacting with people in their environment (Kemp, 1990a). A hearing handicap can be reduced by helping the person to become more comfortable with the condition and with other's

---

PEARL

A disability can be reduced by increasing a person's abilities, in the case of the hearing impaired via hearing aids.

---

reactions to it, and, of course, by communication partners becoming more accepting of and accommodating of the person with a disabling hearing impairment. Thus, family members, the patient, and the hearing health care professional are the agents of change who will determine the outcomes of the rehabilitation process. Family education and support, improvement of functional abilities, psychological support, social integration and acceptance, and empowerment should be our goals as we help older adults with hearing impairments use their hearing aids successfully.

Sorkin (1997) sums up advice from SHHH members to hearing-care professionals very nicely. Her suggestions stem from a survey of SHHH members regarding their needs as hard-of-hearing people. Sorkin (1997, p. 54) notes that: "Hard-of-hearing people become frustrated, confused, even bitter when they realize that a hearing aid is not going to restore normal hearing in the same way that eyeglasses restore vision. When this happens, they become ineffective hearing-aid users or nonusers. Use of amplification is most successful when it is used by people with an understanding of the full range of modifications that a person needs to incorporate hearing loss into their life. People who enjoy such success understand that the effectivenesss of a hearing aid increases with time and with experimentation, that hearing aids work better in certain situations than others and that other assists—used in concert with a hearing aid—can often help someone function more effectively in a range of settings and situations." Her message to audiologists is an important one . . . listen to the patient and make sure that the intervention is adapted to the lifestyle and expresses the needs of the hard of hearing person.

APPENDIX A
Abbreviated Profile of Hearing Aid Benefit (APHAB)

Today's Date

Last Name   *First Name*   *Birthdate*

Address

City   *State*   *ZIP Code*

Home phone   *Work phone*

Hearing Aid Experience:
☐ Less than 6 weeks   ☐ 6 weeks to 11 months   ☐ 1 to 10 years   ☐ Over 10 years

Daily Hearing Aid Use:
☐ Less than 1 hour a day   ☐ 1 to 4 hours a day   ☐ 4 to 8 hours a day   ☐ 8 to 16 hours a day

Employment Status:
☐ Full-time   ☐ Part-time   ☐ Retired, or not employed outside the home

Instructions

Please circle the answer that comes closest to your everyday experience. Notice that each choice includes a percentage. You can use this to help you decide on your answer. For example, if a statement is true about 75 percent of the time, circle "C". If you have not experienced the situation as described, try to think of a similar situation that you have been in and respond for that situation. If you have no idea, leave the item blank.

A. Always (99%)
B. Almost always (87%)
C. Generally (75%)
D. Half the time (50%)
E. Occasionally (25%)
F. Seldom (12%)
G. Never (1%)

	Without My Hearing Aid	*With* My Hearing Aid
1. When I am in a crowded grocery store, talking with the cashier, I can follow the conversation.	A B C D E F G	A B C D E F G
2. I miss a lot of information when listening to a lecture.	A B C D E F G	A B C D E F G
3. Unexpected sounds, like a smoke detector or alarm bell are uncomfortable.	A B C D E F G	A B C D E F G
4. I have difficulty hearing a conversation when I'm with one of my family members at home.	A B C D E F G	A B C D E F G
5. I have trouble understanding dialogue in a movie or at the theatre.	A B C D E F G	A B C D E F G
6. When I am listening to the news on the car radio, and family members are talking, I have trouble hearing the news.	A B C D E F G	A B C D E F G
7. When I am at the dinner table with several people and am trying to have a conversation with one person, understanding speech is difficult.	A B C D E F G	A B C D E F G
8. Traffic noises are too loud.	A B C D E F G	A B C D E F G
9. When I am talking with someone across a large empty room, I understand the words.	A B C D E F G	A B C D E F G
10. When I am in a small office, interviewing or answering questions, I have difficulty following the conversation.	A B C D E F G	A B C D E F G

APPENDIX A (*Continued*)

	Without My Hearing Aid	*With* My Hearing Aid
11. When I am in a theater watching a movie or play, and the people around me are whispering and rustling paper wrappers, I can still make out the dialogue.	A B C D E F G	A B C D E F G
12. When I am having a quiet conversation with a friend, I have difficulty understanding.	A B C D E F G	A B C D E F G
13. The sounds of running water, such as a toilet or shower, are uncomfortably loud.	A B C D E F G	A B C D E F G
14. When a speaker is addressing a small group, and everyone is listening quietly, I have to strain to understand.	A B C D E F G	A B C D E F G
15. When I'm in a quiet conversation with my doctor in an examination room, it is hard to follow the conversation.	A B C D E F G	A B C D E F G
16. I can understand conversations even when several people are talking.	A B C D E F G	A B C D E F G
17. The sounds of construction work are uncomfortably loud.	A B C D E F G	A B C D E F G
18. It's hard for me to understand what is being said at lectures or church services.	A B C D E F G	A B C D E F G
19. I can communicate with others when we are in a crowd.	A B C D E F G	A B C D E F G
20. The sound of a fire engine siren close by is so loud that I need to cover my ears.	A B C D E F G	A B C D E F G
21. I can follow the words of a sermon when listening to a religious service.	A B C D E F G	A B C D E F G
22. The sound of screeching tires is uncomfortably loud.	A B C D E F G	A B C D E F G
23. I have to ask people to repeat themselves in one-on-one conversation in a quiet room.	A B C D E F G	A B C D E F G
24. I have trouble understanding others when an air conditioner or fan is on.	A B C D E F G	A B C D E F G

Page 2

APPENDIX B
The Hearing Handicap Inventory for the Elderly (HHIE)

INSTRUCTIONS: The purpose of this scale is to identify the problems your hearing loss may be causing you. Check YES, SOMETIMES, or NO for each question. Do not skip a question if you avoid a situation because of your hearing problem. If you use a hearing aid, please answer the way you hear without the aid.

Name: _____   Age: _____   Date: _____

	Yes (4)	Sometimes (2)	No (0)
S-1. Does a hearing problem cause you to use the phone less than you would like?			
E-2. Does a hearing problem cause you to feel embarrassed when meeting new people?			
S-3. Does a hearing problem cause you to avoid groups of people?			
E-4. Does a hearing problem make you irritable?			
E-5. Does a hearing problem cause you to feel frustrated when talking to members of your family?			
E-6. Does a hearing problem cause you difficulty when attending a party?			
E-7. Does a hearing problem cause you to feel "stupid" or "dumb"?			
S-8. Do you have difficulty hearing when someone speaks in a whisper?			
E-9. Do you feel handicapped by a hearing problem?			
S-10. Does a hearing problem cause you difficulty when visiting friends, relatives, or neighbors?			
S-11. Does a hearing problem cause you to attend religious services less often than you would like?			
E-12. Does a hearing problem cause you to be nervous?			
S-13. Does a hearing problem cause you to visit friends, relatives, or neighbors less often than you would like?			
E-14. Does a hearing problem cause you to have arguments with family members?			
S-15. Does a hearing problem cause you difficulty when listening to TV or radio?			
S-16. Does a hearing problem cause you to go shopping less often than you would like?			
E-17. Does any problem or difficulty with your hearing upset you at all?			
E-18. Does a hearing problem cause you to want to be by yourself?			
S-19. Does a hearing problem cause you to talk to family members less often than you would like?			
E-20. Do you feel that any difficulty with your hearing limits or hampers your personal or social life?			
S-21. Does a hearing problem cause you difficulty when in a restaurant with relatives or friends?			
E-22. Does a hearing problem cause you to feel depressed?			
S-23. Does a hearing problem cause you to listen to the TV or radio less often than you would like?			
E-24. Does a hearing problem cause you to feel uncomfortable when talking to friends?			
E-25. Does a hearing problem cause you to feel left out when you are with a group of people?			

IMPORTANT: Please go back over the questions to make sure you have not skipped any. Remember, do not skip a question if you avoid a situation because of your hearing impairment. Also, make sure that you answered the way you hear without a hearing aid.

For Clinician's Use Only:

Score:
0–16   = No handicap
17–42   = Mild to moderate handicap
More than 42 = Significant handicap

Total Score: _____

Subtotal E: _____

Subtotal S: _____

Source: Therapy Management Innovations, Inc., Alta Therapies, Healthcare Rehabilitation, 1994. Reprinted with written permission from Weinstein, B. (3/1/93).

APPENDIX C
Hearing Handicap Inventory for the Elderly-Screening version (HHIE-S)

INSTRUCTIONS: The purpose of this questionnaire is to identify the problems your hearing loss may be causing you. Answer YES, SOMETIMES, or NO for each question. To obtain a total score, add up the YES (4 points), SOMETIMES (2), and NO (0) responses. If the score is greater than 10 we recommend that you schedule a hearing test with a certified audiologist at a local hearing clinic.

Name: _____   Date of Screening: _____

	Yes (4)	Sometimes (2)	No (0)
E1. Does a hearing problem cause you to feel embarrassed when you meet new people?			
E2. Does a hearing problem cause you to feel frustrated when talking to members of your family?			
S1. Do you have difficulty hearing when someone speaks in a whisper?			
E3. Do you feel handicapped by a hearing problem?			
S2. Does a hearing problem cause you difficulty when visiting friends, relatives, or neighbors?			
S3. Does a hearing problem cause you to attend religious services less often than you would like?			
E4. Does a hearing problem cause you to have arguments with family members?			
S4. Does a hearing problem cause you difficulty when listening to TV or radio?			
E5. Do you feel that any difficulty with your hearing limits or hampers your personal or social life?			
S5. Does a hearing problem cause you difficulty when in a restaurant with relatives or friends?			

TOTAL SCORE: HHIE-S _____ — **If score is greater than 10, the individual should be referred to an audiologist**

Source: Modified from Ventry and Weinstein, 1983.

APPENDIX D
Hearing Handicap Inventory for the Elderly-Screening version for Spouses (HHIE-SP)

INSTRUCTIONS: The purpose of this questionnaire is to identify the problems the hearing loss may be causing your spouse. Answer YES, SOMETIMES, or NO for each question. To obtain a total score add up the YES (4 points), SOMETIMES (2), and NO (0) responses. If the score is greater than 10 we recommend that your spouse schedules a hearing test with a certified audiologist at a local hearing clinic.

Name: _____   Date: _____

Spouse's Name: _____

	Yes (4)	Sometimes (2)	No (0)
E1. Does a hearing problem cause your spouse to feel embarrassed when meeting new people?			
E2. Does a hearing problem cause your spouse to feel frustrated when talking to members of your family?			
S1. Does your spouse have difficulty hearing when someone speaks in a whisper?			
E3. Does your spouse feel handicapped by a hearing problem?			
S2. Does a hearing problem cause your spouse difficulty when visiting friends, relatives, or neighbors?			
S3. Does a hearing problem cause your spouse to attend religious services less often than he/she would like?			
E4. Does a hearing problem cause your spouse to have arguments with family members?			
S4. Does a hearing problem cause your spouse difficulty when listening to TV/radio?			
E5. Do you feel that any difficulty with hearing limits or hampers your spouse's personal or social life?			
S5. Does a hearing problem cause your spouse difficulty when in a restaurant with relatives or friends?			

TOTAL HHIE-S-SP-SCORE = _____   E = _____ S = _____

Source: Modified from Newman and Weinstein, 1988.

REFERENCES

ABRAHAMSON, J. (1995). Effective and relevant programming. In: P. Kricos & S. Lesner (Eds.). *Hearing Care for the Older Adult.* Boston: Butterworth-Heinemann.

ABRAHAMSON, J. (1997). Patient education and peer interaction facilitate hearing aid adjustment. *Supplement to Hearing Review,* 1:19–23.

ABRAMS, A., HNATH-CHISOLM, T., GUERREIRO, S., & RITTERMAN, S. (1992). The effects of intervention strategy on self perception of hearing handicap. *Ear and Hearing,* 13: 371–377.

BECK, L. (1996). Get a grip on managed care! *Audiology Today,* 8:26.

BERKOWITZ, A., & HOCHBERG, I. (1971). Self-assessment of hearing handicap in the aged. *Archives of Otolaryngology,* 93:25–28.

BESS, F., & HUMES, L. (1995). *Audiology, the Fundamentals,* 2d ed. Baltimore: Williams & Wilkins.

BESS, F., LICHTENSTEIN, M., & LOGAN, S. (1991). Making hearing impairment functionally relevant: linkages with hearing disability and handicap. *Acta Otolaryngol. Suppl.* (Stockholm), 476:226–231.

BESS, F., LICHTENSTEIN, M., LOGAN, S., BURGER, M., & NELSON, E. (1989). Hearing impairment as a determinant of function in the elderly. *Journal of the American Geriatrics Society,* 37:123–128.

BESS, F., LOGAN, S., & LICHTENSTEIN, M. (1990). Functional impact of hearing loss on the elderly. *ASHA Reports,* 19:144–149.

BICKNELL, J. (1984). The psychopathology of handicap. *Annual Progress in Child Psychiatry and Development,* 346–363. In: Van Hecke, M. (1994). Emotional responses to hearing loss. J. Clark & F. Martin (Eds.), *Effective Counseling in Audiology.* Englewood Cliffs, NJ: Prentice Hall.

BINNIE, C. (1991). New perspectives in audiological rehabilitation. In: G. Studebaker, F. Bess, & L. Beck (Eds.), *The Vanderbilt Hearing Aid Report II.* Parkton, MD: York Press.

BINNIE, C. (1994). The future of audiological rehabilitation: overview and forecast. In: J.P. Gagne & N. Tye-Murray (Eds.), Research in audiological rehabilitation: current trends and future directions. *Journal of the Academy of Rehabilitative Audiology, Monograph Supplement,* 27:13–25.

BINNIE, C., & HESSION, C. (1990). A four week communication skillbuilding program. *ADA Feedback,* Winter 1990: 37–41.

BRAMMER, L. (1982). The remediation process: psychologic and counseling aspects. In: J. Alpiner (Ed.), *Handbook of Adult Rehabilitative Audiology,* 2d ed. Baltimore: Williams & Wilkins.

BROOKS, D. (1989). The effects of attitude on benefit obtained from hearing aids. *British Journal of Audiology,* 23:3–11.

BRUMMEL-SMITH, K. (1990). Introduction. In: B. Kemp, K. Smith, & J. Ramsdell (Eds.), *Geriatric Rehabilitation.* Boston: College Hill.

COOPER, J., & GATES, G. (1991). Hearing in the elderly—the Framingham cohort, 1983–1985. Part II. Prevalence of central auditory processing disorders. *Ear and Hearing,* 12:304–312.

COX, R., & ALEXANDER, G. (1995). The Abbreviated Profile of Hearing Aid Benefit. *Ear and Hearing,* 16:176–186.

COX, R., GILMORE, C., & ALEXANDER, G. (1991). Comparison of two questionnaires for patient assessed hearing aid benefit. *Journal of the American Academy of Audiology,* 2:134–144.

DEMOREST, M., & ERDMAN, S. (1986). Scale composition and item analysis of the Communication Profile for the Hearing Impaired. *Journal of the Academy of Rehabilitative Audiology,* 29:515–535.

ERBER, N. (1988). *Communication Therapy for Hearing-impaired Adults.* Abbotsford, Australia: Clavis Publishing.

ERBER, N. & HEINE, C. (1996). Screening receptive communication of older adults in residential care. *American Journal of Audiology,* 5:38–46.

ERDMAN, S. (1993). Counseling hearing impaired adults. In: J. Alpiner & P. McCarthy (Eds.). *Rehabilitative Audiology: Children and Adults,* 2d ed. Baltimore: Williams & Wilkins.

ERDMAN, S. (1994). Self-assessment: from research focus to research tool. In J.P. Gagne & N. Tye-Murray (Eds.), Research in audiological rehabilitation: current trends and future directions. *Journal of the Academy of Rehabilitative Audiology, Monograph Supplement,* 27:67–90.

ERIKSON, E. (1950). *Childhood and Society.* New York: Norton.

FLEXER, C. (1991). Access to communication environments through assistive listening devices. *Hearsay,* 6:9–14.

GAGNE, J.P. (1994). Visual and audiovisual speech perception training: basic and applied research needs. In: J.P. Gagne & N. Tye-Murray (Eds.), Research in audiological rehabilitation: current trends and future directions. *Journal of the Academy of Rehabilitative Audiology, Monograph Supplement,* 27:133–159.

GARSTECKI, D. (1988). Speechreading with auditory cues. *Volta Review,* 90:161–177.

GARSTECKI, D., & ERLER, S. (1996). Use of the Communication Profile for the Hearing Impaired with mildly hearing impaired adults. *Journal of Speech and Hearing Research,* 39:28–42.

GILHOME-HERBST, K., & HUMPHREY, C. (1980). Hearing impairment and mental state in the elderly living at home. *British Medical Journal,* 281:903–905.

GLASS, L. (1990). Hearing impairment in geriatrics. In: B. Kemp, K. Brummel-Smith, & J. Ramsdell (Eds.), *Geriatric Rehabilitation.* Boston: College Hill.

GURLAND, B., KURIANSKY, J., SHARPE, L., SIMON, R., STILLER, P., & BIRKETT, P. (1978). The comprehensive assessment and referral evaluation (CARE)—rationale, development and reliability. *International Journal of Aging and Human Development,* 8:9–42.

HARTKE, R. (1991). Introduction. In: R. Hartke (Ed.), *Psychological Aspects of Geriatric Rehabilitation.* Gaithersburg, MD: Aspen.

HELFER, K. (1998). Auditory and auditory-visual recognition of clear and conversational speech by older adults. *Journal of the American Academy of Audiology,* 9:234–242.

HENOCH, M. (1991). Speech perception, hearing aid technology, and aural rehabilitation: future perspective. *Ear and Hearing, Supplement to 12,* 187S–191S.

HOLMES, A. (1995). Hearing aids and the older adult. In: P. Kricos & S. Lesner (Eds.), *Hearing Care for the Older Adult.* Boston: Butterworth-Heinemann.

HOUSTON, K., & MONTGOMERY, A. (1997). Auditory-visual integration: a practical approach. *Seminars in Hearing,* 18:141–151.

HYDE, M. & RIKO, K. (1994). A decision-analytic approach to audiological rehabilitation. In: J.P. Gagne & N. Tye-Murray (Eds.), Research in audiological rehabilitation: current trends and future directions. *Journal of the Academy of Rehabilitative Audiology, Monograph Supplement,* 27:337– 374.

JENSEMA, C., & LENNOX, D. (1994). Visual alerting and signalling devices. In: M. Ross (Ed.), *Communication Access for Persons with Hearing Loss.* Parkton, MD: York Press.

JERGER, J., CHMIEL, R., FLORIN, E., PIROZZOLO, F., & WILSON, N. (1996). Comparison of conventional amplification and an assistive listening device in elderly persons. *Ear and Hearing,* 17:490–503.

JERGER, J., OLIVER, T., & PIROZZOLO, F. (1990). Impact of central auditory processing disorder and cognitive deficit in the self-assessment of hearing handicap in the elderly. *Journal of the American Academy of Audiology,* 1:75–80.

KANE, R., OUSLANDER, J., & ABRASS, I. (1994). *Essentials of Clinical Geriatrics,* 2d ed. New York: McGraw-Hill.

KAPETYN, T. (1977). Satisfaction with fitted hearing aids II. An investigation in the influence of psycho-social factors. *Scandinavian Audiology,* 6:171–177.

KEMP, B. (1990a). The psychosocial context of geriatric rehabilitation. In: B. Kemp, K. Smith, & J. Ramsdell (Eds.), *Geriatric Rehabilitation.* Boston: College Hill.

KEMP, B. (1990b). Motivational dynamics in geriatric rehabilitation: toward a therapeutic model. In: B. Kemp, K. Smith, & J. Ramsdell (Eds.), *Geriatric Rehabilitation.* Boston: College Hill.

KIRKWOOD, D. (1999). Major survey documents negative impact of untread hearing loss on quality of life. *Hearing Journal,* 52:32–40.

KOTLER, P., & CLARK, R. (1987). *Marketing for Health Care Organizations.* Englewood Cliffs, NJ: Prentice Hall.

KRICOS, P., & HOLMES, A. (1996). Efficacy of audiologic rehabilitation for older adults. *Journal of the American Academy of Audiology,* 7:219–229.

KRICOS, P., LESNER, S., & SANDRIDGE, S. (1991). Expectations of older adults regarding the use of hearing aids. *Journal of the American Academy of Audiology,* 2:129–133.

LAMB, S., OWENS, E., & SHUBERT, E. (1983). The revised form of the Hearing Performance Inventory. *Ear and Hearing,* 4:152–159.

LOEBEL, J., & EISDORFER, C. (1984). Psychological and psychiatric factors in the rehabilitation of the elderly. In: T.F. Williams (Ed.), *Rehabilitation in the Aging.* New York: Raven Press.

MADELL, J., PFEFFER, E., ROSS, M., & CHELLAPPA, M. (1991). Hearing aid returns at a community hearing and speech agency. *Hearing Journal,* 44:18–23.

MASLOW, A. (1954). *Motivation and Personality.* New York: Harper & Row.

MCCARTHY, P. (1991). Clinical observations of self-report and global measures of hearing aid benefit. In: G. Studebaker, F. Bess, & L. Beck, (Eds.), *The Vanderbilt Hearing Aid Report II.* Parkton, MD: York Press.

MONTGOMERY, A. (1991). Aural rehabilitation—review and preview. In: G. Studebaker, F. Bess, & L. Beck (Eds.), *The Vanderbilt Hearing Aid Report II.* Maryland: York Press.

MONTGOMERY, A. (1993). Management of the hearing-impaired elderly. In: J. Alpiner and P. Mcarthy (Eds.), *Rehabilitative Audiology: Children and Adults.* Baltimore: Williams & Wilkins.

MONTGOMERY, A. (1994).Treatment efficacy in adult audiological rehabilitation. In: J.P. Gagne & N.Tye-Murray (Eds.), Research in audiological rehabilitation: current trends and future directions. *Journal of the Academy of Rehabilitative Audiology, Monograph Supplement,* 27:317–336.

MULROW, C., AGUILAR, C., ENDICOTT, J., TULEY, M. (1990). Quality of life changes and hearing impairment: results of a randomized trial. *Annals of Internal Medicine,* 113:188–194.

MULROW, C., AGUILAR, C., ENDICOTT, J., VELEZ, R. (1990). Association between hearing impairment and the quality of life of elderly individuals. *Journal of the American Geriatrics Society,* 38:45–50.

NEWMAN, C., JACOBSON, G., HUG, G., WEINSTEIN, B., & MALINOFF, R. (1991). A practical method for quantifying hearing aid benefit in older adults. *Journal of the American Academy of Audiology,* 2:70–75.

NEWMAN, C., & WEINSTEIN, B. (1988). The hearing handicap inventory for the elderly as a measure of hearing aid benefit. *Ear and Hearing,* 9:81–85.

PALMER, C., & MORMER, E. (1997). A systematic program for hearing instrument orientation and adjustment. *Supplement to Hearing Review,* 1:45–53.

PFEIFFER, E. (1975). A short portable mental status questionnaire for the assessment of organic brain deficit in elderly patients. *Journal of the American Geriatric Society,* 23:433–441.

PICHORA-FULLER, M. (1997). Assistive devices for the elderly. In: R. Lubinski, & D. Higginbotham (Eds.), *Communication Technologies for the Elderly: Vision, Hearing and Speech.* San Diego: Singular Publishing Group.

PRIMEAU, R. (1997). Hearing aid benefit in adults and older adults. *Seminars in Hearing,* 18:29–37.

RAMSDELL, D. (1960). The psychology of the hard of hearing and deafened adult. In: H. Davis and S. Silverman (Eds.), *Hearing and Deafness.* New York: Holt, Rinehart, and Silverman.

RENTZ, D. (1991). The assessment of rehabilitation potential: cognitive factors. In: R. Hartke (Ed.), *Psychological Aspects of Geriatric Rehabilitation.* Gaithersburg, MD: Aspen.

ROSS, M. (1994). Beyond hearing aids: assistance technologies. *Seminars in Hearing,* 18:103–116.

ROSS, M. (1995). Developments in research and technology. *SHHH,* 16:2, 32–34.

ROSS, M. (1996). You've done something about it! Helpful hints to the new hearing aid user. *SHHH Journal,* 17:7–11.

ROSS, M., & LEVITT, H. (1997). Consumer satisfaction is not enough: hearing aids are still about hearing. *Seminars in Hearing,* 18:7–11.

ROTH, E. (1991). The aging process: physiological changes. In: R. Hartke (Ed.), *Psychological Aspects of Geriatric Rehabilitation.* Gaithersburg, MD: Aspen.

SANDRIDGE, S. (1995). Beyond hearing aids: use of auxiliary aids. In: P. Kricos & S. Lesner (Eds.), *Hearing Care for the Older Adult.* Boston: Butterworth-Heinemann.

SCHOW, R., BALSARA, N., SMEDLEY, T., & WHITCOMB, C. (1993). *American Journal of Audiology,* 2:28–38.

SCHOW, R., & NERBONNE, M. (1982). Communication screening profile uses with elderly clients. *Ear and Hearing,* 3:133–147.

SCHUM, D. (1994). Personal adjustment counseling. In: J.P. Gagne & N. Tye-Murray (Eds.), Research in audiological rehabilitation: current trends and future directions. *Journal of the Academy of Rehabilitative Audiology, Monograph Supplement,* 27:223–236.

SCHUM, D. (1997). Evaluation of hearing aid benefit using the shortened hearing aid performance inventory. *Journal of the American Academy of Audiology,* 8:18–26.

SELF HELP FOR HARD OF HEARING PEOPLE, INC. (1996). Position statement on group hearing aid orientation programs. *SHHH Journal,* 17:29.

SORKIN, D. (1997). Consumer and hearing aids: the SHHH perspective. *Seminars in Hearing,* 18:49–56.

STEINFELD, E. (1997). Architecture as a communication medium. In: R. Lubinski & D. Higginbotham (Eds.), *Communication Technologies for the Elderly: Vision, Hearing, and Speech.* San Diego: Singular Publishing Group.

STONE, H. (1990). Hearing health care in the 1990s. *Audiology Today,* July–August: 14–17.

STYPULKOWSKI, P. (1997). Realistic expectations: a key to success. *Supplement to Hearing Review,* 1:56–57.

SWAN, I., & GATEHOUSE, S. (1990). Factors influencing consultation for management of hearing disability. *British Journal of Audiology,* 24:155–160.

TAYLOR, K., & JURMA, W. (1999). Study suggests that group rehabilitation increases benefit of hearing aid fittings. *Hearing Journal,* 52:48–54.

TREZONA, R. (1991). The assessment of rehabilitation potential: emotional factors. In: R. Hartke (Ed.), *Psychological Aspects of Geriatric Rehabilitation.* Gaithersburg, MD: Aspen.

TRYCHIN, S. (1995). Counseling older adults with hearing impairments. In: P. Kricos & S. Lesner (Eds.), *Hearing Care for the Older Adult.* Boston: Butterworth-Heinemann.

TRYCHIN, S. (1997). Coping with hearing loss. *Seminars in Hearing,* 18:77–86.

TYE-MURRAY, N. (1998). *Foundations of Aural Rehabilitation.* San Diego: Singular Publishing Group.

TYE-MURRAY, N., & WITT, S. (1997). Communication strategies training. *Seminars in Hearing,* 18:153–165.

UHLMANN, R., LARSON, E., REES, T., KOEPSELL, T., & DUCKERT, L. (1989). Relationship of hearing impairment to dementia and cognitive dysfunction in older adults. *JAMA,* 261:1916–1919.

VAN HECKE, M. (1994). Emotional responses to hearing loss. In: J. Clark & F. Martin (Eds.), *Effective Counseling in Audiology.* Englewood Cliffs, NJ: Prentice Hall.

VENTRY, I., & WEINSTEIN, B. (1982). The Hearing Handicap Inventory for the Elderly: a new tool. *Ear and Hearing,* 3:128–134.

———. (1983). Identification of elderly people with hearing problems. *American Speech-Language-Hearing Association,* 25:37–42.

WALDEN, B., & GRANT, K. (1993). Research needs in rehabilitative audiology. In: J. Alpiner & P. McCarthy (Eds.), *Rehabilitative Audiology: Children and Adults.* Baltimore: Williams & Wilkins.

WALDEN, B., DEMOREST, M., & HEPLER, E. (1984). Self-report approach to assessing benefit derived from amplification. *Journal of Speech and Hearing Research,* 9:91–109.

WEINSTEIN, B. (1980). Hearing impairment and social isolation in the elderly. Ph.D. diss. New York: Columbia University.

WEINSTEIN, B. (1991). Hearing aids and the elderly: audiologic and psychologic considerations. In: Studebaker, G., Bess, F., & Beck, L. (Eds.), *The Vanderbilt Hearing Aid Report II.* Parkton, MD: York Press.

WEINSTEIN, B. (1996). Treatment efficacy: hearing aids in the management of hearing loss in adults. *Journal of Speech and Hearing Research,* 39:535–543.

WEINSTEIN, B., & AMSEL, L. (1986). Hearing loss and senile dementia in the institutionalized elderly. *Clinical Gerontologist,* 4:3–15.

WEINSTEIN, B., & VENTRY, I. (1983). Audiometric correlates of the Hearing Handicap Inventory for the Elderly. *Journal of Speech and Hearing Disorders,* 48:379–384.

Chapter 9

Hearing Aids and Assistive Listening Devices

Now that my listening problems have finally been solved with my binaural programmable hearing aids, can you help me out with my laptop computer? . . . Then my troubles will be over.

—M.F., 74-year-old musician and retired teacher

It seems to me that my audiologist does the best he can with the knowledge of hearing aids available to him . . . but I have the feeling he knows just how to make his services as financially lucrative to himself as possible with the customer playing second fiddle.

—C.W., 79-year-old woman

There is so much going on in my body that I can't control. It feels good to actually do something positive about one of my problems.

—Tye-Murray, 1998

LEARNING OBJECTIVES

After reading this chapter, you should be able to:

- Understand the nonaudiologic factors that impact on hearing-aid use among older adults.
- Identify the audiologic considerations essential to a successful hearing-aid fitting.
- Detail the beneficial communicative and psychosocial effects of hearing-aid use on the daily life of older adults.
- Recommend the appropriate assistive-listening devices to resolve the needs of older adults with handicapping hearing impairment.

Hearing aids are the intervention of choice for older adults with hearing impairments that are both disabling and handicapping. Recent advances in hearing-aid technology have improved the effectiveness of hearing-aid fittings in individuals with sensorineural hearing loss. The future holds even greater promise with the advent of digital hearing instruments that offer superior performance as compared

with the conventional analog technology. In fact, satisfaction with high performance hearing aids is high at 71%, as compared with 53% for overall customer satisfaction (Kochkin, 1997). Long-term overall satisfaction with hearing aids is critical if audiologists are going to reach those older adults who are potential candidates. For an increasing number of older adults, hearing aids must be supplemented with assistive listening devices (ALDs) if listening needs are truly to be met and end-user satisfaction achieved.

This chapter is organized to develop within the reader an understanding of the impact of the aging process on decisions to be made at each step of the hearing-aid fitting process. The chapter begins with a discussion of the demographics of hearing-aid use and proceeds to a discussion of the impact of aging on aspects of the selection process. A brief overview of current hearing-aid technologies and fitting strategies for use with older adults is offered. The chapter then moves to a comprehensive review of data on the efficacy of hearing aids with older adults and a model for delivering hearing-aid services to older adults. ALDs are discussed in brief as a reminder to the audiologists of the many communication voids to be filled by available auditory technologies. The above organization grows out of the author's belief that texts on hearing aids provide for an understanding of the technological aspects of hearing instruments. The goal of this chapter is to enable the reader to apply information specific to older adults to their working knowledge of hearing aids and assistive listening devices.

DEMOGRAPHY OF HEARING-AID USE

Of the 27 million persons who have hearing difficulty, fewer than 21% use hearing instruments, representing a gap of about 22 million people (Kochkin, 1999). Despite low utilization of hearing aids, there was a significant growth in hearing instrument sales in 1998 with 77% of dispensers reporting a 16% growth in their sales (Skafte, 1999). The year-end Hearing Industries Association (HIA) statistical report for 1998 showed that hearing-aid sales exceeded 1.8 million units sold (Strom, 1999). Hearing-aid penetration varies as a function of age. In 1998, 3% of hearing-aid users were

209

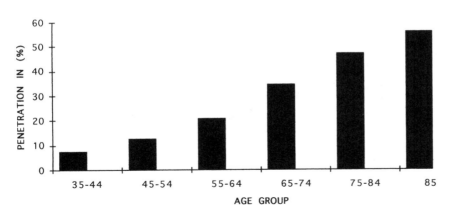

Figure 9–1 Hearing-aid penetration as a function of age. (From Kochkin, 1992.)

between 18 and 29 years and 68% were over 65 years of age (Skafte, 1998). The fact that in 1980 only 48.7% of hearing-aid customers were over 65 years of age suggests that there is an aging client base in the hearing-aid industry (Skafte, 1998). It is noteworthy that in 1998 about 13% of hearing aid users were between 40 and 65, a significant decline since 1980 (Skafte, 1999). Interestingly, as is shown in Figure 9–1 among adults, hearing-aid penetration is greatest among persons over 85 years of age. The percentage of consumers over 65 years seeking hearing health care increased by 8% over the number in 1997 (Skafte, 1999; Strom, 1999).

SPECIAL CONSIDERATION

Hearing-instrument penetration is consistently highest among the old-old and lowest among persons 55 to 64 years (Table 9–1).

As hearing loss severity increases with age, this finding is not surprising.

PEARL

It is of interest that hearing-instrument ownership is highly related to age, even when degree of hearing loss is considered.

TABLE 9–1   Hearing Instrument Penetration in Percent by Age Group: 1984–1992

Age group	1984	1989	1990	1992
55–64 years	22.4	16.3	20.1	20.9
65–74 years	34.0	32.7	31.9	34.4
75–84 years	45.6	45.0	45.7	47.1
85+ years	58.6	51.9	57.8	56.1

Source: Kochkin, 1992.

That is, older adults with severe self-reported hearing loss are more likely to purchase hearing instruments than younger adults with severe self-reported hearing loss. Similarly, older adults with mild self-reported hearing loss are more likely to purchase hearing aids than younger adults with comparable loss (Kochkin, 1992). It is of interest that the average age of new hearing-aid users has not changed over the past few years. In 1989 the average age of new hearing-aid users was 66 years, in 1990 it was 62.9 years, and in 1991 it was 68 years. Geographically, the states selling the largest absolute number of units were California, Florida, New York, and Pennsylvania (Kirkwood, 1998). Arkansas, North Dakota, and Nevada experienced sales gains of 10% over the previous year (Strom, 1999).

According to Kochkin (1995a), the typical hearing-aid owner in the United States who purchased hearing aids in 1993 or 1994 was 68 years of age, had bilateral hearing loss, and wore binaural hearing aids. The primary reason for purchasing hearing aids is the perception that hearing loss has worsened, or the influence of family members, primarily a spouse (Skafte, 1998; Kochkin, 1998). Most hearing aid users are self-referred (Skafte, 1999). It is of interest that 60% of hearing-instrument owners were retired, whereas 51% of owners reportedly have full-time employment (Kochkin, 1992). Further, the majority of hearing-aid owners perceive themselves as having a moderate or severe self-reported hearing loss (Skafte, 1999). One other distinguishing factor between owners and nonowners is that 35% of owners were between 65 and 74 years versus 19% of nonowners. Similarly, 25% of owners were between 75 and 84 years as compared to 8% of nonowners (Kochkin, 1992). Despite the apparent age-related dependence of hearing-aid use, the majority of older adults with hearing loss do not use hearing instruments. According to a variety of surveys, it appears

PEARL

The majority of hearing instrument users are older. The majority of older adults do not use hearing instruments.

that only 18 to 20% of older adults with hearing loss use hearing aids. According to the MarkeTrak III survey of 6000 owners and nonowners, the majority of respondents cited stigma associated with hearing-aid use as the most important reason for not purchasing a hearing instrument (Kochkin, 1992). Interestingly, stigma was more of a deterrent for adults between 35 and 54 years of age than for adults over 55 years of age. Additional deterrents of hearing aid use include the feeling that hearing aids are too noisy, whistle, are limited, break down too much, and cannot be used on the telephone (Kochkin, 1997).

Characteristics of Hearing-aid Owners:

- 48% are first-time users
- 82% bilateral hearing loss
- 59% male
- 65% binaural users
- 15% behind-the-ear (BTE), 41% in-the-ear (ITE), 44% in-the-canal (ITC) users
- 76% had difficulty conversing in noise
- 54% had a moderate loss

As noted above, the major reason persons offer for not purchasing hearing instruments is the stigma associated with use of a "prosthetic device." The following factors have also been isolated as deterrents to hearing-aid use: (1) wearing a hearing aid represents public admission of a hearing loss, (2) hearing aids make people look old, (3) hearing aids make people look disabled, and (4) hearing aids would be embarrassing to wear (Kochkin, 1994). Fino, Bess, Lichtenstein, and Logan (1991) confirmed that hearing-impaired elderly who elected not to pursue amplification believed that they were too conspicuous, too expensive, too noisy, and called attention to one's hearing handicap. It appears that the "stigma effect" is consistent for adults under 65 years such that 47% of persons between 45 and 54 years and 43% of persons between 55 and 64 years reported it as the reason for not purchasing a hearing instrument (Kochkin, 1994). Kochkin (1994) reported that among hearing-instru-

ment owners, 83% of persons younger than 18 versus 13% of persons between 75 and 84 years remain stigmatized by the hearing aid. The fact that the "stigma effect" decreases once older adults begin to use and benefit from hearing aids should be emphasized when counseling resistant older adults regarding the value of hearing aids.

According to a recent series of surveys, the majority of older adults purchase hearing aids from a hearing-instrument specialist rather than a dispensing audiologist (Strom, 1996a; Skafte, 1998). Figure 9–2 shows the breakdown of customers purchasing hearing aids by dispensing practice. It appears that in 1996, 70% of persons 65+ who purchased hearing instruments utilized the services of a hearing instrument specialist whereas 64% obtained their instruments from dispensing audiologists. In contrast, 5% of persons under 18 purchased their instruments from a dispensing audiologist whereas 1% purchased their instruments from a hearing-instrument specialist. Interestingly, the 1998 Hearing Review Survey of Hearing Instrument Dispensers revealed that 61% of persons seeking the services of dispensing audiologists were over 65 years suggesting a slight change from 1996 (Skafte, 1999).

Interestingly, the overall return rate and the return rate for each style hearing aid was relatively comparable for hearing-instrument specialists versus dispensing audiologists. For example, the return rate in 1998 was 8% for dispensing audiologists and 7% for hearing-instrument specialists. Return rates for completely-in-the-canal hearing aids were 10% for dispensing audiologists and 10% for digital signal processing (DSP) hearing instruments (Skafte, 1999). The overall return rate for all hearing aids sold in the United States in 1998 was 18.7%, which is

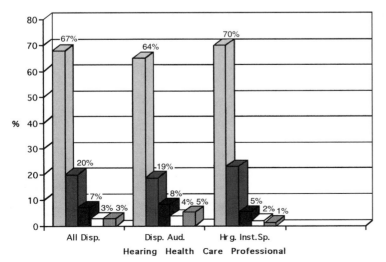
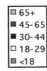

Figure 9–2 Percentage of customers by age, seen by various hearing health care professionals. (Modified from Skafte, 1998.)

slightly higher than the return for credit rate in 1997 (18%) (Strom, 1999).

The fact that hearing-instrument specialists serve the majority of older adults may in part be due to the fact that Florida, the state having the highest proportion of older adults, has a huge share of the hearing-aid market, and perhaps a shortage of certified audiologists. A recent survey of over 2000 hearing-instrument owners revealed that 65% were satisfied and felt that the hearing instrument actually improved their lives (Kochkin, 1992). Eight out of 10 owners indicated that they would recommend a hearing aid to a friend. Consumers were highly satisfied with the ability of hearing instruments to improve hearing in one-on-one situations and while watching TV. However, satisfaction ratings decline in complex or noisy listening environments such as large-group settings and restaurants (Kochkin, 1992). Further, satisfaction is greatest for new hearing aids, declining dramatically as the hearing aid "ages" (Kochkin, 1995a). The latter tendency underlines the importance of long-term follow-up of hearing-aid users. Finally, the data from the National Council on Aging Survey (NCOA) suggest that hearing-aid users are less depressed and more socially engaged than are older adults with comparable hearing loss who do not use hearing aids.

THE HEARING-AID SELECTION AND FITTING PROCESS

The hearing-instrument selection and fitting process should be seen in the context of a comprehensive audiological rehabilitation program. In this context, the responsibility of audiologists involved in audiological rehabilitation is to facilitate the reduction in communication disability and psychosocial handicap associated with a given hearing impairment via an acceptable intervention, such as hearing aids. As is shown in Figure 9–3, the first step in the selection/fitting process is the prefitting,

which entails administering measures that the audiologist uses to describe (audiometrically) and select a hearing-aid candidate. With regard to the former, every attempt should be made to describe the nature of the auditory impairment and its consequences, namely the disability and the handicap. This will serve as the basis for identifying individuals who are likely to use and benefit from hearing-aid technology. It will also help to establish a pretreatment performance baseline against which the outcome of the intervention can be judged. In this era of managed care, the outcome of a treatment relative to baseline will ultimately serve as the green light for third-party payment. An accurate earmold impression is an important part of the prefitting and selection process.

After identifying the candidate for a hearing aid and documenting the person's audiologic profile and communicative needs, the next step is the hearing-aid selection. The purpose of the selection is to identify the most appropriate hearing-aid style and/or type of technology, and to determine the electroacoustic characteristics most likely to optimize performance. Following the selection process, the patient/consumer returns for the hearing-aid fitting, which has as its goal verification that the electroacoustic response of the hearing aid meets the targets chosen during the selection. Above all, the goals must be realistic, patient driven, and adequately reinforced upon completion of each phase of

---

PEARL

At the hearing-aid fitting, baseline information about the disability and handicap, obtained during the audiological evaluation or the prefitting, should be used to establish a set of rehabilitation goals and protocols to be used to achieve a reduction in the problems confronting the hearing-impaired individual.

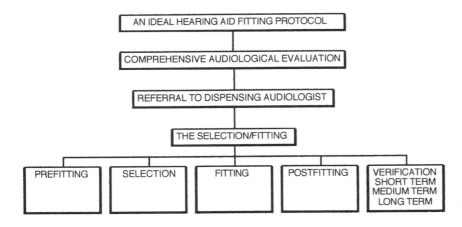

Figure 9–3 The steps included in the selection/fitting process.

the intervention. Following the fitting, a period of accommodation should take place, followed within 3 to 6 weeks by a postfitting session designed to verify the response and to quantify the satisfaction and benefit derived from the hearing aid. If postfitting data suggest that the individual is not deriving adequate benefit, then the response of the hearing aid can be modified and an interval of counseling-oriented rehabilitation instituted. The latter tends to increase the ranks of satisfied hearing-aid users. Of course, if the hearing-impaired consumer continues to be dissatisfied with the recommended unit, a new earmold impression might be taken, a different hearing aid selected, and use of ALDs explored. At this time, the value of ALDs to supplement or complement hearing aids should be discussed with the consumer. The verification phase should continue over 1 year with periodic visits to verify short-term, medium-term, and long-term

benefits. Table 9–2 provides a summary of some of the procedures used during each stage of the selection, fitting and postfitting. Each phase that has special relevance to the older adult is described in the following paragraphs in some detail beginning with the preselection and concluding with the postfitting and verification phase.

PRESELECTION MEASUREMENT

A number of issues must be considered in the preselection process to assure an optimal and successful hearing-aid fitting. Above all, the audiologist should weigh the consumer's expressed needs as they pertain to hearing-aid use. Further, the older adult should be approached from a functional perspective. That is, the hearing impairment

TABLE 9–2 The Hearing-Aid Fitting Process

Components	Steps in the process
1. Preselection or Prefitting: Who is a candidate?	a. quantify impairment, disability, handicap, and listening needs b. screen mental status c. administer tests of peripheral and central auditory processing ability
2. Selection: Determination of electro-acoustic characteristics.	a. selection of the category of instrument, style of instrument, and arrangement using protocols for selecting linear and nonlinear systems b. selection of saturation sound pressure levels using suprathreshold measures of loudness and/or loudness growth measures c. selection of special circuit options
3. Fitting: Setting and verification of real-ear gain frequency-response characteristics and SSPL-90.	a. functional gain b. real-ear measures c. speech-recognition measures d. loudness growth measures e. visual input/output locator algorithm (VIOLA), etc. f. hearing-aid orientation/counseling; realistic expectations
4. Postfitting, performance assessment, or validation.	a. speech-recognition tests b. speech-intelligibility ratings c. judgments of sound quality d. self-report measures e. consider ALD(s) f. modify existing unit(s), change device; additional counseling regarding strategies; AVI training
5. Verification and follow-up after a period of accommodation.	a. outcomes assessment b. counseling c. hearing-aid modifications

Source: Modified from Studebaker, Bess, and Beck, 1991.

TABLE 9–3 Domains of Function to Consider when Selecting Hearing-Aid Candidates

Auditory	Physical	Psychological	Sociological	Environmental
Impairment	Manual dexterity	Motivation	Lifestyle	Safety needs
Disability	Physical health	Cognitive	Familial-support	
Handicap	Visual status	Personality	Financial factors	

should be viewed in the context of the individual's social, psychological, and environmental context. Consideration of five interrelated domains of function will assure that the person with a hearing loss is approached from a functional perspective. These include auditory status, physical status, and sociological, psychological, and environmental status. These factors, which are listed in Table 9–3, are discussed in the following paragraphs as they relate specifically to the elderly.

AUDITORY FACTORS

Audiologic rehabilitation with hearing aids should assist disabled or handicapped individuals to overcome or cope with a measurable hearing impairment. The World Health Organization (WHO) disease response model provides a basis for understanding how various components of disease or disorders inter-relate and serve as a basis for determining hearing-aid candidacy (WHO, 1980). It provides a systems approach to understanding how a pathology at the organ level (i.e., hearing impairment) generates a disability at the personal level that ultimately produces a handicap at the societal level. Each of these domains of function has different descriptors requiring quantification and consideration during the initial phase of the hearing-aid selection.

Impairment or the measurable loss of hearing function is described according to the audiogram that details the extent of hearing loss for pure-tone and speech signals. The problems that result from a hearing impairment, namely the client's predicament, can be described in terms of its disabling or handicapping effects. Disability is the effect of impairment on an individual's auditory functioning in daily life. The severity of the disability is conceived of in terms of the extent of auditory difficulties experienced by the listener and is influenced in part by the auditory demands of a given situation, as well as one's auditory capacity (Hyde & Riko, 1994). It can most validly be measured by self-report of the perception of communication abilities in a variety of daily listening situations. The Abbreviated Profile of Hearing Aid Benefit (APHAB) is a 24-item questionnaire that queries the respondent about the percentage of time that problems hearing in a variety of listening situations are experienced. It can help elicit information about the extent of hearing disability prior to and following a period of hearing-aid use. The Hearing Aid Needs Assessment (HANA) or the Client Oriented Scale of Improvement (COSI) may have potential

as personalized inventories of needs relative to the hearing loss and hearing aids (Dillon & Ginis, 1997; Gatehouse, 1999).

In contrast to disability, handicap represents the social and emotional manifestations of impairment and disability. Handicap represents the nonauditory problems resulting from diminished auditory capacity and the auditory demands of real-life situations (Hyde & Riko, 1994). A given handicap affects the client with the condition, the family/caregiver, and, oftentimes, society. Handicap is typically measured by self-report of the perception of the psychosocial impact of the impairment and disability on everyday function in a variety of situations. Increasingly, audiologists are considering the caregiver or spouse's perception of the handicapping effects of hearing impairment, as well. The Hearing Handicap Inventory for the Elderly (HHIE) and its companion version for spouses (HHIE-SP) are questionnaires that yield information about the emotional and social consequences of hearing loss. Handicap measures can be helpful in deciding on candidacy for a hearing aid, in counseling the candidate and family members regarding realistic expectations from hearing-aid use, and the score serves as a baseline against which to judge outcomes with hearing aids.

The impairment variable that figures most prominently into candidacy is performance on behavioral measures that yield information about the extent and quality of the hearing impairment. Among the impairment measures are pure-tone air and bone-conduction thresholds, loudness judgments, and peripheral and central auditory processing ability. The contribution of data about the hearing impairment to the hearing-aid selection and fitting process is shown in the following list.

Impairment measures in the hearing-aid selection and fitting process:

- Help establish need for medical intervention prior to the hearing-aid fitting
- Help to set realistic expectations regarding auditory and nonauditory benefits of hearing aids
- Help establish and verify electroacoustic characteristics of hearing aids including gain, frequency response, saturation sound pressure level (SSPL-90), etc.
- Assist in decisions regarding hearing-aid style (completely-in-the-canal [CIC] versus in-the-ear [ITE]) and type (analog, programmable, digital)

- Assist in selecting the appropriate hearing-aid arrangement (Binaural, contralateral routing of signal [CROS])
- Help the audiologist decide on the ear to fit (better or poorer)
- Help to verify the hearing-aid fit during the postfitting

To begin with, impairment measures help to determine whether a medical therapy is indicated, that is, does the older adult present with a condition or pathology that can be remediated via medical or surgical intervention? The presence of impacted cerumen is the most likely condition requiring immediate attention. In most cases cerumen management falls within the purview of audiologists. However, I would refer older adults vulnerable to infection, especially those suffering from diabetes and recurrent cancer. If medical contraindication to hearing-aid use presents, referral to a physician, and medical clearance, are necessary steps prior to the selection and fitting.

In the absence of a medically treatable condition, the audiologist next considers the severity of hearing impairment, auditory response area, the hearing configuration, symmetry, and type of hearing loss, or presence of a central auditory processing problem. These variables are not the primary determinants of candidacy for hearing aids, rather they influence decisions regarding the hearing aid style, configuration, arrangement, type, and electroacoustic response. Further, they may determine the benefits to be derived from amplification and can be used to set realistic expectations from hearing use. For example, configuration of hearing loss will influence decisions regarding electroacoustic characteristics of the hearing aid. Symmetry of hearing loss may figure into the decision regarding the arrangement (e.g., monaural or a binaural fitting) rather than about candidacy. Auditory response area and level of impairment may influence the auditory benefits to be derived from hearing aids and can help the audiologist to explain what patients can and cannot expect from hearing aids. Newman, Jacobson, Hug, Weinstein,

SPECIAL CONSIDERATION

Level of hearing impairment does not appear to influence benefit in the handicap domain.

and Malinoff (1991) reported that in their sample of older adults, severity of hearing loss did not appear to influence benefit in the psychosocial domain. Specifically, persons with mild hearing loss derived the same amount of benefit from hearing aids as did individuals with severe hearing impairment. Benefit in their sample was defined according to magnitude of reduction in self-perceived hearing handicap following a short interval of hearing-aid use. Further, according to correlational analyses, hearing-aid benefit (difference between aided and unaided self-assessed psychosocial handicap) bears little relation to pure-tone hearing levels (Taylor, 1993). That is, pure-tone average (PTA) accounted for only a small proportion of the variability in psychosocial benefit.

As the speech-understanding problems experienced by older adults may be central in origin, and the presence of a central auditory deficit compromises benefit from hearing aids, part of the candidate selection process should include a speech test capable of identifying individuals with potential central auditory processing disorders (CAPD). Given the higher prevalence of central auditory processing problems among older adults, I would recommend that all hearing-aid candidates be screened for the presence of CAPD as well as those older adults who currently find their hearing aids ineffective. The ideal central auditory test for screening hearing-aid candidates has not been identified but one that is quick and easy to administer, and free of the confounding effects of mild to moderate peripheral hearing loss makes sense (Musiek & Baran, 1996).

While, the magnitude of benefit cannot be predicted from the severity of hearing loss, the latter may contribute to our understanding of the nature or quality of benefit. For example, restoration of the ability to hear warning signals and environmental sounds is the primary benefit for older adults with profound hearing loss. In contrast, enhanced speech understanding in quiet and noise might be the advantage for persons with mild to moderately severe hearing loss. Similarly, in the case of a high-frequency hearing loss, a hearing aid is expected to restore the audibility cues inherent in high-frequency consonant sounds. For persons with a bilaterally symmetric hearing loss, binaural hearing aids will provide for balanced hearing, improved localization ability, ease of listening, etc. Persons with central auditory processing problems may be expected to experience extreme difficulty understanding in less than optimal conditions as well as on the telephone.

PEARL

When counseling potential hearing-aid users, impairment data should be used to help set realistic expectations.

Hearing and speech measures are critical in decisions regarding hearing-aid candidacy for that segment of the elderly population with postlingual profound hearing loss who are not eligible for conventional amplification because of a limited auditory response area. These individuals should be counseled against hearing aids but should be made aware of data suggesting that prognosis for use of implants in the older adult population with bilateral severe to profound sensorineural hearing loss is impressive. Waltzman, Cohen, and Shapiro (1993) reported that the majority of older adults in their sample (N=20) achieved improved word and sentence recognition with their multichannel cochlear implant. Further, the implant was a significantly better aid to lipreading than conventional amplification.

Swan and Gatehouse (1990) investigated factors that prompt individuals to seek audiological services. They noted that hearing-impaired individuals pursue hearing health care services because of self-perceived hearing disabilities and handicaps that oftentimes do not correspond to the degree of their hearing impairment. That is, most purchasers of hearing instruments are self-motivated because of communication problems (McCarthy, Montgomery, &

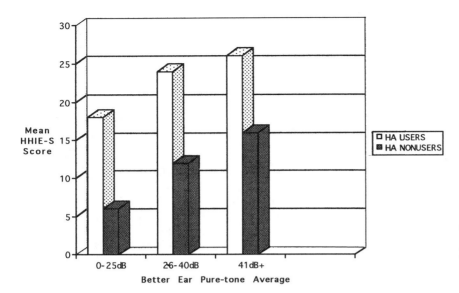

Figure 9–4 HHIE-S scores as a function of hearing loss severity in hearing-aid users and nonusers. (Modified from Fino, Bess, and Lichtenstein, 1991.)

Mueller, 1990). Data are beginning to emerge supporting these conclusions. Fino et al (1991) were among the first investigators to demonstrate that hearing-aid candidacy is directly linked to the prefitting score on a measure of self-perceived handicap, most notably the HHIE. Specifically, they found that the extent of self-perceived hearing handicap on the 10-item screening version of the Hearing Handicap Inventory for the Elderly (HHIE-S) is predictive of hearing-aid candidacy, in that it reliably distinguishes between hearing-aid users and nonusers. At each hearing level category (e.g., mild, moderate, and moderately severe) persons who obtained hearing aids were more handicapped than those who did not. That is, of those with mild hearing loss, persons who obtained higher scores on the HHIE-S, indicative of greater self-perceived handicap, ultimately purchased a hearing aid (Figure 9–4).

Newman et al (1991) reported a link between handicap scores and hearing-aid use. They found that the average prefitting score on the HHIE-S was approximately 18, irrespective of mean hearing level and mean word-recognition scores. Persons with mild and moderately severe hearing levels presented with comparable scores on the HHIE-S (i.e., 18). Similarly, persons with excellent and those with poor scores on a test of word recognition emerged with mean prefitting HHIE-S scores ranging from 16 to 18. Figures 9–5 and 9–6 demonstrate the comparability of pre-fitting HHIE-S scores, irrespective of the severity of hearing loss or severity of speech-understanding problems. It is clear from the data of Newman and his colleagues and Fino and her colleagues that degree of self-perceived hearing handicap is related to hearing-aid candidacy and uptake. Despite the emergence of data supporting the potential of self-assess-

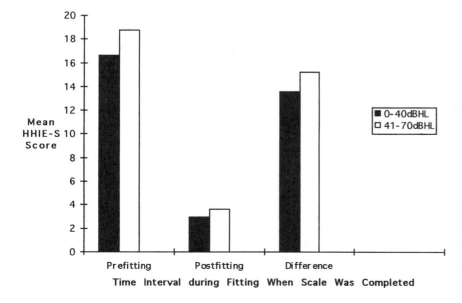

Figure 9–5 Mean pre- and postfitting HHIE-S scores on a sample of hearing-aid users with varying degrees of hearing loss (N = 91). Note: postfitting took place 3 weeks after fitting. (Modified from Newman et al, 1991.)

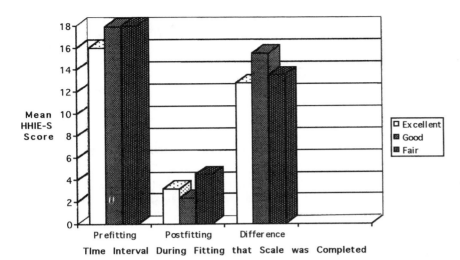

Figure 9–6 Mean pre- and postfitting HHIE-S scores on a sample of hearing-aid users as a function of word-recognition (*N* = 91). Note: postfitting was 3 weeks following the fitting. (From Newman et al, 1991.)

ment scales during the early stages of the rehabilitation process, most audiologists do not use formalized self-assessment inventories (Kirkwood, 1997; Schow, Balsara, Smedley, & Whitcomb, 1993). As psychosocial factors explored through self-report scales influence candidacy, rehabilitation programming, and benefit, especially with older adults, audiologists are encouraged to experiment with the large variety of tools available to the clinician (Cox, 1999).

SPECIAL CONSIDERATION

Available data suggest that self-reported handicap is predictive of hearing-aid benefit, yet most audiologists do not measure perceived handicap.

PHYSICAL FACTORS
Visual Status

The primary physical variables that may influence hearing-aid candidacy include visual status, manual dexterity, ear/ear canal variables, and overall health status. In general, the high prevalence of visual problems in older adults is an important factor in favor of pursuing amplification in the form of hearing aids, ALDs, or a cochlear implant.

PEARL

Loss of one sense heightens the importance of other senses to insure an individual's safety and independence. Severity and nature of the visual problem should influence the hearing-aid arrangement, hearing-aid style, and type of signal processing.

Specifically, the controls should be relatively visible, the hearing aid large enough to see and manipulate, and, of

course, the battery tangible if not visible. Older adults with vision impairment, such as low-vision problems, can benefit from hearing aids that are not necessarily equipped with sophisticated signal-processing capabilities. The ability to hear noises in the environment (e.g., warning signals) may be the sense older visually impaired adults rely on for their safety. In essence, sounds made audible by hearing aids may restore, in part, the sense of safety and security older visually impaired adults have lost. Recall that for older adults with acuity poorer than 20/70, auditory-visual integration training may not be feasible, and more time should be spent counseling, and providing assertiveness and strategies training.

Otologic Considerations

The primary otologic concerns that impact on hearing-aid candidacy relate to conditions in the ear that may preclude hearing-aid use or may render a particular style or arrangement inappropriate. With regard to the outer ear, presence of active infection, unusual growths, atresia, or stenosis of the external ear canal may preclude a canal or deep-canal fitting. If an ear has been surgically altered, the decision to proceed with the fitting should be made in consultation with a physician. Further, inability to obtain a sufficiently deep impression may contraindicate a CIC hearing aid that must be custom made to fit and remain seated in the ear canal. Individuals with abnormal skin sensitivity in the area of the ear canal and persons experiencing excessive cerumen accumulation may not be candidates for microhearing instruments. As the balance between the skin lining the ear canal, the sebacious oils, and glands involved in the production of ear wax is influenced in an unpredictable manner by age, older adults are at risk for dermatologic problems and excessive wax build-up that may interfere with the operation of ITE or canal hearing aids.

To make a determination regarding candidacy and the appropriateness of a particular style unit, the audiologist must examine the shape and dimensions of the external canal to insure compatability with the features of the hearing aid. Older adults with the tendency toward excessive accumulation of cerumen should be acquainted with options for controlling cerumen so that it does not interfere with the operation of hearing instruments. Options include an adhesive wax guard positioned at the end of the hearing aid or a brush and loop to clean the debris. As cerumen contamination compromises the reliability of hearing instruments, and hearing-instrument reliability relates to customer satisfaction, audiologists are urged to consider wax guards for older adults.

Middle ear problems such as active infection or persistent effusion may indicate the need for a bone-conduction receiver. Of course, any indication of retrocochlear involvement should be ruled out prior to the hearing-aid fitting. While older adults can waive the necessity for medical clearance, any individual with significant warning signs of potential medical conditions should be encouraged to see a physician prior to the hearing-aid fitting. Further, older adults with significant medical problems such as diabetes or AIDS should receive medical clearance, for taking an earmold/hearing-aid impression can pose a problem in selected individuals at risk for infection.

Manual Dexterity

The miniaturization of hearing-aid components has allowed for reductions in the dimensions of hearing aids and decreases in the size of their controls. Older adults with manual dexterity problems, compromised wrist or finger mobility, reduced fine motor coordination and/or diminished sense of touch or pain should be encouraged to purchase hearing aids they can manipulate, insert, feel, remove, and adjust independently. When deciding on hearing-aid candidacy, a

---

PEARL

Older adults with arthritic and/or rheumatoid disorders, paralysis, or developmental disabilities are most prone to movement impairments that may interfere with hearing-aid manipulation, and thus may be more suitable candidates for an ALD that has larger controls and can be manipulated independently.

---

dexterity check and an assessment of tactile sensation in the fingers should be used to help determine the style of the hearing aid, the modifications, and the controls to be recommended. Selected hearing-aid manufacturers state specifically that individuals with manual dexterity problems and/or a lack of sensation in the fingers are not candidates for microhearing instruments.

Manual dexterity can be assessed formally using the Nine Hole Pegboard Test, which evaluates fine motor coordination and finger dexterity. The Semmes-Weinstein Monofilaments Test can help to distinguish between light touch, diminished light touch, diminished protective sensation, loss of protective sensation, and deep pressure sensa-

tion. As clinical experience suggests that visual-motor coordination and touch recognition may affect successful use of amplification systems, audiologists are urged to experiment with the latter measures. These tools are easily accessible through occupational or physical therapy departments or professionals. If formal measures of dexterity are not feasible, informal tests of wrist, hand, and finger motion and dexterity should be pursued.

Physical Health Status

Dementia is a general term for mental deterioration that includes loss of memory and intellectual functioning. As indicated in previous chapters, it is a relatively common syndrome among older adults. Auditory problems are prevalent among older adults with dementia and have been shown to both mimic and mask dementing cognitive symptoms (Molloy & Lubinski, 1995). While for some individuals, dementia stands out as a health problem that may preclude hearing-aid candidacy and success, for selected individuals hearing aids have the potential to help maintain the residual assets/strengths and relieve the emotional distress associated with the cognitive decline of dementia. In general, the more severe the dementing illness, the greater the cognitive decline and the less likely the indiviual is to use the hearing aid successfully. Further, a person with severe dementing illness will be less able to learn how to use a new technology such as hearing aids successfully. Simply put, persons with more advanced stages of dementia may (1) have difficulty locating their head to position the unit in the ear, (2) be unable to maintain and adjust the hearing aid, (3) be unable to position and reposition the hearing aid, and (4) be confused by the amplified noise. Experienced hearing-aid users with advanced dementia are more likely to adjust and benefit from amplification than are new hearing-aid users with comparable degrees of dementing illness. For individuals who are not candidates for hearing aids, ALDs, especially hard-wired systems should be considered. These may be used to promote communication on an individual basis and can be used by physicians to aid in reaching a valid diagnosis of dementia. Alerting devices in the home are particularly important for this population especially for persons who do not use

---

PEARL

The audiologist is encouraged to explore the patient's mental status thoroughly prior to making a recommendation for a particular hearing technology and to monitor memory and cognitive function should a hearing aid be pursued.

---

hearing aids yet present with moderate to severe hearing loss. It is advisable that hearing-aid candidates complete a brief screening test of their cognitive abilities using the Short Portable Mental Status Questionnaire (SPMSQ).

Functional health status, including poor general health, reduced mobility, and reduced interpersonal communication, is correlated with degree of hearing handicap and hearing impairment (Bess, Lichtenstein, Logan, Burger, & Nelson, 1989). In fact, mean scores on a measure of physical functional status, such as the Sickness Impact Profile (SIP), increase from 3.3 for older adults with no impairment to 18.9 among those with a hearing impairment in the better ear of 40 dBHL or more (Bess et al, 1989). When physical functional status appears to be reduced and independence is potentially compromised, the contribution of hearing status to the individual's condition should be considered and the possibility of audiologic intervention pursued. On occasion, it is helpful to have the patient complete a standardized questionnaire for assessing sickness-related dysfunction, such as the SIP. Any improvement in the overall score, or in scores on the physical or psychosocial scales can be an important outcome of hearing-aid use. In fact, hearing-aid interventions have been reported to improve the biopsychosocial correlates of hearing impairment, that is reduce the degree of dysfunction. It is incumbent on audiologists to educate primary care physicians and geriatricians about the role hearing aids can play in reversing the declines in physical functional status associated with hearing decrements.

> **PEARL**
>
> Hearing aids are effective in reversing declines in physical functional status in older adults.

PSYCHOLOGICAL VARIABLES

The psychological variables that have been identified by practitioners as potential determinants of hearing-aid candidacy and benefit include motivational level of the patient and caregiver, cognitive status, and personality constellation. The pattern of relationships that have emerged from investigations into the contribution of the above variables to candidacy and benefit does not allow for definitive conclusions regarding the particular role of these variables in selecting hearing-aid candidates (Gatehouse, 1994; Bentler, Niebuhr, Getta, & Anderson, 1993). It is noteworthy that Cox, Alexander, and Gray (1999) did find that the extroversion-introversion dimension of personality does relate to benefit, as does the locus of control. Hence, audiologists should consider assessing personality variables as part of the initial assessment. With regard to cognitive status, the data of Chmiel and Jerger (1996) are of interest.

Chmiel and Jerger (1996) attempted to isolate the extent to which peripheral auditory problems accompanied by cognitive deficits influenced hearing-aid benefit in adults. Cognitive status was defined according to performance on selected neuropsychological tests. Subjects with dementia and other dementing illness were excluded from the study. Benefit was defined according to change in self-perceived handicap following a brief interval of hearing-aid use. They found that individuals with peripheral auditory and cognitive deficits derived significant benefit from hearing aids. The benefit was comparable for those with peripheral problems and

those with peripheral and cognitive deficits. Thus, in their study, age-associated declines in cognitive status did not appear to preclude benefit from hearing aids. Further,

> **PEARL**
>
> Mental status, including short-term memory, should be assessed and figured into the decision regarding hearing-aid candidacy as nearly 10% of persons over 65 years present with some degree of cognitive impairment sufficient to interfere with performance of daily activities.

clinical experience suggests that individuals with significant cognitive declines may not be well served by hearing aids.

Motivation is one of the most important, yet least well-understood, variables that affects adaptation to disability, rehabilitation candidacy, and potential (Kemp, 1990). It explains why behavior is initiated, why behavior persists, and why behavior is attenuated (Kemp, 1990). It is one of the psychological processes that will influence an older adult's resolve regarding hearing-aid use. Motivation is a multivariate

> **SPECIAL CONSIDERATION**
>
> Motivation influences one's capacity to overcome adversity, and one's desire to participate in social activities and to improve function (Kemp, 1990).

process that refers to self-directed behavior. It is defined according to the perception of: (1) what one wants from an intervention; (2) what one expects or believes can be achieved with a given intervention; (3) the relevance of the rewards associated with a given intervention; and (4) associated costs of pursuing an intervention (Kemp, 1990). Motivation to pursue intervention is optimal when an individual knows what he/she wants, expects it can be attained, and believes that the rewards are meaningful and occur at a reasonable cost.

> **PEARL**
>
> Motivation is key to the success of a hearing-aid fitting.

One of the greatest challenges to a dispensing audiologist is motivating an older adult to purchase and continue to use hearing aid(s) once the purchase has been made. The aging process influences one's motivational level especially as regards the purchase of rehabilitation services. Some of the age-related changes that may inhibit one's motivational level for pursuing amplification include the desire to maintain the status quo, fear of risk taking, and fear of failure. It is incumbent on the audiologist to recognize those variables that undermine an individual's motivation to pursue audiologic rehabilitation, in order to counsel the older adult regarding their fears and concerns. An understanding of motivational dynamics as described in Chapter 3, can help the audiologist to insure that lack of motivation does not preclude hearing-aid use and benefit. Oftentimes some motivational counseling at the time of the audiological evaluation or the prefitting will be necessary to convince a person with hearing impairment of the value of hearing aids. When motivating older adults to pursue amplification, it is important to instill realistic expectations as oftentimes client expectations are higher than the actual benefits, thus interfering with success (Schum, 1999).

SOCIOLOGICAL VARIABLES

The primary sociological variables to be considered when selecting candidates for hearing aids include lifestyle, familial support, and financial factors. One's lifestyle (e.g., engagement in physical activities, social interaction, and work-related activities) and the environment in which the individual functions must be explored prior to making any decisions regarding intervention. Consideration of the latter will help in the selection of a device that will optimize communication in the necessary social environments. In addition to impacting on a decision about candidacy, an appreciation for the physical and social environment will impact on decisions regarding hearing-aid style, hearing-aid features, hours of hearing-aid use, and need for assistive devices to supplement hearing-aid use.

The audiologist should explore the candidate's lifestyle from the perspective of the hearing-impaired individual and should seek input from informal or formal caregivers. If responses to a formal or informal interview reveal that the individual has a limited social network then the advantages of part-time hearing-aid use should be discussed, the advantages of early intervention emphasized, and assistive devices considered.

> ### PEARL
> When appropriate, part-time hearing-aid use should be encouraged as ultimately new users gradually come to understand the benefit of hearing aids and increase their use to include a number of listening situations.

Availability of familial support will influence the appropriateness of a hearing aid as an intervention of choice, as well as the audiologist's decision regarding the style of instrument to be recommended. For example, if an individual is relatively independent and does not wish to rely on a family member or a caregiver for hearing-aid insertion or operation then an ITE or a BTE hearing aid may be appropriate. Finally, with regard to financial factors, ability or inability to pay for a hearing aid does not influence benefit and thus should not influence candidacy (Newman, Hug, Wharton, & Jacobson, 1993). Hearing-aid candidates should

understand that persons who pay for hearing aids and those who obtain third-party coverage appear to derive comparable benefit based on improvement in perceived psychosocial handicap. Thus, rather than determining candidacy, financial factors may influence decisions regarding the style of hearing aid to purchase, the fitting arrangement, and the technological sophistication of the unit to be recommended.

> ### PEARL
> Financial factors do not influence psychosocial benefit associated with hearing-aid use.

ENVIRONMENTAL FACTORS

An older person with a hearing impairment who lives alone is an ideal candidate for hearing aid(s) because of the threat to safety and security posed by unremediated hearing loss. It is important that older adults understand the threat to safety posed by an unremediated hearing loss, including inability to hear the smoke alarm, the doorbell, a burglar or fire alarm, or a car horn. They should be counseled about the importance of hearing technologies as an to alert to potential danger in the physical environment. Older adults who ultimately do purchase hearing aid(s) should be encouraged to wear them at home, especially when alone to insure that they can hear warning signals. A recent home visit demonstrated to me the importance of emphasizing to the person with hearing impairment the value of wearing hearing aids indoors especially when alone. A visit to the actual setting in which a device or devices are to be used should be considered when fitting homebound individuals or people who live alone.

> ### SPECIAL CONSIDERATION
> According to Maslow's heirarchy of needs formulation, older adults will pursue a rehabilitative intervention for a chronic condition if in fact it is perceived to be compromising safety at home or outside.

> ### PEARL
> Hearing-aid use can restore the feeling of security and safety compromised by hearing impairment.

In sum, a host of audiologic and nonaudiologic variables combine to determine candidacy and feasibility of hearing-aid use. The audiologist must be mindful of all variables that will determine the appropriateness of a hearing aid for a given individual to insure hearing-aid satisfaction and benefit. Having considered the appropriateness of the individual for a hearing aid, the next step is the actual hearing-aid selection process.

CONSIDERATIONS IN THE HEARING-AID SELECTION PROCESS

The goal of the hearing-aid selection is to select amplification requirements and a hearing-aid arrangement that is electroacoustically, physically, and cosmetically acceptable. It is beyond the scope of this chapter to address in great depth strategies for selecting and verifying the hearing-aid response for older adults. For the most part, the rules and strategies used with younger adults pertain to older adults. The philosophy governing all hearing-aid selections and fittings is that the electroacoustic response of the hearing aid should: (1) maximize audibility and intelligibility, (2) provide good sound quality, and (3) provide an amplified sound that is comfortable and compensates for the loss of loudness resulting from impaired hearing (Bächler, Knecht, Launer, & Uvacek, 1997; McCandless, 1994). Simply put, an optimal hearing-aid fitting is one that makes speech audible without exceeding the listener's loudness discomfort level and restores the normal loudness relations for speech and other environmental sounds (Cox, 1995). Following

PEARL
Above all, for the elderly, the fitting should restore functional independence and promote quality of life.

determination of hearing-aid candidacy and prior to selecting the electroacoustic characteristics of the hearing aid(s), several decisions have to be made. These include determination of the style (e.g., canal) unit; the arrangement (e.g., monaural or binaural); the ear to fit in the case of a monaural unit; and the category of instrument including digital, programmable, or conventional analog device.

Hearing-Aid Style

A variety of hearing-aid styles are available to the hearing-impaired older adult once it is mutually decided that a hearing aid is the appropriate intervention. These include BTE hearing aids and the entire family of ITE units including CIC instruments, canal, and custom ITE aids. Figure 9–7 depicts an example of some hearing aids including in-the-canal (ITC), ITE, and BTE units.

Sale of DSP and programmable hearing instruments grew dramatically in 1998, such that 44% of all instruments sold were of that variety (Skafte, 1999). According to Skafte (1999) 16% of hearing aids sold in 1998 were BTEs, 30% were full-shell ITEs, 27% were ITCs, and 20% were CIC units. Thus, approximately 84% of all hearing aids sold were ITE units (Skafte, 1998). Continuing a 4-year trend, sales to new hearing-aid users were down in 1998, such that only 48% of fittings were to new users (Kirkwood, 1997; Skafte, 1999). The average age of hearing-aid users was 68 years in 1994 (Kochkin, 1996). The 1998 Survey of Hearing Instrument Dispensers revealed that dispensing audiologists tended to fit more BTEs than hearing instrument specialists, who dispensed a higher percentage of ITC instruments (Skafte, 1999). Interestingly, dispensing audiologists sell a higher percentage of programmable and DSP instruments than do hearing instrument specialists (Skafte, 1999). In 1998, the overall return for credit of all hearing aids sold in the United States was 18.7%, with the return rate for CIC instruments being high at 24% (Strom, 1999).

Since their introduction, programmable hearing-aid sales represent an increasingly greater percentage of total domestic hearing-aid sales. For example, a 1994 HIA survey revealed that programmable instruments represented only a small proportion (5%) of the market share. According to Strom (1999), programmable/DSP instruments were projected to comprise 37% of the hearing instrument market in 1999. It is estimated that more than 700,000 programmable/DSP units

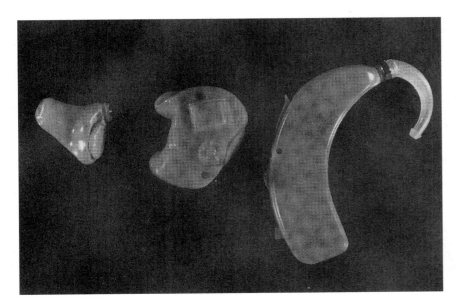

Figure 9–7 Examples of three air-conduction hearing aids. To the left is an ITC hearing aid. In the middle is an ITE hearing aid. To the right is a BTE hearing aid. (From Valente, 1994, p. 256.)

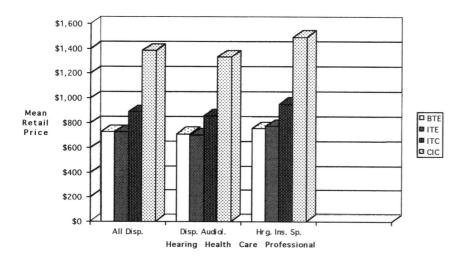

Figure 9–8 Average mean retail price charged per hearing aid by dispenser and style of instrument. Prices are for nonprogrammable units and do not include fees for professional services when those are billed separately. (Modified from Kirkwood, 1997.)

will be sold in 1999, as compared with 323,173 in 1997. Note that nearly one-quarter of all programmable instruments sold in 1998 were returned for credit, with programmable BTEs having the highest return for credit rate and full-shell ITEs the lowest (Strom, 1999).

As noted previously audiologists are more likely to dispense programmable hearing aids than hearing instrument specialists (the gap is closing) with audiologists in private practice dispensing the greatest proportion (Kirkwood, 1997). Audiologists were more likely to dispense hearing aids with automatic signal processing (ASP) than hearing instrument specialists. In light of the above statistics, it seems that older adults wanting to purchase programmable aids or instruments with ASP should be directed to audiologists who have more experience dispensing these products. This type of information should be communicated to patients and referral sources, especially primary care physicians, the entry point into the hearing health care system for most older adults.

Overall, the average price for all hearing aids was $875 in 1996 as compared to $794 in 1995 (Kirkwood, 1997). Overall, in 1997 the average price for hearing instruments reported by dispensing audiologists, was slightly lower than that reported by hearing-instrument specialists (Skafte, 1998). It is noteworthy that the cost of nonprogrammable, standard programmable, and high-end programmable hearing aids differs dramatically by dispenser. Figure 9–8 shows the average price of nonprogrammable instruments by professional and hearing-aid style (Kirkwood, 1997). In each category, the average price of a hearing-aid from a hearing-instrument specialist is slightly higher than from a dispensing audiologist. In 1998, hearing instrument specialists charged more for DSP, programmable, CIC, and ITC units, while dispensing audiologists charged more for BTE and ITE units (Skafte, 1999).

The average prices for hearing instruments sold in 1997 by dispensing audiologists and hearing instrument specialists shown in Figure 9–9 differed somewhat from 1998 prices. The average price for a BTE was $848 versus $897, while the average price for a CIC was $1388 in 1998 versus $1458 in 1997. In contrast, the average price for a DSP unit

was $2402 in 1998 versus $2107 in 1997. The average price for programmable units was $1766 in 1998 versus $1604 in 1997 (Skafte, 1999). In 1998, 80% of all hearing care professionals surveyed said that testing and fees were included in the price of the hearing instrument. However, 35% of dispensing audiologists said charges for testing the instrument were itemized (Skafte, 1999).

With the exception of cochlear implant surgery for severely and profoundly impaired individuals, support for hearing health care is modest or unavailable in most health plans. Interestingly, a majority of dispensers (34% versus 16%) feel that there may be some advantage to managed care in that it may increase the number of patients fit with hearing aids (Kirkwood, 1997). However, most dispensers

---

PEARL

Dispensing audiologists tend to dispense more advanced and more expensive hearing aids than hearing-instrument specialists.

---

fear that because of price restraints, managed care organizations (MCOs) may discourage the sale of high-tech hearing aids (Kirkwood, 1997). Most respondents to the *Hearing Journal* survey feel that managed care will negatively impact the quality of hearing health care services. It is likely that the latter will be the case for older adults in that managed care will decrease the time spent with patients, and will limit rehabilitation and follow-up services so critical to a successful fitting, especially with older adults. Alternatively, some respondents to the *Hearing Journal* survey suggested that MCOs may have their advantages in that it may result in a wider physician base being made aware of the hearing health needs and the value of hearing aids. Interestingly, the 1999 survey conducted by Hearing Review revealed that 24% of patients seen by dispensing audiologists were covered by MCO contracts as compared to 12% for hearing instrument specialists (Skafte, 1999). Overall, there was a decline in the number of dispensing offices that fit hearing aids for MCOs (Skafte, 1999).

Why CICs?

The demand for smaller, less visible hearing aids coupled with miniaturization of hearing-aid components has led to the expansion of the custom hearing-aid market in general and CICs in particular. Custom-fit hearing aids are fitted to the contour of the ear, becoming less and less visible as the insertion point moves deeper into the ear canal. Figures 9–10, 9–11, 9–12, 9–13, and 9–14 clearly show the insertion depth of a typical CIC instrument. ITE aids rest in the entire concha portion of the external ear whereas ITC units terminate at the entrance to the external auditory meatus, and with CIC units the visible end is 1 to 2 mm inside the opening of the ear canal. This is clearly shown in Figures 9–10 to 9–15. Two categories of deep canal or CIC instruments are available. Category A, which includes most CICs, consists of hearing aids that have an ear tip that comes in contact with the second bend of the ear canal, but whose fitting does not involve making contact with the tympanic membrane. Category B are deep-canal instruments whose fitting does include an impression-taking procedure in which the dispenser makes contact with the tympanic membrane (Kirkwood, 1994). According to Mueller (1994), CICs have several potential advantages over other styles of custom instruments. These are displayed in Table 9–4. Investigators are currently attempting to validate the communicative and psychosocial benefits of CIC fittings. These include but are not limited to cosmetics, improved sound localization, increased high-frequency input, reduction in the occlusion effect, less distortion, and better sound quality because of its higher amplifier headroom capabilities (Valente, Valente, Potts, & Lybarger, 1996). Results from a recent survey conducted by Ebinger, Holland, Holland, and Mueller (1995) revealed that overall, CICs significantly reduced the proportion of listening difficulties experienced by older adults. The benefits experienced by older adults in reverberant conditions, background noise, and quiet were comparable to those perceived by a younger adult sample.

While the acoustic and cosmetic advantages are readily apparent, these units were originally designed to penetrate a previously untapped market, namely, younger adults with mild sensorineural hearing loss. However, data on purchase intent by age and hearing instrument (among nonowners) suggest that the percentage of adults between 55 and 74 years who intend to purchase CICs is quite high (30%) as compared to 20 to 25% for adults between 35 and 54 years (Kochkin, 1994). Further, purchase intent is directly proportional to the amount of perceived hearing handicap on the HHIE-S (Kochkin, 1997). Given the manual dexterity and visual problems that are so prevalent among older adults and the cosmetic and acoustic appeal of CICs, candidacy should be determined on an individual basis. Of course, options are

---

SPECIAL CONSIDERATION

The downside of CICs for older adults is difficulty grasping the battery and the aid, difficulty inserting the aid into the ear, and difficulty inserting and removing the tiny batteries that power these units.

---

available to assist with the latter and should be shared with the patient during the orientation.

Older adults who insist on purchasing CIC units should have medical clearance to insure that the ear canal and tympanic membrane are free of visible medical conditions including abrasion, hematoma, dermatologic infections, or visible drainage. Older adults with collapsed ear canals will require considerable effort to fit; those with short canals leave little room for circuitry including the receiver; and persons with straight canals make for difficult acoustic seals (Voll & Jones, 1998). Further, if the bony canal appears to be high in vascularity, as is the case in selected older adults, a deep canal fitting should be discouraged because

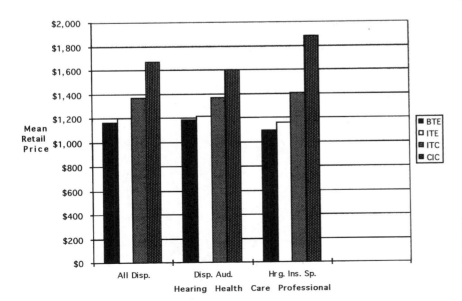

Figure 9–9 Mean retail price charged per hearing aid for standard programmable instruments by style and hearing health care professional. (Modified from Kirkwood, 1997.)

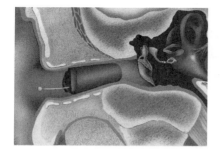 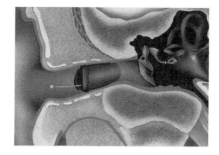

Figure 9–10   Standard CIC (Left).

Figure 9–11   Rexton RX-39XS (Right).

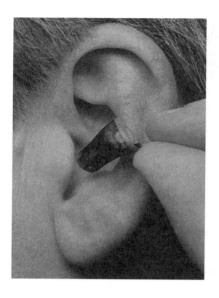 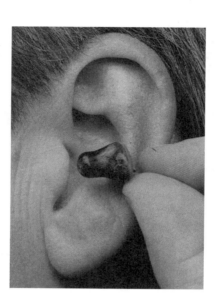

Figure 9–12   Standard CIC (Left).

Figure 9–13   Rexton RX-39XS (Right).

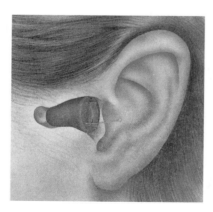 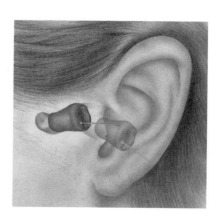

Figure 9–14   The greatest obstacle for a normal CIC is a canal with a sharp bend (Left).

Figure 9–15   The length of the RX-39XS is short enough to pass a sharp bend with minimal insertion or extraction force (Right).

of potential discomfort. The use of video-otoscopy is encouraged with the elderly population given the potential effects of aging on ear canal anatomy. Older adults who ultimately purchase CICs should have extensive hearing-aid orientation with a caregiver to insure adequate insertion of the unit and proper battery insertion. The dispensing audiologist should always keep in mind that key to the success of a CIC fitting is the exactness of fit, a snug fit in the cartilaginous portion of the canal without being too tight in the bony canal. Martin and Pirzanski (1998) suggest that taking

the earmold impression with the jaw open is especially critical, and it is especially important for the second bend of the canal to be present to insure that the canal portion is long enough.

CIC hearing aids should be clearly labeled with proper colors visible to the aging eye (e.g., right ear red, left ear blue). Emphasizing the relative location of the removal cord can facilitate proper placement, as well. The importance of insurance coverage for CICs in particular should be emphasized as, due to their size and the miniaturization

TABLE 9–4 Potential Advantages of CIC Hearing Aids

Advantage	Implication
1. No volume control wheel	Persons with manual dexterity problems will not have difficulty with volume-control adjustments, as automatic gain control circuitry eliminates need for a volume control.
2. Reduction of acoustic feedback	Less need for venting, positioned closer to the eardrum leading to a securer fit.
3. Reduction of occlusion effect	Rests in the bony portion of the canal minimizing the echo and stuffiness associated with the occlusion effect.
4. Ease of removal	A string extending from the faceplate is used for removal making it relatively easy to grasp.
5. Reduced wind noise	The microphone is recessed in the ear canal so it is less affected by wind.
6. Increased high-frequency input	High-frequency input to the microphone is increased because placement deep in the canal allows for natural acoustic effects of the concha and pinna to take place.
7. Improved sound localization	Placement of the hearing-aid microphone in the ear canal allows for the more natural pinna effects, namely improved sound localization.
8. Telephone use	Comfortable when using the phone because it allows the telephone receiver to be placed against the ear. Also, little acoustic feedback when using the phone because of microphone placement.

Source: Mueller (1994).

of components, the potential for loss or damage is great. The acceptance of CIC units is quite apparent when comparing their market share from 1994 to the present. In 1994, CICs captured 7% of the market whereas in 1998 they constituted 20% of the total ITE market (Skafte, 1999). The return rate for nonprogrammable CICs (i.e., 26%) was higher than for programmable CICs, that rate being 21.7% in 1998 (Strom, 1999). These statistics underline the importance of careful prefitting protocols to insure that the patient is right for the instrument, and, of course, for extensive hearing-aid orientation, counseling, and follow-up designed to promote satisfaction and benefit.

Until the 1980s BTE hearing instruments were the most popular among consumers and they remain the hearing aid of choice for persons with severe to profound hearing impairment. It is notable that in 1995 sale of BTE units increased over 1994 presumably because of the appeal of programmable BTEs (Kirkwood, 1996a). Since 1995 sales of BTEs have remained stable, representing 15 to 16% of the market share (Skafte, 1999). Of course, with the advent of programmable ITE and ITC units, this trend has reversed itself. BTEs are

ideal for persons who require high-use gain (50 to 70 dBSPL), output limiting that lies between 120 and 142 dBSPL, and a strong telecoil. Additional advantages include their flexibility, compatability with direct audio input microphones, powerful telecoils, ease of insertion of unit, and larger batteries. Interestingly, some older adults find it easier to insert BTE hearing aids than ITE units and find that smaller and slimmer models are cosmetically acceptable. For the most part, however, smaller custom ITE aids are preferred.

PEARL

Residents of nursing facilities continue to use BTE hearing instruments because of a long history of hearing-aid use. It is important to monitor these individuals to insure that the earmold remains comfortable, rests securely in the ear, and can be inserted and removed.

With regard to earmold style, skeleton and semiskeleton molds provide less bulk and more comfort than shell molds. Valente et al (1996) contend that a semiskeleton is appropriate for patients with manual dexterity problems or a hardened ear texture. Similarly, half-shell molds are good for persons with reduced manual dexterity, as the entire helix is removed making for easier insertion. With regard to earmold materials, the audiologist can choose from eight to nine potential options. Hard materials tend to be more durable whereas softer materials are less susceptible to feedback (Rubinstein, 1997). The possibility of earmolds or custom products that combine soft and hard materials is a nice combination with the soft canal reducing the likelihood of feedback and slippage from the ear (Rubinstein, 1997). In general, if the patient's pinna is hard, soft earmold material may be more appropriate. Soft material is desireable because body heat causes the material to expand to create a tight acoustic seal. Conversely, if the pinna is soft, then a hard earmold material may be preferable (Valente et al, 1996). Many long-time hearing-aid users feel more comfortable with a lucite mold as it tends to be easier to insert. If gain/output requirements of the hearing aid are high, the audiologist might consider ordering an earmold with a hard lucite body with a soft canal portion to provide a better seal and less feedback. If the patient is highly allergic, as many older adults are, polyethylene (hard) or silicone (soft) material should be considered (Valente et al, 1996). New earmolds should be made when the mold routinely becomes unseated or when acoustic feedback becomes a problem. When taking a new impression, keep in mind that older adults tend to prefer the material and style to which they have become accustomed, so discuss any change before ordering the new mold. Also, keep in mind that the cerumen accumulation common in older adults can affect the function of hearing aids so precautions such as manufacturer-installed or disposable wax guards, a belled canal, or receiver tubing extended beyond the end of the aid should be considered.

SPECIAL CONSIDERATION

Cerumen accumulation is a frequent problem for older adults, interfering with hearing aid reliability, so some type of cerumen management strategy should be practiced.

Recently, several companies have incorporated an FM receiver and a conventional hearing aid into a BTE hearing-aid case. The advantage of introducing an FM system is the improved signal-to-noise (SNR) ratio achieved by bringing the microphone closer to the source of sound. Essentially, FM systems bridge the acoustical space between the sound source and the listener by eliminating the detrimental effects on speech perception of distance, noise, and reverberation (Ross, 1995b). By improving the speech-to-noise ratio, one can maximize speech comprehension (Ross, 1996b). The primary advantage of a BTE/FM system over the traditional body-worn FM system is that the single unit worn behind the ear is more convenient to wear. Further, it can be used as

a regular hearing aid, as an FM receiver bringing the signal directly to the user's ear, or as both an FM system and a hearing aid together. It is ideal when driving in the car, when conversing in a noisy environment, when at a lecture, or in a restaurant. The newest model BTE/FM systems have a built-in telecoil, changeable FM channels, and additional electroacoustic features that enhance their flexibility (Ross, 1996a). As of this writing, several companies, including AVR/Sonovation, Telex, and Phonic Ear, manufacture and distribute BTE/FM receivers. Older adults with CAPD who no longer derive benefit from conventional hearing aids should consider a trial period with this technology. If the patient with CAPD is willing, a BTE/FM system may offer advantages over programmable or digital aids in that the negative effects of noise and distance can be overcome. The acoustic advantages may outweigh some of the cosmetic disadvantages. Older adults agreeing to purchase BTE/FM systems must receive some assertiveness training in that they have to be taught to feel comfortable giving different speakers the microphone/transmitter.

One additional point with regard to BTE units relates to the telecoil. In general, for anybody with a moderate to severe hearing loss, a good telecoil used with a compatible telephone is the most effective acoustic method of communication over the telephone (Ross, 1997). A high-power telecoil, which includes a preamplifier in the "T" coil circuit, should be recommended for persons with moderate to severe hearing loss to insure compatability with the telephone and with an ALD coupler. Inclusion of the preamplifier produces an amplified output nearly identical to that obtained with the microphone circuit (Ross, 1995a). The telecoil option is an important one. Self Help for Hard of Hearing People (SHHH) recommends that all hearing-aid dispensers inform their clients of the function and advantages of "T" coils during the selection process and encourage their inclusion in the hearing aid (SHHH, 1996b). The inclusion of a "T" coil affords auditory access to the telephone as well as to ALDs that transmit signals using infrared light, FM radio waves, or an electromagnetic field (SHHH, 1996b). Note that if the person with hearing impairment works in an environment with a good deal of electromagnetic interference, direct audio-input connectors from the telephone to a BTE may be the preferred option (Ross, 1997). Finally, Ross (1995a) recently reported on the availability of a waterproof BTE unit developed in Japan. This arrangement, wherein the body assembly has been made watertight with rubber packing in the seams, may be ideal for older adults who have difficulty removing the earmold/hearing-aid arrangement each time they take a shower, swim, or are caught outdoors in the rain.

High Performance Hearing Aids

Manufacturers have introduced "programmable" and "digital" hearing instruments available as BTE, ITE, ITC, and CIC units. Simply put, programmability allows the parameters of the hearing aid to be changed electronically through programming rather than via screwdriver potentiometers used on conventional hearing aids (Agnew, 1996b). Examples of programmable hearing aids are shown in Figures 9–16,

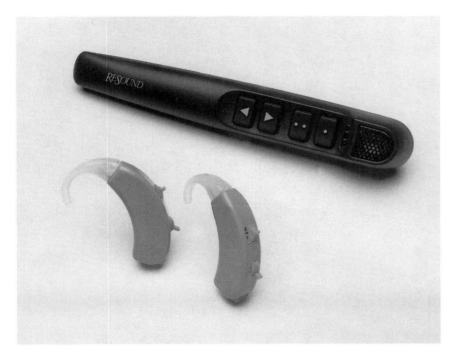

Figure 9–16 Remote control and digitally programmable behind-the-ear hearing aids. (Photograph courtesy of Resound.)

9–17, and 9–18. The units shown in these figures include a remote control. Figure 9–16 shows BTEs with a remote control, Figure 9–17 shows ITEs with a remote, and Figure 9–18 shows CICs with a remote. The remote control, which is optional with certain units, is used to manipulate the parameters of the hearing aid. In essence, programmable hearing aids employ digital technology to shape and manipulate a signal that has been amplified using analog technology (Radcliffe, 1991). According to Agnew, the terms *digital* and *programmable* are frequently used interchangeably, and to remove any confusion the HIA has made an effort to standardize terminology. The term recommended for programmable hearing aids is *digitally controlled analog* (DCA) hearing aids, while the digital units are referred to as DSPs (Agnew, 1996b). The signal path in DCA hearing aids is analog, as in conventional units. However, the control functions

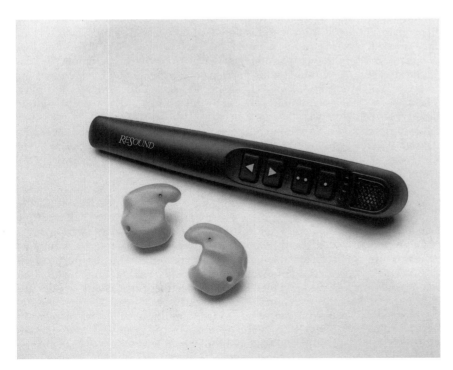

Figure 9–17 Remote control and digitally programmable in-the-ear hearing aids. (Photograph courtesy of Resound.)

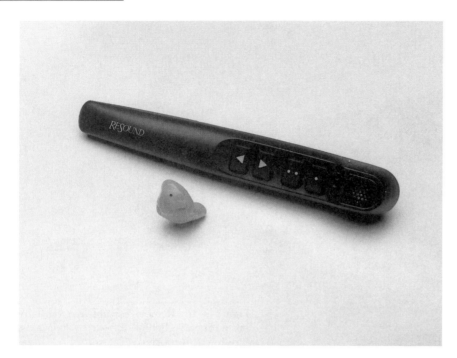

Figure 9–18 Remote control and digitally programmable completely-in-the-canal hearing aid. (Photograph courtesy of Resound.)

used to alter the electroacoustic characteristics are performed by digital circuitry. Specifically, DCA hearing aids use analog amplifiers. According to Northern, DCA hearing aids have greater flexbility and extensive range over all of the traditional frequency and intensity controls (Radcliffe, 1991). In short, the digital nature of the control circuitry, allows for stepped adjustments, with the fineness of the adjustments limited by the number of steps in the adjustment (Agnew, 1996b). Included in all DCA units is an electronic memory associated with the switching, programmed to remember each adjustment position to which the solid-state switches have been adjusted (Agnew, 1996b). In contrast to DCA units, hearing aids that use digital circuitry for both the signal processing and the controlling functions are referred to as DSP hearing aids (Agnew, 1996b). Fully digital hearing instruments statistically analyze the components of the incoming signal over time and modify the signal based on the analysis (Rubinstein, 1997). In truly digital instruments, the input to the hearing aid is digitized, allowing for complex processing of the signal before it is restored to its analog form at the output.

In general, DCA hearing aids employ different circuit options to achieve a variety of sound qualities and performance characteristics. They provide signal processing sophistication with electroacoustic flexibility. The vast majority of instruments must be hooked up to an external programmer and/or computer for adjustment of the electroacoustic characteristics. Some programming devices are proprietary, while many companies utilize a "universal" programmer. In 1999, 25 companies offered programmable aids and 12 companies had launched digital hearing aids (Strom, 1999). As the complexity of hearing aids increases, the number and variety of programmable products and digital units are likely to increase, as well.

DCA instruments offer the user and the dispenser fitting flexibility because of the ability to (1) easily modify or reprogram the instrument's response, and (2) program multiple hearing-aid responses into a single instrument because of the availabilty of a number of memories. Most programmable aids do not offer more than four memories, with two memories being sufficient for most individuals. The availability of multiple memories enables the audiologist to fit different environments into a single hearing aid. For example, the hearing-aid user has the ability to custom tailor the hearing instrument to their lifestyle, enabling them to benefit from amplification in situations in which a previous hearing aid was unusable. The dispenser can adjust the low frequencies independently from the high frequencies depending on the hearing configuration and the nature of the input sound. The dispenser can set one program for quiet, one for noise, one for the telephone, and one for listening to music.

Programmable instruments are often classified according to the number of channels and number of memories available. Using a classification system described by Bray (1997), programmable instruments can be divided into four distinct categories. For example, programmable instruments range from the most simplistic, namely, single channel, single memory, to the more complex multiple channel, multiple memory. What distinguishes a multimemory hearing aid is that the different signal-processing characteristics may be selected manually for use under certain listening conditions. Multimemory hearing aids include those devices that have more than one set of electroacoustic characteristics under the control of the user. In Bray's classification system, the number of memories or multiple memories merely implies that a hearing aid can be programmed to operate in many different environments. It enables the user to change the hearing-aid response to optimize hearing in selected situations and listening environments. In short, multiple memory provides the hearing aid with the capability of storing settings for several different listening situations (Agnew, 1996b). Typically, the primary setting stores the target prescription used for normal communication, whereas the secondary memory is set according to the listening needs of the patient. It may be set for listening in a noisy situation, for communicating in a reverberant setting, or for listening at a group meeting. Agnew (1996b) suggested that for programmable units having three or more switchable memories, some individuals choose to set the third memory on an acoustic telephone setting by limiting the upper end of the bandwidth to 3000 Hz to mimic the frequency response of the typical telephone. Multiple-memory hearing aids contain a switch or other methods to choose between the memory settings, enabling the user access to a number of different amplification characteristics necessary to meet different listening requirements (Keidser, Dillon, & Byrne, 1996). Keidser, Dillon, and Byrne (1996) suggest that those most likely to benefit from a multiple-memory hearing aid are individuals with an average high-frequency loss greater than 55 dBHL, who report a need to optimize listening in a variety of conditions, and can be fitted with more than 5 dB variation in the low-frequency real ear gain.

Programmable instruments, which vary widely in features such as number of memories, number of channels, ease of programming, programmability, and signal processing circuitry, often have features that are unavailable with conventional instruments. Most programmable instruments enable the audiologist to change all adjustable hearing-aid functions. They are typically available as BTE, ITE, ITC, and CIC instruments with amplification capability ranging from mild and moderate to powerful. Some of the adjustable functions, which include the frequency response, compression functions, and on-off switch, are listed in Table 9–5.

To enable manipulation of the hearing-aid parameters, most DCA hearing aids have remote controls. Remote controls vary according to the way in which the signal is transmitted to the hearing aid. Some use ultrasonic signals, others use radio frequency waves, while still others use infrared light to transmit control signals to the hearing aid (Agnew, 1996b). The remote control subserves three functions. One is to change the overall gain of the hearing aid, to turn it on and off and to alter the frequency response of the hearing aid. The second function is to switch between different memories when using a multimemory DCA. This function allows the user the flexibility of switching memories according to the listening environment. Finally, the remote control may serve a combination of the above functions (Agnew, 1996). On some units, the remote control replaces the function of one or several controls such as the gain control, the on-off switch, the noise suppression switch, or the "T" switch. As a remote control often obviates the need for space for selected controls, the size of the hearing aid may be reduced when the unit includes a remote control. While remote controls are intuitively appealing for older adults because the controls are large, easy to manipulate, and easy to visualize, some persons may feel somewhat threatened

by this technologically complex option. To allay anxieties, some audiologists believe that likening the hearing-aid remote control to the television remote control may make it more attractive to the user; in fact this may decrease the appeal. Many older adults in the market for hearing aids today may still be threatened by remote controls used with the television or VCR. If they lose the television remote control, it is likely that they will also lose this user interface. Further,

---

SPECIAL CONSIDERATION

Remote-control hearing instruments may have intuitive appeal. However, for many they are technologically too complex.

TABLE 9–5 Adjustable Functions of Programmable Hearing Aids

Style
BTE, ITE, ITC, CIC

Basic Electroacoustic Parameters
Frequency Response

Overall Gain

Maximum SSPL-90

Resonance peak frequency control

Compression
Compression type: wide dynamic range, compression limiting, or both

Compression ratio: fixed, adjustable, or curvilinear

Compression threshold

Compression time constants: attack/release, fixed/variable

Compression kneepoint: fixed, adjustable

Crossover frequency or frequencies between bands

Miscellaneous Functions
Hearing-aid on-off control

Sleep circuit for reducing battery drain

Options for use with telephone

Remote controls: type of signal, size, number of parameters, ease of use

Microphone: directional, omnidirectional, or both

Data logging

User-operated volume control

Programmer
Dedicated system, PC (with interface), manufacturer, remote control combination

Source: Modified from Agnew, 1996, and Rubinstein, 1997.

remote controls can be troublesome to patients who are forgetful or absentminded, and they do tend to increase the cost of hearing aids, which may be a problem for many older adults (Fabry, 1996). When in doubt, it is not a bad idea to stick with a switch or button on the hearing aid itself.

High performance hearing aids such as programmable units will most likely play an important role in the hearing-aid industry in the next decade and for some older adults may be the option for which they have been waiting. However, make sure to consider the patient type before recommending a multimemory and/or multichannel hearing aid (Kuk, 1993). The majority of older adults, first entering the hearing-aid market may be overwhelmed by the variety and complexity of programmable units. Further, their listening needs may not demand the sophistication inherent in programmable units. The primary determinants of candidacy for programmable hearing instruments are listening needs, whether occupational, social or recreational; hearing-aid history (i.e., experience with hearing aids); and comfort level with technology. In addition to the latter, motivational level and availability for repeat visits should be considered. Should the background history and audiometric profile justify the investment of time and money associated with use of programmable hearing aids, the audiologist should review the options available and allow the candidate an opportunity to "interact with the device." In the case of a multiple-memory hearing aid, for example, the older adults should be given the opportunity to compare the different memories against, perhaps, a conventional device. It is important to insure that the candidate be accompanied by a family member or caregiver through each step of the selection and fitting to facilitate adaptation to the unit. When orienting the older adult, begin slowly, introduce new concepts gradually and allow ample time for trial and error. Allow, enough time to thoroughly explore and learn these devices.

PEARL

The fitting of a programmable unit will be a time-intensive process for an older adult given the numerous unknown variables and their technological sophistication. It is important to schedule additional time and additional sessions when fitting older adults with DCA instruments.

Some final comments with regard to DCA instruments are in order. When fitting a programmable instrument, always keep in mind that for the older adult, the most important features are comfort, ease of operation, and the availability of a program that will assist in their most difficult listening situations. It is critical that the consumer have the opportunity to judge the different signal-processing characteristics with real-life listening materials, allowing adequate time for valid comparisons. Further, older adults may not feel comfortable "having responsibility" for a remote control and this may influence their choice of instrument. Providing the client an opportunity to compare systems with a remote control with those having a device control

can be clarifying. It is often helpful to provide the customer with an opportunity to manipulate the controls and observe the ease or difficulty with which the individual approaches the task. Finally, an increasing number of older adults are demanding objective justification or verification of the value of programmable instruments relative to their cost. Audiologists are urged to involve the consumer in every aspect of the dispensing and decision-making process using objective and subjective measures that enable comparisons of performance in an unaided condition, with their conventional hearing aids and when appropriate, with a programmable instrument. Anecdotal reports suggest that the consumer finds this aspect of the fitting process clarifying as oftentimes the benefits of this technology become readily apparent.

PEARL

Potential advantages of DSP include reduced feedback, improved sound quality, improved audibility and intelligibility, increased flexibility, and improved listener comfort (Valente, 1998).

When I began writing this chapter, hearing instruments incorporating DSP were becoming a reality (Agnew, 1997). At present, several companies are marketing DSP units. The advantage of DSP in hearing instruments is in its ability to perform complex signal processing that cannot be achieved with traditional analog devices (Agnew, 1997). In essence, as the complexity of the signal processing increases, so too does the need for large-memory storage. In the long run, it becomes more efficient and effective to switch to digital processing. With DSP, the incoming signal is converted into a stream of digital bits on which complex mathematical processing takes place. DSP hearing aids therefore have considerable processing power such that an incredible number of manipulations can be performed on the signal to yield an optimum amplified signal (Valente, 1998). In addition, the small and fast microprocessors and transistors operate on low power/voltage, allowing for ear level digital hearing aids with good battery life (Hosford-Dunn, 1997).

SPECIAL CONSIDERATION

DSP hearing aids will produce signals that are cleaner and more natural but not CD sound quality because the hearing-aid response is still limited by the quality of the microphone and receiver (Valente, 1998).

Agnew (1997) suggested that the DSP algorithm can be considered the electronic equivalent of a road map. The word *algorithm* then refers to a set of procedures that tell the processor what to do to the signal and the sequence in which to do it including how the instrument will process incoming signals, the correct settings for the hearing aid, or even how to verify that the desired fitting has been achieved. The processing algorithm represents the manufacturer's interpretation of what is best for the patient and thus what differentiates one digital hearing instrument from the other (Agnew, 1997). As regards the elderly, we need to find the best noise suppression or noise-reduction algorithms available to alleviate the difficulty older adults experience in noise. Also, feedback reduction circuits available in selected DSP hearing aids help to minimize a problem that tends to plague older adult hearing-aid users. Once more diverse methods to process sounds in new ways are available at a reasonable cost (e.g., address outer hair-cell loss rather than inner hair-cell loss), not only as high-end products, DSP instruments will be a strong consideration for older adults (Agnew, 1997). However, we must continue to keep in mind that for older adults "DSP hearing instruments offer high flexibility, but not miracle processing; better sound quality, but not quite true hi-fi sound; more precise fittings but never perfect compensation for everyone; optimal hearing in most, but not all environments; better speech discrimination in noise, but not perfect speech discrimination; automatic adaptation to the auditory environment, but not always optimal processing" (Strom, 1998, pp. 39–40). According to Hosford-Dunn (1997), increasing software control of DSP may lead to improvements in speech-pattern recognition, individual voice-pattern recognition, and improved noise reduction.

PEARL

DSP hearing aids utilize an analog-to-digital converter that converts the sound wave into a binary code. The greater the number of times the digital hearing-aid samples the incoming signal and the greater the number of calculations it performs in manipulating the parameters, the better the reproduction of the signal (Valente, 1998).

Hearing-Aid Arrangement: Monaural Versus Binaural

The term *hearing-aid arrangement* typically refers to a monaural versus binaural fitting. Hearing levels in conjunction with word-recognition scores can be used to decide on the hearing-aid arrangement or, in the case of a monaural unit, the ear to fit. In general, barring medical factors, or the "phenomenon of binaural interference," clinical experience suggests that the only time a hearing aid should not be fit on an ear is when there is no measurable response to sound, or word-recognition ability is virtually nonexistent in a given ear. It is now commonly accepted that binaural fittings are preferable to monaural fittings because of the advantages associated with a binaural fitting (Musiek & Baran, 1996). These advantages include improved localization; binaural summation, improved ability to understand speech in noise; improved hearing at a distance; ease of listening; and a more natural/balanced sound. Given the advantages of a binaural fitting, it should come as no surprise that 68% of all fittings in 1998 were binaural, with hearing instrument specialists fitting binaural more than dispensing audiologists were (Skafte, 1999).

Recently, there has been a flurry of research reporting on auditory deprivation and recovery offered by binaural amplification. These data have been used to further justify binaural amplification for individuals who are deemed audiologically suitable. Silman, Gelfand, and Silverman (1984) were among the first investigators to report on the concept of auditory deprivation associated with failure to amplify an ear with bilaterally symmetrical sensorineural hearing loss. Their data suggest that when speech-recognition scores of subjects with bilateral sensorineural hearing loss who are fit monaurally are compared to those of a comparable group of subjects who are fit binaurally, speech-recognition scores in the unaided ear of the monaurally aided group decline dramatically over a four-to-five-year time period. Most encouraging are reports that some patients with auditory deprivation effects experience clinically significant albeit incomplete recovery following use of binaural amplification (Gelfand, 1995). These aforementioned findings have been replicated by a number of investigators on a variety of populations including older adults with presbycusis. The presence of late-onset auditory deprivation is a compelling reason to fit individuals binaurally. If the phenomenon of late-onset auditory deprivation could be linked to decrements in quality of life associated with failure to fit binaurally, it would provide even more powerful evidence for this fitting strategy. When financial considerations preclude binaural amplification, the possibility of alternating monaural amplification should be explored to minimize the potential for auditory deprivation effects to set in (Gelfand, 1995).

SPECIAL CONSIDERATION

Binaural amplification may not be appropriate for all older adults.

Binaural amplification may not be appropriate for older adults with manual dexterity problems on a particular side; for persons with cognitive or emotional problems; for persons with CAPD; or when binaural performance is impaired by the poorer ear because of the phenomenon of binaural interference (Jerger, Silman, Lew, & Chmiel, 1993). The latter is evident clinically when aided binaural speech-recognition ability is significantly poorer than performance in the better-aided ear. While the exact mechanisms underlying binaural interference are unknown, it does appear that some type of competition is introduced by distortion arising at the peripheral or central auditory system (Musiek & Baran, 1996). While we await electrophysiologic evidence supporting the mechanisms for the apparent "binaural interference," it may be worthwhile to compare aided word-recognition performance in three conditions, namely, monaural right-ear aided, monaural left-ear aided, and binaural aided, when considering a binaural fitting for older adults. If binaural performance is poorer than that of the better ear, one might suspect that the poorer ear may be interfering with the processing of information in the better ear, and a binaural fit may be inappropriate (Jerger et al, 1993). Should an older adult previously fit binaurally come to the clinic reporting a decrement in speech understanding, the audiologist should test the ability to achieve a "fused binaural image." Should evidence emerge suggesting compromised binaural processing, the audiologist might consider removing the hearing aid from the poorer ear or switching to an FM system. Figure 9–19 shows an example of an audiogram and aided speech-recognition scores for a 71-year-old woman showing poorer word-recognition ability for binaurally aided speech than for the better-ear monaurally aided test condition (Musiek & Baran, 1996). It is evident that aided speech-recognition scores were better for the monaurally left-aided test condition.

With regard to CAPD, Stach (1990) provided data demonstrating how the ability to use amplification successfully may be influenced by the presence of a CAPD in one or both ears. In general, his data suggest the following: (1) CAPD adversely affects hearing-aid satisfaction, and (2) hearing-aid satisfaction changes over time as the pattern of the auditory problem progresses from peripheral to central. If one ear shows evidence of CAPD whereas the other does not, the hearing aid should be fit monaurally on the ear with

better peripheral and central auditory processing capabilities. Alternatively, Stach and Stoner (1991) reported that when both ears show evidence of CAPD, an FM system can be successfully used as a supplement to or in lieu of hearing aids. The data recently reported by Chmiel and Jerger (1996) confirmed that elderly persons with central deficits, as measured using dichotically presented sentences (the DSI), show significantly less improvement in self-reported handicap than older adults with a central deficit. Given the latter finding that a CAPD may prevent selected older adults from realizing the full potential of amplification, the hearing-aid selection process should include an estimate of central auditory processing ability to help in deciding on the fitting arrangement and the appropriate amplification system. Musiek and Baran (1996) proposed three potential scenarios for incorporating tests of central auditory processing into the hearing-aid evaluation/process. As depicted in Figure 9–20, one approach could include a central screening test for only those with a positive history of neurological involvement, a second approach could be to include a test of central auditory function for all hearing-aid candidates, and a third would be to conduct a central auditory screen on patients whose hearing aids have become ineffective over time. In my view, both the peripheral and the central auditory systems must be appreciated in the evaluation process. The challenge, of course, is selecting a valid test of central auditory processing ability.

In sum, when the audiogram, speech-recognition data, and physical and financial considerations support a binaural fitting, the older adult should be encouraged to purchase two hearing aids. It is critical to allow time for "physiological and psychological acclimatization" to the hearing aids especially when an ear or ears have been deprived of audi-

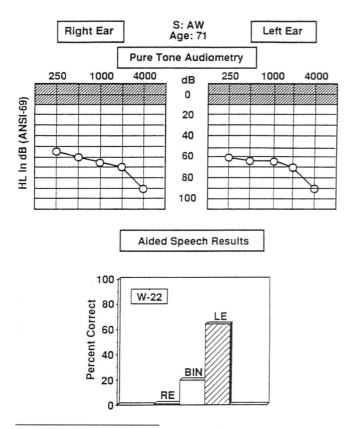

Figure 9–19 Audiogram and aided speech-recognition scores for a 71-year-old woman showing poorer speech-recognition ability for a binaurally aided test condition than for the better-ear monaurally aided test condition. (From Jerger et al, 1993. Reprinted with permission.)

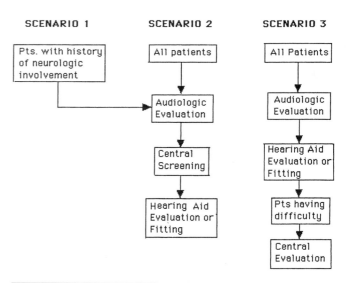

Figure 9–20 Three scenarios demonstrating how central auditory assessment of hearing-aid candidates could be included in the overall evaluation of these clients. (From Valente, 1996, p. 434.)

tory input for an extended period of time. As the typical older adult waits approximately 10 years between first noting

a hearing loss and taking steps toward purchasing a hearing aid, the functional morphology of the auditory system may have been temporarily compromised by acoustic deprivation, necessitating a period of time for the process of adjustment associated with neural plasticity (Musiek & Baran, 1996).

ELECTROACOUSTIC RESPONSE OF THE HEARING AID

In light of technological advances in hearing-aid design, audiologists must make decisions regarding product features that were not, until recently, on the minds of most clinical audiologists. To insure that the frequency-gain characteristics of the hearing aid are shaped to compensate for the loss of audibility, loss of intelligibility, and loss of loudness resulting from impaired hearing, the audiologist has to make a number of technological decisions. These include (1) type of transducer, (2) type of amplifier, (3) circuitry, whether linear or nonlinear, and (4) electroacoustic response of the hearing aid. It is outside the realm of this chapter to present an in-depth discussion of the aforementioned considerations. However, some points relevant to fitting older adults are in order.

Transducer

Transducers, are devices that transform energy in one energy system to energy in another. In essence, transducers function as boundaries between the hearing aid's electrical circuit and the outside world (Madaffari & Stanley, 1996). Transducers used in hearing aids are microphones or telecoils. The model microphone selected by the hearing-aid dispenser can considerably influence the ultimate frequency response of the hearing aid. Some choices available to the dispenser include, but are not limited to, the stepped-response microphone, the omni-directional microphone, the directional microphone, or the well-received dual-microphone directional microphone. In general, the intrinsic microphone-frequency response is essentially flat from the low

frequencies (300 Hz) through the midband to the higher frequencies (4000 to 7000 Hz). The low-frequency response of the internal microphone can generally be modified using an internal microphone vent that, depending on size, reduces the magnitude of low-frequency amplification. Modifications in the frequency response can be introduced through the variety of available options, with the goal generally to compensate for the high-frequency hearing loss that typifies most older adult hearing-aid users. To reiterate, older adults with hearing impairment generally have difficulty separating out the speech signal from background noise. One strategy for improving the SNR is to select a microphone array that can enhance the level of speech relative to the noise.

The stepped-response microphone developed by Killion, is one option. The goal of this microphone design is to achieve a rapid transition in gain as the higher frequencies are approached by avoiding use of a large internal microphone vent that can lead to complete loss of low frequencies. Using a fairly complex structure, the microphone is tailored to produce a relatively constant level at low frequencies and another, higher level, at high frequencies with a rapid transition point in between, typically at 1000 Hz (Madaffari & Stanley, 1996). In contrast, directional-hearing instruments are designed to reduce sound amplification from the rear and sides, rather than amplifying sound from all directions equally, as is the case with omni-directional instruments. In essence, directional microphones are one of the few methods available in hearing instruments for increasing SNR (Preves, 1997). The typical directional microphone is a single microphone with a front and rear port that creates a delay in the time sound (e.g., noise) from the rear reaches of the microphone diaphragm resulting in an improved SNR. While directional microphones have been available for 20 years, they have not gained in popularity because the improvement in speech understanding in difficult listening situations has not been that dramatic. Also, it is only recently that new versions of ITE instruments incorporating directional microphones have become available. They perform as well or better than BTE directional instruments (Preves, 1997).

With the miniaturization of microphones, improved directional microphones are available that use two microphones providing directionality at all frequencies especially high-frequency noise from the rear (Agnew, 1996). Recently, a dual-microphone directional microphone has been introduced that allows the user to select, using a handheld remote control, the dual microphone array or the omnidirectional option. Valente, Fabry, and Potts (1995) recently reported that with the dual-microphone array, the SNR necessary to achieve 50% intelligibility was significantly greater than that achieved with the omnidirectional microphone. Further, mean subjective hearing-aid benefit on the scales of the Profile of Hearing Aid Benefit (PHAB) that assess speech-understanding difficulty in the presence of background noise (BN) or reverberation (RV) was greater than that achieved by the normative group using linear amplification. Their findings suggest that dual microphone arrays may hold promise for older adults whose primary complaint is difficulty understanding speech in the presence of background of noise. In selecting the microphone array, the dispenser should consider the severity of hearing loss, the audiometric configuration, listening difficulties as reported by the client, and, of course, cost and cosmetic concerns. For example, if based on the audiogram, high gain and high output are required, choose the microphone that will deliver high output, free of feedback and distortion. The size of the hearing aid should not be a consideration (Madaffari & Stanley, 1996). ITE instruments that incorporate switch-selectable directional/omnidirectional operating modes should be considered as they may provide more perceived benefit than ITE directional instruments of 20 years ago. In essence, with the switch-selectable ITE, the older adult does not have to be restricted to use of a directional response in all listening situations.

As mentioned earlier, telecoils are a type of transducer used in hearing aids. The two most common uses for telecoils in hearing aids are for telephone pick-up or as the input transducer for a loop system (i.e., assistive device) (Madaffari & Stanley, 1996). As indicated above, because of their larger size, BTE hearing aids easily accommodate a "T" coil if the consumer is willing to assume a slight additional cost. With improved technology, an effective telecoil can now be included in an ITE hearing aid, fulfilling two important functions. First, inclusion of a "T" coil enables persons with more severe hearing loss to use an ITE hearing aid, and second it provides for better overall communication access (Compton, 1996b). The audiologist must ascertain whether the consumer will use the "T" coil for telephone reception, for listening with an ALD, or for both (Compton, 1996b). This information is important as the orientation of the telecoil inside the hearing-aid case differs for hearing aid versus ALD use (Compton, 1996b). For telephone use, a sufficiently sensitive "T" coil can be mounted horizontally (not parallel to the faceplate, however) or vertically. To maximize reception from a room audio-loop installation, the telecoil should be mounted vertically with one end facing skyward and the other end/pole facing the ground (Compton, 1996b). Unless otherwise indicated, hearing-aid manufacturers routinely mount telecoils for telephone use. Some hearing-aid manufacturers include a space on their order forms for the dispenser to indicate whether the "T" coil will be used with a telephone or loop system. Also, to insure that the telecoil is sufficiently sensitive, make sure to note on the form that a preamplifier circuit should be added to the hearing-aid, or merely order a high-power telecoil such as the PowerCoil™ available from Tibbetts Industries (Compton, 1996b). As part of the verification phase of the fitting, the audiologist should make sure, via subjective and objective measurements, that the telecoil is operational. Also, provide ample orientation so that the consumer can maximize their functioning on the telephone and can enjoy access to assistive-listening systems.

While optimally sensitive telecoils facilitate telephone use, the downside is their sensitivity to interference from electromagnetic radiation originating from other electronic equipment such as fluorescent lights, computers, and digital cellular phones (Compton, 1996b). Radiation from sources other than telephone electromagnets and audio loops degrades the speech signal for hearing-aid users. The most difficult problem is created by computer monitors and power transformers that produce intense inductive-radiation fields

making it impossible to use telecoils in their proximity (Compton, 1996b). Compton (1996b) suggests that one can improve the situation by moving away from the computer when using the telecoil option. Similarly, using an incandescent rather than a fluorescent desk lamp can minimize interference, as well. In light of the problems created by inductive interference, it is critical that the orientation session include strategies for overcoming the problems and preparing the hearing aid user for the problems that may eventuate. SHHH and Johns Hopkins have released a video to promote telecoil awareness. It should be made available to consumers during the hearing-aid orientation sessions.

PEARL

Telephone access is critical to older adults so every effort should be made to insure that they can use the telephone effectively.

Amplifier

The amplifier, together with the microphone, receiver, and battery makes up the central core of the hearing instrument (Preves, 1996). In fact, the quality of the signal processing produced by the amplifier, will determine in large part how the individual will do with a given unit. Another important function of the amplifier is to improve the consonant-to-vowel energy ratio so that low-intensity, high-information content consonants may be more easily perceived by hearing-impaired people (Preves, 1996). Amplifiers, which can be single or multiband, consist of three stages: the preamp, the signal processing, and the output stage (Preves, 1996). The preamplifier provides enough gain to amplify incoming signals to a level above the circuit noise of the amplifier. Typically, the amount of gain provided by a preamplifier is relatively low. The signal-processing stage selectively processes the output from the preamp and the output stage further amplifies the processed signals (Preves, 1996). Between stages of amplification, the signal may be filtered or processed in other ways. In most cases, the final signal generally requires an output stage amplifier to provide adequate gain (Fortune, 1996).

Three types of output stage amplifiers are used in current hearing aids with the characteristics of a given hearing loss influencing in part the decision as to which class to recommend. The most common amplifiers are Class A, B, or D. These amplifiers are distinguished from each other according to the manner in which electrical signals are processed and by the efficiency with which battery current is utilized (Fortune, 1996). According to Barry (1998), virtually all hearing-aid preamplifiers operate in Class A. However, Class A is rarely used in the output stage. Contrary to popular opinion, Class A amplifiers are typified by very low distortion, as long as the instrument is operating in the linear range (Barry, 1998). Class A amplifiers are desirable in that they are small in physical size, fit easily into small hearing aids, are reliable, and require little circuitry to operate (Fortune, 1996). The disadvantages of Class A amplifiers include their limited dynamic range and the fact that it continuously draws battery current even when a signal is not present (useful battery life is about 1 to 2 days). Thus, the battery life is low for hearing aids with Class A amplifiers. Class A amplifiers are most appropriate for low gain and low output sound pressure levels (SPLs). Accordingly, individuals with low gain requirements are well suited to Class A amplifiers. Of course, in light of their high battery drain, the high battery costs may be a disadvantage.

PEARL

Class B amplifiers provide low-distortion, high-power amplification in a compact package with greater efficiency than a Class A operation (Barry, 1998).

The Class B or push-pull amplifier consists of two amplifiers, each acting on a different phase of the incoming signal. When the amplifiers are idle, current drain is minimal, yet when high output SPLs and high current are required the amplifiers are capable of generating the necessary signal. In contrast to Class A amplifiers, which produce asymmetrical peak clipping, at high input or gain, Class B amplifiers produce symmetrical clipping. The latter is less objectionable to the listener. The battery life associated with Class B amplifiers is higher than that associated with Class A amplifiers. The Class D amplifier is a more efficient signal processer than Class A amplifiers and operates in a manner distinct from both Class A and Class B amplifiers. Electroacoustically, Class D amplifiers are comparable in many ways to the Class B amplifier. For example, they both produce symmetrical peak clipping upon saturation, and similar gain and SSPL 90 values can be produced with either output stage. Both generate an amplified acoustic signal with efficient use of battery current, but expected battery life is slightly higher with the Class D amplifier (Fortune, 1996). However, a Class D amplifier is 30 to 40% more efficient than a Class B circuit that is projected to equal 4 weeks rather than 3 weeks of useful battery life (Barry, 1998). As compared to Class A amplifiers, mean-aided loudness discomfort level (LDL) ratings for hearing-impaired listeners are approximately 6 dB higher with Class D amplifiers and sound quality ratings are preferable, as well. Overall, it appears that Class B and D amplifiers are less likely to distort and maintain high sound quality as compared to Class A amplifiers.

SPECIAL CONSIDERATION

Most hearing-impaired persons, especially the elderly, are more appropriately fit with Class B or Class D amplifiers due to their efficient use of battery drain, the greater gain and output SPLs associated with these devices, their improved headroom, and better sound quality at higher levels (Fortune, 1996).

While linear instruments with a Class D ouptut stage provide for good sound quality, nonlinear forms of signal processing are gaining in popularity because of their overall superior performance. Nonlinear amplification is less likely to generate saturation-induced distortion than comparable linear aids because they use some form of compression (Fortune, 1996).

Linear Versus Nonlinear

The sensorineural hearing loss characterizing older adults is associated with a decrease in auditory sensitivity as well as a loss of ability to resolve temporal as well as spectral information. Specifically, damage to the inner hair cells affects the cochlea's signal processing ability, while damage to the outer hair cells alters audibility of the signal (Bächler, Knecht, Launer, & Uvacek, 1997). Most important, the hearing loss varies with frequency and the mentioned deficits are often frequency dependent. The task of maximizing audibility and speech-recognition ability through hearing aids is thus considerably challenging in older adults (Fortune, 1996). The goal of restoring audibility and listening comfort in quiet and noise across as wide a range of frequencies can oftentimes be accomplished via careful consideration of the appropriateness of a given circuit type. Accordingly, one of the most important decisions the audiologist must make relates to hearing-aid circuit design. That is, should the circuit be linear or nonlinear? The most commonly used amplifier in hearing aids is the linear amplifier. A linear hearing aid is one that maintains a 1:1 input/output (I/O) function across its unsaturated operating range. For a linear instrument, the I/O curve appears as a straight line sloping upward at a 45°angle. Once the amplifier reaches saturation, the output is limited and it is not possible for the output of the hearing aid to increase beyond its saturation level. Nonlinear amplification implies some type of level dependent processing such that gain at a particular frequency varies with the input level. In essence, gain is reduced as input or output level increases such that the I/O function has a slope of less than 1.0 over some part of the operating range of the hearing aid (Fortune, 1996).

Linear and nonlinear algorithms are designed to perform two basic functions that include amplifying a wide variety of environmental sounds so that they become audible to the hearing-impaired listener without being uncomfortably loud and minimizing the potential for the hearing aid going into saturation (Fortune, 1996). As both functions become increasingly difficult with linear hearing aids for individuals with a small dynamic range, nonlinear hearing aids are theoretically more successful at providing comfortable amplification and are less likely to produce saturation-induced distortion (Fortune, 1996). With regard to the latter, Fortune (1996) suggested that the decision to limit the output of a hearing aid should be based on two interrelated goals, namely, the desire to avoid excessive distortion combined with the desire to insure listener comfort (i.e., prevent loudness discomfort). Listener comfort is an especially important feature to older adults with impaired hearing.

Fortune (1996) suggests that linear amplification is ideal for individuals fitting one of the following profiles. Persons with mild hearing loss who require only small amounts of gain continue to benefit from the sound quality inherent in low-gain linear hearing aids. Further, persons with severe to profound hearing loss who cannot achieve enough gain with nonlinear hearing aids may prefer linear devices due to the improved audibility they provide. Finally, persons who are "accustomed" to linear hearing aids often prefer the sound quality of this form of amplification and thus should be encouraged to "stay the course." In this regard, older adults who have demonstrated the latter form of acclimatization may be best served with linear amplification. The use of Class B or D amplifiers can help to minimize the negative effects of saturation-induced distortion. The advantage of minimizing saturation-induced distortion is that sound quality can be maximized while at the same time allowing for a higher aided LDL (Fortune, 1996).

Nonlinear amplification systems, which are more likely than comparable linear hearing aids to provide comfortable amplification with minimal saturation-induced distortion, are desirable in selected situations. In general, individuals with dynamic ranges of less than 30 dB are the most suitable candidates for nonlinear hearing aids. In these cases, it may not be possible to adjust gain and frequency response in such a way as to provide audibility without discomfort (Fortune, 1996). Compression appears to minimize the need

---

SPECIAL CONSIDERATION

Nonlinear amplification may be desirable with older adults as these systems provide low-distortion limiting, reduce noise, can improve audibility for soft sounds, can normalize loudness perceptions, and can minimize the need for volume-control adjustments (Byrne, 1996). Nonlinear hearing instruments provide maximum gain at low input levels.

---

for volume adjustments making hearing aid usage easier and more comfortable (Byrne, 1996).

Three of the most common types of nonlinear algorithms include (1) algorithms that provide compression (an appropriate alternative to linear hearing aids for individuals having a large dynamic range yet the need to prevent loudness discomfort remains), (2) bass increase at low levels (BILL), and (3) treble increase at low levels (TILL). BILL and TILL are considered categories of amplifiers with level-dependent frequency response (LDFR) (Starkey, 1997). Amplifiers with LDFR provide a different frequency response for different input levels.

Algorithms that provide compression in hearing aids have been designed to compensate for the abnormally rapid growth of loudness that accompanies some sensorineural hearing loss, and often results in a reduced dynamic range. Compression amplifiers are available in three broad categories, namely, automatic gain control (AGC), syllabic compression, and compression limiting (Fortune, 1996). The suitability of one type of compression over the other depends on the client's audiometric profile, especially their

dynamic range and frequency-specific loudness-discomfort levels. For example, compression limiting is well suited to individuals with a wide dynamic range (>30 dB), yet the audiologist wants to prevent loudness discomfort. Thus, as compression limiting provides a buffer for loud sounds while amplifying soft sounds, it may be used to reduce the SSPL-90 for persons with a reduced tolerance to loud sounds. In this case, the output is reduced to keep it below the discomfort level and out of distortion (Starkey, 1997). In contrast, an AGC circuit may be appropriate for an older adult who is frequently exposed to changing sound levels, but is not disturbed by occasional impulsive-type sounds, such as an individual who is semiretired and attends lectures at a variety of facilities including the neighborhood Y, a church, or a local college campus. Finally, syllabic compression may be the circuitry of choice for an individual with a narrow dynamic range (<30 dB) (Fortune, 1996). Fast AGC circuits with low compression thresholds (e.g., wide dynamic range compressions or syllabic compressions) can be used effectively to compensate for recruitment (Bächler, Knecht, Launer, & Uvacek, 1997).

BILL, a LDFR-type circuit, is a form of signal processing that describes the action of hearing aids commonly known as ASP, automatic noise reduction (ANR), or adaptive frequency response (AFR) instruments. BILL-type hearing aids provide a level-dependent frequency response in which low-frequency gain varies with input level (Fortune, 1996). The intent of this signal-processing approach is to reduce amplification of low-frequency background noise as its level increases, thereby reducing the upward spread of masking and ultimately speech intelligibility (Stypulkowski, Raskind, & Hodgson, 1992). In a sense, this form of signal processing responds differently in quiet and in noisy backgrounds and is thus an important option for older adults with complaints of "difficulty understanding speech in noise." It is ideal for older adults exposed to a good deal of environmental noise. Further, this type of circuitry might be recommended for an older adult with a gently sloping or flat configuration loss (Starkey, 1997).

Researchers are currently gathering data to determine the actual advantages of BILL processing over a linear hearing aid. Humes, Christensen, Bess, and Williams (1997) recently completed a study comparing the benefit of well-fit linear hearing aids to instruments with automatic reductions of low-frequency gain, namely BILL-based processing. Subjects of all ages participated but the conclusions are applicable to older adults. Participants presented with symmetrical sensorineural hearing loss that was flat or gently sloping in configuration. Approximately 41 subjects had mild hearing loss, 53 had moderate sensorineural loss, and 16 had severe hearing loss (Humes et al, 1997). Participants were new hearing-aid users fit binaurally with custom ITC hearing aids manufactured by one hearing-aid company. Test hearing aids included an experimental BILL circuit that reduced the amount of gain in the low frequencies as the input intensity increased. It was equipped with a manually adjustable potentiometer that enabled the audiologist to deactivate the BILL circuit. The threshold for activation of the BILL processing was 60 dBSPL. Deactivating the circuit created a linear circuit, which included an output stage characterized by low-distortion peak clipping, reduced low-frequency circuit noise, and low current drain. Hearing-aid benefit was assessed after a 2-month adjustment period to allow for maturation of hearing-aid benefit or acclimatization. Outcome or benefit was assessed using a number of subjective and objective measures. Aided speech-recognition ability using the Connected Speech Test (CST) and the NU-6 word lists presented in a background of noise provided information about improvement in speech understanding. The Hearing Aid Performance Inventory (HAPI) was used to measure the participant's perceptions of the benefit provided by the hearing aid in daily life.

Interestingly, there was significant benefit provided by each hearing-aid circuit, across outcome measures, as compared to unaided listening (Humes et al, 1997). Further, participants reported wearing their hearing aids for approximately 7 to 9 hours per day, suggesting satisfaction with the units. According to responses to the HAPI, participants rated their hearing aids as being beneficial in a variety of listening situations. It is noteworthy that equivalent benefit in speech understanding was measured for the linear and BILL processing circuits. That is, BILL processing did not appear to provide better aided performance on tests of speech understanding in noise than that achieved with the linear circuit. Further, HAPI scores did not differ for the linear or BILL settings, although there was a trend toward a preference for the linear setting across hearing-loss groups. Interestingly, the severe group expressed a notable preference for the linear setting in that the mean HAPI score for the linear setting was 1.88 versus 2.11 for the BILL setting. On the HAPI a rating of "1" suggests that the hearing aid is very helpful whereas a rating of "2" would suggest that the hearing aid is helpful. Their data confirm the beneficial effects of hearing aids, however an advantage of BILL processing over linear circuitry did not emerge.

TILL-type signal processing was first described by Killion, Staab, and Preves (1990). The philosophy behind this approach is that loud sounds do not have to be amplified at all, however quiet sounds do need amplification to be heard by the hearing impaired. This processing scheme provides maximum gain in the high frequencies for low input levels, yet as input level increases there is a reduction in high pass gain, with a goal being unity gain or a flat response. The TILL system is akin to the K-AMP™ hearing aid. TILL-type hearing aids are ideal for older adults with sloping high-frequency hearing loss who require high-frequency gain in quiet yet minimal gain in high-level environments (Fortune, 1996). With TILL circuits, the gain for soft high-frequency sounds is considerable whereas the gain for high-level sounds is minimal (Starkey, 1997).

As indicated in the discussion of programmable hearing aids, compression, TILL- and BILL-type signal processing are not mutually exclusive and a variety of combinations are available through multiband compression circuits. Multiband compression circuits come in a wide variety of forms, some combine linear processing in one band with compression in another, while others combine different types of compression in each band. It is beyond the scope of this chapter to discuss the variety of nonlinear algorithms available in great depth. As they are a consideration for older

adults with compromised speech recognition when the SNR is poor, audiologists working with older adults are encouraged to familiarize themselves with the options available.

Newman and Sandridge (1998) and Humes et al (1999) recently reported that high performance hearing aids do provide benefit over the unaided condition. Kochkin (1997) also reported that high performance instruments yield higher than average ratings on key outcome measures, including overall satisfaction, quality of life, and perceptions of improvement.

SELECTING THE APPROPRIATE ELECTROACOUSTIC RESPONSE OF THE HEARING AID

This chapter will not discuss at any great length strategies for selecting the hearing-aid response for older adults. For the most part, the rules and strategies used with younger adults pertain to older adults. Simply put, an optimal hearing-aid fitting is one that makes speech audible without exceeding the listener's loudness-discomfort level, restores the normal loudness relations for speech and other environmental sounds, and enhances speech intelligibility (Cox, 1995). It goes without saying that the hearing aid should feel comfortable within the user's ears. The leading complaint of older adults rejecting hearing aids is that they make sounds too loud and that they amplify speech and noise to the same extent, which interferes with understanding. Carefully selecting hearing-aid parameters that amplify a wide range of environmental sounds so that they are audible without being uncomfortably loud is an important challenge for audiologists. Similarly, providing comfortable amplification without generating saturation-induced distortion is critical to insure the satisfaction of the user (Fortune, 1996).

Prescriptive formulas used for selecting frequency-gain characteristics and setting the SSPL-90 are typically based on threshold measures and suprathreshold judgments of comfort and discomfort at each ear. Prescriptive formulas like the National Acoustic Laboratory–Revised (NAL-R) and Prescription of Gain/Output (POGO) provide widely accepted guidance for selecting gain and frequency response for use with linear hearing instruments (Studebaker, Bess, & Beck, 1991). Frequency-specific tests of suprathreshold loudness discomfort should be used to help set the SSPL-90 thereby preventing the loudness discomfort associated with overamplification, so common among older adults. Threshold-based strategies for adjusting gain and frequency response are not well suited to fitting nonlinear hearing aids as they do not provide for a way to fit level-dependent signal processing where gain varies as a function of input levels to the device or output from the device (Fortune, 1996). That is they do not take into account level-dependent gain requirements (Starkey, 1997).

In response to the shortcomings associated with conventional prescriptive formulas, quantification of suprathreshold information, such as loudness growth, or "fitting by loudness strategies (FBL)" may be more appropriate for achieving the loudness-based objectives of nonlinear amplification (Ricketts & Van Vliet, 1996). Formulas for fitting nonlinear hearing aids have emerged as this form of amplification is seen as an acceptable approach to fitting hearing-impaired persons requiring audibility without discomfort. By design, target gain must be established for soft and loud speech as well as average speech. Multiple targets are necessary to enable the audiologist to correctly fit hearing aids that best match compression parameters with overall gain settings (Mueller, 1996). These formulas, which are used to select targets for nonlinear hearing devices and for selecting special circuit options, are based on comparisons of the hearing-impaired person's perception of loudness to the normal perception of loudness (Starkey, 1997). For the most part, these strategies either attempt to restore normal loudness impression or a normal dynamic range (Ricketts & Van Vliet, 1996). As of this writing, the generic prescription formula for fitting nonlinear hearing aids includes the Visual Input-Output Locator Algorithm (VIOLA) based on the Contour test procedure recommended by the International Hearing Aid Fitting Forum (IHAFF), the Desired Sensation Level Formula (DSL I/O), the NAL-NL1 (version 1) and FIG 6 (Cox, 1999). These programs, each of which is referenced to a different value, can be helpful as a starting point for selecting the appropriate electroacoustic response for a given hearing aid, including the ideal SPL targets for a variety of inputs, and frequency-specific compression ratios (Mueller, 1996).

VIOLA requires clinical measures of loudness growth using the loudness growth test. The loudness perception data is obtained at the prefitting using the Contour test procedure (Cox, 1999). The IHAFF philosophy is that compression amplification should normalize the relationship between environmental sounds and loudness perception (Cox, 1995). IHAFF software is a DOS program intended for an IBM or compatible PC. Recently, Cox (1999) suggested that computerized loudness testing is prone to error, so she advocates computer scoring with loudness testing administered by a "human being"! FIG 6 described by Killion assumes average loudness growth data (Ricketts & Van Vliet, 1996). FIG 6 is a threshold-based formula that relies on average loudness growth data for normal and hearing-impaired listeners. Software is available from Etymotic Research. Finally, the objective of the DSL I/O formula which is based on the Desired Sensation Level Formula is to place amplified speech sounds within a listener's dynamic range. It relies on threshold levels and measured or predicted thresholds of discomfort. The goal of DSL I/O is to amplify all sounds occurring in the normal dynamic range into the hearing-impaired dynamic range so that the output of the

SPECIAL CONSIDERATION

Algorithms for fitting nonlinear hearing aids have gained widespread use despite the lack of validity data.

hearing aid falls between the hearing-impaired threshold and discomfort levels. Software is available from the Hearing Health Care Research Unit at the University of Western

Ontario. Ricketts and Van Vliet (1996) provide a useful update on fitting strategies, referred to as FBL, which obtain and use suprathreshold information for obtaining prescriptive gain and compression parameters for nonlinear versus linear amplification.

It is important to note that while the above formulas have recently been advocated by a number of clinical and research audiologists, they have not been validated. Further, certain of these procedures may be difficult for some older adults. The use of frequency-specific loudness-discomfort levels, speech uncomfortable levels/most comfortable levels (UCL/MCL) should not be abandoned. Frequency-specific UCL data in combination with threshold data, for example, can be used to assure that the output of the hearing aid falls between the hearing-impaired threshold and discomfort levels. Most older adults will have no problem following the directions and making the loudness judgments necessary for a frequency-specific map of loudness-discomfort levels. The loudness categories should be written out in large print and reviewed with the patient. The seven-point loudness rating scale described by the IHAFF (1994) group can be used. Loudness categories range from very soft, to soft, to comfortable but slightly soft, to comfortable, to comfortable but slightly loud, to loud but okay, to uncomfortably loud. Older adults should be given the opportunity to practice the procedure used during tests of loudness evaluation. While the most common use of probe-microphone measures is to compare actual gain with a prescriptive target, use of broadband noise at different input levels ranging from 50 to 90 dBSPL when selecting nonlinear hearing aids should be considered (Starkey, 1997; Fabry, 1996). Real ear measures in conjunction with compression amplifiers can be used successfully to estimate the overall gain level and frequency response shape using various input levels (Starkey, 1997).

VERIFYING THE HEARING-AID FIT

Once the electroacoustic response has been selected, the target met, and the hearing aid dispensed, it is the responsibility of the audiologist to verify that the goals of the hearing-aid fitting are achieved. That is: (1) are the variety of speech inputs to which the client is exposed audible, comfortable, and tolerable across as wide a frequency range as possible; (2) do the electroacoustic characteristics necessary to achieve target produce maximum speech recognition and sound quality; and (3) have the communication and psychosocial handicaps associated with hearing loss been adequately addressed?

The procedures used during the verification phase of the hearing-aid fitting should be closely tied to the preselection and selection process. Further, the verification visits should be scheduled over a 1-year time interval to monitor short-term, medium-term, and long-term adaptation to the hearing aid. Monitoring the response of the hearing aid over time allows for acclimatization and adjustment. In short, it enables the audiologist to modify the response of the unit in reaction to the client's amplification experiences and their changing expectations as exposure to amplified sound increases. At each follow-up visit the client should be actively involved to enable the audiologist to make the fine adjustments conducive to a comfortable and acceptable fitting (Studebaker, Bess, & Beck, 1991). Fine-tuning the instrument to better match the client's auditory preferences is especially important when fitting nonlinear amplification systems, multichannel, and noise-reduction systems (McCandless, 1994).

The 1990 Consensus Statement for "Recommended Components of a Hearing Aid Selection Procedure for Adults," suggested that verification strategies incorporate the individual's perceptions about the adequacy of their amplification system. In a sense, the latter relates to the concept of

---

SPECIAL CONSIDERATION

It is incumbent on the audiologist to see how the older client is doing with the hearing aid, and to determine if the client likes the fit as much as the audiologist does (Mueller, 1996).

---

treatment efficacy. The Office of Technology Assessment (1978, p. 16) defines treatment efficacy as the "probability of benefit to individuals in a defined population from a medical technology applied for a given medical problem under ideal conditions of use." The term *treatment efficacy* addresses several questions related to quality (Are we meeting the client's expectations?), treatment effectiveness (Do hearing aids work?), and treatment effects (In what way does the use of hearing aids alter behavior?) (Olswang, Thompson, Warren, & Minghetti, 1990).

Hearing-aid benefit is inferred from scores on outcome measures that identify and quantify the overall advantage attributable to the intervention (Montgomery, 1994). Benefit must be expressed with respect to a frame of reference (e.g., baseline information) and relative to a specific significance level (e.g., 95% confidence intervals). In the arena of the hearing-aid fitting and audiologic rehabilitation, benefit is being quantified in terms of performance on self-assessment tools that measure two important domains of function, namely, disability and/or handicap. The recent proliferation of disability and handicap questionnaires enables the clinician to quantify objectively treatment efficacy (Hyde & Riko, 1994). According to McCarthy (1996), most of the measurement tools used to date to measure benefit are disorder specific and of the self-report variety.

Available disability and handicap questionnaires focus attention on what the patient is telling the audiologist rather than on what audiometric test results suggest. One reason for more widespread acceptance of asking the hearing-impaired consumer to judge how he or she feels about a given hearing impairment and their function in the presence of the condition, is the availability of measures that are reproducible, valid, and responsive. An additional factor is the advent of newer, more costly hearing-aid technologies that demand justification of the value of an intervention. Thus, the impact of a particular device on audibility of pure-tone and speech signals (impairment), communication in se-

lected situations (disability), and corresponding well being and psychosocial function (handicap) is of utmost importance. Data are beginning to emerge demonstrating that as criterion measures, self-report measures yield information on the ability of hearing aids to reduce the communicative disability and psychosocial handicap associated with hearing impairment in older adults.

The HHIE and a companion scale, the HHIE-S (Appendices B and C, Chapter 8), are widely used clinical tools for measuring self-reported outcomes with hearing aids in older adults because of their reliability and validity and because benefit in the handicap domain can be measured quickly and efficiently. Approximately half of the items assess the self-perceived emotional (E) consequences of hearing loss, and half assess the social/situational consequences (S). The HHIE contains 25 items whereas the HHIE-S is much shorter, having only 10 items. Scores range from 0 to 100% on the HHIE and from 0 to 40% on the HHIE-S, the higher the score the more handicapped the individual. Differences between unaided and aided scores on each scale enable the audiologist to infer benefit. The 95% confidence interval (or critical difference value) associated with the HHIE is 18.7, while the 95% confidence interval for the HHIE-S is 10. Thus, if prior to obtaining a hearing aid an older adult obtained a score of 60 on the HHIE-S and following 3 weeks of hearing-aid use the score improved to 30, significant benefit has been achieved, albeit some residual handicap remains.

The APHAB (Appendix A, Chapter 8) consists of 24 items scored on four 6-item subscales including ease of communication, background noise, reverberation, and aversiveness of sound. Respondents complete the APHAB under both aided and unaided conditions following the hearing-aid fitting. The response format entails indicating the percent of time the individual experiences problems hearing under the situations described in the questionnaire. Hearing-aid benefit in the disability domain is operationally defined as a change score indicative of hearing problem reduction. Further, a respondent's score on each scale can be compared to equal percentile profiles for APHAB subscales developed by Cox and Alexander (1995) on a sample of successful hearing-aid users. Norms for the the APHAB are based on responses obtained at one sitting with the respondent rating frequency of difficulty in a given listening condition twice, once without their hearing aid and once with their hearing aid. It is recommended that older adults respond to the APHAB on two occasions, at the time of the audiological evaluation and during the postfitting or verification phase. This separation in time will probably be less demanding and will likely increase the validity of responses. Additional outcome measures, although not designed specifically for older adults, include the Client Oriented Scale of Improvement, the Glasgow Hearing Aid Benefit Profile, the Satisfaction with Amplification in Daily Life (SADL), and the Expected Consequences of Hearing Aid Ownership (Cox, 1999). The Perception of Aided Loudness (PAL) developed by Mueller and Palmer (1998) assesses self-reported benefit in the loudness domain.

A number of studies have recently been conducted using the above scales for quantifying benefit in the disability

TABLE 9–6 Focus of Hearing-Aid Outcome Studies

- Short-term benefit from hearing aids in new users using disorder-specific quality-of-life measures
- Medium-term benefit from hearing aids in new users using disorder specific quality-of-life measures
- Long-term benefit of hearing aid aids in new users using disorder-specific quality-of-life measures
- Benefit from hearing aids using disorder-specific versus generic quality-of-life measures
- The influence of counseling based audiologic rehabilitation on hearing-aid benefit in the handicap domain
- The influence of listening training on hearing-aid benefit in the disability domain
- Acclimatization to hearing aids in the psychosocial domain
- Audiologic and nonaudiologic correlates of hearing-aid benefit using disorder-specific quality-of-life measures
- Cost benefit of hearing aids
- Personality correlates of benefit

and/or handicap domains. The majority of subjects in the studies have been older adults as this is representative of the vast majority of hearing-impaired individuals who own hearing aids. According to the studies, the majority of hearing-instrument owners are well served by their hearing instruments. Table 9–6 summarizes the focus of the outcome studies conducted on older hearing-aid users. The outcomes on the studies in each of the areas are summarized in the following paragraphs.

BENEFITS ASSOCIATED WITH HEARING AIDS

Short-Term Benefits from Hearing Aids

A number of studies have been conducted to determine whether in fact the benefits associated with hearing aids, namely, improvement in communication function and reduction in psychosocial handicap emerge within 3 weeks of first using a hearing aid. Interestingly, the subjects in most

PEARL

The overwhelming majority of studies in this area have demonstrated that hearing aids worn by new or experienced users do in fact improve speech communication ability in general and psychosocial handicap in particular.

of the studies demonstrating short-term benefit were older, fit monaurally, and received only 45 to 60 minutes of hearing-aid orientation/counseling at the time of the fitting.

Benefit, as defined by the difference between aided and unaided performance, was demonstrable in some of the studies in nearly 70 to 80% of subjects fit with hearing aids. Most notable among the studies was that conducted by Malinoff and Weinstein (1989), Newman et al (1991), and Primeau (1997) using the HHIE or HHIE-S as the dependent variable, namely, benefit in the handicap domain.

In the study by Malinoff and Weinstein (1989) each of the 45 subjects had mild to moderate bilateral sensorineural hearing loss, were fit with ITE hearing aids, and were recruited from the hearing-aid dispensary at an eye, ear, and throat hospital in a major metropolitan area. Following a rather brief period of hearing-aid use, there was a statistically and clinically significant reduction in self-perceived hearing handicap in the emotional and social domains of function. Nearly 80% of subjects in this study had mean scores differing by more than 18%, the value that reflects the 95% confidence interval for a true change attributed to intervention (Weinstein, Spitzer, & Ventry, 1986).

In a larger scale study ($N = 91$), Newman et al (1991) explored the short-term benefits of hearing aids. Once again, the majority of subjects had mild to moderate sensorineural hearing loss. Mean scores on the total, emotional, and social subscales of the HHIE-S improved dramatically and significantly after short-term hearing-aid use. Using 10 points as the 95% confidence interval for computing a true change in HHIE-S scores, 78% of subjects demonstrated a true change/reduction in perceived hearing handicap, whereas 7% of subjects did not reach the criterion for a significant change in handicap (Newman et al, 1991). The remaining proportion of subjects (i.e., 15%) had total handicap scores that were less than the confidence interval of 10, and thus were not eligible to be included in this computation. The authors concluded that these data confirm the beneficial effects of hearing-aid use among older adults.

Primeau (1997) reported on the efficacy of hearing aids worn by a population of 233 veterans ranging in age from 27 to 97 years, with a mean age of 65.5 years. The majority of subjects had mild to moderately severe, adult onset, bilaterally symmetric, sensorineural hearing losses and were fit binaurally with ITE hearing aids. Prior to obtaining the hearing aid(s) and each of the 6 weeks following the initial fitting, patients completed the screening version of the Hearing Handicap Inventory for Adults (HHIA-S) or the screening version of the HHIE to determine the short-term benefit of hearing aids. Of the 233 individuals obtaining hearing aids, 181 (77.7%) experienced a significant reduction in self-perceived handicap with hearing-aid use. It was of interest that young and older adults were similar in the amount of perceived psychosocial handicap experienced prior to and following hearing-aid use and hence in the magnitude of benefit in the psychosocial domain. In addition, new and experienced hearing-aid users were comparable in terms of the magnitude of perceived benefit in the psychosocial domain.

Cox and Alexander (1995) demonstrated that hearing aids provide a statistically significant short-term benefit in a variety of listening situations according to improvements in scores on selected scales of the APHAB following 3 months of hearing-aid use. In their sample of 22 older adults who were new hearing-aid users, significant improvement in communication ability in various daily life situations emerged for the majority of respondents. Despite dramatic benefit in the disability domain, a number of subjects still chose to return their hearing aids. In their view, the benefit may not have been sufficient to warrant the purchase (Cox & Alexander, 1995). It was notable that all persons choosing to keep their hearing aids scored higher on the EC, RV, and BN subscales than those choosing to return their aids. Their data, albeit based on a research group, suggest that a

> ## SPECIAL CONSIDERATION
>
> **In light of their findings, the authors tentatively concluded that the amount of reported benefit in the disability domain (i.e., difference scores on the APHAB) is not always enough to make the hearing-aid purchase worthwhile for the hearing-impaired individual.**

number of variables contribute to the decision to purchase amplification and that scores on individual scales as well as overall benefit should be considered.

Humes, Halling, and Coughlin (1996) followed a sample of 20 older adults with mild to moderately severe, bilaterally symmetrical, high-frequency sensorineural hearing loss with various hearing-aid use histories (e.g., some subjects were new users, some were experienced). Subjects were fit with binaural multiple memory ITE hearing aids. A close match to NAL-R target was achieved, and verified over time, for the majority of subjects, with NAL targets reduced by 5 dB at all frequencies for both ears to allow for binaural loudness summation (Humes, Halling, & Coughlin, 1996). Subjects completed the Hearing Aid Performance Inventory (HAPI) and the HHIE at several intervals including 20, 40, 60, 80, and 180 days postfitting. The HAPI is considered a measure of auditory disability and the HHIE is considered a measure of psychosocial handicap. Overall, subjects experienced significant amounts of benefit in the disability domain and the handicap domains following even a brief interval of hearing-aid use, namely 2 to 3 weeks postfit. It was notable that short-term benefit was comparable to long-term benefit suggesting little acclimatization with the multiple-memory hearing aids.

In sum, it is clear from the studies above that positive outcomes with hearing aids emerge soon after the initial fitting. The selected studies reviewed in the following paragraphs suggest that benefit over time may vary. Some studies show changes in benefit scores in either a positive or negative direction over time, while others show no change in benefit over time. The variability in benefit may reflect the timing at which outcomes were measured or subject factors such as the magnitude of initial benefit derived from the hearing aid.

Medium-Term Benefits from Hearing Aids

In an attempt to determine whether hearing-aid benefit changes over time as the client learns to make use of newly available speech cues made audible by the hearing instrument, a number of investigators have explored the time course of hearing-aid benefit (Turner, Humes, Bentler, & Cox, 1996). As part of their investigation into the impact of financial outlay on self-perceived hearing-aid benefit, Newman et al (1993) evaluated the short- (3-week) and long-term (6-month) benefit of hearing aids on a sample of adults 65 to 85 years of age. Subjects were new hearing-aid users with essentially mild to moderate sensorineural hearing loss, approximately half of the subjects paid privately for their hearing aids and an age-matched group had a health insurance policy that paid for the hearing aid. Each group of subjects demonstrated a statistically and clinically significant reduction in perceived emotional and social handicap following short- and long-term hearing-aid use. It was of interest however, that for both groups short-term benefit in the psychosocial domain was somewhat greater than medium-term benefit. That is, while statistically and clinically significant, the magnitude of the benefit score (aided—unaided HHIE score) was greater at 3 weeks than at 6 months. This finding suggests that perhaps exposure to the variety of listening situations afforded by amplification may lead to some form of psychosocial acclimatization over time. Accordingly, the client may continue to feel some advantage in the psychosocial domain. However, some of the inherent limitations in hearing-aid technology may temper enthusiasm.

The data of Taylor (1993) corroborate the findings of Newman et al (1993). The majority of the 58 subjects were older, had mild to moderate sensorineural hearing loss, were first-time hearing-aid users, and purchased ITE hearing aids. Performance of subjects on an objective speech-recognition test, namely, the NU-6 monosyllabic word lists, and on the more subjective HHIE, was monitored over time at baseline, 3 weeks, 3 months, 6 months, and 1 year following hearing-aid use. As in previously described studies, most of the subjects (78%) demonstrated statistically and clinically significant reductions in HHIE scores after 3 weeks of hearing-aid use. Taylor (1993) found significant differences in HHIE scores at baseline, 3 weeks, 3 months, 6 months, and 1 year following the initial hearing-aid fitting. The most dramatic reduction in social and emotional function emerged just 3 weeks after hearing-aid use. Interestingly, mean scores on the HHIE rose significantly after 3 months of hearing-aid use but stabilized after 6 months and 1 year, suggesting some form of acclimatization in the psychosocial domain. In contrast, no significant change in aided word-recognition ability in quiet or noise were noted over time. These data corroborate that a period of accommodation or adaptation tends to occur within the first several months of hearing-aid use most notably in the psychosocial domain (Taylor, 1993). In this form of psychosocial acclimatization following exposure to varied listening experiences, the patient experiences some of the limitations inherent in hearing-aid technology, but continues to feel the advantage in the psychosocial domain over their unaided hearing. Their study did not support the concept of acclimatization when monitoring outcomes with monosyllabic word lists such as the NU-6s.

The most comprehensive, randomized, controlled clinical trial of the short- and medium-term benefits of hearing aids was conducted on a sample of male veterans (Mulrow, Aguilar, Endicott, Tuley, Velez, Charlip, Rhodes, Hill, &

Denino, 1990). One hundred ninety-four older adults with mild to moderately severe sensorineural hearing loss participated. Half of the subjects were assigned to a hearing-aid group and the other half to a waiting list group. Each group was matched on important demographic and clinical characteristics. Ninety-eight percent of individuals in the hearing-aid group received monaural ITE hearing aids. Hearing-aid benefit was defined as a multidimensional phenomenon, according to the amount of improvement in scores on a variety of quality-of-life measures. The domains of function that were tapped included the social, emotional, cognitive, physical, and psychological. Responses to items on the disorder-specific HHIE provided data on the perceived emotional and social effects of hearing loss. The other disorder-specific outcome measure was the Denver Scale of Communication Function (DSCF) that provided an estimate of perceived communication function. Subjects completed each of these disorder-specific quality-of-life measures at baseline and at 6-week and 4-month follow-up visits. Mean scores on each of these measures were comparable at baseline between subjects in the control (waiting list) and experimental (hearing-aid recipients) groups.

Hearing-aid treatment effects were noted on each of the disorder-specific quality-of-life outcome measures for the experimental group at both the 6-week and 4-month follow-ups. While dramatic improvements in social and emotional function as assessed by the HHIE emerged in the hearing-aid group, mean scores for the control group remained the same. Similarly, the hearing-aid group demonstrated significant improvement in communication function as measured on the DSCF, whereas no change in communication function was noted for the waiting-list group. Of interest was the finding that benefit, according to the difference between unaided and aided responses to items on the HHIE and the DSCF, emerged 6 weeks after receipt of the hearing aid was sustained at the 4-month follow-up (Mulrow et al, 1990). That is, hearing-aid benefit at 4 months following hearing-aid use was comparable to that obtained as early as 6 weeks following the initial fitting. The authors concluded that their study established that hearing aids do in fact improve the quality of life of persons with hearing loss and that short- and medium-term effects are most pronounced when using disorder-specific quality-of-life instruments. In this study, psychosocial acclimatization is not evident. This may be because of the time intervals at which benefit was measured, namely 6 weeks and 4 months following the initial hearing-aid fitting.

Tesch-Romer (1997) recently completed a quasi experimental study of the medium-term benefits (i.e., 6 months) of hearing-aid use. Outcomes were assessed in a number of domains of functioning including psychosocial well being as measured by score on the German version of the HHIE. Seventy individuals were assigned to the "aural rehabilitation group—those obtaining hearing aids," 42 to the hearing-impaired control group, and 28 to the normal-hearing control group. The average age of participants was 71.2 years. While similar with regard to sociodemographic and health characteristics, the two hearing-impaired groups differed slightly in mean hearing levels and mean baseline HHIE scores. The majority of subjects in the experimental group purchased one ITE hearing aid. The majority of respondents judged themselves to be satisfied with their hearing aids using them on the average of 418 minutes per day at baseline and 396 minutes per day at follow-up. Statistical analysis revealed an intervention effect of hearing aids in the domain of self-perceived hearing handicap for the experimental group whereas for the control groups mean HHIE scores remained stable over time. To compensate for the differences between the experimental and control group in baseline PTA and HHIE scores, a matched subsample was created such that the hearing-impaired control group was comparable to the hearing-impaired experimental group. In the subsample as well, an intervention effect of hearing aids was noted. The authors concluded that high hearing-aid use at baseline reliably led to lowered self-perceived hearing handicap at follow-up (Tesch-Romer, 1997). This study does not speak to an acclimatization effect, as benefit was assessed 6-months postfitting, it does however support the fact that hearing aids continue to provide benefit in the psychosocial domain as much as 6 months after the initial fitting. Tesch-Romer (1997) found no effect of hearing-aid use on satisfaction with social activities, well-being, or cognitive function.

Crandell (1998) completed a small study of the relationship between functional health status and hearing-aid use over time. Twenty older adults with mild to severe degrees of sensorineural hearing loss participated in the study. Subjects ranged in age from 65 to 91 years with a mean age of 75. Subjects were new hearing-aid users fit binaurally with Oticon Microfocus or Multifocus hearing aids. Outcome measures completed prior to the hearing-aid fitting, 3 months, and 6 months following the fitting included the APHAB and the SIP. As discussed in Chapter 8, the SIP is a measure of functional health status and absolute scores bear a relation to hearing loss severity. The higher the score on the physical or psychosocial scales of the SIP the greater the functional disability in that arena. Scores on the physical and psychosocial scales of the SIP decreased (improved) after 3 months of hearing-aid use and remained stable from 3 to 6 months following the fitting. This finding confirms the benefit of hearing aids in both the physical and the psychosocial domains of function and confirms that after 3 months, acclimatization to hearing aids takes place.

Bridges and Bentler (1998) reported on a small survey they completed on the relation between well being, hearing status, and hearing-aid use in a sample of older adults. Two hundred fifty-one older adults or 26% of individuals receiving the survey completed it. The questionnaire included items about depression (Geriatric Depression Scale—GDS) and life satisfaction (Satisfaction with Life Scale—SWLS) along with a personal data form. Thirty percent of respondents were male, 70% were female, and the majority of subjects lived by themselves or with a spouse in a private home. Respondents ranged in age from 53 to 93 years. Interestingly, half of respondents reported a hearing loss while half indicated that they did not feel they had hearing difficulties. Only 21% of respondents reportedly wore hearing aids successfully while 95% wore contact lenses or eyeglasses. Of the subjects who owned hearing aids, 78% considered themselves to be successful users. It was noteworthy that subjects reporting success with their hearing aids exhibited higher ratings of life satisfaction than those who currently wore hearing aids but did not report success. Also of interest was the observation that the mean score on the GDS for respondents who had worn hearing aids but do not wear them successfully now was higher (more depressed) than the mean score for individuals wearing hearing aids successfully now. While this study was only a survey, and audiometric data were not available for respondents, I think the findings are valuable to audiologists who find themselves having to justify hearing aids to their clients or to managed care agencies. The data can certainly be used to suggest that "hearing aids are necessary, not only for improved communication, but also for enhanced sense of well-being" (Bridges & Bentler, 1998, p. 44). The data from the 1999 National Council on Aging study confirm that hearing-aid use has a positive impact on quality of life, including a reduction in affective symptoms. That is, higher rates of depression, anxiety, and anger were found among older adults who do not use hearing aids yet have comparable self-reported hearing loss than those who do use hearing aids (Kirkwood, 1999).

In sum, the above studies clearly demonstrate that the psychosocial, communicative, and functional benefits from hearing aids are sustainable up to 6 months following the initial fitting.

SPECIAL CONSIDERATION

It appears that some form of psychosocial acclimatization may take place arguing in favor of long-term follow-up, yet the timing of it is not clear.

Long-Term Benefits from Hearing Aids

Newman and Weinstein (1988) were among the first investigators to assess the efficacy of the HHIE as an index of long-term hearing aid benefit in the psychosocial domain. Eighteen male veterans with ages ranging from 66 to 84 years and a mean pure-tone average of 43 dBHL in the better ear and 56.6 dBHL in the poorer ear were fit with hearing aids. Subjects responded to the HHIE at baseline and 1 year following the fitting. Significant others also responded to the significant others version of the HHIE (HHIE-SO) prior to and 1-year following hearing-aid use. Differences between scores on the initial and follow-up administration of the HHIE and HHIE-SO were statistically significant on the total, emotional, and social/situational subscales. The mean difference score on the HHIE was rather large (27.7) exceeding the 95% confidence interval that defines a clinically significant change due to the intervention.

Using a randomized controlled clinical trial, Mulrow et al (1990); Mulrow, Michael, and Aguilar (1992); and Mulrow, Tuley, and Aguilar (1992) conducted a series of studies documenting that the benefit of hearing aids can be sustained up to 1 year following the initial fitting. Subjects were new hearing-aid users with sensorineural hearing loss. Approximately half of the subjects were assigned to the experimental group and fit with monaural ITE hearing aids while the other half comprised the control group. Groups were matched for hearing loss, age, physical status, educational level, etc. The majority of subjects in the experimental group wore their hearing aids for more than 4 hours daily at the 4-month, 8-month, and 12-month follow-up. In general, 70 to 80% of the 162 subjects reported being quite satisfied with their units over the 1-year period during which they were followed. Mean scores on the HHIE improved after 6 weeks of hearing-aid use and were sustained at 4, 8, and 12 months, concluding that the benefits of hearing aids in the psychosocial and communicative domains of function are sustainable over a period of 1 year. In their study, absolute and relative benefit in the psychosocial domain at 6 weeks was comparable to that at 4 months, 8 months, and 1 year.

It is of interest that the findings of Malinoff and Weinstein (1989) confirmed the findings of Mulrow and her colleagues (1992) that hearing-aid benefit is sustainable out to 1 year following the initial fitting. In contrast, however, the potential for some form of psychosocial acclimatization to hearing aids did emerge. Subjects in their study were older adults with mild to moderate sensorineural hearing loss. Twenty-five subjects were followed over a period of 1 year to determine whether benefit in the psychosocial domain could be sustained. In their study, hearing-aid benefit was notable at 3 weeks, 3 months, and at 1 year following the initial fitting. Benefit at 3 weeks (mean difference score of 29. 6) was more dramatic than that which emerged at 3 months and 1 year (difference score of ~15 points). The data of Taylor (1993) corroborate the findings of Malinoff and Weinstein (1989). In the Taylor study, hearing-aid benefit relative to baseline was notable at 3 weeks, 3 months, 6 months, and at 1 year. The most dramatic reduction in social and emotional function emerged just 3 weeks after the initial hearing-aid fitting. Interestingly, the mean score on the HHIE rose significantly after 3 months of hearing-aid use but stabilized after 6 months and 1 year, suggesting once again some form of acclimatization in the psychosocial domain.

It appears that in their sample as in Taylor's (1993), benefit may stabilize at 3 months such that it is comparable and sustainable after 1 year of use. The longitudinal study of Malinoff and Weinstein (1989) corroborated the data of Taylor (1993) as well as the findings of Newman et al (1993). Based on the pattern of findings described, it appears that a period of accommodation, adaptation, or acclimatization may occur within the first several months of hearing-aid use such that the magnitude of benefit in the psychosocial domain may change somewhat over time, with reality and exposure to a variety of listening situations, moderating the initial euphoria some people feel after the initial hearing-aid fitting. In fact, Malinoff and Weinstein (1989) reported that one of their clients actually captured the experience of hearing-aid use quite aptly. He explained that once you have worn a hearing aid for a while you suddenly become more aware of the sounds you were missing and of the different sounds you are now hearing causing a total readjustment in your auditory reality base. As such, the benefits of hearing aids become self-evident as do their limitations.

The findings from the longitudinal studies on long-term benefit in the psychosocial domain concur with the observations made by Gatehouse (1992) who used speech-recognition materials. In the Gatehouse study, benefit was defined according to change in scores on speech tests presented in a background of noise following selected intervals of hearing-aid use. He also found that improvements in speech-recognition ability continued over a 12-week period of hearing-aid use allowing for adjustments in the volume control setting within the first 5 weeks of the hearing-aid fitting. The acclimatization effect, as evidenced by changes in the magnitude of objective and subjective benefit over time, appeared to be complete at about 3 months after the initial fitting. It may in fact be due to "perceptual learning" wherein the client gradually adjusts to the newly audible speech cues (Turner et al, 1996). The perceptual learning may translate into an improvement in scores on objective tests of speech-recognition ability over time but a decrease in scores on subjective measures of benefit over time. With regard to the latter, for some individuals the newly audible sounds may not match with client expectations reducing somewhat the perceived psychosocial advantage of hearing-aid use.

SPECIAL CONSIDERATION

The longitudinal studies on benefits associated with hearing-aid use underline the importance of following clients over time at least for 3 months as problems seem to arise that can be remedied through counseling and/or hearing-aid modification.

Interestingly, the psychological literature is replete with studies demonstrating that 3 months is a key time frame for adaptation or acclimatization in a variety of domains. Schum (1999) concurred that expectations influence benefit such that satisfaction may be compromised if expectations are too high.

Table 9–7 summarizes the benefits of hearing aids as perceived by the consumer. Clinical experience suggests that audiologists should use this information as a "report card" on hearing aids by sharing with potential consumers available data demonstrating the value of hearing aids from the perspective of the consumer.

PEARL

Older adults do experience short-, medium-, and long-term benefit from hearing aids in the disability and handicap domains of function.

AUDIOLOGIC CORRELATES OF HEARING-AID BENEFIT

A number of studies conducted in a variety of settings have explored the relationship between audiologic variables and hearing-aid benefit in the psychosocial domain. The audio-

TABLE 9–7 Perceived Benefits from Hearing Aids as Reported by Older Adults with Impaired Hearing

Improvements in communication*
1. Improved communication in easy-listening conditions 2. Easier to communicate 3. Improved speech understanding in reverberant conditions, with background noise, and with reduced visual cues

Improvements in psychosocial function
1. Improved emotional function** 2. Improved social function** 3. Improved psychosocial function as perceived by the spouse of the hearing impaired** 4. Improved cognition*** 5. Improved affect****

*Assessed using the PHAB and the Intelligibility Rating Scale (IRIS) post hearing-aid fitting (Cox, Alexander, & Gilmore, 1991).
**Assessed using the HHIE (pre and post hearing-aid fitting).
***Assessed using the SPMSQ (pre and post hearing-aid fitting).
****Assessed using the GDS (pre and post hearing-aid fitting).

logic variables that have been studied include the relation between aided functional gain and hearing aid benefit; the relation between hearing loss severity and hearing aid benefit; the relation between word-recognition ability and hearing aid benefit; and, finally, the extent to which real ear insertion gain measures correlate with self-perceived benefit derived from hearing aids. It appears that for the most part, audiologic variables, while integral to the selection and fitting process, may not contribute to our understanding of the individual variability in perceived benefit from hearing aids.

PEARL

Audiologic variables do not bear a strong relation to subjective measures of hearing-aid benefit.

As noted earlier, Newman et al (1991) reported on the beneficial effects of short-term hearing-aid use in their large sample of new hearing-aid users. As an adjunct to their study, they explored the relation between hearing loss severity, word-recognition ability, and benefit in the handicap domain. They found that severity of hearing loss, and word-recognition ability, did not influence the absolute handicap perceived by subjects in their sample. Similarly, the amount of improvement in the psychosocial domain associated with hearing-aid use was not influenced by the latter audiometric variables. Subjects with mild and those with moderate to severe sensorineural hearing loss presented with comparable mean prefitting HHIE-S scores (e.g., 16 to 18) and postfitting HHIE score (e.g., 3). Similarly, subjects with excellent word-recognition ability perceived their handicap to be comparable to those with fair to poor performance on the monosyllabic word-recognition task (Newman et al, 1991). As irrespective of hearing loss severity and word recognition ability, the mean HHIE-S score of subjects in the sample was approximately 18; this score may in fact be indicative of need for a hearing aid. These data are shown in Figures 9–5 and 9–6.

Mulrow, Tuley, and Aguilar (1992) also explored the audiologic correlates of hearing-aid use and benefit in a sample of older adults with moderate sensorineural hearing loss. Benefit was assessed at 6 weeks and following 4 months of hearing-aid use. The average functional gain in the high frequencies was reportedly 26 to 30 dB. The majority of subjects experienced over a 50% improvement in social and emotional function as assessed by the HHIE. As would be expected, the satisfaction rate was quite high; nearly 70 to 80% reported being very satisfied with their units. Amount of functional gain in the high frequencies and gain in the Speech Reception Threshold (SRT) following hearing-aid use accounted for less than 11% of the variance in hearing-aid success as defined by improvements in HHIE scores. Thus, audiometric data were not considered predictive of benefit in the psychosocial domain. The data of Taylor (1993) corroborated their findings in that in their study functional gain was minimally correlated with the magnitude of benefit in the psychosocial domain (i.e., according to difference scores on the HHIE).

With regard to word-recognition ability, investigators have considered the relation between performance on a variety of speech-recognition tests and hearing-aid benefit in the handicap domain. Overall, it seems that the beneficial treatment effects of hearing aids depend upon the speech materials used, the presentation level, and whether in fact individuals present with peripheral or CAPD. Hnath-Chisolm and Abrams (1993) investigated the relation between improvement in speech-recognition performance and improvement in self-perceived handicap among new hearing-aid users. Speech-recognition performance was assessed at baseline and at 2-week intervals over a period of 4 sessions. Speech-recognition ability was assessed with the CUNY Topic Related Sentence Test presented in the presence of multiple-talker babble. Changes in auditory and auditory-visual word-recognition ability were assessed over time. The HHIE was completed at baseline and at the final test session approximately 6 to 8 weeks following the initial hearing-aid fitting. While large individual differences in performance on the word-recognition tasks emerged, significant differences between unaided and aided performance did not emerge on any of the word-recognition tasks. Significant changes did however emerge in the perception of handicap such that the mean HHIE score at approximately 2 months after the fitting revealed a clinically and statistically significant reduction in self-perceived emotional/ social handicap associated with the hearing impairment. As would be expected, only a minimal correlation emerged between subjective (HHIE) and objective (speech) measures. According to the authors, their findings are consistent with the data of Cox, Alexander, and Gilmore (1991) who reported that significant changes in speech-recognition performance in the presence of a background of noise did not emerge following hearing-aid use in a sample of older adults. They did, however, note a relation between objective benefit using speech measures and more subjective benefit in the disability domain according to scores on the Profile of Hearing Aid Benefit (PHAB). Hnath-Chisolm and Abrams (1993) concluded that perhaps other auditory abilities not tapped by the speech-recognition materials employed in their study may account for the reductions in hearing handicap noted. It may also be surmised that performance on the speech-recognition tasks with hearing aids may impact more on perceived function in the auditory/communicative domain than in terms of psychosocial handicap.

Chmiel and Jerger (1996) evaluated the impact of hearing aids on the quality of life of older adults with or without CAPD. Subjects who had primarily high-frequency sensorineural hearing loss, were classified into two groups according to scores on the DSI test. The DSI-normal group (n = 42) had comparable audiograms to those in the DSI-abnormal group (n = 21). The subjects who were closely matched for age with a mean age of 72 for the former group and of 70 for the latter group were fit monaurally with either a Siemens Triton 3000 or a 3M Memory Mate digital/analog hybrid instrument. Their data suggested that treatment effects varied as a function of group membership. Persons in the DSI-normal group derived significant benefit from their hearing aids as evidenced by the reduction in HHIE scores following 6 weeks of hearing-aid use. Subjects in the DSI-abnormal group, namely those considered to have CAPD, did not derive clinically significant benefits from hearing aids in the psychosocial domain of function, as evidenced by the comparability of scores on the HHIE at baseline and following 6 weeks of hearing-aid use. In short, the apparent central auditory deficit appeared to attenuate the self-perceived improvement in quality of life afforded by amplification. It was of interest that informal caregivers, however, perceived benefits in the psychosocial domain attributable to hearing-aid use in older adults with CAPD. Caregiver ratings of psychosocial handicap experienced by subjects with CAPD revealed statistically significant reductions in scores on the HHIE-SO. That is, even when the patient with CAPD did not report a reduction in hearing handicap with hearing-aid use, the significant other often reported a reduction in handicap as a result of hearing-aid use. The latter finding suggests that hearing-aids may reduce the stress on communication partners despite the fact that the respondent with CAPD does not necessarily judge hearing aids to be effective in reducing their psychosocial handicap. Audiologists are urged to consider using the HHIE-SO as a pre- and post-fitting measure, as it is sensitive to short-term and long-term differences achieved with hearing-aid use (Newman & Weinstein, 1988). Further, the information can be helpful during counseling sessions when a caregiver or significant other is present. Data from the National Council on Aging survey of hearing-aid users and nonusers confirms that input from significant others is an important outcome indicator (Kirkwood, 1999).

The final audiologic correlate to be studied in relation to hearing-aid benefit in the handicap domain is that of real ear data. As real ear measures are used by the majority of dispensing audiologists to select the electroacoustic characteristics of hearing aids and to verify their performance, it is important to know the extent to which these measures relate to perceived benefit in the handicap and/or disability domain. Nerbonne, Christman, and Fleschner (1995) fit 51 adults and older adults with linear amplification using the NAL-R prescription formula. One to 4 months following the fitting, subjects completed the HHIE or HHIA (depending on the subject's age) to determine perception of aided performance with the newly acquired hearing aid. The authors computed the amount of "fitting error" or deviation from target found in real ear insertion gain (REIG) relative to NAL-R target values. For the most part, fitting errors resulted in less gain than prescribed by the NAL-R formula. The correlation between REIG-fitting error values and aided scores on the HHIE/HHIA were weak and nonsignificant on the total, emotional, and social subscales of the HHIE/HHIA. Their conclusion, that no obvious relationship appears to exist between degree of REIG-fitting error and self-perceived benefit from amplification, underlines the importance of measuring each. Real ear data may be viewed as evidence of improved audibility with amplification and as a way of verifying the desired electroacoustic response of the hearing aid. In contrast, change in HHIE/HHIA scores serve as an estimate of the amount of reduction in perceived handicap associated with hearing-aid use. With linear hearing aids it appears that closeness of fit to target may not influence magnitude of benefit. With the advent of nonlinear hearing aids, the question becomes whether restoration of the loudness function correlates with benefit in the disability and handicap domains. It is probable that the relation is imperfect and that the protocol for fitting nonlinear devices should incorporate a measure of benefit in the disability or handicap domain as in the IHAFF protocol as well as judgments of loudness perception.

NONAUDIOLOGIC CORRELATES OF HEARING-AID BENEFIT

One myth surrounding hearing aids is that older adults use their hearing aids less consistently and derive less benefit from hearing aids than do younger adults. A series of recent studies have demonstrated that this conclusion cannot be substantiated empirically. Bender and Mueller (1984) compared younger and older adults in their subjective judgments of hearing-aid use, satisfaction, and benefit. After 1 year of hearing-aid use, responses of older adults were comparable to those of younger adults. In fact, the vast majority of older adults reported more than a moderate degree of benefit and satisfaction with amplification. Kochkin (1992) also reported that there were no statistically significant differences by age group in overall mean satisfaction ratings. Ebinger et al (1995) found that older and younger adults reported comparable benefit in the disability domain from CIC hearing aids. Specifically, according to responses to the APHAB, the percent of aided problems in various listening conditions was comparable for older and younger adults. Further, the CIC units reduced the percent of listening problems experienced by older and younger adults to below the

50th percentile of the norms established by Cox and Alexander (1995). Finally, Primeau (1997) reported that older and younger adults were comparable in the magnitude of perceived benefit in the psychosocial domain that emerged on the HHIE/HHIA.

PEARL
There appears to be little difference between older and younger adults in the magnitude of self-rated benefit.

Cost is another factor that has been considered a variable influencing hearing-aid benefit. Newman et al (1993) explored the impact of financial outlay on self-perceived hearing-aid benefit. As noted above, the older adults comprising the sample had essentially mild to moderate sensorineural hearing loss. Individuals who paid privately for their hearing aids had comparable hearing levels and prefitting HHIE scores, and were age matched to the group of subjects whose health insurance paid for the hearing aid. The magnitude of hearing-aid benefit at 3 weeks and 6 months was comparable for the insured and uninsured groups. That is, each group demonstrated a statistically and clinically significant reduction in perceived emotional and social handicap following short- and long-term hearing-aid use.

SPECIAL CONSIDERATION
Financial outlay for a hearing aid does not appear to influence perceived hearing-aid benefit in the psychosocial domain.

SUMMARY OF STUDIES ON HEARING-AID BENEFIT

In sum, using various disability and handicap measures as the gold standard the following conclusions can be drawn for older adults using hearing aids: (1) beneficial treatment effects from hearing aids emerge as early as 3 to 6 weeks after the initiation of treatment; (2) the benefit of hearing aids is demonstrable and sustainable in the handicap domain throughout a 1-year period; (3) accommodation or adaptation to hearing aids may take approximately 3 months and can be sustained out to 1 year; (4) nearly 70 to 80% of older adults appear to experience significant reductions in psychosocial handicap associated with hearing-aid use; (5) the audiologic variable that appears to influence the magnitude of benefit is central auditory processing ability; and (6) nonaudiologic variables such as cost and age do not appear to influence hearing-aid benefit. Table 9–8 summarizes the beneficial effects of hearing aids in the handicap domains. Despite the apparent psychosocial and communicative benefits associated with hearing-aid use, the high cost of hearing aids continues to deter potential candidates from pursuing amplification.

TABLE 9–8   Outcomes with Hearing Aids in the Handicap Domain

- Beneficial treatment effects from hearing aids emerge as early as 3 weeks after the initiation of treatment.

- The overwhelming majority (70 to 80%) of experienced or new hearing-aid users experience dramatic reductions in the extent of psychosocial handicap after only 3 weeks of hearing-aid use.

- The benefit of hearing aids is demonstrable and sustainable in the handicap domain over a 1-year time interval.

- Audiometric data bear little relationship to benefit with the exception of central auditory processing ability.

- Age, financial status, and neuropsychologic status bear little relation to benefit in the handicap domain.

- Counseling-oriented rehabilitation can influence benefit.

- Hearing-aid benefit is more pronounced using disorder-specific rather than generic quality-of-life measures.

- Listening training is effective in reducing auditory disabilities over and above that achieved with hearing aids alone.

Source: Primeau, 1997; Malinoff and Weinstein, 1989; Taylor, 1993; Newman et al, 1993; Newman et al, 1991; Mulrow et al, 1990; Kricos and Holmes, 1996.

The cost-effectiveness estimates generated by Mulrow et al (1990) suggest that when the cost of a hearing evaluation, hearing-aid selection, and fitting are compared against the functional and quality-of-life benefits of amplification, hearing aids actually represent an inexpensive intervention for the amount of benefit gained. These data should be used by audiologists to convey the value of hearing aids relative to their cost. In light of the increasing penetration of DCA and DSP hearing aids, cost-benefit may actually become an outcome audiologists are asked to produce.

An Ideal Hearing-Aid Fitting Protocol for Older Adults

Based on this discussion, the hearing-aid fitting protocol shown in Figure 9–3 is recommended when dispensing a hearing aid to an older adult. The protocol is lengthy, however it contains all of the components this author believes are critical to a successful fitting. Note there is considerable overlap with the most recently proposed Guidelines for Hearing Aid Fitting for Adults (ASHA, 1998).

The Comprehensive Audiological Evaluation or Assessment (AE)

The AE should enable the audiologist to obtain a complete picture of the three distinct domains of hearing function, namely, impairment, disability, and handicap. In-depth exploration of each of these domains will help the clinician to determine the most appropriate intervention for a given individual. That is, information garnered from the AE helps to identify candidates for a hearing aid. The case history and otoscopic examination are precursors to the audiologic assessment, and will help to determine need for medical/surgical referral as well as need for medical clearance as outlined by the Food and Drug Administration (FDA) (ASHA, 1998). Recall that the following conditions necessitate referral to a physician prior to dispensing hearing aids: (1) visible congenital or traumatic deformity of the ear, (2) history of active drainage from the ear within the previous 90 days, (3) history of sudden or rapidly progressive hearing loss within the previous 90 days, (4) acute or chronic dizziness, (5) unilateral hearing loss of sudden or recent onset within the previous 90 days, (6) air bone gap in excess of 15 dB, (7) visible evidence of cerumen impaction, or (8) a foreign body in the ear canal (Staff, 1997).

The pure-tone and speech evaluation should provide a complete picture of the client's auditory status, including peripheral and central auditory processing ability. Assessment of communication disability will yield information on the individual's auditory functioning in daily life. Keidser, Dillon, and Byrne (1996) suggest that the extent of difficulty understanding speech in different listening environments is an indicator of need for a multiple-memory hearing aid. Thus, a comprehensive inventory of situational handicaps may influence the fitting recommendation. Quantification of handicap will provide information about the perceived effects of impairment and disability on nonauditory aspects of daily life including social and emotional issues. Handicap as well as disability information will serve as a baseline against which outcomes with hearing aids can be judged. As there is an imperfect relationship between the extent of impairment, disability, and handicap, it is incumbent on the audiologist to explore each area. As the audiological evaluation is the occasion for selecting hearing-aid candidates, each of the domains of function listed in Table 9–3 should be informally assessed and considered when arriving at a rehabilitation plan.

In addition to selecting candidates for a particular intervention, it is at this stage of the process that audiologists may have to persuade a reluctant individual to consider the purchase of a hearing aid. Motivational counseling can assist in encouraging older adults to attempt a trial period with hearing aids. Motivational dynamics are discussed extensively in other sections of the text including Chapters 3 and 8. Further, informational counseling may take place during this phase of the evaluation. This consists of a discussion of hearing-aid styles, arrangements, types, and cost of amplification systems. The more extensive the exchange, the better positioned the older adults will be to make an informed decision about hearing aids.

> **PEARL**
>
> A client-centered approach that considers audiometric and nonaudiometric variables is required for a successful hearing-aid fitting.

The Prefitting or Preselection

The goal of the prefitting or preselection is to obtain baseline information necessary to a successful fit. During the preselection, the audiologist should gather nonaudiologic and audiologic information that will help in decisions regarding the most appropriate amplification system and electroacoustic characteristics. The audiologic variables should include measures of audibility (e.g., pure-tone thresholds, audibility index), measures of speech understanding (e.g., using a conversion chart—the audibility index (AI) can be used to estimate the percentage of speech that is understandable), thresholds of discomfort using frequency-specific stimuli, and/or measures of suprathreshold loudness (e.g., using a wide range of input levels and frequency-specific loudness measures). Mueller (1996) also recommends that a measure of disability and handicap be included in this stage of the process if it has not been incorporated into the routine audiological evaluation. This is important as self-perceived disability does have a strong impact on the decision to purchase hearing aids (Kochkin, 1998). Unfortunately only 14% of audiologists report administering formalized self-assessment inventories (Kirkwood, 1997).

At this stage of the process, telecommunication needs should be addressed. Members of SHHH feel strongly that telecoils are integral components of hearing aids (Sorkin, 1997). Hearing-aid users report that telecoils give them clearer reception on the telephone and enable them to use the telephone more comfortably (Sorkin, 1997). According

---

SPECIAL CONSIDERATION

The positive impact of telecoil use increases with increasing hearing loss (Sorkin, 1997).

---

to SHHH members, they have to make a strong case to dispensers to include a strong coil in their hearing aid (Sorkin, 1997). This should not be the case. The data on the positive impact of telecoil use underscore the importance of recommending the telecoil option to the hearing-aid users who frequently find themselves on the telephone (Sorkin, 1997).

Nonaudiologic factors that will impact on the success of the fitting include lifestyle considerations, activity level, physical status, social factors, psychological health, cognitive variables, and stage of denial (Kochkin, 1998). The Client Oriented Scale of Improvement (COSI), a measure of communication improvement, should be considered a potential tool for identifying selected nonaudiologic variables that can impact on the hearing-aid fitting (Dillon, James, & Ginis, 1997). In a sense, the COSI enables the audiologist to indirectly consider the patient's lifestyle as a factor in selecting, fitting, and verifying the hearing aid. The COSI enables the patient to decide on and record the five situations that are most important to them and in which they would like to cope better. At the postfitting, for each situation, the respondent rates how much better (or worse) the patient can now hear with the hearing aid and the ease with which communication exchanges now take place. The COSI

is an attractive tool as it is easy to elicit the necessary input from older adults, administration time is brief, and scoring and interpretation is straightforward. In keeping with the recommendations of Keidser, Dillon, and Byrne (1996), information from the COSI can help in a decision regarding candidacy for multiple-memory hearing aids as well as serving as an index of benefit.

Other nonaudiologic factors such as financial considerations, may not impact on benefit but will influence the type of system recommended as well as the arrangement. Older adults who commit to a hearing-aid purchase should be encouraged to purchase a system that will give them the best yield for their pocketbooks. Always remember, that purchasing a hearing aid can represent a short-term financial setback that older adults will find acceptable if they are satisfied with their purchase. Counseling, follow-up, and encouragement will be especially important to benefit and satisfaction. Cognitive factors can also influence the amplification system recommended. Audiologists should consider administering a test of cognitive function such as the Short Portable Mental Status Questionnaire (SPMSQ), a widely used screening tool, described by Pfeiffer (1975). A failing score on the SPMSQ may steer the audiologist toward a conventional ITE or BTE hearing aid or perhaps even assistive devices depending on the extent of involvement. At this time, an informal or formal test of manual dexterity should be administered to assist in a decision regarding the most appropriate unit given fine-motor considerations. It is often helpful to ask an older adult to insert a battery into and remove a battery from a different hearing aid with the audiologist observing the patient's potential for independent control over this function. In short the preselection is the foundation upon which subsequent evaluations and fittings are built. The more comprehensive and individualized the process, the greater the probability of a successful match between the individual and the device. At the conclusion of this session a joint decision (i.e. audiologist, client, and family/caregivers) is made regarding the virtues of proceeding with the hearing-aid selection. The decision should be made with the full knowledge on the part of the user and his/her family of the potential benefits, limitations, and costs associated with hearing-aid use. This is especially important given the increasing popularity of high performance hearing aids.

The Hearing-Aid Selection

Ultimately, the challenge to the audiologist is to select a hearing aid that best meets the needs of patients with hearing impairment. The audiologist must arrive at a hearing-aid configuration that reflects the electroacoustic characteristics likely to meet the unique requirements of a particular hearing-impaired older adult (Seewald, 1994). During the selection process, audiologists must define, distinguish, and maximize those factors most likely to contribute to a successful hearing-aid fitting (Fortune, 1996). The task is inherently complex because of the large number of relevant audiometric and nonaudiometric variables that must be considered (Seewald, 1994). At the selection, the audiologist uses information from the audiological evaluation and the prefitting to reach a decision about physical characteristics of the hearing aid, about hardware options, and a variety of technical decisions, as well (Seewald, 1994). Physical characteristics include the type and style of hearing aid; hardware options include microphone type, telecoil, direct audio-input; technical decisions include type of signal processing (e.g. DSP, DCA, BILL, and TILL), gain, frequency response, and output limiting characteristics; and, of course, the arrangement to be recommended (e.g., monaural or binaural) (Seewald, 1994).

Of course, electroacoustic parameters must be chosen at the selection. It is important to emphasize that there is no universally accepted method for expressing the appropriate physical and electroacoustic characteristics of the desired hearing aids for a particular individual (ASHA, 1998). In general, specifications should be in keeping with the client's auditory characteristics and personal needs (ASHA, 1998). When fitting linear hearing aids, frequency-gain characteristics are typically generated using one of several formulas incorporated into commercially available software and implemented in many real-ear analyzers (ASHA, 1998). Potential formulas include the NAL-R, the POGO, the Berger procedure, and the Memphis State University procedure (ASHA, 1998). It is important to remember that frequency-gain characteristics will need to be expressed in a 2 cm³ coupler and should be calculated for conversational inputs of 60 to 70 dBSPL (ASHA, 1998).

Output sound pressure level with a 90 dB input or SSPL90 targets should be generated, as well. Frequency-specific SSPL90 targets should be derived from loudness-discomfort levels using one of the available prescribed procedures such as that described by Hawkins, Walden, Montgomery, and Prosek (1987). The maximum ouput of the hearing aid should be no more than 10 dB below the targets developed from threshold of discomfort data at each octave frequency from 500 Hz through 4000 Hz.

In contrast to linear hearing aids, where calculation of the desired frequency/gain characteristics and SSPL90 defines the input/output characteristics, for nonlinear hearing aids the audiologist must prescribe a series of different gain and frequency-response prescriptions for different input levels and spectra (Byrne, 1996; ASHA, 1998). Multiple signal levels will provide an estimate of linear gain, target gain, and saturation gain, and an estimate of the dynamic processing of the ear. One of the prescriptive methods for fitting nonlinear hearing aids can be attempted, although none have been validated on older adults. Ross and Levitt (1997) suggest that for multiple-memory hearing aids, the optimum electroacoustic characteristics for the patient's most commonly encountered situations should be programmed into the hearing aid.

Throughout the selection process, the audiologist must regularly get feedback from the client regarding the comfort level, quality, and tolerability level of the amplified signal. User's judgments of sound quality are considered by audiologists to be an important part of the fitting/selection process (Kirkwood, 1997). Ross and Levitt (1997) suggest that comparing different types of hearing aids as well as different signal-processing schemes will enable patients to make informed decisions. For example, the audiologist might con-

sider comparing a single-band CIC aid with a 2-band multiple-memory BTE.

Difficulty understanding speech in noisy and reverberant conditions is often instrumental in an older adult's decision to pursue amplification. Further, customer satisfaction ratings are always lowest when the listening environment is less than optimal. To maximize aided speech recognition in less than optimal conditions, the hearing-aid selection process should include speech recognition testing in a variety of noisy conditions and at a variety of listening levels, including soft conversation (Humes et al, 1999). Speech tests in noise can help to fine tune the hearing-aid fitting and can help to clarify the value of a recommended amplification system. For example, the advantage of noise-reduction circuitry, or the flexibility of a programmable unit over a more conventional hearing aid can be made readily apparent. Chmiel and Jerger (1995) recently described a randomization test for evaluating different hearing-aid styles and circuits using a variety of speech in noise tests. It has considerable application to older adults, but an effort must be made to keep test sessions as abbreviated and focused as possible.

Finally, during the selection process decisions regarding "add-ons" should be made such as remote control versus screw-adjust volume control, removal notches, raised volume controls, telecoil, directional/multiple microphones, wax guards, etc. Hearing aids with larger battery doors should be considered for patients with visual or manual-dexterity problems. Of course, each patient should be given the instrument owner's manual, warranty, loss, and damage information. The correct type and size battery should be listed on any literature given to the patient. Also, a diary to enable the patient to keep a record of their listening experiences is often helpful to the adaptation process. Similarly, it is often helpful to assess the client's ability to operate the hearing aid and its conventional controls and then make a decision about the importance of controls that will make the aid easier to operate independently. Remember the key is independent use and a reliable instrument.

PEARL

Every effort should be made to enable the patient to feel comfortable with the fit of the hearing aid and to independently operate each component.

THE POSTFITTING, VERIFICATION, AND VALIDATION PHASE

The verification phase is tied to both the preselection and selection with the goal being to "see how the client is doing with his or her hearing aids" (Mueller, 1996, p. 22). ASHA (1998) guidelines suggest that the term *verification* refers to measures made to determine whether the hearing aid(s) meet a set of standards. The standards range from electroacoustic performance to cosmetic appeal, ease of insertion/removal, and comfort level. Objective measures provide evidence that the fitting goals for gain and output have been met, namely the input is audible, the amplified signal is comfortable, and high-level inputs are tolerable, not exceeding the threshold of discomfort (Table 9–9) (ASHA, 1998). Match to target should be verified with insertion gain measurements (Cox, Alexander, Taylor, & Gray, 1996). The fitting goals should be as close a match to target through 3000 Hz, and presumably above this frequency, if possible. Mueller (1996) recommends that real-ear insertion gain should fall within 10 dB of the target gain curve at all octave frequencies below 4000 Hz and within 14 dB at 4000 Hz. Cox et al (1996) suggested that relatively small deviations from NAL-R recommendations at higher frequencies are unlikely to have dramatic effects on speech understanding or on acclimatization. For nonlinear amplification, the audiologist wants to verify that soft sounds are audible, conversational level sounds are comfortable, and loud sounds are acceptable (Starkey, 1997).

PEARL

Signal audibility, intelligibility comfort, and tolerance comprise the verification stage designed to ensure electroacoustic performance; self-report measures are integral to the validation phase to assess the impact of the intervention (ASHA, 1998).

Speech recognition ability should be assessed informally or formally once the electroacoustic reponse of the hearing aid has been selected. Theoretically this information enables the audiologist to predict actual performance with hearing aid(s) in the real world but in reality it merely reflects improvement in audibility and recognition over the unaided condition. With regard to audibility we want to verify that the hearing aid circuitry allows good aided audiblity without making average and loud speech inputs too loud. With regard to intelligibility, we want to check to insure that a significant portion of speech is understandable in a variety of listening conditions. Routine tests of aided versus unaided speech understanding using monosyllabic words or sentence materials should be considered. Calculating the AI using probe-microphone systems or available paper and pencil charts is an expedient way to assess audibility and the percentage of speech understandable with the hearing aid can be estimated from the AI using available conversion charts (Mueller, 1996).

The most simplistic method for deriving improvement in AI associated with hearing-aid use, is using the count-the-dot audiogram developed by Mueller and Killion (1990). Simply put, the number of dots included by the aided result, predicted by the fitting strategy, compared with the unaided AI is equivalent to the improvement with the hearing aid or the AI percentage change. Sharing AI information with the patient is often quite a powerful way of confirming the value of hearing aids in improving word recognition. Software packages, built into probe-microphone systems automatically conduct AI calculations for both aided and unaided conditions. Mueller (1996) recommends that the

volume control wheel should be set to use-gain when conducting AI calculations to obtain face valid estimates.

SPECIAL CONSIDERATION

Speech understanding tests should not be sacrificed because of the availability of real ear measures. They can be indispensable with the elderly especially with binaural amplification (Chmiel, Jerger, Murphy, Pirozzolo, & Tooley-Young, 1997).

While providing verification of the prescribed response, objective measures such as tonal and speech data may not be predictive of real-world function with or acceptance of hearing aids. Self-assessment scales that assess benefit in the disability (APHAB) and handicap (HHIE) domains will help to validate whether the patient is actually deriving adequate "real-world benefit." That is, these latter measures serve to validate the impact of the hearing aid/audiologic intervention (ASHA, 1998). Benefit in the disability and handicap domains should be assessed using the the same scales used to obtain baseline information (e.g., APHAB, HHIE-S, and COSI). The data gathered during the audiological evaluation or the preselection should serve as a baseline against which to verify benefit from the hearing aid. The confidence intervals associated with significant benefit should be applied to determine if the benefit achieved by a given client is clinically significant. If in fact the patient is not deriving clinically and statistically significant benefit from hearing aids, hearing-aid modification, replacement, or additional counseling should be explored. Extensive discussion with the patient regarding options and expectations is very helpful at this stage.

A multidimensional measure of satisfaction should be administered at the postfitting to determine the client's level of satisfaction with hearing-aid features and with the professional services. The satisfaction survey developed by Kochkin at Knowles Electronics has been used in a series of large-scale studies, and is a good starting point, as is the recently described SADL. Of course, at the postfitting, the audiologist should make sure that the hearing-aid quality and fit are satisfactory. For DCA and DSP hearing aids, it is important to follow the trouble-shooting guidelines included in the operation manuals of most professional fitting systems. Do not assume that everything is okay because the patient has not complained. Ask specific questions to elicit responses that will enable you to make the necessary adjustments. The questions and solutions included in Table 9–9 can be helpful during the postfitting.

Medium- and Long-Term Verification and Validation

The objective and subjective measures used to verify and validate the fitting should be administered at 3 weeks, 3 months, and approximately 1 year after the initial fitting. The verification and validation phase should take place over time to allow for acclimatization of benefit to take place (Cox et al, 1996). The latter implies that there is an increase in the

TABLE 9–9   Troubleshooting at the Postfitting or Verification Phase

Questions for the patient	Possible solutions
Questions pertaining to the fit of the hearing aid or earmold:	
1. Is the hearing aid too loose?	a. Build up shell, new impression
2. Is the hearing aid too tight?	a. New impression, grind or buff areas that may be causing tightness
3. Does the hearing aid cause any allergic reactions like a rash?	a. Coat shell with hypoallergenic nail polish, make a lucite mold, or a mold with hypoallergenic material
Questions pertaining to the amplified sound:	
1. Does your own voice sound hollow as if in a barrel or plugged?	a. Reset low cut control to a higher value b. Increase crossover frequency if it is a programmable device c. Bell the bore d. Widen the diameter of the vent e. Provide a deep canal fit f. Reset gain control to a higher value, as there may be too much gain
2. Does the hearing aid sound tinny or harsh?	a. Insert filter in receiver or microphone b. Shift high frequencies with a resonant peak control c. Reduce low-frequency gain or reset low cut control to a lower value d. Reduce high-frequency output or gain e. Reduce crossover frequency f. Increase compression ratio
3. Is their acoustic leakage/feedback?	a. Reset gain control as there may be too much gain b. Reset high cut control as the high-frequency peak may be the problem c. Build up the shell/earmold as it may be too loose, take a new impression d. Reduce vent size e. Build up or lengthen canal f. Check for excessive cerumen g. Reduce canal length because the tip, may be against the canal wall
4. Are sounds too loud?	a. Reduce output, gain b. Insert filter in receiver c. Reset the compression ratio d. Reset compression knee-point, reset compression threshold e. Shorten canal tip to reduce gain
5. Are sounds too soft?	a. Check the battery b. Check for cerumen c. Check microphone d. Increase low-frequency gain e. Increase overall gain f. Decrease compression ratio, reset compression threshold to a lower value g. Check receiver tube for debris h. Check for moisture

TABLE 9–9   Troubleshooting at the Postfitting or Verification Phase (continued)

Questions for the patient	Possible solutions
6. Is the sound intermittent?	a. Replace volume control b. Replace receiver/microphone c. Check for moisture build-up
7. Is the sound clear?	a. Increase high-frequency output b. Replace microphone c. Circuit may need repair d. The canal portion may be against the wall of the external auditory canal
8. Is wind noise a problem?	a. Use windscreen or windhood b. Place foam in the microphone port c. Decrease high-frequency gain or output
9. Is there too much noise or bass?	a. Make vent wider b. Reduce low-frequency gain c. Increase crossover frequency

Source: Modified from Valente, 1994 Chapters 6–10.

ability to recognize newly amplified speech due to a phenomenon known as perceptual learning (Turner et al, 1996). Cox and her colleagues suggest that the acclimatization effect may be a result of general refinement abilities. Patients should understand that daily practice with the hearing aid can lead to significant improvements beyond those seen within the first week of use (Cox et al, 1996). The audiologist should monitor this effect using a variety of subjective and objective outcome measures. Cox and her colleagues found a small acclimatization effect for speech intelligibility in noise in a small sample of older adults. That is, during the time interval between 6 and 9 weeks postfitting a significant improvement in aided intelligibility emerged.

In addition to tracking word-recognition ability in noise over time, extent of benefit in the handicap and/or disability domain should be plotted. Some individuals may not show improvement in speech understanding over time as was demonstrated in the study by Taylor (1993), yet will show dramatic change in the extent of psychosocial benefit over time. In fact, using the HHIE-S, the psychosocial benefit over time is the reverse of the growth benefit for speech. It appears that initial benefit in the handicap domain is much greater than benefit achieved after 3 months yet medium-term benefit is comparable to long-term benefit. Benefit data should be shared with the patient as a way of demonstrating the cost-benefit of hearing aids.

If outcomes with the hearing aid are favorable, where the client is benefiting and is satisfied, then the audiologist should consider the job complete. If in fact, the client is not benefiting in one or both of the domains being assessed, then some form of intervention beyond hearing aids should be introduced. This should include additional client-centered rehabilitation and ALDs for situations in which hearing aids are not proving beneficial.

BEYOND HEARING AIDS

ALDs

Successful use of hearing aids by older adults can be hampered by a number of nonaudiologic and audiologic variables. The nonaudiologic variables that contraindicate hearing-aid use in the elderly and argue in favor of alternative devices include cognitive impairments such as dementia; financial factors; manual-dexterity problems; and lifestyle considerations. The presence of central auditory processing problems is the primary audiologic factor that interferes with successful hearing-aid use. Even hearing aids that are digital, programmable, have special circuitry, or use directional microphones, do not provide for the easy or clear listening one desires in communication environments characterized by noise and reverberation (Kaplan, 1996). It is often helpful to perform a needs assessment of the patient's hearing ability in a number of specific listening situations to determine the need for an ALD in lieu of or to supplement hearing aids. Table 9–10 includes sample items from a listening questionnaire described by Sandridge (1995). The listening questionnaire should be administered prior to a hearing-aid fitting to insure that the hearing aid will meet all listening needs, and/or after a brief interval of hearing-aid use when it becomes evident during the verification sessions that the hearing aid is not providing adequate assistance in listening situations important to the client. It is imperative that the audiologist ask specific questions about hearing-related difficulties to jog the patient's memory about specific problems experienced along the way (Ross, 1997).

Alternative hearing technologies, hearing-assistance technologies, or ALDs, have proven invaluable in overcoming some of the environmental barriers to successful com-

TABLE 9–10   Needs Assessment for Hearing Aid Technologies

Without a hearing aid	YES	NO

Do you have difficulty hearing:

   a. over the telephone

   b. in the theater

   c. the television

   d. in a small group

   e. at a conference table

   f. at a restaurant

   g. when someone is calling from a distance or from a separate room

   h. when the room is noisy

   i. at lectures

   j. at religious services

With a hearing aid	YES	NO

Do you have difficulty hearing

   a. over the telephone

   b. in the theater

   c. the television

   d. in a small group

   e. at a conference table

   f. at a restaurant

   g. when someone is calling from a distance or from a separate room

   h. when the room is noisy

   i. at lectures

   j. at religious services

Source: Modified from Sandridge, 1995.

munication with or without hearing aids. These devices can overcome the communication problems created by noise or distance by use of a remote microphone that is placed within 3 to 6 inches from the sound source. While, with a hearing aid, the microphone is located at the ear of the listener, with a remote microphone arrangement the speech is processed in such a way that it reaches the listener's ear directly without attenuation or interference by noise (Kaplan, 1996). To explain, the major reason for the lack of a clear acoustic signal in selected situations is that the speech signal (S) is much louder than the background noise (N) yielding an unfavorable S/N ratio (Flexer, 1991). People with normal hearing require the signal to be twice as intense as background noise for speech to be intelligible, whereas people with hearing loss require the primary signal to be 10 times more intense than background sounds to enable them to detect word/sound distinctions. Well-fit hearing aids can provide a favorable S/N if the environment is free of distractions and if the speaker is close to the person with hearing impairment. For the most part, however, the hearing-aid microphone at the listener's ear is typically some distance from the sound source making speech difficult to understand. In essence, the further away from the sound source one is, the softer the sound pressure and the less clear the speech signal (Flexer, 1991).

SPECIAL CONSIDERATION

For the most part, the listening environments we live in are demanding. Hearing aids alone are insufficient to access auditory events that are not close to the person who is hearing impaired.

Generally, hearing aids can interface with assistive devices. Four categories of devices are available to supplement or to be used in lieu of a hearing aid. The categories of devices include (1) sound-enhancement technology, (2) television-enhancement technology/media devices, (3) telecommunications technology, and (4) signal-alerting technology. In this chapter the first three technologies will be described to insure that the reader considers these options for clients whose potential is not maximized through hearing aids.

Sound enhancement technologies enable a person with hearing impairment to understand speech clearly when the speaker is at a considerable distance from the listener. Sound enhancement technologies vary in terms of how the signal is picked up, how the signal is transmitted, and how the signal is delivered Table 9–11. In essence, sound-enhancement technologies require signal pickup close to the sound source (within 6 inches), signal transmission via one

TABLE 9–11   Characteristics of Auxiliary Aids or ALDs

1. How signal can be picked up
   - Microphone
   - Direct connection
   - Induction pick-up

2. How signal can be transmitted
   - Hard-wired systems
   - Wireless systems: FM radio waves, Infrared light waves (IR), or electromagnetic energy (induction loop systems)

3. How signal can be delivered
   - Auditory mode (e.g., earphones)
   - Visual mode (e.g., captioning)
   - Tactile mode (e.g., vibrators)

Source: Modified from Sandridge, 1995.

of several modes, and signal delivery to the listener's ear(s). The most common input device is a remote microphone, placed close to the sound source. By far the most versatile mode of transmission is via radio waves. The most efficient mode of delivery is via the auditory mode. Thus, an ideal system might consist of a remote microphone that converts the acoustic signal into an electrical signal that is carried to the transmitter; a transmitter that transduces the electrical signal into an FM signal that is transmitted via a radio-frequency carrier to a receiver; and a receiver that demodulates and amplifies the signal and sends it directly to an ouput device such as an earphone or headphone (Sandridge, 1995). With regard to the latter, several good FM systems can be interfaced with hearing aids using induction or direct audio input.

Hardwired systems that use a direct electrical connection in the delivery of the signal are commercially available, are relatively inexpensive (i.e., under $50), are portable, have good sound quality, and are ideal in one-on-one situations as in a physician's office, or when being interviewed by a nurse or social worker. They are limited in that the speaker has to be tethered to the listener. By far the most versatile technology for improving the SNR, and hence speech understanding in a background of noise, is an FM system. Behind-the-ear/FM (BTE-FM) hearing aids have recently been introduced and represent a cosmetically appealing way to enhance speech understanding in a noisy backgound using an ear-level array (otherwise FM systems require a body-worn receiver that connects in one of several ways to a personal hearing aid). In the BTE-FM arrangement, the FM receiver and a conventional hearing aid are both incorporated in a BTE case such that the BTE-FM system can be used as a regular hearing aid, as an FM receiver, or as both. The person with hearing impairment merely uses the switching option that allows the device to be used as a personal hearing aid, an FM unit, or an FM unit with an environmental microphone. The transmission range of personal FM systems is 150 to 200 feet (Kaplan, 1996).

FM systems have several distinct advantages that may make them worth the investment. They can facilitate speech understanding in large and small group situations, and in the presence of a background of noise such as in restaurants, at lectures, or at noisy receptions. FM systems can be used outdoors, when the speaker and listener are even in different rooms, with radio or television. When an older adult is on a trip or at a lecture the speaker can use the microphone/transmitter of the personal FM system enabling the person with hearing loss to follow the entire discussion. BTE-FM systems are an important innovation for cosmetic reasons and because they are more convenient than having to use a personal hearing aid as well as a separate assistive device (Kaplan, 1996).

Jerger, Chmiel, Florin, Pirozzolo, and Wilson (1996) recently completed a study comparing FM systems to conventional amplification systems in their ability to enhance speech understanding and reduce the psychosocial handicap associated with hearing impairment. Subjects in the study were older adults with primarily high-frequency sensorineural hearing loss. Their data suggested that an FM system, or an FM system coupled to a hearing aid provided dramatic improvements in speech understanding over and above that afforded by a programmable hearing aid. In contrast, hearing aids were comparable to the FM system in

their positive impact on self-perceived hearing handicap associated with the hearing impairment. Similarly, despite the superiority of both the FM system and the hearing aid and FM system on speech-recognition tasks, subjects overwhelmingly chose the conventional hearing aid as a system they would prefer to use in daily life. Interestingly, the hearing aid was used by subjects approximately 11 hours per day whereas the FM system was used about 1 hour a day. The FM system was considered cumbersome and intrusive. The authors suggested that, should FM systems become more user friendly and be more common among elderly hearing-impaired individuals, perhaps it may become a more acceptable technology. Compton (1996a) has reported success with a pressure zone microphone (PZM) developed by Centrum Sound that can be attached to any FM transmitter and placed in the center of a reflective table top eliminating the need for a lapel microphone to be passed around. It can also be coupled successfully to the television so that hearing-impaired individuals can understand both the TV and the speaker. Compton (1996a) indicated that she has recommended the PZM microphone to a 92-year-old gentleman with a moderate hearing loss and central auditory processing problems that preclude successful hearing-aid use, and he and his wife of 70 years are using it successfully.

Finally, infrared sytems use invisible light, the wavelength of which is outside the range of human visibility to transmit signals indoors in a single room from the speaker to the listener. They are not as flexible as FM systems and are more complicated to install as they require an alternating-current power source rather than a battery. Further,

---

SPECIAL CONSIDERATION

FM systems have a positive impact on self-perceived handicap yet older adults prefer conventional hearing aids.

---

infrared light is absorbed by dark or dull surfaces and reflected by shiny surfaces thus are best used in rooms without windows or in rooms that do not have shiny reflecting walls (Sandridge, 1995). In view of these disadvantages, infrared systems are more appropriate for use with the television or in large areas such as the theater rather than for small group communication. These are discussed in greater detail in the section on media devices.

Finally, telecommunication technology can augment or be used in place of a hearing aid when communicating over the telephone. Table 9–12 classifies the telecommunication

---

PEARL

Older adults often rely on the telephone to communicate with family members as well as friends, to make contacts with health professionals, and to make emergency contacts. Therefore, it is imperative that older adults with hearing aids who continue to have difficulty using the phone be made aware of the options that exist.

TABLE 9–12   Telecommunication Options

Amplifying the system through
Portable couplers
Handset amplifiers
In-line amplifiers
Amplified telephones
Interpersonal listening devices

Visual representation of the signal through
Computer modems
Fax
TTY or TDD

Source: Sandridge, 1995.

options available to the hearing impaired. It is noteworthy that the advent of the Americans with Disabilities Act (ADA—1990), which mandates telephone accessibility for all individuals with telephones, actually minimizes the need for portable devices, however in-home use of the available options remains important for older adults.

Devices that provide auditory enhancement of the signal may be preferable to those that visually represent the signal, although the latter options should not be ruled out. The devices providing auditory enhancement have distinct differences that should be clear to the audiologist and ultimately the consumer. As is shown in Table 9–12, the first option is a portable coupler. These are available in two varieties, namely as acoustic couplers or inductive couplers. Acoustic couplers, which are available for use on a variety of phones, attach to the receiver of the handset by an elastic or detachable strap. Acoustic couplers can be used with or without a hearing aid on all telephones including cellular and car phones. They make all telephones hearing aid compatible, if necessary. Acoustic couplers can be used with a

telecoil (T switch) because an electromagnetic field is produced during the transduction of energy (Sandridge, 1995). Acoustic couplers pose difficulties for older adults with poor manual dexterity because of the need to attach and remove the coupler each time the phone is used. Also, older adults may forget to turn the battery off, draining the battery and requiring the need to replace it, which can become costly. Induction couplers, while less costly than acoustic couplers, provide slightly less acoustic gain than an acoustic coupler. Similarly, they are restricted to persons with a hearing aid equipped with a telecoil.

The next option is a handset amplifier that primarily increases the loudness of the incoming signal, providing between 20 and 30 dB of gain. Handset amplifiers can only be used with modular telephones. That is, phones wherein the handset can be detached from the part of the phone that contains the dialing mechanism. Older adults wedded to their old trimline phones cannot use a handset amplifier. Similarly, selected electronic telephones may not be compatible with certain amplifier handsets. Finally, less expensive telephones may not be compatible with an amplifier handset because they may not provide enough power to drive the amplifier. In short, prior to recommending a handset amplifier, the audiologist must obtain very specific information about the client's telephone to insure that he/she is giving the correct recommendation. If a handset amplifier is recommended, a touchbar volume control is the preferred option for older adults. They are easier to manipulate than the rotary wheel, and amplification is disengaged when the handset is placed back on the cradle of the phone. This minimizes the chance of overamplification when the next user, who may not have a hearing loss, picks up the phone. Using a touchbar, the intensity is increased or decreased by depressing the top or bottom of the bar.

In-line amplifiers are interfaced between the body of the telephone and the handset. They operate on the same principle as the amplified handset with fewer restrictions. They have several advantages over handset amplifiers as is evident from Table 9–13. Amplified telephones are the most expensive option for the hearing impaired because of the variety of available options. Prices range from $100 to $350

TABLE 9–13   In-Line Amplifiers Versus Handset Amplifiers

In-line amplifiers	Handset amplifers
Can be used on a variety of telephones including electronic phones	Can only be used with modular phones
Are portable, and compatible with most phones	Lack of compatibility limits portability
Can use rotary-wheel or sliding-bar volume control as there is little difference between the two	Touchbar volume control is preferable
Less costly	Initially more costly
Provide up to 25 dB of gain under optimal conditions (some only provide 10 dB of gain)	Provide approximately 20 dB of gain under optimal conditions although some provide as much as 30 dB of gain

Source: Sandridge, 1995.

depending on where the phone is purchased. They are fully functioning telephones equipped with large dialing buttons for persons with manual-dexterity problems and with adjustable volume controls located on the base of the telephone allowing for excellent visibility. Amplified telephones are available with the following options (Sandridge, 1995): (1) cordless, (2) circumaural earpiece, (3) variable gain depending on the hearing loss, (4) programmable memory, (5) lighted ringer indicators for those who cannot hear the ringer, (6) amplified or low-frequency audible ringers for persons with adequate hearing in the lower frequencies, and (7) return to normal volume when hung up. The latter option is available so that there is less of a risk of overamplification for users with normal hearing.

The final auditory enhancement device available to the hearing impaired is an interpersonal listening aid that can be interfaced with the telephone through a specialized connecting device. These devices enable the hearing impaired to use their personal ALD with the telephone, such that the telephone signal can be routed through and controlled by the listening device. In sum, a number of telecommunication devices that use auditory enhancements are available to the hearing-impaired consumer to augment or replace the personal hearing aid. The audiologist is encouraged to become well versed in the variety of available options and to apprise hearing-aid users of their advantages and disadvantages. Telecommunication is an important activity of daily living for older adults as auditory access allows for communication with family members, friends, relatives, and health professionals. For more detailed information about telecommunication options, the reader is referred to the Sandridge chapter titled "Beyond Hearing Aids: Auxiliary Aids" in the text by Kricos and Lesner (1995).

Amplification devices such as the ones described may not provide adequate amplification for individuals with severe to profound hearing loss or for persons with extremely poor speech-recognition ability. A variety of visual systems are available to promote telephone access. Telecommunication options include facsimiles (fax) machines, electronic-mail (e-mail), and text telephones known as telecommunication systems for the deaf (TDD) or teletypewriters (TTYs). TDDs have their basis in TTY technology, merely transmitting visual signals over the standard telephone line. They rely on Baudot (TTY language). TTYs are invaluable to persons with severe to profound hearing loss for whom it is impossible to discriminate speech over the telephone. TTYs are about the size of a typewriter. Individuals communicating over the telephone merely type in their message, or use a relay operator who types in a message, and it is displayed across the listener's TTY. Thanks to the ADA—1990, the telephone company provides relay service free of charge for persons wishing to speak with a TTY user.

For older adults wishing to invest in a TTY, Compton (1996) recommends the Ameriphone "read and talk" telephone, the Dialogue VCO. This telephone has a built-in LCD display so it can be used as a TTD and it can also be used as a regular phone. By making voice carry-over (VCO) calls toll free through the local relay service, the hard-of-hearing individual can read what the caller is saying as the relay operator types the caller's words onto a computer. In turn, the text is sent to the client's phone where it appears on an LCD display. The listener simply talks back to the caller through the telephone as usual. The phone also has a built-in answering machine so that all messages appear as text on the built-in screen. If the presence of a third party is bothersome, the Ultratec Uniphone 1140 is ideal as a voice/text phone. This phone, which must be used by third parties, allows direct communication between people who are deaf, hard-of-hearing, and/or speech impaired. The phone is quite versatile such that it can be used as an amplified, hearing-aid–compatible voice phone to call another hard-of-hearing person. When necessary, messages can be typed into the phones to clarify what was said by voice. That which is typed appears on the LCD on the other person's phone (Compton, 1996a). In sum, the Ultratec-Uniphone represents what some consider to be an unbeatable combination namely the TTD, telecommunications relay service, and VCO. According to Danielson, (1995, p. 12) the opportunity to use one's own voice again during telephone calls, is "a true blessing . . . not so much a change as a return to a previous, more natural, and greatly satisfying life skill."

Older adults with severe to profound hearing loss who are computer users may prefer to use their computer as a text phone rather than a traditional TTY. For these individuals, Futura software in combination with a smart modem, will allow the computer to operate as a TTY. The modem and software cost less than a free-standing TTY, however the client must have some training to understand how to operate the computer when a call comes into the TTY phone line (Compton, 1996a). Finally, older adults who are not scared away by technological advances should consider an alpha-numeric pager as a way of communicating with others. An alpha-numeric pager can be an efficient way to access messages.

Fax or e-mail are also excellent forms of telecommunication technology for persons with hearing impairment unable to communicate comfortably over the telephone. More and more individuals have invested in fax machines and computers, making these forms of technology less expensive, and user friendly to persons of all ages with and without disability.

Media/Television Devices

A major reason older adults obtain audiologic intervention is because of difficulty hearing the television. A frequent complaint of family members is that persons with hearing loss turn the volume up on the television to an uncomfortably loud level. Even when wearing a hearing aid, older adults still find that the signal is not sufficiently amplified (Pichora-Fuller, 1997). The difficulty lies in the fact that extraneous noise in the environment, distance between the TV and viewer, and reverberation combine to distort the signal from the television. Media devices, which enhance the SNR for the listener, are ideal for home or apartment use. Four amplification devices are available for television, each delivering the auditory signal to the listener's ear in a different way. These devices are (1) infrared systems (IR); (2) FM systems; (3) hardwired systems; and (4) magnetic loop systems

(Davis, 1994). While the devices differ in how the sound source from the television is delivered to the listener's ears, they each effectively reduce the impact of distance, noise, and reverberation on the intelligibility of the signal.

IR systems, are wireless systems that utilize invisible infrared light beams to transmit the TV sound signal. IR systems are commercially available, portable, easy to install, and have excellent sound quality. They work best for persons with mild to moderately severe hearing impairment (Compton, 1989). IR systems consist of a microphone and amplifier, and a transmitter that is placed on top of the television set facing the listening area. The transmitter, which is plugged into an AC power source, has an emitter panel with an array of light-emitting diodes LEDs. The person with hearing impairment wears a receiver (available in a number of varieties), which uses a detector that decodes the signal from the emitter/transmitter, amplifies it, and directs it to the listener's ears (Davis, 1994). The person wearing the receiver must be in the same room and must always face the transmitter. Further, the path between the transmitter and receiver must be uninterrupted, as light rays do not travel through solid surfaces. Receivers are battery powered and lightweight with one of the most common ones being the stethoset receiver with an output jack for attaching additional ALDs, neck loops, etc. The IR system allows the TV to be heard at the desired volume by everyone in the room and the person with hearing impairment merely adjusts the volume on the receiver to a comfortable listening level.

FM systems are also wireless, easy to install, portable, and battery powered. They are the most flexible of the television systems. The listener does not have to be confined to the room for listening; signals can be transmitted almost 200 feet; systems can be used indoors and outdoors; and people with all levels of hearing impairment can benefit (Davis, 1994). The FM system also contains a transmitter, microphone, receiver, and some device to couple sound to the listener's ears (Davis, 1994). The FM system works in much the same way as the IR system, however the transmitter, which is attached to the microphone, transduces the audio signal that is picked up from the TV and transmits it through the room as a frequency-modulated signal. The receiver picks up the signal, demodulates it, and delivers it directly to the ear. The receiver directs the sound to the ear via a neckloop, earbud, headphone, silhouette, or direct audio input. The volume of transmission can be controlled at the television or at the FM reciever (Davis, 1994; Pichora-Fuller, 1997). Some systems allow the TV signal to be broadcast to a free-standing speaker. For residents of nursing facilities, who may have difficulty managing headsets, an FM receiver and amplifier integrated into a self-powered loudspeaker may be helpful (Ross, 1997). These can be placed in a convenient location, such as a table close to the resident. It is noteworthy that newer FM systems allow for each ear to be controlled separately, and some systems are built especially for television use providing stereophonic and monophonic sound at both high- and low-frequency emphasis (Davis, 1994).

Hardwired systems are portable, easy to install, battery-operated, and relatively inexpensive. However, the listener is tethered to the wire, thus limiting their mobility, and the sound quality is not as good as with the IR or FM systems. Personal hardwired systems consist of an amplifying unit with a microphone placed near the television speaker. The signal from the television is picked up by the microphone, changed into an electrical signal, amplified, and changed back into sound at the earpiece. The earpiece is typically a headset such as the one used with a Sony Walkman. Some people who wear BTE hearing aids may choose to connect their hearing aid to the TV by direct audio input, wherein a wire connected to the television plugs into the hearing aid. With direct audio input, the television connection can be wired so that viewers without hearing problems can hear the signal from the TV loudspeaker (Pichora-Fuller, 1997). Finally, viewers may choose to wear earphones that connect directly into the audio-output jack on the TV.

Induction loop systems that use the principle of electromagnetic induction can be used by hearing-aid wearers to transmit the television signal. TV loop systems do not have some of the advantages inherent in the FM or IR systems in that they are not as portable; require some installation; and transmission distance is limited to within or close to the loop. Sound quality depends on the listener's location relative to the loop such that signal strength is strongest when closest to the loop wire and weakest when the person is located within the center of the looped area (Davis, 1994). With these systems, sound is picked up by a microphone at the television, converted into an electrical signal, amplified, and directed to a wire that is looped around the listening area (Davis, 1994). The receiver is typically a hearing aid with a T-coil that converts the electromagnetic signal from the wire loop back into sound (Davis, 1994). For persons not having a hearing aid with a T-coil, the signal can be picked up through a headset receiver with a T-coil.

Finally, some older adults may not be able to understand the audio signal from the television even with the above technology, because of the severity of loss or auditory-processing difficulties. Closed-captioned television is an excellent alternative and since July 1993, all new television sets, with screens greater than 13 inches, made or sold in the United States include a decoder chip with the capability to access closed captioning (Ross, 1997). Thus, for persons purchasing new televisions, separate decoders are not necessary. Persons with older televisions must purchase separate decoder boxes as the Television Decoder Circuitry Act of 1990 does not require older televisions to be retrofitted. With captioning, a written version of what is said is added like a subtitle along the bottom of the TV image (Pichora-Fuller, 1997). Television listings indicate which shows are captioned by a code or symbol such as "CC." It is important to inform all patients of the closed-captioning option, as people with all levels of hearing impairment can enjoy the increased access to television programming afforded by closed captioning (Ross, 1997).

In sum, a wide variety of assistive devices are available to persons with handicapping hearing impairments. Available devices can be used as stand-alone systems or in conjunction with hearing aids; can help to communicate messages visually; and can facilitate communication over the telephone. Meeting all of the communication needs of the hearing impaired will insure that expectations are met and that the consumer leaves the office a satisfied client. Appendix A includes a list of device vendors.

CONCLUDING REMARKS

This chapter is lengthier than I had originally anticipated, however it seemed appropriate to include information on hearing aids and ALDs together, given their combined purpose of enhancing communication function for older adults with handicapping hearing impairments. It is apparent from the preceding review that hearing aids, whether analog, digital controlled analog, or "true" digital are effective treatments for the communication disabilities and psychosocial handicaps that attend presbycusis. Persons with hearing impairment, however, must be convinced of the value of hearing aids in the face of the negative press and exorbitant cost. It is incumbent on audiologists to insure that older adults are informed of the value of hearing aids in overcoming the communication difficulties that attend hearing loss, and of the importance of ALDs and audiologic re-

habilitation as adjuncts to hearing aids. Audiologists must remember to look beyond the technology at the individual and remember that the hearing-aid fitting should be driven by the expressed needs of the older patient. The hearing premises enumerated by McSpaden (1996) say it all:

- Patients do not come into a dispenser's office because their audiogram is abnormal. They come in because their perception indicates a loss, a decrease in sensitivity, a change, or simply a social "failure" that they impute to their hearing.
- Patients do not care about numbers. What is important is their perception of what the numbers mean.
- To the extent that we improve the patient's communicative efficiency, what we have done will be worth it. If we do not improve communicative efficiency, yet achieve good aided thresholds and higher discrimination scores, whatever we have done is not worth it.
- No one listens to anything at threshold. Everyone wants to listen to everything at MCL without ever exceeding LDL. This is true for every signal.
- It is not about hearing any kind of signal, it is about understanding and decoding.
- The patient is the one with the symptoms.
- We must stop anthropomorphizing the audiogram. The audiogram is merely a graph of auditory behavior, elicited on a given day, at a given time. It is not the hearing impaired person.
- Make every effort to meet the needs of the patient, and stop trying to make the patient's needs fit our understanding.
- It's about the patient!

APPENDIX A
Name and Address of Vendors of ALDs

American Loop Systems
43 Davis Road, Suite 2
Belmont, MA 02178

AT&T National Special Needs Center
2001 Route 46
Parsippany, NJ 07054

Audio Enhancement
12613 South Redwood Road
Riverton, UT 84065

Audiometrics
5145 Avenida Encinitas, Suite B
Carlsbad, CA 92008

Centrum Sound
215809 Stevens Creek Blvd.,
Suite 209
Cupertino, CA 95014

Custom All Hear Systems
20833 67th Ave. West, Suite 101
Lynnwood, WA 98036

Hal-Hen
P.O. Box 6077
Long Island City, NY 11106

Harris Communications
15159 Technology Drive
Eden Prairie, MN 55344

Hear You Are
4 Musconetong Ave.
Stanhope, NJ 07874

Hearing Aid Center (HAC) of America
HARC Mercantile LTD.
3130 Portage Rd.
P.O. Box 3055
Kalamazoo, MI 49003-3055

Hi-Tec Group International
801 N. Cass Avenue #021
Westmont, IL 60559

Lifeline Amplification Systems
55 South 4th Street
Platteville, WI 53818

Phonic Ear, Inc.
3880 Cypress Drive
Petaluma, CA 94954-7600

Precision Controls, Inc.
14 Doty Road
Haskell, NJ 07420

Radio Shack
Fort Worth, TX 76102

Siemens Hearing Instruments Inc.
Piscataway, NJ 08855-1397

Silent Call Corporation
P.O. Box 16348
Clarksont, MI 48016

Sonic Alert
209 Voorheis
Pontiac, MI 48053

Telex Communications, Inc.
9600 Aldrich Avenue South
Minneapolis, MN 55420

Ultratec, Inc.
6442 Normandy Lange
Madison, WI 53719

Wheelock, Inc.
273 Branchport Ave.
Long Branch, NJ 07740

REFERENCES

ABRAMS, H., CHISOLM, T., GUERREIRO, S., & RITTERMAN, S. (1992). The effects of intervention strategy on self-perception of hearing handicap. *Ear and Hearing,* 13:371–377.

AGNEW, J. (1996a). Directionality in hearing . . . revisited. *Hearing Review,* 3:20–29.

———. (1996b). Hearing aid adjustments through potentiometer and switch options. In: M. Valente (Ed.), *Hearing Aids: Standards, Options and Limitations.* New York: Thieme Medical Publishers.

———. (1997). An overview of digital signal processing in hearing instrument. *Hearing Review,* 4:11–18, 66.

AMERICAN SPEECH-LANGUAGE HEARING ASSOCIATION. (1994). Audiology Update, 13, 17.

———. (1998). Guidelines for hearing aid fitting for adults. *American Journal of Audiology,* 7:5–13.

BÄCHLER, H., KNECHT, W., LAUNER, S., & UVACEK, B. (1997). Audibility, intelligibility, sound quality and comfort. *Supplement to Hearing Review,* 2:31–37.

BARRY, S. (1998). Review of hearing aid amplification circuits. *Journal of the American Academy of Audiology,* 9:105–111.

BENDER, D., & MUELLER, H.G. (1984). Factors influencing the decision to obtain amplification. *ASHA,* 26(10):120.

BENTLER, R. (1994). Future trends in verification strategies. In: M. Valente, (Ed.), *Strategies for Selecting and Verifying Hearing Aid Fittings.* New York: Thieme Medical Publishers.

BENTLER, R., NIEBUHR, D., GETTA, J., & ANDERSON, C. (1993). Longitudinal study of hearing aid effectiveness. II: Subjective Measures. *Journal of Speech and Hearing Research,* 36:820–831.

BESS, F., LICHTENSTEIN, M., LOGAN, S., BURGER, M., & NELSON, E. (1989). Hearing impairment as a determinant of function in the elderly. *Journal of the American Geriatrics Society,* 37:123–128.

BRAY, V. (1997). Classification system for programmable hearing instruments. In: B. Weinstein (Ed.), *Seminars in Hearing,* 18:57–62.

BRIDGES, J., & BENTLER, R. (1998). Relating hearing aid use to well-being among older adults. *Hearing Journal,* 51:39–44.

BYRNE, D. (1996). Hearing aid selection for the 1990s: where to? *Journal of the American Academy of Audiology,* 7: 377–395.

CARTER, T. (1994). Age-related vision changes: a primary care guide. *Geriatrics,* 49:37–47.

CHMIEL, R., & JERGER, J. (1995). Quantifying improvement with amplification. *Ear and Hearing,* 16:166–175.

CHMIEL, R., & JERGER, J. (1996). Hearing aid use, central auditory disorder and hearing handicap in elderly persons. *Journal of the American Academy of Audiology,* 7:190–202.

CHMIEL, R., JERGER, J., MURPHY, E., PIROZZOLO, F., & TOOLEY-YOUNG, C. (1997). Unsuccessful use of binaural amplification by an elderly person. *Journal of the American Academy of Audiology,* 8:1–10.

COMPTON, C. (1989). *Assistive Devices: Doorways to Independence.* Washington, DC: Gallaudet University.

———. (1996a). Innovations in assistive technology: a potpourri of exciting approaches. *Hearing Journal,* 49:10–20.

———. (1996b). Fact or fairy tale? You can get a good telecoil in an In-the-Ear Hearing Aid. *SHHH Journal,* 17:8–17.

COX, R. (1995). Page ten: a hands on discussion of the IHAFF approach. *Hearing Journal,* 48:10, 39–44.

———. (1997). Administration and application of the APHAB. *Hearing Review,* 50:32–48.

———. (1999). Five years later: an update on the IHAFF fitting protocol. *Hearing Journal,* 52:10–18.

COX, R., & ALEXANDER, G. (1995). The Abbreviated Profile of Hearing Aid Benefit. *Ear and Hearing,* 16:176–186.

COX, R., ALEXANDER, G., & GILMORE, C. (1991). Objective and self-report measures of hearing aid benefit. In: G. Studebaker, F. Bess, & L. Beck (Eds.), *The Vanderbilt Hearing Aid Report II.* Parkton, MD: York Press.

COX, R., ALEXANDER, G., & GRAY, G. (1999). Personality and the subjective assessment of hearing aids. *Journal of the American Academy of Audiology,* 10:1–13.

COX, R., ALEXANDER, G., TAYLOR, I., & GRAY, G. (1996). Benefit acclimatization in elderly hearing aid users. *Journal of the American Academy of Audiology,* 7:428–441.

CRANDELL, C. (1998). Hearing aids and functional health status. *Audiology Today,* 10:20–23.

DANIELSON, J. (1995). An unbeatable combination: the text telephone, telecommunications relay service, and voice carry-over. *SHHH Journal,* 16:12–13.

DAVIS, D. (1994). Television amplification devices. In: M. Ross (Ed.), *Communication Access for Persons with Hearing Loss.* Parkton, MD: York Press.

DILLON, H. (1996). Tutorial—Compression? Yes, but for low or high frequencies, for low or high intensities, and with what response times? *Ear and Hearing,* 17:287–307.

DILLON, H., & GINIS, J. (1997). The Client Oriented Scale of Improvement (COSI) and its relationship to several other measures of benefit and satisfaction provided by hearing aids. *Journal of the American Academy of Audiology,* 8: 27–43.

DILLON, H., JAMES, A., & GINIS, J. (1997). Client Oriented Scale of Improvement (COSI) and its relationship to several other measures of benefit and satisfaction provided by hearing aids. *Journal of the American Academy of Audiology,* 8:27–43.

EBINGER, K., HOLLAND, S., HOLLAND, J., & MUELLER, G. (1995). Using the APHAB to assess benefit from CIC hearing aids. Poster session presented at the Annual Meeting of the American Academy of Audiology.

FABRY, D. (1996). Clinical applications of multimemory hearing aids. *Hearing Journal,* 49:10, 53–56.

FINO, M., BESS, F., LICHTENSTEIN, M., & LOGAN, S. (1991). Factors differentiating elderly hearing aid wearers and nonwearers. *Hearing Instruments,* 43:6–10.

FLEXER, C. (1991). Access to communication environments through assistive listening devices. *Hearsay*, 6:9–14.

FORTUNE, T. (1996). Amplifiers and circuit algorithms of contemporary hearing aids. In: M. Valente (Ed.), *Hearing Aids: Standards, Options and Limitations*. New York: Thieme Medical Publishers.

FRANKS, J., & BECKMAN, N. (1982). Rejection of hearing aids: attitudes of a geriatric sample. *Ear and Hearing*, 6:161–166.

GATEHOUSE, S. (1992). The time course and magnitude of perceptual acclimatization to frequency responses: evidence from monaural fitting of hearing aids. *Journal of the Acoustical Society of America*, 92:1259–1268.

———. (1994). Components and determinants of hearing aid benefit. *Journal of the American Academy of Audiology*, 15:30–49.

———. (1999). Glasgow Hearing Aid Benefit Profile. Derivation and validation of a client-centered outcome measure for hearing aid services. *Journal of the American Academy of Audiology*, 18:80–103.

GELFAND, S. (1995). Long-term recovery and no recovery from the auditory deprivation effect with binaural amplification: six cases. *Journal of the American Academy of Audiology*, 6:141–149.

HAWKINS, D., WALDEN, B., MONTGOMERY, A., & PROSEK, R. (1987). Description and validation of an LDL procedure designed to select SSPL-90. *Ear and Hearing*, 8:162–169.

HEARING INDUSTRIES ASSOCIATION. (1998). *Quarterly Statistics Report for Fourth Quarter 1997*. Washington, DC: HIA.

HNATH-CHISOLM, T., & ABRAMS, H. (1993). Adaptation to the use of amplification in the elderly. *FLASHA Journal*, 2:7–21.

HOSFORD-DUNN, H. (1997). Your questions answered on digital hearing aids. *Hearing Journal*, 50:10–21.

HUMES, L. (1996). Evolution of prescriptive fitting approaches. *American Journal of Audiology*, 5:19–23.

HUMES, L., CHRISTENSEN, L., BESS, F., & WILLIAMS, A. (1997). Comparison of the benefit provided by well-fit linear hearing aids and instruments with automatic reductions of low-frequency gain. *Journal of Speech and Hearing Research*, 40:666–685.

HUMES, L., CHRISTENSEN, L., THOMAS, T., BESS, F., WILLIAMS, A., & BENTLER, R. (1999). A comparison of aided performance and benefit provided by a linear and two channel wide dynamic range compression hearing aid. *Journal of Speech, Language and Hearing Research*, 32:65–79.

HUMES, L., & HALLING, D. (1994). Overview, rationale and comparison of suprathreshold based gain prescription methods. In: M. Valente (Ed.), *Strategies for Selecting and Verifying Hearing Aid Fittings*. New York: Thieme Medical Publishers.

HUMES, L., HALLING, D., & COUGHLIN, M. (1996). Reliability and stability of various hearing aid outcome measures in a group of elderly hearing aid wearers. *Journal of Speech and Hearing Research*, 39:923–936.

HYDE, M., & RIKO, K. (1994). A decision-analytic approach to audiological rehabilitation. In: J.P. Gagne & N.T. Murrary (Eds.), Research in audiological rehabilitation: current trends and future directions. *Journal of the American Academy of Rehabilitative Audiology, Monograph Supplement*, 27:337–374.

JERGER, J., CHMIEL, R., FLORIN, E., PIROZZOLO, F., & WILSON, N. (1996). Comparison of conventional amplification and an assistive listening device in elderly persons. *Ear and Hearing*, 17:490–504.

JERGER, J., SILMAN, S., LEW, H., & CHMIEL, R. (1993). Case studies in binaural interference: converging evidence from behavioral and electrophysiologic measures. *Journal of the American Academy of Audiology*, 4:122–131.

KAPLAN, H. (1996). Assistive devices for the elderly. *Journal of the American Academy of Audiology*, 7:203–211.

KEIDSER, G., DILLON, H., & BYRNE, D. (1996). Guidelines for fitting multiple memory hearing aids. *Journal of the American Academy of Audiology*, 7:406–418.

KEMP, B. (1990). The psychosocial context of geriatric rehabilitation. In: B. Kemp, K. Brummel-Smith, & J. Ramsdell (Eds.), *Geriatric Rehabilitation*. Boston: College Hill.

KILLION, M., STAAB, W., & PREVES, D. (1990). Classifying automatic signal processors. *Hearing Instruments*, 41:24–26.

KIRKWOOD, D. (1994). HJ Report. *Hearing Journal*, 47:7–8.

———. (1996a). Resurgent hearing aid market nearing record-high level. *Hearing Journal*, 49:13–20.

———. (1996b). Dispensers report expanding practices, predict additional growth in 1996. *Hearing Journal*, 49:13–23.

———. (1997). Survey finds dispensers mostly positive but not about mangaged care. *Hearing Journal*, 50:3, 23–31.

———. (1998). Hearing aid sales increase 7.5% in 1997: expansion expected to continue. *Hearing Journal*, 51:21–28.

———. (1999). World of Hearing conference seeks to raise awareness of hearing loss, care. *Hearing Journal*, 52:49–52.

KOCHKIN, S. (1992). MarkeTrak III: higher hearing aid sales don't signal better market penetration. *Hearing Journal*, 45(7):2–7.

———. (1993). MarkeTrak III: the billion dollar opportunity in the hearing instruments market. *Hearing Journal*, 46:35–38.

———. (1994). Optimizing the emerging market for completely-in-the-canal instruments. *Hearing Journal*, 47:1–6.

———. (1995a). Customer satisfaction and benefit with CIC hearing instruments. *Hearing Review*, 2:16–26.

———. (1995b). MarkeTrak IV norms: subjective measures of satisfaction and benefit. Presented at the American Academy of Audiology Convention, March 1995.

———. (1996). MarkeTrak IV: 10-year trends in the hearing aid market—has anything changed? *Hearing Journal*, 49:23–33.

———. (1997). MarkeTrak IV: what is the viable market for hearing aids? *Hearing Journal*, 50:31–39.

———. (1998). MarkeTrak IV: correlates of hearing aid purchase intent. *Hearing Journal*, 51:30–41.

———. (1999). "Baby boomers" spur growth in potential market, but penetration rate declines. *Hearing Journal*, 52:1.

KRICOS, P., & HOLMES, A. (1996). Efficacy of audiologic rehabilitation for older adults. *Journal of the American Academy of Audiology*, 7:219–229.

KUK, F. (1993). Clinical consideration in fitting a multimemory hearing aid. *American Journal of Audiology*, 2:23–27.

MADAFFARI, P., & STANLEY, W. (1996). Microphone, receiver and telecoil options: past, present and future. In: M. Valente (Ed.), *Hearing Aids: Standards, Options and Limitations*. New York: Thieme Medical Publishers.

MALINOFF, R., & WEINSTEIN, B. (1989). Measurement of hearing aid benefit in the elderly. *Ear and Hearing*, 10:354–356.

MARTIN, R., & PIRZANSKI, C. (1998). Techniques for successful CIC fittings. *Hearing Journal*, 51:72–74,

McCANDLESS, G. (1994). Overview and rationale of threshold based hearing aid selection procedures. In: M. Valente (Ed.), *Strategies for Selecting and Verifying Hearing Aid Fittings*. New York: Thieme Medical Publishers.

McCARTHY, P. (1996). Hearing aid fitting and audiologic rehabilitation: a complementary relationship. *American Journal of Audiology*, 5:24–28.

McCARTHY, P., MONTGOMERY, A., & MUELLER, G. (1990). Decision making in rehabilitative audiology. *Journal of the American Academy of Audiology*, 1:23–30.

McSPADEN, J. (1996). Thirty-six hearing premises. *Hearing Review*, 3:8–10.

MOLLOY, D., & LUBINSKI, R. (1995). Dementia: impact and clinical perspectives. In: R. Lubinski (Ed.), *Dementia and Communication*. San Diego: Singular Publishing Group.

MONTGOMERY, A. (1994). Treatment efficacy in adult audiological rehabilitation. In: J.P. Gagne & N.T. Murray (Eds.), Research in audiological rehabilitation: current trends and future directions. *Journal of the American Academy of Rehabilitative Audiology, Monograph Supplement*, 27:317–337.

MUELLER, G. (1994). Small can be good too! *Hearing Journal*, 47:11.

———. (1996). Hearing aids and people: strategies for a successful match. *Hearing Journal*, 49:13–28.

MUELLER, G., & KILLION, M. (1990). An easy method for calculating the articulation index. *Hearing Journal*, 43:14–17.

MUELLER, C., & PALMER, K. (1998). The Profile of Aided Loudness: a new "PAL" for '98. *Hearing Journal*, 51:10–19.

MULROW, C., AGUILAR, C., ENDICOTT, J., TULEY, M., VELEZ, R., CHARLIP, W., RHODES, M., HILL, J., & DENINO, L. (1990). Quality of life changes and hearing impairment: results of a randomized trial. *Annals of Internal Medicine*, 113:188–194.

MULROW, C., MICHAEL, T., & AGUILAR, C. (1992). Correlates of successful hearing aid use in older adults. *Ear and Hearing*, 13:108–113.

MULROW, C., TULEY, M., & AGUILAR, C. (1992). Sustained benefit of hearing aids. *Journal of Speech and Hearing Research*, 35:1402–1405.

MUSIEK, F., & BARAN, J. (1996). Amplification and the central auditory nervous system. In: M. Valente (Ed.), *Hearing Aids: Standards, Options and Limitations*. New York: Thieme Medical Publishers.

NERBONNE, M., CHRISTMAN, W., & FLESCHNER, C. (1995). Comparing objective and subjective measures of hearing aid benefit. Poster presentation at the 1995 Convention of the American Academy of Audiology, St. Paul, MN, March 1995.

NEWMAN, C., HUG, G., WHARTON, G., & JACOBSON, G. (1993). The influence of hearing aid cost on perceived benefit in older adults. *Ear and Hearing*, 14:285–289.

NEWMAN, C., JACOBSON, G., HUG, G., WEINSTEIN, B., & MALINOFF, R. (1991). Practical method for quantifying hearing aid benefit in older adults. *Journal of the American Academy of Audiology*, 2:70–75.

NEWMAN, C., & SANDRIDGE, S. (1998). Benefit from satisfaction with and cost-effectiveness of three different hearing aid technologies. *American Journal of Audiology*, 7:115–128.

NEWMAN, C., & WEINSTEIN, B. (1988). The Hearing Handicap Inventory for the Elderly. *Ear and Hearing*, 9:81–85.

OFFICE OF TECHNOLOGY ASSESSMENT. (1978). Assessing the efficacy and safety of medical technologies. Washington, DC: Congress of the United States, Office of Technology Assessment, OTA-11–75.

OLSWANG, L., THOMPSON, R., WARREN, S., & MINGHETTI, N. (1990). *Treatment Efficacy Research in Communication Disorders*. Rockville, MD: American Speech-Language-Hearing Foundation.

PFEIFFER, E. (1975). A short portable mental status questionnaire for assessment of organic brain deficit in elderly patients. *Journal of the American Geriatrics Society*, 23:433–441.

PICHORA-FULLER, M.K. (1997). Assistive listening devices for the elderly. In: R. Lubinski & D. Higginbotham (Eds.), *Communication Technologies for the Elderly*. San Diego: Singular Publishing Group.

PREVES, D. (1996). The role of the hearing aid instrument amplifier. *Hearing Review*, 3:34–38.

———. (1997). Directional microphone use in ITE hearing instruments. *Hearing Review*, 4:21–27.

PRIMEAU, R. (1997). Hearing aid benefit in adults and older adults. *Seminars in Hearing*, 18:29–36.

RADCLIFFE, D. (1991). Programmable hearing aids: digital control comes to analog amplification. *Hearing Journal*, 44:9–12.

RAMSDELL, J. (1990). A rehabilitation orientation in the workup of general medical problems. In: B. Kemp, K. Brummel-Smith, & J. Ramsdell (Eds.), *Geriatric Rehabilitation*. Boston: College Hill.

RICKETTS, T., VAN VLIET, D. (1996). Updating our fitting strategies given new technology. *American Journal of Audiology*, 5:29–35.

ROSS, M. (1995a). Developments in technology. *SHHH Journal*, 16(1), 25–26.

———. (1995b). Developments in research and technology. *SHHH Journal*, 16(2), 32–34.

———. (1996a). Developments in research and technology. *SHHH Journal*, 17:34–37.

———. (1996b). You've done something about it! Helpful hints to the new hearing aid user. *SHHH Journal*, 17:7– 11.

———. (1997). Beyond hearing aids: hearing assistance technologies. *Seminars in Hearing,* 18:103–116.

ROSS, M. & LEVITT, H. (1997). Consumer satisfaction is not enough: hearing aids are still about hearing. *Seminars in Hearing*, 18:7–13.

RUBINSTEIN, A. (1997). Hearing aid fitting and management. *Seminars in Hearing,* 18:87–101.

SANDRIDGE, S. (1995). Beyond hearing aids: use of auxiliary aids. In: P. Kricos & S. Lesner (Eds.), *Hearing Care for the Older Adult.* Boston: Butterworth-Heinemann.

SCHOW, R., BALSARA, N., SMEDLEY, T., & WHITCOMB, C. (1993). Aural rehabilitation by ASHA audiologists: 1980–1990. *American Journal of Audiology,* 2:28–38.

SCHUM, D. (1992). Validation of self-assessment scales as outcome measures in hearing aid fitting. *Seminars in Hearing,* 14:326–337.

———. (1999). Perceived hearing aid benefit in relation to perceived needs. *Journal of the American Academy of Audiology,* 10:40–45.

SEEWALD, R. (1994). Current issues in hearing aid fitting. In: J.P. Gagne & N. Tye-Murray (Eds.), Research in audiological rehabilitation: current trends and future directions. *Journal of the American Academy of Rehabilitative Audiology, Monograph Supplement,* 27:93–113.

SELF HELP FOR HARD OF HEARING PEOPLE, INC. (1996a). Position statement on group hearing aid orientation programs. *SHHH Journal,* 17:29.

———. (1996b). Position statement on telecoils. *SHHH Journal,* 17:29–30.

SILMAN, S., GELFAND, S., & SILVERMAN, C. (1984). Late onset auditory deprivation: effects of monaural versus binaural aids. *Journal of the Acoustical Society of America,* 76:1357–1362.

SKAFTE, M. (1996). The 1995 hearing instrument market—the dispenser's perspective. *Hearing Review,* 3:16–34.

———. (1997). The 1996 hearing instrument market—the dispenser's perspective. *Hearing Review,* 4:8–36.

———. (1998). The 1997 Hearing instrument market—the dispenser's perspective. *Hearing Review,* 6:6–26.

———. (1999). The 1998 hearing instrument market—the dispenser's perspective. *Hearing Review,* 6:6–32.

SORKIN, D. (1997). Consumers and hearing aids: the SHHH perspective. *Seminars in Hearing,* 18:49–57.

STACH, B. (1990). Hearing aid amplification and central processing disorders. In: R.E. Sandlin (Ed.), *Handbook of Hearing Aid Amplification: Vol. II. Clinical Considerations and Fitting Practices.* Austin: Pro-Ed.

STACH, B., & STONER, R. (1991). Sensory aids for the hearing-impaired elderly. In: D. Ripich, (Ed.), *Handbook of Geriatric Communication Disorders.* Austin: Pro-Ed.

STAFF. (1997). Hearing aid devices: professional and client labeling and conditions for sale. *Federal Register,* 42:9286–9297.

STARKEY (1997). *The Compression Handbook,* 2d ed. Eden Prairie, MN: Starkey Labs, Inc.

STROM, K. (1996a).Understanding the senior market: a statistical profile. *Hearing Review*, 3:8, 12, 16–18, 66.

———. (1996b). An analysis of 1995 hearing instrument sales. *Hearing Review,* 5:8–36.

———. (1998). A review of the 1997 hearing instrument market. *Hearing Review,* 5:8–16, 72.

———. (1999). The 1998 hearing instruments market and what's ahead in '99. *Hearing Review,* 6:8–68.

STUDEBAKER, G., BESS, F., & BECK, L. (1991). *The Vanderbilt Hearing Aid Report II.* Parkton, MD: York Press.

STYPULKOWSKI, P. (1994). *Differentiating between Programmability and Performance.* St. Paul, MN: 3M Hearing Health Series.

STYPULKOWSKI, P., RASKIND, L., & HODGSON, W. (1992). 3M programmable hearing instruments and fitting systems. *Seminars in Hearing,* 13:135–142.

SWAN, I., & GATEHOUSE, S. (1990). Factors influencing consultation for management of hearing disability. *British Journal of Audiology*, 24:155–160.

TAYLOR, K. (1993). Self-perceived and audiometric evaluatons of hearing aid benefit in the elderly. *Ear and Hearing,* 14:390–395.

TESCH-ROMER, C. (1997). Psychological effects of hearing aid use in older adults. *Journal of Gerontological Behavioral Psychological Social Science,* 52:127–138.

TURNER, C., HUMES, L., BENTLER, R., & COX, R. (1996). A review of past research on changes in hearing aid benefit over time. *Ear and Hearing,* 17:14S–28S.

TYE-MURRAY, N. (1998). *Foundations of Aural Rehabilitation.* San Diego: Singular Publishing Group.

VALENTE, M. (1994). *Strategies for Selecting and Verifying Hearing Aid Fittings.* New York: Thieme Medical Publishers.

———. (ED.). (1996). *Hearing Aids: Standards, Options, and Limitations.* New York: Thieme Medical Publishers.

———. (1998). Responses to manufacturers' claims of digital technology in hearing aids. *Hearing Loss,* 19:12–15.

VALENTE, M., FABRY, D., & POTTS, L. (1995). Recognition of speech in noise with hearing aids using dual microphones. *Journal of the American Academy of Audiology,* 6:440–449.

VALENTE, M., POTTS, L., & VALENTE, M. (1997). Development of a clinical protocol in an attempt to improve user satisfaction with hearing aids. *Seminars in Hearing,* 18:19–29.

VALENTE, M., VALENTE, M., POTTS, L., & LYBARGER, S. (1996). Options: earhooks, tubing and earmolds. In: M. Valente (Ed.), *Hearing Aids: Standards, Options, and Limitations.* New York: Thieme Medical Publishers.

VENTRY, I., & WEINSTEIN, B. (1982). The Hearing Handicap Inventory for the Elderly: a new tool. *Ear and Hearing,* 3:128–134.

VOLL, L., & JONES, C. (1998). CICs: five years later, what have we learned? *Hearing Review,* 5:8–14.

WALTZMAN, S., COHEN, N., & SHAPIRO, B. (1993). The benefits of cochlear implantation in the geriatric population. *Otolaryngology Head Neck Surgery*, 108:329–333.

WEINREB, R., FREEMAN, W., & SELEZINKA, W. (1990). Vision impairment in geriatrics. In: B. Kemp, K. Brummel-Smith & J. Ramsdell (Eds.), *Geriatric Rehabilitation.* Boston: College Hill.

WEINSTEIN, B., SPITZER, J., & VENTRY, I. (1986). Test-retest reliability of the Hearing Handicap Inventory for the Elderly. *Ear and Hearing*, 6:295–299.

WORLD HEALTH ORGANIZATION. (1980). *International Classification of Impairments, Disabilities and Handicaps (ICIDH).* Geneva: World Health Organization.

Health Care Delivery

Health Promotion Strategies for Identifying Older Adults with Handicapping Hearing Impairment

No one would suggest that the quality of life of all old deaf people can be improved by the most comprehensive audiological service, but large-scale screening would undoubtedly reveal very large numbers of people who could be helped.

—A.L. Cochrane, 1971

LEARNING OBJECTIVES

After reading this chapter, you should be able to:

- State the epidemiological principles underlying health promotion activities.
- Explain the reasons for screening older adults for the presence of handicapping hearing loss.
- Utilize the approaches available for screening older adults for handicapping hearing impairment.

HEALTH PROMOTION STRATEGIES FOR IDENTIFYING OLDER ADULTS WITH HANDICAPPING HEARING IMPAIRMENTS

Preventive health care for older adults is an area of active concern in geriatric medicine. Older adults are frequently the target of activities designed to identify persons with unrecognized remediable conditions because of the high incidence of chronic conditions that often pose a threat to quality of life. Further, early identification can help reduce the cost of caring for persons burdened by disabilities. Interest-

ingly, a number of medical and governmental agencies have highlighted the need for improved and more efficacious hearing screening programs (Weinstein, 1992). The purpose of this chapter is to provide a background justifying selected screening activities designed to identify older adults with handicapping hearing impairment and alleviating the conditions so as to improve or maintain functional health status. In this connection, functional health status implies the ability of older adults to relate to the outside world (e.g., family, friends, and business associates) in leisure and social activities (Williams, 1998).

PEARL

The demographic changes in the United States and abroad are leading to increased proportions of older adults with increased levels of disability who require preventive activities to reduce the burden of the condition(s).

Healthy People 2000 is a government initiative designed to improve the health of citizens throughout the United States (U.S. D.H.H.S., 1992). The particular goals of Healthy People 2000 include (1) increasing the span of healthy life for Americans; (2) reducing health disparities among Americans; and (3) achieving access to preventive services for all Americans. As part of the initiative, the U.S. Public Health Service categorized, planned, and evaluated activities for systematically improving the nation's health. The report growing out of the Healthy People 2000 initiative detailed 22 priority areas that

267

must be targeted if in fact citizens will be able to achieve their potential to live full, active lives (U.S. D.H.H.S., 1992). The priority areas can be divided into three broad categories, namely, health promotion, health protection, and preventive services. Health promotion strategies relate to individual lifestyle—personal choices made in a social context that can have an influence on one's prospects for good health. Health promotion activities include any combination of health education and related organizational, environmental, and economic interventions designed to promote health. Priority areas listed in the report include physical activity and fitness, nutrition, family planning, tobacco, alcohol and other drugs, mental health, and mental disorders.

Health protection strategies are those related to environmental or regulatory measures that ultimately protect large population groups (U.S. D.H.H.S., 1992). Targeted areas include unintentional injuries, occupational safety and health, environmental health, food and drug safety, and oral health. Community-wide efforts are a necessary aspect of all health protection initiatives. Finally, preventive health services imply key services that can be delivered by health poviders in an effort to promote quality of life and prevent disability. Preventive activities can either be primary, secondary, or tertiary (Williams, 1998). Tertiary prevention, or the early recognition and seeking out of individuals with conditions that tend to go underreported so that treatment can be instituted to reduce potential functional deficits, is the basis for preventive activities targeting older adults with handicapping/disabling hearing impairments. In the latter connection, even if the impairment is not amenable to treatment, the preventive process should be concerned with preventing disability and handicap (Williams, 1998). For tertiary prevention to be successful, health care professionals must be educated about the chronic conditions to which older adults are susceptible so they can become partners in detection activities. Preventive services include counseling, screening, immunization, or chemoprophylactic interventions for individuals in clinical settings. According to the Public Health Service, priority areas for preventive strategies include maternal and infant health, heart disease and stroke, cancer, diabetes and chronic disabling conditions, HIV infection, and infectious diseases.

With regard to older adults, an important goal of Healthy People 2000 is to maintain health and quality of life as we move into the 21st century. That is to say, improving the functional independence, not just the length of life, is seen as an important element in promoting the health of individuals over 65 years of age. According to the Healthy People 2000 report, chronic problems such as arthritis, osteoporosis, and visual and hearing impairments are priority areas because of their significant impact on daily life. The report goes on to emphasize that "we must prevent the ill from being disabled and help people with disabilities preserve function and prevent further disability" (U.S. D.H.H.S., 1992, p. 24). The report from Healthy People 2000 emphasizes that primary health-care providers are necessary partners in the maintenance of good health and functional independence. The report suggests that providers play an important role in identifying people at risk for chronic conditions for which efficacious interventions are available. It is incumbent on

health care providers to ensure appropriate screening, to make the appropriate referrals for services, and to counsel and supply information about conditions prevalent among older adults (U.S. D.H.H.S., 1992). In addition to primary care providers, community support networks were encouraged to provide services to help older adults maintain independence.

Three health promotion and disease prevention initiatives pertain to hearing health care for older adults. One important health status objective is to reduce the prevalence of significant hearing impairment among people aged 45 and older from a rate of 203 per 1000 to a prevalence of no more than 180 per 1000. Self-reported hearing impairment is the proxy measure for significant hearing impairment. An important service and protection objective is to increase to 60% the proportion of primary care providers for older adults who routinely evaluate people aged 65 and older for urinary incontinence and impairments of vision, cognition, and functional status. Finally, an important educational and community-based health promotion objective is to increase to at least 90% the proportion of people aged 65 and older who participated during the previous year in at least one organized health promotion program through a senior center or other community-based setting serving older people. Potential channels for preventive or health promotion efforts include senior centers, lifecare facilities, retirement villages, and clubs and organizations that meet regularly in the community. As of this writing, many of the goals of Healthy People 2000 that related to hearing have not been met. It is hoped that Healthy People 2010, which builds on the initiatives of Healthy People 2000, will include objectives relating to hearing health care (Healthy People 2010, 1999).

The appendix of the Healthy People 2000 report lists recommendations of the U.S. Preventive Services Task Force (U.S. P.S.T.F.) for individuals age 65 and over. This 20-member, non-Federal, multidisciplinary expert panel studied the evidence for 169 preventive interventions, reviewed over 2500 relevant clinical trials and epidemiologic studies and developed a report recommending screening for certain conditions in asymptomatic persons having no clinical evidence of the target condition (U.S. P.S.T.F., 1989). Under screening guidelines for individuals 65 and over, it was recommended that part of the physical exam include a "hearing and hearing aid screen." Specifically, the U.S. P.S.T.F. (1989) and the American Academy of Family Physicians (1993) recommend that elderly patients be periodically evaluated regarding their hearing status, counseled regarding the availability of hearing aids, and referred appropriately should any abnormalities be detected. Interestingly, these authorities state the following:

> it is unclear that benefits are sufficient to justify the substantial cost of audiometric screening of the nearly 30 million Americans over age 65. A more practical but unproven strategy might include a careful historical evaluation of hearing in older individuals, a simple otoscopic examination for cerumen and other findings, and patient education regarding the availability of efficacious hearing aid devices.

—U.S. D.H.H.S., 1994, P. 173

It is likely that the U.S. P.S.T.F. based the above recommendations (i.e., historical evaluation, otoscopic and patient education) on opinions of respected authorities, reports of expert committees, and descriptive studies due to the lack of evidence from well-designed controlled trials that support pure-tone screening as the most efficacious preventive-care protocol for older adults.

Additional clinical recommendations for screening for hearing impairment come from the Canadian Task Force on the Periodic Health Examination (1984) and the American College of Obstetricians and Gynecologists (1993). The former group contends that there is justification for screening for hearing loss as part of the periodic health examination for adults while the latter group recommends that women 65 years and older be evaluated for hearing loss. Finally, the American Speech-Language-Hearing Association (ASHA) (1997a) recently developed a set of guidelines that recommend screening adults for impairment and disability at three-year intervals after age 50. The ASHA provides no evidence from clinical trials for their recommendations.

Principles of Screening

Screening, counseling, and immunizations are three major types of preventive care. Prior to discussing the principles that underlie screening and counseling programs, a working definition of screening is a necessary foundation. Screening, is a form of early diagnosis, wherein members of the general public are invited to undergo tests to separate them into those with higher and lower probabilities of having the disorder . . . the former group is then urged to seek medical attention for definitive diagnosis (Sackett, Haynes, & Tugwell, 1985). The greater the potential burden a disease represents to the individuals and society, the greater the impetus to screen. For a screening program to be successful, there must be a clear and measurable definition of the condition one is attempting to identify.

SPECIAL CONSIDERATION

The ideal screening program is one that is quick, easy, inexpensive to administer, and employs a test that is accurate (i.e., high in sensitivity, specificity, and predictive value) (Sackett, Haynes, & Tugwell, 1985).

In addition, a screening program can only be considered effective if diagnostic and treatment services are available, effective, and utilized by those undergoing the screen and when treatment recommendations are shown to alter the natural history of the disease, and, of course, are complied with (Cadman, Chambers, Feldman, & Sackett, 1984; ASHA, 1997a). Unfortunately, persons with chronic conditions demonstrate poor compliance with recommended therapies. Historically, hearing screening programs for adults have a high yield with low compliance with recommended therapies, as well. As will be discussed later in the chapter, hearing screening programs must incorporate compliance-improving strategies to insure their efficacy. Compliance

with recommended treatments is critical because of the economic implications of mounting a screening program (Weinstein, 1992).

CRITERIA FOR SELECTING A SCREENING PROTOCOL

Based on a review of epidemiologic literature, seven criteria exist for evaluating the legitimacy of a screening program (Mulrow & Lichtenstein, 1991; Cadman et al, 1984). The criteria are listed as follows along with circumstances that must exist for a screening test to be useful. A brief discussion of how handicapping hearing impairment measures up to each of the conditions follows.

Criteria

1. Does the burden of suffering posed by the condition warrant screening efforts?
2. Are there good screening tests?
3. Are efficacious treatments available?
4. Do persons with positive screenings comply with advice and interventions?
5. Has the effectiveness of the program been demonstrated in a randomized trial?
6. Can the health care system cope with the program?
7. Does the program reach those who could benefit?

Circumstances

1. The condition must have a significant effect on the quality and quantity of life.
2. Acceptable methods of treatment must be available.
3. The condition must have an asymptomatic period during which detection and treatment reduce morbidity and mortality.
4. Tests that are acceptable to patients must be available at a reasonable cost, to detect the condition in the asymptomatic period.
5. The incidence of the condition must be sufficient to justify the cost of screening.

How do handicapping hearing impairments rate against these basic epidemiologic questions?

The answer to the first question, Does the burden of suffering warrant screening? is "yes." It is clear from existing prevalence data and the discussion of effects of hearing loss on general well-being, physical, cognitive, emotional, and social function that unremediated hearing loss can be detrimental. Interestingly, the adverse effects of hearing loss on a diversity of functions remains when adjusting for degree of hearing loss, age, education, and comorbid diseases (Mulrow & Lichtenstein, 1991).

The answer to the second question, Are there good screening tests? is "yes" and "no." In order to answer this question, one must be familiar with the concepts of sensitivity, specificity, and predictive value as consideration of these issues is critical when evaluating and selecting screening tests. The terms *sensitivity* and *specificity* relate to the ability of the test to identify correctly both those with and those without the disease (U.S. D.H.H.S., 1994). Specifically, *sensitivity* refers to the proportion of persons with a condition who correctly test positive when screened, whereas *specificity* refers to the proportion of persons without the condition who correctly test negative when screened. Thus, sensitivity is the percentage labeled positive on the screening test of all those who truly have the target condition. Thus, a test with poor sensitivity will miss cases and will produce a large proportion of false-negative results. In contrast, specificity is the percentage labeled negative on the screening test of all those who truly are free of the target condition. A test with poor specificity will result in healthy persons being told they have the condition (false-positives). Persons who receive false-negative results may experience important delays in diagnosis and management. Likewise, false-positive results may lead to follow-up testing that may be expensive, uncomfortable, and even life threatening.

The test performance (sensitivity and specificity) together with the percentage of the population with the disease (disease prevalence) determine predictive values (ASHA, 1997a). Predictive values vary with disease/disorder prevalence and they determine rates of over-and-under referral for diagnosis. The positive predictive value is the proportion of persons with a positive test who have the condition. It is directly related to the prevalence of the disease and the specificity of the test. Typically, most target conditions for screening are relatively uncommon and most screening tests have imperfect specificity. Accordingly, the positive predictive value of screening tests is often low, ranging from 10 to 30% (U.S. D.H.H.S., 1994). That is to say, many patients will have positive screening tests yet will not actually have the disease. The negative predictive value (NPV) is the ratio of the number of persons scoring negative who truly do not have the disease to the number of all those scoring negative on the test. The NPV is closely tied to the under-referral rate. Thus, the under-referral rate is the proportion of those not referred who do not have the disease (1-NPV).

With regard to the question, Are good screening tests available? audiologists presently have at their disposal physical diagnostic tests (e.g., otoscopic, pure-tone audiometry using a portable audiometer or the portable Audioscope™, self-administered questionnaires, or an approach that combines both). The basic difference between these two approaches is the purpose of the screen or the expected outcome. Physical diagnostic tests are designed to identify people likely to have a hearing disorder or a hearing impairment. A disorder is any anatomic abnormality or pathology that may or may not result in a change in function of a given organ or organ system that requires referral and/or a condition in the ear that may require medical evaluation (WHO, 1980). Hence when screening for a hearing disorder the goal is to identify older adults most likely to have ear or other related conditions that require medical evaluation (ASHA, 1997a). In contrast, an impairment is any loss or abnormality of psychological or physiological function. It implies that some functional aspect of an organ, system, or mechanism is outside the normal range (WHO, 1980). Thus when screen-

ing for hearing impairment, we are attempting to identify those older adults at risk for a hearing impairment that requires an audiologic referral. When screening for hearing impairment the question becomes, What is the fence one should use as the cutoff for the presence of an impairment? Stated differently, What should the pass/refer criterion be for an individual over 65 years of age?

Self-administered/assessment questionnaires are used to identify individuals who perceive themselves to have a hearing disability or a hearing handicap and thus require referral to an audiologist. According to the World Health Organization (WHO), a disability is any restriction or lack of ability (resulting from an impairment) to perform an activity in a manner or within the range considered normal for a human being. In contrast, a handicap is the disadvantage experienced by an individual resulting from an impairment or disability that limits or prevents the fulfillment of a role that is normal for the individual. It may occur as a function of barriers (e.g., communication, structural, or attitudinal), lack of accommodations, and/or lack of appropriate auxiliary aids and services (e.g., hearing aid/assistive-listening device) (WHO, 1980). Subjective reports from the client provide the key information that determines whether in fact a referral is necessary. As pertains to hearing, we are seeking to identify those older adults with disabilities or handicaps that may interfere with their social, emotional, communicative, vocational, or educational performance (ASHA, 1997a).

When screening to identify individuals likely to have a medical condition of the ear most audiologists would agree that an otoscopic examination should be combined with a brief case history. The purpose of the otoscopic examination should be to visually inspect the ear, looking for conditions, such as impacted cerumen, that may warrant medical referral. Individuals having access to video-otoscopy may consider this as an alternative but remember a key aspect of screening is that it is quick and easy to administer and above all inexpensive. Immittance measures are not recommended because of the low incidence of active middle-ear disease in older adults. The point of the brief case history should be to ask questions designed to identify those individuals who may have a significant medical condition. Sample questions are shown in Table 10–1. Above all, the questionnaire should be brief including those questions that will help identify older adults with a medical condition of the ear requiring referral to a primary care physician or an otolaryngologist. Typically, the older adult should be referred if the oto/videoscopic reveals any outer- or middle-ear abnormality or cerumen impaction. In addition, any positive responses to the case history warrant medical referral. In my opinion, the screen for hearing disorders should be an essential part of any screening protocol.

The hearing impairment screen requires decisions regarding the frequency and intensity characteristics of the signal as well as the pass/fail criteria. Interestingly, a great deal of controversy surrounds the selection of the intensity characteristics of the pure-tone stimuli used during an impairment screen. At the heart of the debate is whether normal hearing defined audiometrically as "hearing levels better than 25 dBHL" should be adopted as the fence, irrespective of the age, activity level, and ultimate compliance

TABLE 10–1 Sample Case History Questions

Question	Answer	
1. Do you have a hearing loss in one or both of your ears?	One ear	Both ears
2. Was your hearing loss sudden in onset?	Yes	No
3. Do you have any recent discharge or drainage from your ear(s)?	Yes	No
4. Do you have any pain, fullness, or discomfort in the ears?	Yes	No
5. Do you have any ringing or noises in your ears?	Yes	No

with the recommendation deriving from the screening program. Current ASHA guidelines for adults (age 18 years and older) specify a 25 dB screening level at 1000, 2000, and 4000 Hz, with no response at any frequency in either ear constituting a failure (ASHA, 1997a). The majority of those over 65 years of age screened with this protocol may fail and because of this some authorities have recommended a higher intensity screen.

Ventry and Weinstein (1983) were among the first investigators to suggest elevating the fence to 40 dBHL at 1000 and 2000 Hz for community-based individuals 65 years and older. They offered two simple explanations for selecting 40 dBHL. First, 90% of older adults with hearing levels in excess of 40 dBHL perceive themselves as being handicapped by their impairment. Second, while a number of individuals with hearing levels less than 40 dBHL obtain hearing aids, the majority of older adults complying with the recommendation for audiologic intervention (e.g., hearing aids) have hearing levels in excess of 40 dBHL. The epidemiologic literature suggests that the higher compliance with audiologic recommendations associated with use of a higher fence is integral to defining the efficacy of any screening program. Opponents of a 40 dBHL hearing screening level are concerned that such a high fence suggests that persons with lesser hearing impairments are not handicapped, and that persons with lesser impairments do not need hearing aids. The latter reasoning is a misinterpretation of Ventry and Weinstein's (1983) rationale for recommending 40 dBHL for older adults, which was to set the level high enough to assure a higher compliance rate. Finally, by way of compromise Schow and Longhurst (1986) advocated a fence of 25 dBHL at 1000 and 2000 Hz, and of 30 dBHL at 4000 Hz, with inability to hear one frequency in either ear constituting a failure.

SPECIAL CONSIDERATION

While acknowledging that a 25 dBHL screening level will likely have a high referral rate associated with it, the ASHA (1997a) guidelines for audiologic screening advocate a screening level of 25 dBHL at 1000, 2000, and 4000 Hz. This panel contends that a uniform screening level should be adopted because hearing impairment exceeding 25 dBHL can affect communication, regardless of age.

It is important to emphasize that ASHA's recommendation for impairment screen awaits validation whereas the studies advocating a higher screening level (e.g., 40 dBHL) have high sensitivities, specificities, and likelihood ratios (Lichtenstein, Bess, & Logan, 1988).

With regard to frequencies, most advocates of screening incorporate 1000 and 2000 Hz at the very minimum, with 500 and 4000 Hz as an option. The former are important frequencies to include because of the strong relationship between the hearing level at these frequencies and speech perception. Further, anyone who fails a screening at 1000 and 2000 Hz will likely fail at 4000 Hz. While 4000 Hz is an important frequency at which to screen, the rate of hearing impairment increases as a function of age. The high prevalence of hearing loss at 4000 Hz substantially increases the risk of over-referrals (i.e., false-positives) (Gates, Cooper, Kannal, & Miller, 1990). To avoid the latter, a reasonable hearing level such as 35 to 40 dBHL should be selected. Again the philosophy underlying the elevated screening level is to insure that everyone who fails ultimately has a hearing impairment that requires audiologic follow-up. An individual who only fails a hearing screen at 30 dBHL at 4000 Hz in the right ear may not be a candidate for a referral whereas an older adult who is screened at 35 dBHL at 4000 Hz and is unable to hear the tone in each ear may be a more likely candidate for a referral. While 500 Hz may have some advantages as a frequency at which to screen, it is not typically included because of the confounding effects of ambient noise and because of the low incidence of middle-ear disease in older adults. Interestingly, screening specificity (using conventional audiometry as the gold standard) tends to be lowest at 500 Hz (ASHA, 1997a).

While there is little agreement on the frequencies and fences to be used in screening, most recognize that the more frequencies included and the stricter (lower) the levels, the greater the possibility for referral and failure. It is well accepted that a screening protocol yielding a failure rate of 90% would not be practical from a clinical or an economic point of view, albeit some audiologists might appreciate the referrals and the opportunity to educate older adults about the interventions available to alleviate the handicapping effects of hearing impairment.

When conducting screenings for hearing impairment, the setting is an important consideration. It is of utmost importance that the screening take place in a clinical or natural environment that is conducive to obtaining reliable and valid outcomes (ASHA, 1997a). Thus, the ambient noise levels should be low enough to allow for accurate screening.

The instrumentation used during routine screening is important, as well. Limited-range or narrow-range audiometers should be calibrated to ANSI S3.6-1996 specifications, and should be biologically calibrated daily. The Welch Allyn Audioscope™, a handheld otoscope with a built-in audiometer has been shown to be a reliable and valid alternative to a portable screening audiometer. The Audioscope is capable of delivering into the external auditory canal a 20, 25, or 40 dB tone at frequencies of 500, 1000, 2000, and 4000 HZ. The Audioscope has a conditioning tone built in to allow for a trial period prior to the actual test. This is especially helpful with older adults, enabling the audiologist to verify that the patient knows what is expected. To use the Audioscope, an appropriate size ear speculum is placed within the external auditory canal to achieve an adequate seal. The tympanic membrane must be visualized before the testing begins. A tonal sequence is presented by pushing a button on the Audioscope, and the patient merely raises a hand or finger to signify that the tone has been heard. Once the tone goes away the patient should quickly put the finger or hand down again to await the next signal presentation.

While the Audioscope and the portable audiometer have similar operating characteristics, the Audioscope has some advantages (Mulrow & Lichtenstein, 1991). For example, it may be less costly than a screening audiometer, it is more portable, and it enables the clinician to view the external auditory meatus prior to the screening to determine whether in fact cerumen is present, potentially invalidating screening adults. Additionally, an Audioscope screen can be completed in approximately 33 seconds (McBride, Aguilar, Mulrow, & Tuley, 1990). Welch Allyn Corporation sends out mailing boxes and labels to persons purchasing the Audioscope to enable the company to calibrate the Audioscope annually. Turnaround time is excellent. A final consideration when conducting an impairment screen is the issue of personnel. ASHA (1997a) suggests that screening practitioners be limited to audiologists and speech-language pathologists with a Certificate of Clinical Competence from ASHA as well as a state license where applicable. In my opinion, primary care physicians, geriatricians, family practitioners, and geriatric nurse practitioners should receive proper instruction in the use of the Audioscope and should be encouraged to routinely screen older adults as part of annual physical exams. As part of the screen, those individuals who fail should be referred to an audiologist for an evaluation.

PEARL

For audiologists providing the training to health care professionals outside the fields of speech-language pathology and audiology, it is important to specify the hearing levels to be used (e.g., 25 dBHL verses 40 dBHL) along with the advantages and disadvantages associated with each.

When conducting screening for hearing disability, self-assessment measures with high internal consistency and test-retest reliability should be chosen. Commonly used screening instruments include the Hearing Handicap Inventory for the Elderly-Screening Version (HHIE-S) (Ventry & Weinstein, 1983) and the Self Assessment of Communication (SAC) (Schow & Nerbonne, 1982). Each of these questionnaires contains 10 simple questions that query the respondent about the handicap or disability associated with hearing loss. The items on the HHIE-S tap into the emotional and social effects of hearing loss whereas the SAC questions delve into the respondent's self-perceived communication problems. The test-retest reliability of the HHIE-S is 0.84 and of the SAC is 0.80. On the HHIE-S, patients answer questions about circumstances related to hearing by stating whether the situation represents a problem. A "no" response scores 0, "sometimes" scores 2, and "yes" scores 4. Total scores range from 0 to 40, with a score less than 10 indicating no handicap and a score greater than 24 indicating moderate to severe handicap (Mulrow & Lichtenstein, 1991). Persons obtaining scores equal to or greater than 10 should be referred for an audiologic evaluation. Individuals with scores in excess of 18 on the HHIE-S are likely to purchase and benefit from hearing aids. The HHIE-S can be completed in a little over 2 minutes (McBride et al, 1990). The SAC uses a Likert Scale, with responses recorded on a scale ranging from "almost never" (1) to "practically always" (5). A percentage score is calculated by multiplying the raw score by 2, subtracting 20 and multiplying by 1.25. On the SAC, a score equal to or greater than 19 suggests the need for a referral to an audiologist. For each of these questionnaires, the higher the cut-off score, the more favorable the likelihood ratios (Schow, Smedley, & Longhurst, 1990).

The operating characteristics against pure-tone audiometry have been established for each of the aforementioned questionnaires. According to a study conducted using a sample of older adult community volunteers and the Ventry and Weinstein criteria of 40 dBHL, the likelihood ratio for hearing impairment ranged from 0.36 using a cutoff of 0 to 8 on the HHIE-S, rising to 12 when the cutoff on the HHIE-S was between 26 and 40 (Lichtenstein, Bess, & Logan, 1988). The overall accuracy in identifying people with and without hearing impairment is 75%. Using a cutoff on the SAC of 0 to 18, the likelihood ratio of hearing impairment according to Ventry and Weinstein's definition of impairment, is 0.19, rising to 4.25 when the cutoff is raised to 19 to 100 (Mulrow & Lichtenstein, 1991; Schow, Smedley, & Longhurst, 1990).

Screenings for disability or handicap should take place in a quiet environment. I prefer a face-to-face interview in lieu of paper-pencil in that it is more personal, it enables the audiologist to establish a rapport with the respondent, and responses tend to be somewhat more reliable. It is always helpful to have a hardwired or FM system available during the screening to insure that the respondent understands the questions being asked. Upon completion of the screen, responses to the items should be discussed briefly and an appropriate referral made, when indicated. It is recommended that individuals conducting screenings for disability or handicap also incorporate a screen for medical disorders.

In an effort to address the question pertaining to screening efficacy, a few studies have been conducted that consider this very important issue. It is critical to emphasize that it is difficult to evaluate the performance of a particular screening test/protocol, as the gold standard against which to judge its characteristics remains somewhat elusive. It is certainly easy to judge the efficacy of a screening protocol designed to identify individuals with medical disorders. In this case, the gold standard should be the presence of a medical condition in the ear diagnosed by a physician at the time of follow-up. When conducting an impairment screen, should the gold standard be the presence of a hearing impairment in one ear, in both ears, at one frequency, or at two or more frequencies? What level should be used for defining hearing impairment? Typically, we use 25 dBHL or age-adjusted norms that suggest a decrement in hearing sensitivity in the high frequencies. When conducting a disability or handicap screen, should the gold standard be presence of impaired hearing, hearing-aid uptake, or the presence of a hearing handicap on a more extensive self-administered questionnaire? When validating a disability or impairment screen, the studies that use a presence of hearing impairment as their gold standard have more favorable sensitivities, specificities, and predictive values than studies that use hearing-aid uptake, for example. However, when individuals undergoing a hearing screening are followed longitudinally through the audiological evaluation, the hearing-aid selection, and the hearing-aid fitting the proportion of individuals ultimately purchasing hearing aids is very low—only about 5 to 10%. Thus, the yield from the screen is quite low.

One might argue that the gold standard against which to validate a screen (i.e., disorder, impairment, or disability) should merely be compliance with the recommendation to see an audiologist to evaluate an impairment and/or disability, or compliance with the recommendation to see a medical doctor in the case of a disorder screen. As will be discussed later in the chapter, compliance with recommendations is integrally intertwined with the client's internal perceptions about their condition and with their belief regarding the feasibility of remediating the condition for which they have undergone a screening.

Unfortunately there is no right or wrong answer in terms of what the gold standard should be. For example, if audiologists merely want to screen to identify people with hearing levels in excess of 25 dBHL, then presence of a hearing impairment should be the gold standard. If audiologists merely want to screen to identify individuals with medical disorders requiring intervention, then using otoscopic examinations and medical diagnosis should be the gold standard. Similarly, if audiologists want to screen to identify individuals who perceive themselves to be handicapped by their hearing loss and hence want to purchase hearing aids to reduce the devastating consequences of hearing loss, then the gold standard should be hearing-aid use. It is important to reiterate that in addition to meeting certain performance criteria (e.g., adequate sensitivity and specificity) any screening protocol should be quick and easy to administer, inexpensive, comfortable to the client, and brief in duration.

One of the few studies designed to test the efficacy of pure-tone screening was conducted by Lichtenstein, Bess, and Logan (1988). Lichtenstein and his colleagues screened a large sample of older adults in a primary care setting using the Welch Allyn Audioscope, a handheld instrument with excellent between-location and between-subject reliability (Bess, 1995). In their study, screenings were conducted at 40 dBHL at 1000 and 2000 Hz. The sensitivity and specificity of the screen were judged against specific criteria for hearing impairment, namely, presence of a 40 dB hearing loss in both ears at either 1000 or 2000 Hz, or presence of a 40 dB hearing loss in either ear at both 1000 and 2000 Hz. According to Lichtenstein, Bess, and Logan (1988), the Audioscope performed quite well, with sensitivities ranging from 87 to 96% and specificities ranging somewhat lower from 72 to 90%. Bienvenue, Michael, Chaffinish, and Ziegler (1985) also found that using a 25 dBHL screening level, the Audioscope performed well against a hearing impairment criteria of >/= 30 dBHL. In their sample of adults 51 to 81 years, sensitivities were as high as 93% and specificities were on the order of 70%. Frank and Peterson (1987) screened a large sample of older adults at 40 dBHL comparing the outcome on the Audioscope against hearing impairment criteria >/= 45 dBHL at 500 to 4000 Hz. Overall sensitivity was high, on the order of 90%, as was the specificity of the Audioscope (i.e., 90%). Using thresholds =/> 40 dBHL as the gold standard, McBride et al (1990) also reported high sensitivities and specificities with the Audioscope on a sample of older adults at Veteran's Administration Centers and community clinics.

The next epidemiologic criterion against which to judge a screening initiative is whether efficacious treatments are available. Stated differently, if a medical condition is detected, are adequate treatments available? If a hearing impairment or handicap is verified at the follow-up examination are there treatments available to remediate the problem? The answer to both questions, of course, is a resounding "yes." The efficacy of hearing aids purchased by older adults has been clearly established in well over 20 studies conducted across the country, using a variety of populations and using subjects recruited from diverse settings. These studies have been reviewed in Chapter 9 on hearing aids.

The next epidemiologic criterion is whether persons with positive screening results comply with advice and interventions. That is, even if individuals have documented hearing impairments and disabilities, will they obtain further evalu-

---

SPECIAL CONSIDERATION

When choosing a screening test, the audiologist must first consider what he/she wants to accomplish through the screening and then select a test that has been compared against that particular gold standard.

ation and purchase hearing aids or assistive listening devices if so advised? Various rates of compliance with recommended interventions have emerged from the few studies in this area. Unfortunately, it appears that as few as 5 and as many as 50% of individuals who undergo follow-up audiologic evaluations actually take the next step, namely, purchasing hearing aids. Not surprisingly, the more successful rates have occurred in studies where hearing evaluations and/or hearing aids were provided at no cost.

There are several reasons for the low compliance with advice and interventions. Hearing-impaired individuals have identified a number of significant barriers to following recommendations regarding further audiologic evaluation or hearing-aid use. These include the high cost of hearing aids, lack of insurance coverage for the evaluation and/or the hearing aid, myths about hearing aids (e.g., amplify noise, not appropriate for persons with sensorineural hearing loss), the belief that hearing aids call attention to the handicap (i.e., stigma associated with hearing loss and use of hearing aids), ageism (e.g., belief that hearing loss is a normal concomitant of the aging process), and the false impression that hearing aids are not effective in remediating the psychosocial and communicative consequences of hearing loss.

SPECIAL CONSIDERATION

In my opinion, a major reason that the majority of people who fail a screening test do not follow advice concerning the need for audiologic testing and hearing aids is the design of the preventive-care protocol.

In short, preventive care (i.e., screening protocols) is not implemented in a context which will ensure that the patient is armed with information that will enable them to take an active role/interest in preventive care. Further, counseling is not typically a part of screening because of the time involved and the lack of reimbursement for counseling services. The U.S. P.S.T.F. has developed a list of 10 principles of patient education and counseling that all audiologists should consider when designing a hearing screening program. Some of the principles are listed in Table 10–2.

SPECIAL CONSIDERATION

Screening protocols which do not include an educational component are associated with low compliance rates.

These principles are inextricably intertwined with the Health Belief Model described by Jenz and Becker (1984) and the Stages-of-Change Model described by Prochaska, DiClemente, and Norcross (1992). The Health Belief Model, which is based on cognitive theories of behavior, was developed to predict participation in health-prevention programs

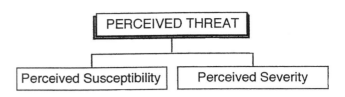

Figure 10–1 Perceptual components of perceived threat.

(Becker, 1974). According to the Health Belief Model, health-related behaviors are determined and can be predicted by (1) perceived threat of disease or illness, (2) perceived benefits/ barriers associated with engaging in particular behaviors, and (3) self-efficacy or the belief that one is capable of acting upon professional recommendations. These three behavioral determinants of the Health Belief Model should influence the design of any preventive-care protocol if in fact it is desirable for patients to comply with screening recommendations.

The Health Belief Model suggests that behavior is dependent on the value that an individual places on a desired outcome and the belief that if a behavior is performed it will result in a desired outcome (Noh, Gagne, & Kaspar, 1994). As is shown in Figure 10–1, perceived threat is a function of two interrelated perceptual components, namely, perceived susceptibility and perceived severity (Noh, Gagne, & Kaspar, 1994). Perceived susceptibility refers to an individual's view regarding their risk of contracting a health condition such as handicapping hearing loss. According to this model, the likelihood of engaging in appropriate health behavior increases as the level of perceived susceptibility increases. Thus, as pertains to screening outcomes for example, a person who fails a screen and

TABLE 10–2   U.S. Preventive Services Task Force: Principles of Patient Education and Counseling (U.S. P.S.T.F., 1989)

1. Develop a therapeutic alliance.
2. Counsel individuals who have been screened.
3. Ensure that patients understand the relationship between behavior and health.
4. Work with patients to assess their readiness to change their health-related behaviors and to establish barriers to behavior change.
5. Gain commitment from patients to change their behavior with assistance if appropriate.
6. Involve patients in selecting risk factors to change.
7. Use a combination of strategies to change the patient's health-related behavior.
8. Monitor patients through follow-up contacts.
9. Involve office staff. Staff may be able to help patients gain access to follow-up services. They should be knowledgeable about agencies in the community, etc.

has a positive diagnostic test, is likely to agree to wear a hearing aid if he/she accepts the diagnosis and recognizes that they can develop the devastating psychosocial and communication problems associated with hearing loss (Noh, Gagne, & Kaspar, 1994). Perceived severity refers to the subjective evaluation that if left untreated, a disorder, an impairment, or a disability, will have devastating consequences such as handicapping an individual or reducing the quality of life.

SPECIAL CONSIDERATION

In the context of screening, willingness to seek hearing health care services depends on perceptions of susceptibility to hearing loss and on personal evaluations of the seriousness of the consequences associated with hearing loss.

While perceived threat influences engagement in preventive health behavior in that it could influence a person to take action, the choice of behavioral options depends on the individual's perceptions of benefits. According to proponents of the Health Belief Model, an individual's choice of behavioral options depends on their perceptions of the effectiveness of the intervention in reducing the consequences of the condition (i.e., benefits) and on the obstacles or negative outcomes associated with the available interventions (i.e., barriers such as cost). When perceived barriers outweigh benefits that may ensue from audiologic intervention, compliance is impeded (Noh, Gagne, & Kaspar, 1994). So if, as a result of a positive screening, an individual is referred for an audiologic evaluation and possible hearing-aid use, compliance may be increased if at the time of the screen the individual is made aware of the fact that hearing aids have proven useful in reducing the burden of disease. The information obtained at the screening may assist the patient in conducting an informal cost-benefit analysis (i.e., will the outcome with hearing aids outweigh some of the inconveniences of actually making the purchase such as the high cost, the need to make several return visits, etc?).

PEARL

The person undergoing the screen must come to understand that there is a course of action available to remediate hearing loss using hearing aids and assistive-listening devices, delivered in the context of an audiologic rehabilitation program.

Finally, self-efficacy refers to the belief in one's capabilities to succeed. That is, does the person feel competent enough to implement the change and succeed? In the case of handicapping hearing impairment, self-efficacy may not be as important at the screening stage, it will come into play when a decision is made to purchase and use hearing aids for the long term.

SPECIAL CONSIDERATION

In the context of audiologic screening and audiologic rehabilitation, the Health Belief Model holds that people must feel threatened by their condition (handicapping hearing loss), they must believe that there will be psychosocial and communicative benefits associated with engaging in a particular behavior (audiologic evaluation, hearing aid purchase), and they must feel competent to adjust to the demands of hearing aid use (Noh, Gagne, & Kaspar, 1994).

Audiologists conducting hearing screening should also consider the patients' readiness to change their health-related behaviors as a potential obstacle to compliance and build in mechanisms that move patients from one stage of readiness to the next. The Public Health Service emphasizes that sensitivity to stages of change is important to health. Once the correct stage is reached, the individual will follow the advice of the clinician doing the screening or the follow-up. Provision of information and counseling are the ways to move people from one stage to the next. It is essential that the information be appropriate to the stage the individual is at, is culturally appropriate, and is at the level of comprehension and learning skills of the patient (U.S. D.H.H.S., 1994).

SEQUENCE OF STAGES

According to Prochaska, DiClemente, and Norcross (1992) individuals go through a sequence of stages before they are actually ready to change their health-related behaviors (e.g., follow the advice of an audiologist or a physician or a spouse to obtain a hearing test and purchase hearing aids). According to the Transtheoretical Stages-of-Change Model espoused by Prochaska, Norcross, and DiClemente (1984) the processes individuals undergo as they make personal changes include precontemplation, contemplation, preparation, action, maintenance, and termination.

Precontemplation

The individual cannot see the problem and thus has no intention of changing his/her behavior. These individuals are considered deniers. Often family and friends can see the problem clearly . . . hence the patient wants everyone around them to change. A large number of older adults with mild hearing loss are most likely to fit into this category. These individuals are not yet ready for the audiologist. They can, however, benefit from information that can move them into the next stage.

Contemplation

These individuals acknowledge that they have a problem and are willing to begin to think seriously about solving it. They struggle to understand their problem, to see its causes, and to wonder about solutions. They have definite plans to take action within a 6-month period of time. These individuals also need information at the time of the screen. The information should direct the person being screened to a particular professional who in turn should be prepared to counsel the individual about options.

Preparation

These people are planning to take action within a month. They are making the final adjustments before they begin to change their behavior. They talk about it with others and have already begun to make small behavioral changes. They will keep their appointments if you schedule them at the time of the hearing screening. Of course, these individuals require information about hearing loss, hearing aids, etc. To reiterate, it is helpful if these individuals are scheduled for their follow-up appointments at the time of the hearing screen, as in this group you have a captive audience.

Action

People in this stage make the move for which they have been preparing. They see the audiologist for a test. They still, however, need encouragement and support. These are probably the individuals who regard themselves as having a considerable handicap and are motivated to purchase audiologic services. Individuals in this category who fail the screen are the most likely to comply with the recommendation to see an audiologist. These individuals need information, support, and follow-up as they move through the hearing health-care system (U.S. D.H.H.S., 1994).

The latter two stages apply to people who have already purchased audiologic services, including hearing aids, and they will require the services of a caring, supportive, and well-trained audiologist!

Maintenance

Here the person must work to maintain the progress they have made and not give up if they experience setbacks. In the case of hearing aids, they have to continue to see the audiologist for counseling and to ask the questions that tend to come up within the first three months of hearing-aid use.

Termination Stage

Patients are happy with their hearing aids, wear them, use them, are satisfied and benefit from them. Interestingly, these individuals can be helpful when trying to modify the behaviors of older adults who are not yet ready to change their behaviors.

PEARL

Key components of patient behavior change are information and counseling, "more counseling tends to be better counseling, and any counseling, no matter how brief, is better than none at all" (U.S. D.H.H.S., 1994, p. 29).

SPECIAL CONSIDERATION

In order for screening to be successful, which is to say that individuals comply with recommendations to pursue hearing health-care services, persons undergoing the screen must be at a stage wherein they are prepared and ready to change their behavior.

Pushing individuals prematurely to act is one of the most common reasons for low rates of follow-up with audiology appointments and hearing-aids. In my view, individuals organizing screening programs should recognize that most older adults undergoing the screen are probably in the "contemplation stage" and thus they must design a screening protocol that takes this into account. Self-report questionnaires in combination with educational material that describes hearing impairment, its effect on psychosocial function, and interventions that are successful at alleviating its consequences are probably the approach that would yield the highest follow-through rates. In the next section of this chapter, I will propose two approaches to hearing screening that take into account the Health Belief Model and the Stages-of-Change Model.

Now let us return to the fifth criterion against which to judge the value of screening for hearing loss. Has the effectiveness of the program been demonstrated in a randomized trial? Unfortunately, randomized trials have not been attempted to document the effectiveness of a given screening protocol. One reason is the lack of agreement among audiologists over the condition to be screened for, the components of a screening protocol, and the pass-fail criteria. It is hoped that the principles outlined and the protocol proposed in this chapter will serve as a stimulus to action. I feel strongly that routine screening when embedded in an educational context is the ideal way for hearing-impaired older adults to reach audiologists.

The two final criterion against which to judge the value of screening for hearing loss in older adults is whether the program reaches those who could benefit and whether the health care system can cope with the referrals. Unfortunately, the answer to the first concern is "no," but fortunately the answer to the second is "yes." With regard to the former, the most efficacious way to reach the majority of older adults is to involve primary care physicians, family practitioners, and geriatricians in the process. After all, these professionals are the entry point into the health care system (e.g., in 1991 there were about 5.6 physician contacts per person) (NCHS, 1993). Abrams, Beers, and Berkow (1995) recommend strongly that physicians screen all elderly persons for hearing loss. Unfortunately, less than 10% of physicians screen older adults for hearing loss. In my opinion, audiologists are obliged to educate physicians about the value of hearing screening and about effective screening protocols as most older adults see a primary care physician on a regular basis, providing opportunities for case finding in their general practice. According to Fujikawa and Cunningham (1989), patients often prefer it if physicians rather than audiologists perform the initial screen as they regard the recommendation of a physician as important.

The answer to the question about caseload capabilities is a resounding "yes." In short, relative to the large number of older adults with hearing impairment, these individuals constitute a small proportion of the audiologist's caseload. The breakdown is as shown in Table 10–3. Interestingly, while the proportion of older adults with hearing loss is much greater than the proportion of people under 17 years of age, these groups constitute equivalent proportions of our caseload. The principle of supply and demand would

> ## SPECIAL CONSIDERATION
>
> **The fact that only 18 to 20% of older adults with hearing loss own hearing aids further attests to the under-utilization of hearing health-care services by older adults, as does Kochkin's (1997) projection that the viable market for hearing aids should be 12.7 million rather than the current size of 5.6 million.**

suggest that if more individuals with hearing loss would purchase audiologic services in the form of evaluation or rehabilitation, the cost of services including hearing aids is likely to go down. Further, if managed care organizations better understood the value of our services, perhaps cost would no longer remain a barrier to many older adults who could benefit from our services.

In sum, the bulk of the evidence suggests that it is reasonable to screen the ears of older adults. Unfortunately, the protocols to be used, the time frame for screening, and the appropriate professional to do the job remain the subject of considerable debate. According to my review of the epidemiologic literature, it may not be cost effective for audiologists to conduct screenings at senior citizen centers, because of the low yield from screening the generally healthy and vigorous older adults who take advantage of these services. I do however, believe that audiologists should consider participating in health promotion activities sponsored by community agencies. I also think that efforts should be

TABLE 10–3 Monthly Caseload of Audiologist by Age

Age group	Proportion of caseload overall	Hospitals
Birth to 2 years	9.3%	16.0%
3 to 5 years	12.4%	15.0%
6 to 11 years	10.3%	8.8%
12 to 17 years	6.2%	4.9%
18 to 21 years	4.9%	4.1%
22 to 64 years	21.8%	20.9%
65 to 84 years	27.3%	23.1%
85 years and older	7.9%	7.0%

Source: ASHA, 1997b.

expanded to educate older adults about hearing health care as this is an important component of any screening endeavor. An ideal way to reach older adults is through the Internet, primary care physicians, or health promotion activities in the community. In fact, materials are currently available that allow for offsite or onsite screening without the audiologist having to be actively involved (i.e., I believe it is not cost effective for audiologists to devote their time to screening activities, but screening is important).

What follows are two alternative approaches to hearing screening that were developed with the Health Belief Model and the Stages-of-Change Model in mind. These strategies are alternatives to the routine pure-tone screen, self-assessment screen, or the combined approach advocated by ASHA (1997a). They allow screening to be accomplished in a variety of settings without the active involvement of the audiologist.

THE MULTIMEDIA HEARING HANDICAP INVENTORY (MHHI)

In weighing the recommendations of the U.S. P.S.T.F., and in consideration of the principles of the Health Belief Model, I believe the HHIE-S presented in an educational context is the ideal approach to preventive activities designed to identify older adults with handicapping hearing impairment. The HHIE-S has high test-retest repeatability, and very adequate sensitivity and specificity. In fact, Bess (1995) contends that the HHIE-S can be an invaluable screening tool for the hearing professional. In my view, this tool must be presented in an educational context as patient education has proven successful in altering compliance with therapeutic regimens that target chronic conditions (Mazzuca, 1982). Patient education that teaches about the disease and its treatment is designed to place individuals in a better position to participate in their own health care, hence maximizing the potential therapeutic benefit (Mazzuca, 1982). Patient education should be considered by audiologists as a process of "influencing patient behavior, producing changes in knowledge, attitudes and skills required to maintain or improve health. The process begins with the imparting of factual information, and includes interpretation and integration of the information in such a manner as to bring about attitudinal or behavioral changes which benefit the person's health status" (Vogt & Kapp, 1987, p. 273).

In consideration of the role patient education plays in compliance with screening activities, Punch and Weinstein (1996) introduced a multimedia version of the Hearing Handicap Inventory (MHHI). This tool enables the clinician to administer a reliable and valid screening test in an educational and counseling context—elements critical to a successful screening program. The authors hope that this format will promote compliance with recommendations that grow out of the handicap/disability screen (Punch & Weinstein, 1996). A pilot study I recently completed revealed that scores on the MHHI are comparable to scores on the paper-pencil and face-to-face versions of the HHIE-S. We are currently establishing the test-retest reliability and predictive validity of the MHHI, as well.

TABLE 10–4 Major Features of the MHHI

Section 1:	Program overview
Section 2:	Computer introduction
Section 3:	Overview of anatomy of normal hearing and hearing impairment
Section 4:	HHI questionnaire
Section 5:	Treatments for hearing loss
Section 6:	Hearing profiles

The MHHI combines video, text, graphics, and sound in an interactive format. The software program, which is contained on a CD-ROM, runs on a personal computer equipped to handle multimedia applications. The system requirements include a mouse; a minimum of 16 MB of available RAM for software (24 MB preferred); 4 MB free disk space; a CD-ROM drive; Sound Blaster-compatible sound card; monitor capable of 256 colors; system connected to a local or remote printer; Pentium grade processor 100 MHz or higher; Windows® 95/98 operating system; Quick Time 2.1.2 or later; and volume-controlled speakers. The program uses large, open-captioned text, and is narrated by male and female professional radio broadcasters. The respondent has the opportunity to select the gender of the speaker based on the vocal characteristics that the individual judges to be most intelligible.

The program has several interactive features. For example, the respondent is asked to indicate a preference for a male or female talker and is prompted to adjust the volume of the selected voice to a comfortable level. The respondent is asked to indicate his/her range and thus the correct version of the Hearing Handicap Inventory (HHI) is administered, that is, the HHIE-S or the Hearing Handicap Inventory for Adults-Screening version (HHIA-S). The individual has the opportunity to indicate whether the questionnaire is being completed by a hearing-aid user (i.e., aided condition) or by a nonhearing-aid user (i.e., unaided condition). Finally, the respondent is asked to indicate whether or not

parts of the program have been viewed previously. If so, the respondent can ask to skip specific parts of the program (i.e., the educational piece about hearing impairment). The program is self-administering once the examiner enters in the identifying information and the respondent clicks the start button. The authors feel that by designing a program that is automated, the application is appropriate for respondents having a wide range of computer skills. As we move into the 21st century, more and more older adults are embracing computers, hence the increasing use of CD-ROMs in health promotion activities.

Table 10–4 displays the six major sections of the program. The program overview orients the respondent to the program and informs the patient that he/she will be completing a questionnaire that assesses hearing handicap as opposed to hearing impairment and that at the end an individualized hearing profile based on his/her responses will be provided, including a recommendation regarding the next step in the hearing health-care system. The monitor displays a generic handicap questionnaire with a simple answer key and states that "the main purpose of the program is to evaluate the degree of any handicap caused by hearing loss, using the Hearing Handicap Inventory." This is shown in Figure 10–2.

The next section includes an introduction to the basic components of the computer including the spacebar, the mouse, the monitor, and the printer. The respondent is given the opportunity to practice with the mouse and spacebar to make sure they understand what is required. This section is simple enough so that even people who are completely unfamiliar with computers can learn about the essential components by following the on-screen instructions. Figure 10–3 shows the monitor and the practice exercise with the computer mouse.

Next is the introduction to hearing and hearing impairment. It provides an educational context for the questionnaire, touching on the important points necessary to raise respondents' awareness about the prevalence, severity, and consequences of untreated hearing loss. Specifically, the common problems experienced by persons with hearing impairment are listed. In addition, the respondent is given a

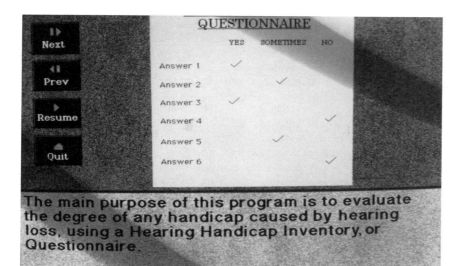

Figure 10–2 Screen depicting basic purpose of the program: use of a questionnaire to determine degree of self-perceived hearing handicap.

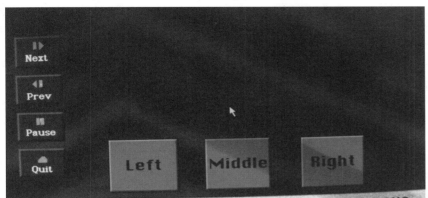

Figure 10–3 Practice exercise using the computer mouse.

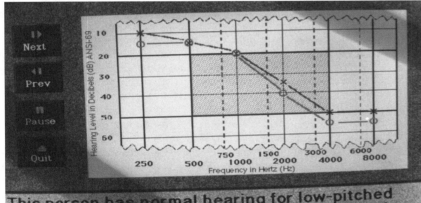

Figure 10–4 Sample audiogram displayed on the MHHI.

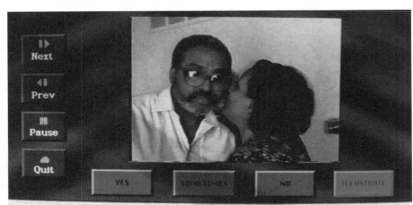

Figure 10–5 Example of the HHI screen depicting the illustrate function.

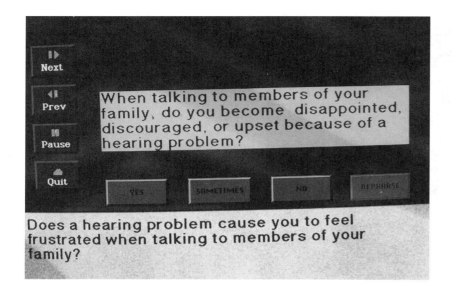

Does a hearing problem cause you to feel frustrated when talking to members of your family?

Figure 10–6   Example of the HHI screen depicting the rephrase function.

simplistic overview of the ear and how we hear, and there is a brief discussion of how hearing sensitivity is charted on the audiogram. Sample audiograms (e.g., mild hearing loss, high frequency hearing loss) are displayed providing the respondent with a feel for how to read and understand what the audiogram is telling them. This is displayed in Figure 10–4. If the respondent has already viewed the educational piece, he/she has the option to skip to the next section on the MHHI questionnaire. This is the actual screening test where an age-appropriate screening version of the questionnaire (e.g., HHIA-S or HHIE-S) is administered. The MHHI can be administered in either an aided or unaided situation. The multimedia questionnaire offers a degree of flexibility not available in pencil-paper or interview formats (Punch & Weinstein, 1996). For example, each of the social-situational questions is accompanied by an illustrate button that allows the respondent to visualize the type of situation referred to in the specific question. As is depicted in Figure 10–5, this gives the respondent a feel for the situation being described. Respondents who would like one of the questions on the emotional effects of hearing loss to be restated can click on the rephrase button if the original question is unclear. Of course, use of these buttons is optional. Figure 10–6 displays the prompt following the standard question on the HHIE: "Does a hearing problem cause you to feel frustrated when talking to members of your family?" We are currently field testing the relationship between scores on the MHHI when the rephrase and illustrate functions are used, and scores on the MHHI when these functions are not accessed.

The next section of the multimedia version discusses treatments available for hearing loss including medical, surgical, and audiologic options. Once again, with the tenets of the Health Belief Model in mind, we discuss such treatment options as hearing aids, assistive listening devices, and counseling, and emphasize that available research has demonstrated that these interventions are successful in reducing the handicapping effects of hearing loss as perceived by older adults. It is hoped that information on treatment options will motivate respondents to comply with a recommendation to seek professional assistance. The respondent

has the opportunity to visualize the variety of available hearing aids when worn within the ear of an individual with hearing impairment. The photos are intended to help the person overcome their cosmetic concerns about hearing aids. It should be clear from the photos that hearing aids are small and for the most part inconspicuous.

The final section of the MHHI is the Hearing Profile. After completing the questionnaire, the respondent is prompted to click a special button to produce a printed copy of their hearing profile. The Profile consists of a one-page printed description of the respondent's hearing handicap status and follow-up recommendations that derive directly from the score. The Profile is individualized based on (1) the total hearing handicap score, (2) whether or not the questionnaire has been completed previously, and (3) whether the responses were based on unaided or aided hearing. For a given respondent, one of eight profiles is generated. Sample profiles are depicted in Appendices A–H. It is worth noting that on the multimedia version, scores ranging from 0 to 8 are considered a pass, whereas scores of 10 or greater are considered a fail. This is the cut-off established by Ventry and Weinstein (1983) and Lichtenstein, Bess, and Logan (1988). Appendices A and C are indicative of the need for routine follow-up (unaided condition); Appendices B and D indicate the need for routine follow-up of respondents who use hearing aids; Appendices E and G indicate the need for a hearing evaluation and possible hearing-aid candidacy; and Appendices F and H indicate unsatisfactory aided performance, suggesting the need to consider hearing-aid adjustment, repairs, replacement, and counseling. Of course, the printed profile contains a disclaimer indicating that recommendation and referral information are based, in part, on a comparison of the respondent's questionnaire with that of averaged scores obtained from a sample population having known characteristics and do not directly identify hearing impairment or ear pathology (Punch & Weinstein, 1996).

It is worthwhile noting that data collected are stored and can serve as the basis for interpreting absolute self-perceived hearing handicap, for monitoring change in scores over time (e.g., unaided versus aided listening), and for developing individualized recommendations in the form of Hearing Profiles. The data are stored on the hard drive as comma-delimited text, making it simple to import to a database, a spreadsheet, or a word-processing application of the examiner's choice.

The authors are optimistic that delivering a screening test embedded in an educational context will have considerable appeal to a variety of health care professionals. They feel that this type of screening tool can be used while in the waiting room of a doctor's office, can be installed in the waiting room of a hearing health-care clinic or a private practice, or can be used as part of a community health promotion program. In fact, it has great potential for helping to realize some of the important educational objectives of Healthy People 2000, and most likely of Healthy People 2010. These include increasing the proportion of people aged 65 and older who participate in at least one organized health promotion program through a senior center, lifecare facility, or other community-based setting that serves older adults; focusing preventive efforts on modifiable risk behaviors matched to the leading problems of older adults and addressing these health issues through multiple strategies including education, counseling, and screening; insuring that providers identify patients at risk for a condition such as handicapping hearing impairment, for which interventions may be appropriate; and developing educational services that will enable patients and their families and friends, when appropriate, to make informed decisions about their health (U.S. D.H.H.S., 1992). Assuming a multimedia personal computer is available, the MHHI can be used to help realize most of these objectives.

SPECIAL CONSIDERATION

Multimedia technology is an ideal medium for educating and screening purposes. However, information transfer can also be accomplished using pamphlets, videotapes, or lectures. The end result should always be the same presentation of medical facts and treatment principles intended for persons with a chronic condition such as hearing impairment (Mazzuca, 1982).

When the use of multimedia technology is not an option, audiologists are urged to consider the following patient education guidelines should they choose to administer a hearing screening protocol in an educational context (Vogt & Kapp, 1987): (1) use terms the client/patient can understand, (2) recall that patients generally remember only three to four points so remember to present only the important information, (3) be specific when giving instructions and explanations, (4) provide written information, (5) sit down when providing informational counseling—this gives the perception that you are willing to take time to explain all the important information, and (6) reinforce or review the information you have presented to make sure it is understood and the individual will act on it. In recognition of the value of education and of the time-consuming nature of counsel-

ing as part of a screening program, Punch and Weinstein have developed a Web site for hearing screening.

Advances in telecommunications are revolutionizing the way in which society functions, leading Punch and Weinstein to take advantage of these changes to help to increase the numbers of hearing-impaired persons receiving appropriate hearing health care. Specifically, the Internet has left the realm of research laboratories and is being used to promote wellness in many segments of the health-care delivery system. Specifically, health care professionals are developing Web sites to educate and screen older adults for selected disorders. We adapted the MHHI, developing and copyrighting a Web site on which any adult with English reading skills and Internet access can complete a self-administered questionnaire that will effectively screen for hearing handicap.

The Web site can be accessed by dialing www.Ph.D.msu.edu/hearing. Prior to completing the HHI on the Web, a brief overview distinguishing among impairment, handicap, and disability is provided. Following this, the respondent should click on "questionnaire" and based on the respondent's selection of their age range, the adult or older adult version of the HHI is administered. Once each of the questions has been answered, the respondent clicks the mouse and their hearing handicap score is calculated. It can be viewed immediately and a set of follow-up recommendations based on the score is printed. To facilitate compliance with the recommendation, respondents will be able to obtain information indicating the location of a nearby ASHA-accredited audiology program where they can receive the services they need. For this purpose and with ASHA's permission, we have linked our Web site with ASHA's Web pages containing the names of Professional Service Board (PSB)-accredited programs. Linkages with the ASHA Web site will likely increase the number of consumers referred to audiologists who agree to participate in the program. Based on the scores, the Web-based version recommends that the respondent visit his or her audiologist when the score exceeds 18. Respondents, of course, use the Web HHI free of charge and there is no charge for the link to PSB-accredited programs, thus it is like free nationwide advertising for audiology services. In our view, the Web HHI is another way of educating and reaching the large, unserved hearing-impaired population and encouraging them to seek out audiologic services.

CONCLUDING REMARKS

According to the National Center for Health Statistics, hearing loss defined audiometrically or according to self-report, is the third most prevalent chronic condition affecting adults over the age of 65. The functional impact of hearing loss includes interference with communication, as well as the social, psychological, emotional, and vocational domains of function. Despite the "lesions" and "barriers" created by acquired hearing loss, it is difficult for most aged hearing-impaired persons to acknowledge a sensory loss such as a hearing deficit. Despite technological advances in hearing aids, and the satisfaction aged hearing-handicapped individuals derive from amplification, only 13 to

TABLE 10–5   Screening Options for Noninstitutionalized Older Adults

Condition	Options	Fail criteria
1. Medical disorder	Video-otoscopy, otoscopic	Wax, redness, discharge, etc.
2. Impairment	Pure-tones, Audioscope (1000, 2000, 4000 Hz)	40 dBHL
3. Handicap	HHIE-S, SAC	HHIE-S: 10 or 18 SAC: 19
	Multimedia HHI	10
	Web version, HHI	18

Note: Counseling and compliance-inducing strategies should be incorporated into every screening to insure that individuals who fail the screen actually pursue follow-up services.

20% own a hearing aid, highlighting the gap between prevalence and service utilization. As hearing loss is prevalent, affects quality of life, and is amenable to intervention, it is an ideal target of early identification efforts according to the U.S. D.H.H.S. (1994).

A number of screening protocols have been proposed for identifying aged individuals with hearing loss requiring audiologic assistance. Despite differences across protocols in terms of such variables as pass-fail criteria, hearing levels, and frequencies for screening, the sensitivity, specificity, and predictive accuracy of most proposals tend to be uniformly high and acceptable. Notwithstanding the adequacy of available reliability and validity data, hearing-impaired aged individuals demonstrate poor compliance with recommended therapies. As screening programs can only be considered effective if available diagnostic and treatment services are utilized by those undergoing the screen and when treatment recommendations are complied with, selected professionals are rethinking the value and efficacy of traditional screening programs that target hearing loss in aged individuals.

Alternatives to pure-tone screening have been developed with the principles set forth by the U.S. Public Health Service in mind. The Public Health Service suggests that when implementing health promotion activities, information and services should be provided at a level of comprehension consistent with the age and learning skills of the patient, using terminology consistent with the patient's language and communication style. In addition, they recommend the use of short questionnaires that can quickly assess patient needs for follow-up services. Questionnaires about hearing loss

TABLE 10–6   Hearing Handicap Inventory for the Elderly-Screening Version

INSTRUCTIONS: The purpose of this questionnaire is to identify the problems your hearing loss may be causing you. Answer YES, SOMETIMES, or NO for each question. To obtain a total score add up the YES (4 points), SOMETIMES (2), and NO (0) responses. If your score is greater than 10 we recommend that you schedule a hearing test with a certified audiologist at a local hearing clinic.

	YES (4)	SOMETIMES (2)	NO (0)
E1. Does a hearing problem cause you to feel embarrassed when you meet new people?			
E2. Does a hearing problem cause you to feel frustrated when talking to members of your family?			
S1. Do you have difficulty hearing when someone speaks in a whisper?			
E3. Do you feel handicapped by a hearing problem?			
S2. Does a hearing problem cause you difficulty when visiting friends, relatives or neighbors?			
S3. Does a hearing problem cause you to attend religious services less often than you would like?			
E4. Does a hearing problem cause you to have arguments with family members?			
S4. Does a hearing problem cause you difficulty when listening to TV or radio?			
E5. Do you feel that any difficulty with your hearing limits or hampers your personal or social life?			
S5. Does a hearing problem cause you difficulty when in a restaurant with relatives or friends?			
TOTAL SCORE: HHIE-S _____ Refer if score > 10			

should contain items that attempt to identify communication problems, and social and emotional handicaps stemming from hearing loss. Counseling and education should be integral to any health promotion activity and resources such as computers, Web sites, pamphlets, posters, and books should be used to create a milieu that reinforces healthy behavior. In this chapter, I describe the MHHI and the Web version of the HHI. I consider these good alternatives to more traditional screening protocols as they can reach a wider audience, and the educational components can theoretically increase compliance with recommendations to seek follow-up.

PEARL

When selecting a screening protocol, the audiologist should always consider what they are screening for (e.g., disorder, impairment, disability, handicap) and should keep in mind that the goal should be to correctly identify individuals at risk who are likely to follow-up with the recommendation to seek assistance.

Table 10–5 summarizes screening options for noninstitutionalized older adults and Table 10–6 contains items from the HHIE-S that can be an extremely valuable tool for the hearing health professional (Bess, 1995). It is my hope that the discussion in this chapter will be used by audiologists to launch screening programs that will help to close the gap between the number of hearing-impaired older adults in general and the number who purchase audiologic services to help improve the quality of their lives.

GLOSSARY OF TERMS

A Screening Test High in Sensitivity*: a test that yields a high proportion of individuals who actually have the disorders.

A Screening Test High in Specificity*: a test that yields a normal result in a high proportion of those who do not have the disorder.

A Screening Test with a High Predictive Value*: a test that results in a high proportion of those with and without the disorder among those with abnormal and normal test results, respectively.

Effective Screening Program*: a screening program can only be considered effective when available diagnostic and treatment services are used by screened individuals and when the treatment recommendations provided by the services are complied with.

Handicap**: a disadvantage for a given individual resulting from an impairment which limits or prevents the fulfillment of a role that is normal for the individual.

Impairment**: any loss or abnormality of psychological, physiological, or anatomical structure or function.

*Sackett, Haynes, and Tugwell, 1985
**WHO, 1980

APPENDIX A
HEARING PROFILE:
HEARING HANDICAP INVENTORY
(Protocol 1)

(IF the current score is 0 to 9, AND a previous test result IS NOT found in the database for this individual, AND the listening condition is Unaided, print the following:)

Examinee Name:
Examinee ID:
Listening Condition: Insert Unaided or Aided here
Date:
Time:

Interpretation: Scores indicate degree of hearing handicap; the higher the number, the greater the perceived handicap associated with hearing impairment. The highest possible handicap score for a given administration of the questionnaire is 40. Scores between 0 and 8 should be interpreted as no perceived handicap, and scores between 10 and 40 represent varying degrees of perceived handicap.

Hearing Profile: Your hearing handicap score today was (insert score here). A score in this range suggests either that there is no hearing loss, or if present, hearing loss is not interfering substantially with communication or other activities in your daily life.

Recommendations: It is recommended that you return to complete this Hearing Handicap Inventory in 1 year, or sooner if you should notice a change in your hearing. If you have any medical problems such as pain or discharge from your ears, ringing or other sounds in your ears, or dizziness, you should schedule an appointment with your primary care physician.

If you have any questions about this Hearing Handicap Inventory or its interpretation, please contact:

Disclaimer: This has not been a direct test of your hearing. Recommendations and referral information are based, in part, on a comparison of your questionnaire score with average scores obtained from a sample of people having known hearing characteristics, and do not directly identify hearing impairment or ear pathology.

APPENDIX B
HEARING PROFILE:
HEARING HANDICAP INVENTORY
(Protocol 2)

(IF the current score is 0 to 9, AND a previous test result IS NOT found in the database for this individual, AND the listening condition is Aided, print the following:)

Examinee Name:
Examinee ID:
Listening Condition: Insert Unaided or Aided here
Date:
Time:

Interpretation: Scores indicate degree of hearing handicap; the higher the number, the greater the perceived handicap associated with hearing impairment. The highest possible handicap score for a given administration of the questionnaire is 40. Scores between 0 and 8 should be interpreted as no perceived handicap, and scores between 10 and 40 represent varying degrees of perceived handicap.

Hearing Profile: Your hearing handicap score today was (insert score here). A score in this range suggests that your hearing loss is not interfering substantially with communication or other activities in your daily life, and that you are receiving ample benefit from your hearing aid(s).

Recommendations: It is recommended that you return to complete this Hearing Handicap Inventory in 1 year, or sooner if you should notice either a change in your hearing or in the performance of your hearing aid(s). If you have any medical problems such as pain or discharge from your ears, ringing or other sounds in your ears, or dizziness, you should schedule an appointment with your primary care physician.

If you have any questions about this Hearing Handicap Inventory or its interpretation, please contact:

Disclaimer: This has not been a direct test of your hearing. Recommendations and referral information are based, in part, on a comparison of your questionnaire score with average scores obtained from a sample of people having known hearing characteristics, and do not directly identify hearing impairment or ear pathology.

APPENDIX C
HEARING PROFILE:
HEARING HANDICAP INVENTORY
(Protocol 3)

(IF the current score is 0 to 9, AND a previous test result for this individual IS found in the database, AND the listening condition is Unaided, print the following:)

Examinee Name:
Examinee ID:
Listening Condition: Insert Unaided or Aided here
Date:
Time:

Interpretation: Scores indicate degree of hearing handicap; the higher the number, the greater the perceived handicap associated with hearing impairment. The highest possible handicap score for a given administration of the questionnaire is 40. Scores between 0 and 8 should be interpreted as no perceived handicap, and scores between 10 and 40 represent varying degrees of perceived handicap.

Hearing Profile: Your hearing handicap score today was (insert score here). A score in this range suggests either that there is no hearing loss, or if present, hearing loss is not interfering substantially with communication or other activities in your daily life. Your previous score on (insert date of last test here) was (insert last test score here). A difference in that score and today's score of less than 10 suggests no real change in perceived handicap, while a difference of 10 or more suggests a possible change in perceived hearing handicap.

Recommendations: It is recommended that you return to complete this Hearing Handicap Inventory in 1 year, or sooner if you should notice a change in your hearing. If you have any medical problems such as pain or discharge from your ears, ringing or other sounds in your ears, or dizziness, you should schedule an appointment with your primary care physician.

If you have any questions about this Hearing Handicap Inventory or its interpretation, please contact:

Disclaimer: This has not been a direct test of your hearing. Recommendations and referral information are based, in part, on a comparison of your questionnaire score with average scores obtained from a sample of people having known hearing characteristics, and do not directly identify hearing impairment or ear pathology.

APPENDIX D
HEARING PROFILE:
HEARING HANDICAP INVENTORY
(Protocol 4)

(IF the current score is 0 to 9, AND a previous test result for this individual IS found in the database, AND the listening condition is Aided, print the following:)

Examinee Name:
Examinee ID:
Listening Condition: Insert Unaided or Aided here
Date:
Time:

Interpretation: Scores indicate degree of hearing handicap; the higher the number, the greater the perceived handicap associated with hearing impairment. The highest possible handicap score for a given administration of the questionnaire is 40. Scores between 0 and 8 should be interpreted as no perceived handicap, and scores between 10 and 40 represent varying degrees of perceived handicap.

Hearing Profile: Your hearing handicap score today was (insert score here). A score in this range suggests that your hearing loss is not interfering substantially with communication or other activities in your daily life, and that you are receiving ample benefit from your hearing aid(s). Your previous score on (insert date of last test here) was (insert last test score here). A difference in that score and today's score of less than 10 suggests no real change in perceived handicap, while a difference of 10 or more suggests a possible change in perceived hearing handicap.

Recommendations: It is recommended that you return to complete this Hearing Handicap Inventory in 1 year, or sooner if you should notice either a change in your hearing or in the performance of your hearing aid(s). If you have any medical problems such as pain or discharge from your ears, ringing or other sounds in your ears, or dizziness, you should schedule an appointment with your primary care physician.

If you have any questions about this Hearing Handicap Inventory or its interpretation, please contact:

Disclaimer: This has not been a direct test of your hearing. Recommendations and referral information are based, in part, on a comparison of your questionnaire score with average scores obtained from a sample of people having known hearing characteristics, and do not directly identify hearing impairment or ear pathology.

APPENDIX E
HEARING PROFILE:
HEARING HANDICAP INVENTORY
(Protocol 5)

(IF the current score is 10 or more, AND a previous test result for this individual IS NOT found in the database, AND the listening condition is Unaided, print the following:)

Examinee Name:
Examinee ID:
Listening Condition: Insert Unaided or Aided here
Date:
Time:

Interpretation: Scores indicate degree of hearing handicap; the higher the number, the greater the perceived handicap associated with hearing impairment. The highest possible handicap score for a given administration of the questionnaire is 40. Scores between 0 and 8 should be interpreted as no perceived handicap, and scores between 10 and 40 represent varying degrees of perceived handicap.

Hearing Profile: According to your responses to the questionnaire, your hearing handicap score today was (insert score here). Research has shown that individuals with scores of 10 or greater are likely to have measurable hearing impairment. Many people who are considering using hearing aids for the first time have scores of 18 or greater, irrespective of severity of hearing loss. In addition, 3 to 4 weeks after these people have purchased hearing aids, their perception of hearing difficulties is dramatically reduced. This outcome suggests that hearing aids have helped them in problematic situations.

Recommendations: It is recommended that you contact a local audiologist to arrange for a hearing evaluation and possibly a trial period with hearing aids. If you have any medical problems such as pain or discharge from your ears, ringing or other sounds in your ears, or dizziness, you should schedule an appointment with your primary care physician.

If you have any questions about this Hearing Handicap Inventory or its interpretation, please contact:

Disclaimer: This has not been a direct test of your hearing. Recommendations and referral information are based, in part, on a comparison of your questionnaire score with average scores obtained from a sample of people having known hearing characteristics, and do not directly identify hearing impairment or ear pathology.

APPENDIX F
HEARING PROFILE:
HEARING HANDICAP INVENTORY
(Protocol 6)

(IF the current score is 10 or more, AND a previous test result for this individual IS NOT found in the database, AND the listening condition is Aided, print the following:)

Examinee Name:
Examinee ID:
Listening Condition: Insert Unaided or Aided here
Date:
Time:

Interpretation: Scores indicate degree of hearing handicap; the higher the number, the greater the perceived handicap associated with hearing impairment. The highest possible handicap score for a given administration of the questionnaire is 40. Scores between 0 and 8 should be interpreted as no perceived handicap, and scores between 10 and 40 represent varying degrees of perceived handicap.

Hearing Profile: According to your responses to the questionnaire, your hearing handicap score today was (insert score here). This score suggests that you may have some residual disability associated with your hearing loss, even though you wear hearing aids. Recent research has shown that many people who are considering using hearing aids for the first time have scores of 18 or greater, irrespective of severity of hearing loss.

Recommendations: If you are experiencing difficulty with your hearing aid(s), such as whistling, need for frequent repair, or poorer-than-expected performance, it is recommended that you contact the professional who fitted your hearing aid(s). If you have any medical problems such as pain or discharge from your ears, ringing or other sounds in your ears, or dizziness, you should schedule an appointment with your primary care physician.

If you have any questions about this Hearing Handicap Inventory or its interpretation, please contact:

Disclaimer: This has not been a direct test of your hearing. Recommendations and referral information are based, in part, on a comparison of your questionnaire score with average scores obtained from a sample of people having known hearing characteristics, and do not directly identify hearing impairment or ear pathology.

APPENDIX G
HEARING PROFILE:
HEARING HANDICAP INVENTORY
(Protocol 7)

(IF the current score is 10 or more, AND a previous test result for this individual IS found in the database, AND the listening condition is Unaided, print the following:)

Examinee Name:
Examinee ID:
Listening Condition: Insert Unaided or Aided here
Date:
Time:

Interpretation: Scores indicate degree of hearing handicap; the higher the number, the greater the perceived handicap associated with hearing impairment. The highest possible handicap score for a given administration of the questionnaire is 40. Scores between 0 and 8 should be interpreted as no perceived handicap, and scores between 10 and 40 represent varying degrees of perceived handicap.

Hearing Profile: According to your responses to the questionnaire, your hearing handicap score today was (insert score here). Research has shown that individuals with scores of 10 or greater are likely to have measurable hearing impairment. Many people who are considering using hearing aids for the first time have scores of 18 or greater, irrespective of severity of hearing loss. In addition, 3 to 4 weeks after these people have purchased hearing aids, their perception of hearing difficulties is dramatically reduced. This outcome suggests that hearing aids have helped them in problematic situations. Your previous score on (insert date of last test here) was (insert last test score here). A difference in that score and today's score of less than 10 suggests no real change in perceived handicap while a difference of 10 or more suggests a possible change in perceived hearing handicap.

Recommendations: It is recommended that you contact a local audiologist to arrange for a trial period with hearing aids. If you have any medical problems such as pain or discharge from the ears, ringing or other sounds in your ears, or dizziness, you should schedule an appointment with your primary care physician.

If you have any questions about this Hearing Handicap Inventory or its interpretation, please contact:

Disclaimer: This has not been a direct test of your hearing. Recommendations and referral information are based, in part, on a comparison of your questionnaire score with average scores obtained from a sample of people having known hearing characteristics, and do not directly identify hearing impairment or ear pathology.

APPENDIX H
HEARING PROFILE:
HEARING HANDICAP INVENTORY
(Protocol 8)

(IF the current score is 10 or more, AND a previous test result for this individual IS found in the database, AND the listening condition is Aided, print the following:)

Examinee Name:
Examinee ID:
Listening Condition: Insert Unaided or Aided here
Date:
Time:

Interpretation: Scores indicate degree of hearing handicap; the higher the number, the greater the perceived handicap associated with hearing impairment. The highest possible handicap score for a given administration of the questionnaire is 40. Scores between 0 and 8 should be interpreted as no perceived handicap, and scores between 10 and 40 represent varying degrees of perceived handicap.

Hearing Profile: According to your responses to the questionnaire, your hearing handicap score today was (insert score here). This score suggests that you may have some residual disability associated with your hearing loss, even though you wear hearing aids. Recent research has shown that many people who are considering using hearing aids for the first time have scores of 18 or greater,

irrespective of severity of hearing loss. Your previous score on (insert date of last test score here) was (insert last test score here). A difference in that score and today's score of less than 10 suggests no real change in perceived handicap, while a difference of 10 or more suggests a possible change in perceived hearing handicap.

Recommendations: If you are experiencing difficulty with your hearing aid(s), such as whistling, need for frequent repair, or poorer-than-expected performance, it is recommended that you contact the professional who fitted your hearing aid(s). If you have any medical problems such as pain or discharge from your ears, ringing or other sounds in your ears, or dizziness, you should schedule an appointment with your primary care physician.

If you have any questions about this Hearing Handicap Inventory or its interpretation, please contact:

Disclaimer: This has not been a direct test of your hearing. Recommendations and referral information are based, in part, on a comparison of your questionnaire score with average scores obtained from a sample of people having known hearing characteristics, and do not directly identify hearing impairment or ear pathology.

REFERENCES

ABRAMS, W., BEERS, M., & BERKOW, R. (1995). *The Merck Manual of Geriatrics*, 2d ed. Whitehouse Station, NJ: Merck Research Laboratories.

AMERICAN ACADEMY OF FAMILY PHYSICIANS, COMMISSION ON PUBLIC HEALTH AND SCIENTIFIC AFFAIRS. (1993). *Age Charts for Periodic Health Examination*. Kansas City, MO: American Academy of Family Physicians.

AMERICAN COLLEGE OF OBSTETRICIANS AND GYNECOLOGISTS. (1993). *The Obstetrician-Gynecologist and Primary Preventive Health Care*. Washington, DC: American College of Obstetricians and Gynecologists.

AMERICAN SPEECH-LANGUAGE-HEARING ASSOCIATION PANEL ON AUDIOLOGIC ASSESSMENT. (1997a). *Guidelines for Audiologic Screening*. Rockville, MD: American Speech-Language-Hearing Association.

AMERICAN SPEECH-LANGUAGE-HEARING ASSOCIATION. (1997b). *1997 Omnibus Survey Reports*. Rockville, MD: American Speech-Language-Hearing Association.

BECKER, M. (1974).*The Health Belief Model and Personal Health Behavior*. Thorofare, NJ: Charles B. Slack.

BESS, F. (1995). Applications of the Hearing Handicap Inventory for the Elderly-Screening Version (HHIE-S). *Hearing Journal*, 48: 10, 51–55.

BIENVENUE, G., MICHAEL, P., CHAFFINISH, J., & ZIEGLER, J. (1985). The Audioscope: a clinical tool for otoscopic and audiometric examination. *Ear and Hearing*, 6: 251–254.

CADMAN, D., CHAMBERS, L., FELDMAN, W., & SACKETT, D. (1984). Assessing the effectiveness of community screening programs. *JAMA*, 251: 1580–1585.

CANADIAN TASK FORCE ON THE PERIODIC HEALTH EXAMINATION. The periodic health examination: 2, 1984 update. *Canadian Medical Association Journal*, 130: 1278–1285.

COCHRANE, A. (1991). Effectiveness and efficiency: random reflections on health services. In: C. Mulrow & M. Lichtenstein (Eds.), Screening for hearing impairment in the elderly: rationale and strategy. *Journal of General Internal Medicine*, 6: 249–258.

FRANK, T., & PETERSON, D. (1987). Accuracy of a 40 dBHL Audioscope and audiometer screening for adults. *Ear and Hearing*, 8: 180–183.

FUJIKAWA, S., & CUNNINGHAM, J. (1989). Practices and attitudes related to hearing: a survey of executives. *Ear and Hearing*, 10: 357–360.

GATES, G., COOPER, J., KANNAL, W., & MILLER, N. (1990). Hearing in the elderly: the Framingham Cohort, 1983–1985. *Ear and Hearing*, 11: 247–256.

Healthy People 2010. (1999). Home page. Available at: http://www.health.gov/healthy people/. Accessed November, 1999.

Jenz, N., & Becker, M. (1984). The Health Belief Model: a decade later. *Health Education Quarterly*, 11: 1–47.

Kane, R., Ouslander, R., & Abrass, I. (1994). *Essentials of Clinical Geriatrics*, 3d ed. New York: McGraw-Hill.

Kirby, K. (1993). Impairment, disability and handicap. In: J. DeLisa & B. Gans, (Eds.), *Rehabilitation Medicine: Principles and Practice*, 2d ed. Philadelphia: Lippincott Company.

Kochkin, S. (1997). MarkeTrak IV: what is the viable market for hearing aids? *Hearing Journal*, 50: 31–39.

Lichtenstein, M., Bess, F., & Logan, S. (1988). Validation of screening tools for identifying hearing-impaired elderly in primary care. *Journal of the American Medical Association*, 259: 2875–2878.

Mader, S., & Ford, A. (1992). History and physical examination of the geriatric patient. In: E. Clakins, A. Ford, & R. Katz (Eds.), *Practice of Geriatrics*, 2d ed. Philadelphia: W. B. Saunders.

Mazzuca, S. (1982). Does patient education in chronic disease have therapeutic value? *Journal of Chronic Disease*, 35: 521–529.

McBride, W., Aguilar, C., Mulrow, C., & Tuley, M. (1990). Screening tests for hearing loss in the elderly. *Clinical Research*, 38: 707A.

Mulrow, C., & Lichtenstein, M. (1991). Screening for hearing impairment in the elderly: rationale and strategy. *Journal of General Internal Medicine*, 6: 249–258.

National Center for Health Statistics. (1993). *Health United States 1992 and Healthy People 2000 Review*. DHHS Pub. No. (PHS) 93-1232. Hyattsville, MD: U.S. Public Health Service.

Noh, S., Gagne, J.P., & Kaspar, V. (1994). Models of health behaviors and compliance: applications to audiological rehabilitation research. In: J.P. Gagne & N. Tye-Murray (Eds.), Research in audiological rehabilitation: current trends and future directions. *Journal of the American Academy of Rehabilitative Audiology, Monograph Supplement*, 27: 375–389.

Prochaska, J., DiClemente, C., & Norcross, J. (1992). In search of how people change: applications to addictive behaviors. *American Psychologist*, 47: 1102–1114.

Prochaska, J., Norcross, J., & DiClemente, C. (1984). *Changing for Good*. New York: Morrow.

Punch, J., & Weinstein, B. (1996). The Hearing Handicap Inventory: introducing a multimedia version. *Hearing Journal*, 49: 35–49.

Sackett, D., Haynes, R., & Tugwell, P. (1985). *Clinical Epidemiology: A Basic Science for Clinical Medicine*. Boston: Little Brown.

Schow, R., & Nerbonne, M. (1982). Communication Screening Profile: use with elderly clients. *Ear and Hearing*, 3: 134–147.

Schow, R., Smedley, T., & Longhurst, T. (1990). Self-assessment and impairment in adult/elderly hearing screening—recent data and new perspective. *Ear and Hearing*, 11: 17S–27S.

Siu, A., Reuben, D., & Moore A. (1994). Comprehensive geriatric assessment. In: W. Hazzard, E. Bierman, J. Blass, W. Ettinger, & J. Halter (Eds.), *Principles of Geriatric Medicine and Gerontology*, 3d ed. New York: McGraw-Hill.

U.S. Department of Health and Human Services. (1992). *Healthy People 2000: National Health Promotion and Disease Prevention Objectives*. Boston: Jones and Bartlett Publishers.

———. (1994). *The Clinician's Handbook of Preventive Services*. Alexandria: International Medical Publishing, Inc.

U.S. Preventive Services Task Force. (1989). Screening for hearing impairment. *Guide to Clinical Preventive Services*. Baltimore: Williams & Wilkins.

Ventry, I., & Weinstein, B. (1983). Identification of elderly people with hearing problems. *American Speech-Language-Hearing Association*, 25: 37–42.

Vogt, H., & Kapp, C. (1987). Patient education in primary care practice. *Postgraduate Medicine*, 81: 273–278.

Weinstein, B. (1992). Hearing screening in the elderly: what to do? *American Speech-Language-Hearing Association, Reports*, 21: 112–114.

Williams, I. (1998). Preventive and anticipatory care. In: R. Tallis, H. Fillit, & J. Brocklehurst (Eds.), *R. Brocklehurst's Textbook of Geriatric Medicine and Gerontology*, 5th ed. London: Churchill Livingstone.

Williams, T. (1992). Comprehensive geriatric assessment. In: E. Clakins, A. Ford, & R. Katz (Eds.), *Practice of Geriatrics*, 2d ed. Philadelphia: W.B. Saunders.

World Health Organization. (1980). International classification of impairments, disabilities, and handicaps. Geneva: Author.

Chapter 11

Long-Term Care Services

Long-term care's day has not yet come, but it will come very shortly because of the millions of baby boomers. The weight of the need for long-term care solutions is so heavy that it has to be faced.

—C.E. Koop, 1998

LEARNING OBJECTIVES

After reading this chapter, you should be able to:

- Understand the long-term care continuum.
- Explain how long-term care is organized.
- State characteristics of individuals eligible for long-term care.
- Deliver audiologic services in nursing facilities.
- Understand the role of audiologists in home care settings.

The purpose of this chapter is to provide audiologists with a brief perspective on the long-term care continuum in general and on audiologic services for the recipients of long-term care in particular. There are a number of institutional and community-based long-term care facilities in which audiologists are increasingly becoming involved, thus it is imperative that audiologists gain some insight into this continuum of services. Portions of the section on nursing facilities were borrowed from the American Speech-Language-Hearing Association (ASHA) guidelines which I was integrally involved in developing and disseminating (ASHA, 1997a).

Long-term care is a broad term that encompasses a wide range of populations, services, and funding sources. While there is no uniform definition, the following description encompasses the continuum of services: "a wide range of health and health-related support services provided on an informal or formal basis to people who have functional disabilities over an extended period of time with the goal of maximizing their independence" (Evashwick, 1996, p. 4). Long-term care has also been defined as an array of health and social services provided inside or outside of institutions over an extended period of time to individuals who have chronic, long-term, and complex conditions, are functionally impaired, and for the most part, elderly (Evashwick, 1993). The broad range of services may be continuous

or intermittent but are generally delivered for a sustained period of time to people who are limited in their ability to function independently. The functional disabilities may be permanent or temporary, physical or mental (Evashwick, 1993). Functional dependency is typically defined in terms of the ability to perform essential activities of daily living (ADLs) (e.g., eating, dressing, or getting out of bed) or activities necessary to remain independent, known as instrumental activities of daily living (IADLs). IADLs include shopping, cooking, housekeeping, and managing household finances.

PEARL

The essential element in defining the need for long-term care is functional capacity. Long-term care implies the dependence of an individual on the services of another person (Kane, Ouslander, & Abrass, 1994).

SPECIAL CONSIDERATION

It is important to emphasize that long-term care services can be provided by formal or informal arrangements.

While 60% of long-term care clients currently reside in nursing facilities, over 70% of adults with chronic conditions and functional disability receive long-term care services in their homes from family and friends, or in the community (Richardson, 1998; Evashwick, 1996; Kane, Ouslander, & Abrass, 1994). Hence, for the most part, services are provided through informal systems. Informal care can be provided by family members, friends, or neighbors. When circumstances require more assistance than through informal networks, individuals must opt for the formal care system. This entails a variety of health and health-related support services including home health, mental health programs, social services, institutional services in nursing homes, rehabilitation facilities

289

---

or residential settings (Richardson, 1998; Kane, Ouslander, & Abrass, 1994).

RECIPIENTS OF LONG-TERM CARE

The largest group of potential users of long-term care is individuals over the age of 75 years. However, recipients of long-term care may be of any age but, for the most part, they are frail and suffer from a multiplicity of acute and chronic conditions. Estimates of the size of the long-term care population vary. It has been projected that approximately 2.1 million older adults in the United States are long-term care clients. The need for long-term care is expected to increase dramatically as we move into the 21st century during which time the absolute number of older adults will increase dramatically as will the percentage of persons over 65 years of age who will be over 85 years of age.

The high prevalence of chronic conditions, the frailty of advanced age, coupled with acute episodes with long recovery place older adults at risk for developing functional disabilities that require long-term care services (Evashwick, 1996). Functional disabilities rather than a specific disease or condition is the primary reason for long-term care (Evashwick, 1996).

SPECIAL CONSIDERATION

Functional ability or disability is the primary indicator of need for long-term care. Ability to perform ADLs and IADLs is the primary index of functional disability.

Typically the magnitude of the functional disability depends on the individual's ability to perform ADLs and IADLs. These are listed in Table 11–1. The prevalence of functional disability, defined according to ability to perform the ADLs, increases dramatically with age. Of those 65 to 74 years, 14% are disabled, rising to 58% for individuals aged 85 and older. Functional disabilities and chronic illness (e.g., hearing impairment) are interrelated and both increase in prevalence with age (Evashwick, 1993). Chronic diseases such as arthritis, hypertension, and hearing loss tend to be accompanied by functional disabilities.

Consumers of long-term care can be divided into two types, those needing shorter term care and those requiring longer term or permanent long-term care (Evashwick, 1993). Persons requiring short-term care tend to be those with acute injury or illness or individuals who require extended time periods for convalescence. The traditional long-term care population includes individuals with ongoing and multiple health, mental health, and/or social problems who are unable to care for themselves. Individuals requiring short-term care and those requiring longer term care often require the assistance of an audiologist to determine their unique hearing health-care needs given their lifestyles. Home visits can be an essential with the long-term care population.

TABLE 11–1 Activities of Daily Living and Instrumental Activities of Daily Living

Basic activities of daily living: self-care tasks

1. Feeding
2. Dressing
3. Ambulation
4. Toileting
5. Bathing
6. Transferring
7. Continence
8. Grooming
9. Communication

Instrumental activities of daily living (IADL): activities necessary to live independently in the community

1. Writing
2. Reading
3. Cooking
4. Cleaning
5. Shopping
6. Doing laundry
7. Climbing steps
8. Using the telephone
9. Managing medication
10. Managing money
11. Ability to travel (use public transportation)

Source: Kane, Ouslander, and Abrass, 1994.

PEARL

The goal of long-term care is to enable individuals to maintain the maximum level possible of functional independence. For many, the expectation is not a cure, rather to maximize the ability to do the most for oneself given health status considerations (Evashwick, 1996).

The ideal system of long-term care has been referred to as the long-term care continuum by Evashwick (1993). A continuum of care is "a client oriented system composed of both services and integrating mechanisms that guides and tracks patients over time through a comprehensive array of health, mental health and social services spanning all levels and intensity of care" (Evashwick, 1993, p. 183). More than 80 distinct services constitute a complete continuum of care. For the sake of simplicity, Evashwick (1993) grouped the services into distinct categories that include (1) extended care, (2) ambulatory care, (3) home care, (4) outreach and linkage, (5) wellness/health promotion, and (6) housing. Table 11–2 lists the services offered under each of the categories of care. A continuum of care includes mechanisms for

TABLE 11–2 Selected Long-Term Care Services

Extended care	Outreach
Nursing facilities	Screening
Step-down units	Information and
Swing beds	referral
Nursing home follow-up	Telephone contact
	Transportation
	Meals on Wheels
	Senior membership
	programs

Ambulatory	Wellness/health promotion
Outpatient clinics	Educational programs
Physician's offices	Exercise programs
Day hospitals	Recreational and social
Adult day care centers	programs
Mental health clinics	Senior volunteers
Satellite clinics	Congregate meals
Psychosocial counseling	Support groups
Alcohol and substance abuse	

Home care	Housing
Home health—Medicare	Continuing-care retire-
Home health—private	ment communities
Hospice	Independent senior
High-technology home	housing
therapy	Congregate care
Durable medical equipment	facilities
Home visitors	Adult family homes
Home-delivered meals	Assisted-living
Homemaker and	facilities
personal care	Intermediate-care
Caregivers	facilities for
Respite care	mentally retarded
	individuals

Source: Evashwick, 1996.

organizing those services and operating them as an integrated system (Evashwick, 1993).

These categories represent the basic services older adults may need over time during periods of wellness and illness. A brief description of each follows with more lengthy discussion of the services that pertain to audiologists later on in the chapter. Extended care services are for people who are functionally disabled and therefore require nursing and support services delivered in a formal health-care institution. The majority of extended care facilities are referred to as nursing facilities (Evashwick, 1996). Acute care is hospital care for older adults with acute illnesses or injury. Ambulatory care services, which are provided for in the context of a formal health-care facility, encompass a wide variety of services including those which are preventive, maintenance,

diagnostic, and recuperative. Recipients can be healthy, may be recuperating from hospitalization, or may require ongoing monitoring for chronic conditions (Evashwick, 1996). In contrast, home care encompasses a broad array of nursing, therapeutic, and support services provided to individuals and their families in the home (Richardson, 1998). Home health programs range from formal organizations providing skilled nursing care to informal networks arranging housekeeping for friends. Outreach programs make health care services available in a variety of places including health fairs, senior centers, etc. Selected community organizations like Meals on Wheels can reach homebound individuals, as well (Evashwick, 1996). Mobile hearing vans are examples of an attempt to take audiologic services to individuals in the community rather than staying within the walls of a big institution. Wellness programs are for healthy individuals who want to maintain their health and learn how to do so. Wellness programs include health-education classes, health screenings and exercise programs (Evashwick, 1996). Finally, housing for older adults increasingly includes health and support services with the variety increasing daily.

SPECIAL CONSIDERATION

Long-term care services can be provided to people irrespective of their location or residence. That is they can be provided in either institutional or home settings and there tends to be an exchange between these two venues.

CATEGORIES OF LONG-TERM CARE
Nursing Facilities

Nursing facilities are a critical component of health care for persons needing intensive, 24-hour medical care. They are highly regulated, subject to federal Medicare and Medicaid rules, with all states using licensing and inspection systems. Each state licenses nursing facilities, having its own reimbursement policies, classification systems, and terminology (Evashwick & Langdon, 1996). The term *nursing home* is broad, referring to a wide spectrum of facilities that ranges from small, privately owned, adult residential-care homes to 1200-bed government-operated institutions (Evashwick, 1993). The National Center for Health Statistics (NCHS) defines a nursing home as "a facility with three beds or more that is either licensed as a nursing home by its state, certified as a nursing facility under Medicare or Medicaid, identified as a nursing care unit of a retirement center or determined to provide nursing or medical care." While many nursing facilities have combinations of beds that are for residents needing skilled nursing, specialty, or personal care, the common thread across facilities is that they are for people who are unable to remain home due to physical health problems, mental health problems, or functional disabilities (Evashwick & Langdon, 1996). Nursing homes may be either freestanding, units of a hospital, or components of multilevel retirement centers (Evashwick & Langdon, 1996). In general, three levels of care are provided by nursing homes: (1) basic care, (2) skilled care, or (3) sub-acute care. Many facilities offer multiple levels of care while some may offer only one level of service. Irrespective of the level of nursing care required, it is always under the direction of a physician. Nursing facilities must be certified and meet specific conditions of participation, if they are to be reimbursed by Medicare and Medicaid.

Nursing facilities must provide or arrange for the provision of the services listed in Table 11–3. According to the rules and regulations governing the long-term care facilities that are listed in the Federal Register, nursing facilities are obliged to provide or obtain from an outside resource the rehabilitative service (e.g., audiology) if they are required as part of the resident's comprehensive plan of care. Audiologic services certainly fall under the purview of specialized rehabilitative services to attain or maintain the highest practicable physical, mental, and psychosocial well-being. Audiologists working in nursing facilities must think of themselves as rehabilitation specialists as well as diagnosticians. It is important to emphasize that each state licenses long-term care facilities, and has its own licensing policies, governing regulations, reimbursement policies, terminology, and classification systems (Evashwick, 1993). Over 75% of nursing homes are owned by proprietary organizations, 5% are government owned, and the remaining 20% are owned by voluntary groups or hospitals. In 1985, nearly 50% of nursing homes were operated by a chain, for-profit organization that operates a group of facilities (Evashwick, 1993). Nursing facilities are institutions that provide skilled nursing care and related services for residents who, because of their mental or physical condition, require medical or nursing care or rehabilitation services on a regular basis through an institutional facility.

Prior to admission to a nursing home, a preadmission screen is necessary and performance on the screen is con-sidered along with the individual's medical needs to determine the case mix. For the most part, the screen is based on an individual's ability to perform the ADLs, which include bathing, dressing, toileting, transferring, bladder and bowel control, and eating. Simply put, the case mix refers to the amount of care the individual will require. Admission to nursing facilities can be of several types: short-term recovery and rehabilitation from surgery or acute illness; terminal care; or long-term residency based on physical or mental inability to function (Evashwick & Langdon, 1996). Hence, nursing home residents can be characterized broadly on the basis of their length of stay: "short," one to six months; versus "long," over six months. Short-term stayers or those eligible for short-term long-term care enter for short-term rehabilitation after an acute illness such as stroke or hip fracture, or if they are medically unstable or terminally ill. In contrast, long-term stayers (i.e., long-term long-term care) fall into one of the following categories: (1) primary cognitive impairments; (2) primary physical impairments, such as severe arthritis or end-stage heart disease; or (3) both cognitive and physical impairments (Ouslander, Osterweil, & Morley, 1991). Both categories of residents require audiologic services, however, the extent of involvement is dictated by health status, economics, and time constraints.

PEARL

The typical American nursing home is a privately owned and operated free-standing facility with the majority having between 50 and 100 beds.

About 1.8 million or 5% of America's population over 65 are receiving care in one of 19,100 nursing homes (Ouslander, 1998). Almost 90% of residents are 65 years and older while 35% are aged 85 years and older. Interestingly, despite the growth in the number of adults over 65 years, there has been only a slight increase in the number of nursing home residents and a slight decline in the occupancy rate. Residents are predominantly white (88%) and female (72%). According to the 1985 survey conducted by the NCHS, the median age of residents was 81 years. Forty-five percent of residents were over 85 years of age, 39% were between 74 and 85 years, and 16% between 65 and 74 years. Elderly white people are more likely to reside in a nursing home than elderly black individuals. It is noteworthy that in 1997 1% of persons aged 65 to 74 years lived in nursing homes, compared to 20% of persons aged 85 years and older (NCHS, 1999). The primary diagnoses of nursing home residents are circulatory disorders, mental disorders, and disorders of the nervous system. While not necessarily the primary diagnosis, a high proportion of residents have some type of mental disorder with the number of people presenting with Alzheimer's disease increasing. Specifically, about 63% of elderly nursing home residents exhibit disorientation or memory impairment with nearly half being diagnosed with some form of senile dementia (Kane, Ouslander, & Abrass, 1994).

TABLE 11–3   Services Offered by Nursing Facilities

1. Nursing and related services and specialized rehabilitative services to attain or maintain the highest practicable physical, mental, and psychosocial well-being of each resident
2. Medically related social services to attain or maintain the highest practicable physical, mental, and psychosocial well-being of each resident
3. Pharmaceutical services
4. Dietary services
5. Ongoing programs, directed by a qualified professional, of activities designed to meet the interests and the physical, mental, and psychosocial well-being of each resident
6. Routine dental services
7. Treatment and services required by mentally ill and mentally retarded individuals

> ### SPECIAL CONSIDERATION
>
> **Individuals residing in nursing homes tend to be mentally and physically frail with high levels of functional dependency.**

The majority of nursing home residents have some degree of hearing loss, with only about 20% of residents having normal hearing status. Among nursing home populations, the incidence of hearing loss is over 80% with a range from 30 to 97% (Schow & Nerbonne, 1980; Garahan, Waller, Houghton, Tisdale, & Runge, 1992). Some investigators have reported that approximately 92% of persons residing in health care facilities possess hearing impairment of sufficient degree to interfere with the communication process (Hull, 1995). The high prevalence of disabling hearing loss is primarily due to the fact that the majority of residents are over 80 years of age, and, as discussed in previous chapters, there is a direct correlation between age and hearing loss severity. Hearing loss among nursing home residents is typically moderate to moderately severe, whereas in the noninstitutionalized population the hearing loss tends to be mild to moderate. Many of the residents possess auditory processing problems that tend to be more severe than the hearing impairment would suggest. Garahan et al (1992) reported that 52% of residents they evaluated had moderate to severe hearing loss (average of 1000 to 2000 Hz). The majority of residents with moderate to severe hearing impairment perceived themselves to be handicapped. Interestingly, nurses tended to underestimate the extent of handicap relative to the resident's judgments. This is not surprising given the limited interpersonal contact nurses tend to have with residents. The latter finding suggests that the validity of nurses' judgments of hearing status is questionable, underlining the importance of audiologists or speech-language pathologists in the identification process. Interestingly, nearly half of the residents with moderate to severe hearing impairment did not have a record of documented hearing impairment.

In 1987 Congress passed the Omnibus Budget Reconciliation Act (OBRA), requiring nursing homes certified for Medicare coverage to screen all newly admitted residents for hearing loss. While OBRA does not specify the professional needed to assess hearing status of newly admitted residents, most facilities contract with audiologists in private practice or hearing instrument specialists (Bloom, 1994). OBRA (1987) is relevant to audiologists in that it requires a structured resident assessment and care plan including consideration of hearing status and communicative function. Specifically, it mandates a uniform assessment strategy for all nursing home residents and is structured to trigger consideration of selected functional health problems that will ultimately lead to care planning for the resident. The use of a uniform geriatric assessment tool has been found to increase the rate at which residents' care problems are addressed. Incorporated into the OBRA was the Nursing Home Reform Act, which is a series of amendments to the federal budget that changed the focus of long-term care from process evaluations to an emphasis on patient care outcomes, the caring process, and resident feelings (Evashwick, 1993). Hearing status correlates with functional health status and is thus an important consideration in nursing facilities.

Home Care

Home care, a cost-effective alternative to hospital or institutional care, entails a broad spectrum of health care and social services provided in the home or other residential settings (Richardson, 1998). Home health care involves at least two basic types of care delivered in a person's home: medically related services often referred to as "home health care" and services related to personal care or social needs (e.g., homemaking and chore services) (Richardson, 1998; Kane, Ouslander, & Abrass, 1994). Home health-care services consist of visits by health care professionals and include (1) nursing care, (2) physical, occupational, or speech therapy, (3) medical social services, and (4) home health-aide services. Physician services are also offered by most agencies. For medically related services, a plan of care must be prescribed by a physician and the care provided in the home must be supervised by a professional (e.g., a nurse). In contrast, personal care services, usually referred to as "home care," are semiskilled or nonskilled services that are designed to assist with the tasks of bathing, grooming, light housekeeping, meal preparation, laundry, and grocery shopping. This classification of home health services includes help with the IADLs, whereas medically related services include assistance with ADLs (Richardson, 1998). Home health services are provided by a home health aide.

According to the National Association for Home Care, there are approximately 12,000 home care agencies across the United States, including 6129 Medicare-certified home-health agencies; 1110 certified hospices; and 5258 noncertified home-health agencies, home care aide organizations, and hospices that do not participate in Medicare (Richardson, 1998). Interestingly, only recently, when Medicare included home-health services as a benefit, did the number of Medicare-certified home-health agencies rise to 6000. Medicare-certified home-health agencies must meet several conditions of participation including certain policies, training requirements, record-keeping practices, etc. (Richardson, 1998). Visiting Nurse Association (VNA) is an example of a well-known Medicare-Certified Home Health Agency (CHHA). Proprietary certified home-health agencies represent 32% of all CHHAs whereas VNAs presently represent only 10% of all proprietary CHHAs (Richardson, 1998). In 1967, 37% of CHHAs were VNAs and none were proprietary. This change is due in large part to the implementation of the Diagnostic Related Group method of hospital reimbursement that effectively broadened the home health benefit as an alternative to the cost of remaining in the hospital for a long period of time to recuperate (Richardson, 1998). Table 11–4 outlines the home care classification system established by the Health Care Financing Administration.

According to a survey conducted by Altman and Walden (1993), 2.5% of the civilian noninstitutionalized population received some type of home health service in 1987. Utilization of home care services is partially associated with age

TABLE 11–4   Agencies Providing Home Care Services

Agency type	Ownership, control, tax status
1. Hospital-based	Operated as part of a hospital, such as a department within a hospital
2. Visiting nurse association	Nonprofit organization governed by a board of directors and financed by tax-deductible contributions as well as by earnings
3. Government agencies	Sponsored by a state, county, city, or other unit of local government (e.g., a public health department)
4. Proprietary agencies	These are for profit institutions that range from single agencies owned by an individual to large chains
5. Private nonprofit	Privately developed, governed, and owned nonprofit agency

Source: National Association for Home Care, 1991. *Basic Statistics about Home Care—1991.* Washington, DC.

such that in 1987, 31% of those 85 and older received home health services as compared to 7% of persons between the ages of 65 and 74 (Richardson, 1998). For the most part, home care users differ substantially from nursing home residents. For example, just over 50% of persons receiving home care services were over 65 years in 1987 while persons under 40 years of age received almost 30% of home health visits. Further, a recent survey of home care providers conducted by the NCHS revealed that service users had a mean age of 70 years and an average of 1.7 ADL impairments (U.S. D.H.H.S., 1993). In contrast, of the 1.3+ million residents of nursing facilities, 84% were over 74 years of age with the median age being 81 years (NCHS, 1991). Functional dependence is quite high among nursing home residents and the average number of functional dependencies (i.e., requiring assistance with the ADLs) was 3.9 according to a recent report from the NCHS (Hing, 1989). In contrast, nearly 50% of persons receiving home health services were not limited in their ADLs or IADLs (Altman & Walden, 1993). Interestingly, for every person in a nursing home, two equally ill people reside at home, cared for by family and friends (Evashwick & Langdon, 1996). It is noteworthy that by 2018, the number of people receiving home care, including Medicare beneficiaries, could grow to as many as 6 to 8 million.

Health-related services provided by home health agencies differ dramatically from those offered by nursing facilities, primarily due to the case mix. Skilled home-health services include skilled nursing care; skilled therapies including speech, occupational, and physical therapy; medical social work; and nutritional counseling, with skilled nursing care accounting for the bulk of the reimbursable visits (Hughes, 1993). Oftentimes, several services are offered to one patient requiring use of a multidisciplinary team. Team members visit the patient at different times yet coordinate the paperwork required on each patient (Evashwick, 1993). In contrast to home health-care services, homemaker care tends to consist of personal care, bathing and grooming, meal preparation, shopping, transportation, household chores, etc. Eligibility for home health coverage by Medicare depends on the following: (1) client must be homebound, (2)

client must be capable of improvement, and (3) client must require short-term, intermittent nursing care, physical therapy, or speech therapy (Evashwick, 1993). All services *must* be formally prescribed by a physician.

Private home health agencies are not bound by Medicare rules although they do offer the same professional services with the addition of numerous others (Evashwick, 1996). Noncertified agencies provide 24-hour care and daily care, as well as specialty services. Of course, these agencies also offer homemaker care services including meal preparation, home repair, shopping, housekeeping, etc. Physician prescription is not required for these services. Private home-care agencies are staffed by a pool of health care professionals, home health aides, or homemakers who, for the most part, work on an as needed basis. These agencies charge hourly rates, and typically a minimum number of hours is required.

For the most part, audiologists do not work for home health agencies yet many recipients of home health care have handicapping hearing impairments. It is incumbent on audiologists to educate the registered nurses, speech-language pathologists, and home health aides (i.e., these professionals account for the majority of all staff in Medicare-certified agencies) about symptoms of hearing loss and referral criteria so that their clients are referred for the hearing health care services from which they can benefit.

I recently did some consulting work for a visiting nurse service and in that capacity was responsible for identifying individuals requiring audiologic services. My decisions were to be based on my impressions from the client's medical records. This was an impossible task as there was little evidence regarding hearing status in the charts. Hence I developed a brief checklist to be used by home health personnel to identify individuals with potentially handicapping hearing loss. Table 11–5 lists some of the questions I developed. If the answer to any of these questions is "yes," I would recommend a referral for audiologic services.

Finally, whenever feasible financially and geographically, I feel that one home visit is necessary for individuals identified as having a hearing impairment, as certain environmental modifications may be necessary to make sure

TABLE 11–5   Hearing Impairment Checklist for Individuals Eligible for Home Health Care Services

Name:		
Date of screening:		
Status: _____ Homebound: _____ Date of discharge: _____		
Hearing aid: _____ Yes _____ No		

Item	YES	NO
1. Does the patient have the television volume raised to a very loud level?	☐	☐
2. Does the patient ask you to repeat yourself when you speak?	☐	☐
3. Does the patient answer when the doorbell rings, the telephone rings, or when someone knocks on the door?	☐	☐
4. Does the patient misunderstand when spoken to by professionals or visitors?	☐	☐
5. Do family members report that the patient frequently does not hear or misunderstands what they say?	☐	☐
6. Does the patient complain of difficulty hearing/understanding?	☐	☐
7. Does the patient own a hearing aid that he or she does not wear?	☐	☐
8. Does the patient have impacted cerumen in one or both ears?	☐	☐
Recommendation and disposition:		

that the home is safe. Assistive listening devices that might be installed include an amplified telephone, a telecommunication device for the deaf (TDD), and alerting devices such as a visible smoke alarm, a vibrating or flashing alarm clock, and/or a visual display device that attaches to the door and emits a flashing light when someone knocks. If a home visit is not possible, a comprehensive assessment of the client's lifestyle, living arrangements, and listening difficulties should be completed to assist in decisions regarding installation of auxiliary assistive devices in the home.

PEARL

Homebound patients with hearing impairments and hearing aids must be reminded to wear their hearing aids at home to enable them to hear environmental and warning sounds. It is important for their safety. We, as professionals, must communicate this to the professionals working with the homebound.

Adult Day Care (ADC)

ADC is a long-term care alternative that offers older adults the option of remaining at home while taking advantage of an array of services available in a group setting. According to guidelines developed by the National Institute on Adult Daycare (NIAD), adult day care is a community-based group program designed to meet the needs of functionally impaired adults through an individual plan of care (NIAD, 1984). It is a day program of nursing care, rehabilitation services, and socialization that helps the frail elderly to stay at home as long as possible (Evashwick, 1993). According to

the NIAD, all 50 states and the District of Columbia sponsor adult day-care programs as a long-term care alternative. The majority of ADC programs are operated by nonprofit organizations. ADC participants differ from clients receiving home health services. Because of physical or mental conditions, participants cannot remain alone during the day, yet have caregivers who can take care of them when not at an ADC facility (Tedesco, 1996).

ADC has become an integral component of the continuum of health care for older adults as evidenced by the rise in the number of programs across the country. Whereas before 1975 fewer than 100 centers were in operation, as of 1989, more than 2100 centers were operating, providing services to nearly 42,000 persons per day (Evashwick, 1993). ADC centers can be freestanding or operate as part of a parent organization such as a nursing home, multipurpose senior center, or even a hospital. The majority of ADC programs are nonprofit organizations, depending in large part on philanthropy, volunteers, and in-kind contributions (Evashwick, 1993). A recent National Adult Day Care Census revealed that the average age of participants is 76 years, with 50% of participants having cognitive impairments and 33% having a diagnosis of Alzheimer's disease or a related disorder. Typical services offered through adult day-care programs may include nursing, personal care, assistance in activities of daily living, physical therapy, occupational therapy, social services, recreation, medical assessment and treatment, family counseling, and transportation (Evashwick, 1993).

The majority of participants attend ADC programs for the long term. Medicare does not pay for ADC, yet some programs do take Medicaid participants. Medicaid is the largest single payor for ADC services with the second largest source being fees paid by patients and family members (Evashwick, 1993). ADC programs are typically licensed by states that tend to require selected licensed personnel including, but not limited to, recreational, physical, and occupational therapists; registered nurses; and social workers. State licensing regulations may require a prescribed number of hours per month of a geropsychiatrist/geropsychologist, a speech pathologist, and perhaps even a physician acting in the capacity of a medical director (Tedesco, 1996). Referrals to ADC programs generally come from home health agencies, discharge planners at hospitals, primary care physicians, senior centers, community agencies, or employee assistant programs.

Once again, audiologists are not generally on the staff of ADC programs. However, it is likely that the majority of participants have some degree of hearing impairment, which in many cases may be handicapping to the individual and family members. Audiologists must educate referral sources about the importance of hearing status to the maintenance of functional abilities and independence, and arrange for program participants to take advantage of audiologic diagnostic and rehabilitative services. Offering hearing screening programs embedded in an educational context at ADC programs is an excellent way of reaching older adults who require the services of audiologists.

ADC programs generally fall into one of two categories, namely, the health-rehabilitative model (adult day health care) or the social psychological model (social day care) (Tedesco, 1996). The adult day health care serves individuals recovering from acute episodes of illness, such as stroke; persons who are suffering from physically or neurologically degenerative diseases including Parkinson's disease; or individuals suffering from chronic conditions such as diabetes or cardiovascular disease (Tedesco, 1996). These individuals tend to be recipients of intense medical, nursing, and therapeutic services. ADC programs offer speech, physical and occupational therapy, psychosocial services, and caregiver support services. In contrast, the social day care is suitable for individuals who do not need ongoing health monitoring or physical therapy, but are suffering from dementia, for example, and because of this mentally debilitating condition require therapeutic recreation, personal care, a midday meal, or caregiver support, etc.

Selected services are common to both the social and the ADC models. Therapeutic recreation is an important part of both the social and health-day care models. Group socialization and therapeutic recreation programs are designed to encourage socialization through a variety of group activities (Tedesco, 1996). The rehabilitation therapies can help in the restoration or maintenance of functional abilities. Caregiver support is integral to both models, providing respite for caregivers needing time to "catch-up," relax, and tend to their own needs; as well as support groups for caregivers. Registered nurses play a key role in the adult day health care model as they monitor health status and educate participants and their families about important lifestyle or medical decisions.

Supportive Housing Options

As people are living longer and tend to stay at home there is an increasing demand for dwelling units that provide support such as supervision or companionship. Accordingly, housing is recognized as an important part of the continuum of long-term care services for older adults (Richardson,

1998). A number of options are available including board and care homes, assisted living, and continuing care retirement communities. As of 1996, between one and two million older adults live in some form of supportive housing setting. The term *assisted-living community* is often used interchangeably with *adult living facilities, adult foster-care facilities,* or *community-based retirement facilities.* Assisted living, which provides a special combination of residential housing, personalized supportive services, and healthcare, is designed to meet the individual needs of older adults who require help with activities of daily living, but not necessarily skilled medical care. It is the fastest growing type of supportive housing (Richardson, 1998). Assisted living offers individualized personal care in a homelike setting that offers dignity, space, and privacy. Assisted-living communities can be freestanding, affiliated with a nursing home, or part of a Continuing Care Community that provides independent, assisted, and nursing care. Assisted living varies across states in terms of the target population, admission and retention practices, services and staffing requirements, sponsorship, and size (Richardson, 1998). According to Richardson (1998), the most common assisted-living options include: congregate living, board-and-care homes, or continuing care communities. Table 11–6 describes the features of the assisted-living options. It is clear that individuals residing in assisted-living environments are likely candidates for audiologic rehabilitation services.

DELIVERY OF AUDIOLOGY SERVICES IN SELECTED LONG-TERM CARE SETTINGS
Nursing Facilities

According to the 1997 ASHA Omnibus Survey, only 1.1% of certified audiologists reported working in a nursing home setting (ASHA, 1997b). Audiologists working in nursing facilities must conduct diagnostic and therapeutic services on a heterogeneous population in a nontraditional test environment. The procedures comprising the audiologic assessment and intervention must be moderated by the overall goals of nursing home care, the residents' length of stay (short stay or long stay), and the requirements of the OBRA. The focus of care at all times must be on maintaining the resident's functional independence, autonomy, quality of life, comfort, and dignity (Kane, Ouslander, & Abrass, 1994). To be eligible for Medicare and Medicaid funding, nursing homes must provide care that will help residents attain the highest practicable physical, mental, and psychosocial wellbeing. The Nursing Home Reform Act of 1987 requires a comprehensive assessment of functional status, using a standardized, comprehensive, functional assessment tool for nursing facilities (OBRA, 1987).

The comprehensive assessment tool mandated by the Nursing Home Reform Act guides individualized care planning (Lubinski & Frattali, 1993). The Resident Assessment Instrument (RAI) consists of a multidimensional assessment known as the Minimum Data Set (MDS). The RAI must be used by most nursing homes participating in Medicare and Medicaid. The RAI has two sections: the MDS and the Resident Assessment Protocols (RAPs). MDS assessment items

TABLE 11–6 Assisted-Living Options for Older Adults

Assisted-living options	Characteristics
1. Congregate living	Includes group living and supportive service arrangements, typically occurring in multiunit apartment complexes. Residents may need assistance with routine activities of daily living.
2. Board-and-care homes	Covers adult foster-care homes, sheltered care facilities, halfway houses, and adult homes. These facilities offer meals, as well as help with ADLs. Residents tend to pay for services or receive Supplemental Security Income (SSI).
3. Continuing care communities	Have three levels of living: independent, assisted, and nursing home care. These communities are costly given their entrance fees and monthly charges.

Source: Richardson, 1998.

cover dimensions ranging from cognition and physical function to mood and well-being with checklists for common geriatric diagnoses, symptoms, and syndromes. The 16 sections of the MDS require assessment of communication/hearing patterns and psychosocial well-being, among other areas of function. Depending upon responses to items on the MDS, residents are "triggered" into a RAP as potentially having a related problem, risk factor, or potential for improved function. The RAPs are designed to guide nursing facility staff in identifying and developing care plans for patient problems (Phillips, Hawes, Mor, Fries, & Morris, 1998). OBRA (1987) requires a registered nurse to coordinate the assessment with the MDS, with appropriate input from health professionals including speech-language pathologists and audiologists (Lubinski & Frattali, 1993).

While the standard/traditional protocol for audiological evaluation and management requires an acoustically treated test environment in accordance with American National Standards Institute (ANSI) guidelines governing calibration of instrumentation and the environment, alternative test environments and protocols are the rule rather than the exception when providing audiologic services in nursing homes (ASHA, 1997a). The approach to the delivery of audiologic services should be outcome oriented with the role of the audiologist at every stage being to gain an understanding of the resident's function, perceived needs, abilities, and limitations. The challenge to the audiologist is to apply standard procedures to a typically frail older adult in non-standard settings to attain a complete picture of hearing status and audiological rehabilitation needs.

The first step in the delivery of hearing health-care services to residents of nursing facilities is a hearing screen. In my view, the goal of hearing screening procedures in a nursing facility is to identify residents with impaired hearing and/or a hearing disorder in need of audiologic and/or otolaryngologic services in order to ensure their health, safety, and maximal level of functioning in that particular setting (Ammentorp, Gossett, & Euchner, 1991).

According to OBRA (1987), hearing screening and referral for hearing health care services should occur within the first two weeks following entry into the long-term care system. The referral can be made by hospital discharge plan-

ners, nurses, social workers, speech-language pathologists, audiologists, physicians, or home health-care providers. The screening results and any referrals should be documented in the patient's medical record. The initial "screening" in nursing facilities is typically through the MDS administered routinely to all residents to obtain a comprehensive approach to assessment, problem identification, and individualized care planning. Included in the MDS is Section C, "Communication/ Hearing Patterns," which contains two questions that are used to determine the functional adequacy of the resident's hearing. Item C-1 requires the examiner to rate hearing ability (with a "hearing appliance," if used) and item C-2 asks the examiner to indicate whether the resident has and/or uses a hearing aid. Preferably, an audiologist, but more typically a speech-language pathologist is responsible for completing Section C. For each RAP, the audiologist/speech-language pathologist must indicate if the plan is to proceed with a particular care plan. If so, an appropriate care plan must be completed and updated accordingly. A registered nurse must sign and certify completion of the entire assessment (Lubinski & Frattali, 1993). Table 11–7 lists the behaviors one should consider when completing items C-1 and C-2. Consideration of these behaviors will ensure at the bare minimum that ratings on the MDS and RAP reflect the point of view of the resident's functional, medical, mental, and psychosocial status.

The MDS must be completed annually, and a full reassessment is necessary when a change in resident status is noted. Quarterly reviews are mandated in 11 areas, including the ability to understand others, cognitive skills, and the ability to make oneself understood. These quarterly reviews assure that the resident status is monitored between the annual assessments. In my view, hearing status may influence the latter behaviors and it is therefore incumbent on audiologists to emphasize this during inservice training sessions.

A recent study conducted by Phillips et al (1998) wherein they sampled 254 nursing facilities in a variety of metropolitan areas across the country, revealed changes in the prevalence of key care processes over the first three years OBRA (1987) was in effect. Specifically, in 1990, prior to use of the RAI, 80% of residents reportedly had a hearing loss but did not have or use hearing aids whereas in 1993 the percentage

TABLE 11–7 Indicators for Referral for Audiologic/ Otolaryngologic Services

1. Does the resident require repetition of verbal questions, instructions, or messages?
2. Has a family member or caregiver voiced concern about the adequacy of the individual's hearing?
3. Does the resident complain of current or past history of difficulty hearing or understanding?
4. Does the resident complain of current or past history of head noise, ear pain, or ear discharge?
5. Is there any discharge visible from the ear(s)?
6. Does the resident say "what" often or misunderstand what is being said?
7. Does the resident own a hearing aid but rarely uses it?
8. Is the resident's hearing aid malfunctioning?

dropped to 70%. Similarly, residents were less likely to deteriorate functionally and cognitively during the initial period the RAI was in use. The authors concluded that comprehensive functional assessment data alerted staff to the need for selected interventions and led to improvements in selected areas of function. Audiologists must maintain their visibility in nursing facilities and do ongoing in-service training sessions to remind the staff of the importance of assessing hearing status, recognizing individuals with hearing problems, and assisting and encouraging residents in the use of amplification devices.

Individuals requiring hearing health care will ultimately undergo an audiologic assessment. The purpose of this assessment is to determine hearing status, the candidacy and need for otologic and/or audiologic rehabilitative intervention, and to identify residents with hearing loss who have been misdiagnosed as "senile" or "depressed." With regard to the latter, identifying and managing hearing loss can often reverse the diagnosis or lessen the severity of a confusional state.

PEARL

Keep in mind that many residents are not eligible for audiologic services because of their medical or cognitive status, but they can certainly benefit from use of devices to improve communications with medical staff, other residents, and family members.

Typically, decisions about the severity and nature of hearing loss can be reached using routine behavioral audiometry and immittance tests. If additional diagnostic evaluations are indicated (e.g., auditory brainstem response testing) the residents should be referred to an off-site agency. The components of the audiologic assessment should take into account the patient's functional status, cognitive ability, physical status, and lifestyle. The ideal diagnostic audiology protocol might include:

1. An otoscopic or videoscopic examination of the external ear canal and tympanic membrane prior to the pure-tone evaluation. The audiologist should make sure to study the features of the outer ear given the susceptibility of residents to collapsed canals, impacted cerumen, and tumorous growth. In my view, cerumen management should not be attempted in nursing homes given the frail status and complexity of medical conditions characterizing most residents.

2. Air-conduction (AC) testing should be conducted at 250, 500, 1000, 2000, 3000, 4000, and 6000 Hz. Insert earphones are recommended when a sound-treated booth is not available. In a non–sound-treated environment, the clinician may wish to omit 250 and 500 Hz if acoustic immittance testing is accomplished. The purpose of AC testing is to determine hearing loss type and severity, to identify residents with dementia who have underlying hearing loss that may exacerbate the cognitive problems, and to identify candidates for intervention. It is important to emphasize that the diagnosis of senile dementia may be confounded by the presence of hearing loss and that ruling hearing loss in or out is critical for these individuals.

3. Bone conduction testing (BC) should be conducted at 250 to 4000 Hz. In the event that an unexplained high-frequency air/bone gap presents, the audiologist should check carefully for collapsed canals.

4. Speech recognition or detection thresholds should be established to determine a recognition level for speech information and to determine reliability of test results. Test reliability may be jeopardized in residents with cognitive problems. Oftentimes, a speech detection threshold is the only measure of speech recognition that can be obtained because of compromised cognitive status.

5. Suprathreshold word-recognition testing should be conducted when feasible using face valid materials such as sentence materials or simple questions presented in quiet and/or noise. Functionally relevant test materials should be used to assess the adequacy of the resident's functional-communication capacity as the primary purpose of word-recognition testing for residents of nursing facilities is to insure that hearing/understanding is adequate for communication with other residents, caregivers, and staff members. A secondary goal is to identify those persons in need of assistive technology, including hearing aids. The final purpose of speech-recognition testing is to uncover any peripheral or central auditory processing difficulties. Tests of central auditory processing are not appropriate for this population although speech-in-noise testing may be helpful for hearing aid candidates.

6. Assessment of uncomfortable listening levels if the individual is considered a hearing-aid candidate.

7. Immittance testing when air/bone gaps are present or valid bone-conduction thresholds could not be established.

8. A reliable and valid scale that assesses functional communication status. The scale should have been standardized on institutionalized individuals. A simple questionnaire regarding communicative abilities could be completed by a formal or informal caregiver when the resident is too confused to respond.

9. The audiologist should monitor hearing status annually to determine whether any significant change has taken place, or more frequently when symptoms arise.

10. The audiologist should document audiometric findings in the resident's chart.

Referral and Intervention Options

Following the audiologic assessment, the audiologist has one of two referral options (ASHA, 1997a). The first is a medical referral. If otoscopic examination and/or audiometric tests are indicative of a possible medical condition requiring treatment, immediate referral to an otolaryngologist is indicated. If medical clearance is necessary for a potential hearing-aid fitting, referral to the physician should take place prior to the hearing-aid evaluation session. The second option is referral for audiologic rehabilitation if audiometric findings, and cognitive, physical, and psychosocial conditions suggest that the resident can use and benefit from a hearing aid or assistive device. The decision regarding candidacy for rehabilitation should take into account the audiologist's data, input from the nursing and rehabilitative staff, input from the resident, and input from family members. Audiologic rehabilitation with hearing aids should be restorative and maintenance oriented, using a holistic approach that takes into account physical, sociological, psychological, cognitive, and communicative capabilities. Restoration as applied in long-term care settings implies assisting residents to do as much as they can, as well as they can, for as long as they can (Hegner & Caldwell, 1994). Maintenance is aimed at preventing further fuctional loss and limitation and assisting the resident in achieving as high a level of wellness and independence as possible (Hegner & Caldwell, 1994). Properly fit hearing aids or assistive-listening devices can achieve these latter goals.

Hearing-Aid Assessment and Fitting

As discussed in Chapter 9, hearing aids can have a positive effect on an older adult's physical health, psychological well-being, and cognitive status (Mulrow, Tuley, & Aguilar, 1991; NCOA, 1999). A successful fit will depend on consideration of the audiologic and nonaudiologic factors shown in Table 11–8. With regard to physical factors, older adults who are very frail and who are not ambulatory may not be ideal hearing-aid candidates. Further, older adults with central auditory processing deficits (e.g., difficulty understanding speech in noise) may be candidates for assistive-listening devices given their beneficial effects in overcoming the effects of unfavorable signal-to-noise ratios. Wax buildup is a problem, especially for residents fit with hearing aids. Audiologists must be alert to residents with this problem and establish a system for monitoring hearing-aid users with problems in this area.

TABLE 11–8 Audiologic and Nonaudiologic Factors to be Considered when Fitting Hearing Aids to Residents of Long-Term Care Facilities

Physical
General health
Audiometric status—Peripheral, central
Visual status
Manual dexterity
Functional health status
Cerumen

Psychological
Mental status
Motivational level
Affect
Expectations
Level of independence
Availability of formal or informal caregivers

Socio-economic variables
Lifestyle
Financial factors
Cosmetics
Physical/social environment
Caregiver availability

SPECIAL CONSIDERATION

Hearing-aid malfunction due to cerumen is a major problem in nursing homes. Wax guards are especially important for this population.

With regard to psychological factors, I typically administer the Mini-Mental Status Examination (MMSE) or the Short Portable Mental Status Questionnaire (SPMSQ) during the hearing-aid assessment (with and without amplification) to gain a feel for the client's cognitive status. Of course, information from the resident's chart regarding mental status also figures into my decision regarding intervention options. The MMSE provides brief questions and tasks that sample orientation, immediate and delayed word recall, attention and calculation, naming, repetition, responses to verbal and written commands, writing, and visuoconstructional abilities (Folstein, Folstein, & McHugh, 1975). By administering the MMSE with and without amplification (hardwired system), the audiologist can quickly gain insight into whether amplification impacts on the resident's orientation and mental status. I have worked with a number of residents with undiagnosed severe hearing loss for whom the quality of their responses to the items on the MMSE differed dramatically once my voice was made audible. Many of these residents may not be candidates for hearing aids, but certainly should be using a hardwired assistive-listening device when communicating with staff, family members, or other residents. Motivational level is an important consideration when fitting hearing aids, but the audiologist must make sure to distinguish between poor motivation and a depressed affect. Interestingly, use of amplification can improve the affect and hence residents often become motivated to hear again. Assistive devices rather than hearing aids may be the route to go.

Finally, with regard to socio-economic factors, willingness on the part of the nursing staff or a family member to assist the resident with every aspect of hearing-aid use is a critical consideration. The nursing staff should be responsible for working with the audiologist to develop a system to minimize the number of lost hearing aids and should establish a schedule for putting the hearing aid on in the morning and retrieving it in the evening. Financial arrangements for the purchase of hearing aids vary from state to state, and facility to facility. The private-pay residents tend to pay for the device out-of-pocket. However, Medicaid residents do not have funds to purchase hearing aids. Selected states do have Medicaid programs that pay for hearing aids so the audiologist must make the appropriate inquiries. Once the decision is made regarding amplification options, the next step is to select an appropriate device.

The appropriate electroacoustic characteristics of the hearing aid should be determined at the time of the prefitting using standard procedures (e.g., audiometric data; real ear measures, when available; and loudness judgments). Care should be taken to recommend an earmold or hearing aid that can be easily maintained, inserted, and removed by the resident or staff members. While completely-in-the-canal (CIC) hearing aids may be acoustically appropriate and do not require the manipulation of a volume control, for individuals with decreased visual acuity or limited manual dexterity, they may be difficult to manipulate, insert, and remove. Battery placement will be virtually impossible for the majority of residents given the size of the batteries. In addition, the small size of CICs and canal hearing aids make them a higher risk for damage or loss. Older adults with reduced tactile sensation in the ear canal may not even feel when the hearing aid mistakenly falls out of the ear. High performance hearing aids are not necessary for the listening needs of most residents of nursing facilities. Zinc air batteries are less toxic than mercury batteries and have a longer battery and shelf life, and thus should be routinely recommended. Extended warranties and/or supplemental insurance for loss and damage should be considered.

PEARL

A successful hearing-aid fitting depends in large part on the resident's level of dependency and the availability of a caregiver to assist the resident in inserting and adjusting to the hearing aid.

The caregiver should be included in the rehabilitation process, and should be encouraged to attend the hearing aid orientation sessions to insure that the he/she understands how hearing aids operate, and their advantages and disadvantages. It is especially important to emphasize the limitations of hearing-aid use and to instill realistic expectations. Suggestions for how best to communicate with the hearing-impaired resident, such as those contained in Table 11–9 should be emphasized.

At the time of the hearing-aid fitting, it is important for the audiologist to verify the hearing-aid response. The approaches described in Chapter 9, including real ear measures of insertion gain and output and speech recognition testing are acceptable procedures. Informal conversations between the resident and a staff member or between residents are a powerful way to verify the adequacy of the hearing-aid fit. New hearing-aid users should be scheduled for a postfitting session, within one week of the fitting. The goal is to determine if in fact the resident is deriving communicative, psychosocial, and functional benefit from the hearing aid(s). When the perceived benefit is at odds with real-ear data, the audiologist must make a decision as to the adequacy of the response, paying attention to the input from the resident and caregiver as well as the real-ear data. The resident should be seen on a weekly basis for approximately one month before a determination is made as to the value of the hearing aid(s) for the resident. At each session, the fit

TABLE 11–9 Tips for Communicating with Hearing-Impaired Residents to Be Explained to the Resident and Caregiver

- Get the resident's attention by gently touching the shoulder or raising a finger.
- Face the resident. Do not walk away while talking, do not talk from outside the resident's room.
- Eliminate distractions: no food, cigars, or cigarettes when speaking.
- Rephrase what you have said if repetitions do not clarify.
- Speak using a slightly slower rate and pause between lengthy sentences.
- Supplement communication with gestures, reading, and writing modalities.
- Use a hardwired amplification system when speaking to residents who do not use hearing aids.
- Enunciate difficult words.
- Pay attention to the resident for puzzled looks that may suggest that there was a communication breakdown.
- Speak slightly louder than normal.
- Make sure the hearing aid is turned on and that batteries are working.
- Slow down but do not exaggerate when you speak.
- *Speak* to the hearing impaired, do not *shout*—this distorts the sound and look of speech.
- *Do not* underestimate the resident's intelligence.
- Keep your hands away from your face when talking.
- Recognize that hard-of-hearing people recognize less when they are tired or ill, so be patient and understanding.

should be verified, and the resident should be counseled about the operation and use of the hearing aid, and how best to communicate with others. In short, these ongoing hearing-aid orientation sessions are important to optimize the benefits of hearing-aid use. As discussed earlier, staff, a caregiver or a family member should participate in the orientation and counseling sessions when feasible to ensure carryover of information into daily life. It is critical that the orientation sessions be client-centered with particular attention being paid to the resident's communication needs within the given facility or listening environment. Hearing-aid users should be given a set of large-print instructions describing hearing-aid care, maintenance, use, insertion, removal, and operation. Some helpful hints for adjusting to hearing aids and communicating with others should be distributed and posted in the resident's room (Table 11–10). The latter should be reviewed with the resident and caregiver at each session.

Safety and infection-control procedures should be in effect before, during, and after the hearing-aid fitting. Audiologists are encouraged to wear latex gloves when handling hearing aids and earmolds. However, their use should be discouraged when taking silicone earmold impressions. Finally, the audiologist should maintain a list of residents obtaining hearing aids. The list should include the resident's name, hearing-aid model, serial number, battery type, ear(s) fit, and date of fitting. The hearing aid(s) should be imprinted with the resident's name in the event of loss.

SPECIAL CONSIDERATION

Hearing-aid loss and damage are a major problem in nursing homes but can be obviated by vigilance.

TABLE 11–10 Helpful Hints for Adjusting to Hearing Aids

- Be patient and allow time to adjust to hearing aids. Hearing aids do require time for adaptation and to attain maximum performance potential.
- Take advantage of services offered by the audiologist.
- Do not get discouraged if the hearing aid does not restore hearing to normal. Return to the audiologist for reassurance and counseling regarding realistic expectations. Understand that hearing aids *will not* restore hearing capabilities to normal.
- Gradually adjust to loud, incoming signals by first using the hearing aid in quiet and in small groups, later moving to larger, less favorable listening situations.
- Understand the audiogram in terms of the particular speech sounds and words that may be problematic and in terms of the effect of noise on speech understanding. This will help make sense of some of the misunderstandings.
- Understand that hearing aids will not filter out all background noise and certain listening environments will continue to present a significant listening challenge.
- Tell people you have a hearing loss and ask for repetition if the speech of others is unclear.

The majority of residents of nursing facilities do not use hearing aids and are not candidates for hearing aids. Interestingly, only 5 to 10% of residents at any one time use hearing aids. A number of nonaudiologic factors account for the latter statistic. Nonaudiologic factors include lifestyle variables, financial considerations, manual dexterity, listening needs, and cognitive status. Cognitive impairment associated with dementia or depression may render residents dysfunctional and unable to use hearing aids. Further, older residents who are withdrawn, isolated, and rarely interact with others may be adverse to hearing-aid use. Finally, the structure and staffing of nursing facilities is an additional reason for limited utilization of hearing aids in nursing facilities. Residents tend to be reliant on nurses and aides for insertion, removal, and maintenance of hearing aids. If these professionals are not available or are unwilling to assist residents, hearing aids cannot be utilized. Among the audiologic factors that account for the lack of hearing-aid use in nursing facilities is the probable high incidence of central auditory processing disorders (CAPD) in this population coupled with the fact that individuals with CAPD tend to derive minimal benefit from hearing aids. That is to say, there is an important place for assistive listening devices

PEARL

Personal amplifiers are less costly than hearing aids and may provide sufficient auditory benefit for individuals with limited financial resources or who don't warrant full-time hearing-aid usage.

or "rehabilitation technology" in nursing facilities. Sound-enhancement devices available as hardwire, wireless, FM, or audio-induction systems are ideal for one-on-one (e.g., when talking to nursing staff), large or small group situations (e.g., recreational therapy), and television or radio listening. In particular, hardwire systems can facilitate resident-to-resident, resident-to-staff, or informal caregiver-to-resident interactions. These inexpensive systems are, durable, easy-to-use, and make communication exchanges easier and more meaningful. An additional advantage of hardwire systems is that they represent a visible symbol of hearing loss signaling to other residents and staff that it is necessary to modify communication techniques to ensure understanding. This will minimize misunderstandings and the tendency for people who have significant hearing loss to be ignored.

Wireless devices are ideal for residents who enjoy television viewing. If the lounge area within the nursing facility is equipped with a television, the facility should make sure to include a transmitter along with several receivers to enable residents to enjoy television viewing. Infrared systems have been installed successfully in large listening areas such as auditoriums, activity rooms, and places for religious observance, enabling large numbers of residents to follow the speaker free of noise and free of the disadvantage posed by distance.

A variety of telecommunication technologies that enhance speech understanding over the telephone are ideal for use in nursing facilities, as well. In-line amplifiers installed in each resident's telephone is often the way to go given the high prevalence of hearing impairment in nursing facilities. Staff members in regular contact with residents, family members, or potential residents should also have in-line amplifiers installed in their telephones. All telephones should be compatible with hearing aids. All coin-operated telephones should be hearing-aid compatible and contain in-line amplifiers. At least one coin-operated telephone should incorporate a text telephone. Access to text telephones is especially important for residents who do not have sufficient hearing to use a regular telephone with an amplifier or have a speech impairment that precludes use of standard telephones. Availability of telecommunication technology is critical to the quality of life of residents of nursing facilities as it facilitates contact with loved ones. Finally, alerting devices should be used throughout the nursing facility, especially in large areas where residents congregate. Telephone alerting devices and smoke detectors with strobe lights or vibrotactile stimulation should be in rooms with persons with hearing impairment. Convenient sources for assistive-listening devices are listed in Table 11–11.

Individuals with hearing loss, nursing facility staff, family members, and administrators should be informed of the availability and advantages of rehabilitation technology. The fact that these devices can be used to bring facilities into compliance with the Americans with Disabilities Act of 1990 helping to create a barrier-free environment for the hearing impaired should be emphasized.

SPECIAL CONSIDERATION

Audiologists should consult with the nursing facility administration to ensure that it is in compliance with the Americans with Disabilities Act. It is our professional responsibility to insure this law is implemented so that residents who are hard-of-hearing and deaf have equal access to services in nursing facilities.

TABLE 11–11   Sources for Assistive Technology

Hal-Hen Co.
14-33 24th Street
Long Island City, NY 11577
800-242-5436

HARC Mercantile Ltd.
P.O. Box 3055
Kalamazoo, MI 49003-3055
800-445-9968

National Hearing Aid Distributors, Inc.
145 Tremont Street
Boston, MA 02111
800-627-9930

Williams Sound Corp.
10399 West 70th Street
Eden Prairie, MN 55344-3459
800-843-3544

Hearing-Aid Maintenance Program

The hearing-aid maintenance program is a system in place for insuring that hearing aids given to residents are used on a regular basis, are maintained, and are secured when not on the resident's ear(s). This is especially important because of the high rate of hearing-aid loss and damage in nursing facilities. The hearing-aid maintenance program for each nursing home resident with hearing loss should be included in the comprehensive care plan (CCP). As part of the plan, the extent of assistance from nursing staff/caregivers should be specified (See Table 11–12). Reporting the extent of assistance is critical so that staff are made aware of their ongoing responsibilities vis à vis the hearing aid. A hearing-aid fitting can only be successful if the nursing staff is made aware of and is willing to accept responsibility for the units (ASHA, 1997a).

A list that includes the (1) resident's name and room number, (2) hearing-aid model and serial number, (3) battery type, (4) ear(s) fit, and (5) need for notification in the event of emergency should be posted at the nursing station to provide a quick and easy reference. When a resident receives a hearing aid, they should automatically be placed on a maintenance program. This program includes periodic checks conducted by the audiologist, a nurse's aide, or a volunteer to ensure that the aid remains clean and in good working order, is worn on a regular basis, has a working battery, and is turned on when worn by the patient. Typically, residents will either not have the hearing aid on or will not have it turned on.

Documentation is especially important in nursing facilities. All contacts with the resident, information about the dispensed product, canceled appointments, and rescheduled appointments should be noted in the chart. Instructions for the staff should be specified as well. An effort should be made to incorporate an index of the quality of service provided to the resident. For example, document if the

---

TABLE 11–12   Ratings of Degree of Assistance Required by Nursing-Home Residents

1. INDEPENDENT
Resident is responsible for insertion, removal, daily care, and maintenance of hearing aid. Resident can manipulate hearing-aid controls, insert, remove, and change battery. Resident is responsible for reporting any problems with the hearing aid or loss of hearing aid to the audiologist.

2. PARTIAL ASSISTANCE
Resident is responsible for daily care and maintenance of hearing aid. Resident needs assistance with batteries. Nursing staff is responsible for reporting any problems with or loss of hearing aid.

3. FULL ASSISTANCE
Hearing aid is stored by the nursing staff. Nursing staff is responsible for insertion, removal, daily care, and maintenance of hearing aid, routine battery checks, and changing batteries. Nursing staff is responsible for reporting damage/loss of hearing aid to audiologist.

Source: Modified from American Speech-Language-Hearing Association, 1997a.

resident uses an assistive-listening device on a regular basis when communicating with family members. Similarly, include as a chart entry whether the resident is able to use the hearing aid independently and seems to be more coherent and communicative (ASHA, 1997a).

PEARL

Documenting the value of audiologic services is important as it demonstrates to the facility the importance of contracting with an audiologist for hearing health-care services.

Caregiver Education

The audiologist should provide regular and periodic inservices for the entire nursing-home staff to provide carryover about hearing-aid use into the daily lives of the residents (Hull, 1995). In-service programs should be scheduled periodically and regularly to ensure that all staff members (e.g., aides, recreational therapists, and social workers) have the opportunity to attend. Most of the hands-on care in nursing homes is provided by nurse's aides who are typically poorly educated, poorly paid, and speak a limited amount of English. Nursing homes employ very few registered and licensed nurses (Ouslander, 1998). Hence aides are the primary targets of our in-service efforts. Recall, that shifts for aides and nurses can be 12 hours or 8 hours, requiring the need for in-service programs to be scheduled during the day and in the evening. Further, turnover in nursing facilities is quite high, underlining the importance of regularly scheduled sessions. Audiologists are encouraged to take advantage of technology such as videotape playback units and computers as these devices can be used to demonstrate important points and to reinforce them as well. Software packages such as the multimedia version of the Hearing Handicap Inventory for the Elderly or commercially available videotapes can be invaluable. Similarly, talking about par-

---

PEARL

I have videotaped residents actually inserting, operating, and removing their hearing aids and have found this helpful. When staff members see residents struggling with hearing aids they tend to remember the problems encountered as well as the solutions.

---

ticular residents often helps the hospital staff to remember important points about hearing-aid use and operation and a particular resident's experience with amplification. Hands-on experience with hearing aids and interactivity is important as well. The sessions should be practical and relevant to the attendees. Finally, I find that applying the Health Belief Model when outlining the content of the inservice session is important. Thus, it is important to emphasize the following:

1. Residents of nursing facilities are particularly susceptible to hearing loss because of their age (e.g., briefly discuss etiologies of hearing loss experienced by older adults).
2. Hearing impairment experienced by older adults has been documented to be handicapping in terms of the ability to communicate with family, caregivers, and other residents.
3. Unremediated hearing impairment can have significant psychosocial consequences including depression, confusion, isolation.
4. Amplification devices including hearing aids and assistive-listening devices can reverse the negative consequences of hearing impairment.
5. Amplification devices can make it easier for staff members when communicating with the hearing impaired.
6. The role of amplification in the diagnosis of cognitive status and during a routine intake. Social workers, physicians, nurses, etc. should be encouraged to use hardwired systems when communicating with residents. This will certainly promote easier communication.

In addition to the preceding list, the following issues about hearing aids should be discussed:

1. styles, parts, and functions of hearing aids,
2. batteries (storage, dangers of battery ingestion, types, and insertion),
3. hearing-aid maintenance and troubleshooting procedures (Table 11–13),
4. feedback: causes and prevention,
5. realistic expectations about hearing aids,
6. methods to facilitate communication, and
7. procedures to report lost hearing aids.

At the beginning or end of each in-service session it is important to emphasize that staff members are key to realizing the functional communication potential of hearing-impaired residents and that hearing aids and assistive

---

TABLE 11–13 Hearing-Aid Maintenance Tips

- Hearing aid should be kept dry preferably in a hearing-aid dehumidifier at night.
- Hearing aid should not be worn in the shower, when applying hair spray, or when sleeping.
- Battery should be removed when hearing aid is taken out of resident's ear and checked before reinserting.
- Hearing aid should be stored in a safe place and in the same place each night, preferably in a drawer.
- Prior to inserting hearing aid, check opening for wax build-up. If present, clean opening with a wax pick and arrange to have resident's ear checked for impacted cerumen.
- The earmold from behind-the-ear hearing aids should be disconnected from the hearing aid, washed, and dried thoroughly on a regular basis using a blower supplied by the audiologist.

devices are designed to enable residents to (1) maintain hearing abilities; (2) effectively communicate their needs and requests, and (3) participate in social communication. If the latter is accomplished, the quality of life for nursing-home residents will be enhanced indirectly impacting positively on the morale and functioning of nursing facilities.

PEARL

Periodic in-service sessions are key to the success of any hearing health-care program in place in nursing facilities. Cooperative and informed staff members make the difference for hearing-impaired residents.

Garahan et al (1992) recommend designating one nurse at each nursing facility as the "hearing health-care specialist." Responsibilities would include insuring that residents needing hearing assessment are scheduled and evaluated. Other responsibilities might include otoscopics/cerumen management, hearing-aid management and maintenance, staff training, and distribution of assistive listening devices. I concur with Garahan et al (1992) that training a single nurse would most likely result in an increase in hearing-aid/assistive-listening device utilization and promote communication among residents and staff.

In sum, in my view hearing health care is critical to the quality of life of residents of nursing facilities. To accomplish this, the audiologist should be involved in the assessment of the resident's continuing care and contribute to a written plan for meeting communicative needs. Audiologists should work closely with speech-language pathologists as oftentimes the speech-language pathologist will be responsible for following up on residents in the absence of the audiologist. Finally, aides, nurses, and therapists should be considered important partners as well. These professionals help to ensure carryover of information and inclusion of recommendations into the daily lives and routines of the residents.

DELIVERY OF AUDIOLOGIC SERVICES FOR OLDER ADULTS ELIGIBLE FOR HOME HEALTH CARE

Demand for home care has increased dramatically over the past several years especially among Medicare enrollees 85 years and older. Therapeutic services provided by home health agencies typically involve skilled therapies including physical, occupational, or speech (Hughes, 1996). Audiologic services for homebound individuals are only covered to the extent that Medicare covers diagnostic services. Hence, audiologists typically do not usually do home visits but do have a role to play in home care (0.4% of respondents to the ASHA 1997 Omnibus Survey reported home health care as a primary setting) especially when one considers that registered nurses and home health-aides account for approximately 65% of all staff in Medicare-certified home health agencies (Hughes, 1996). In my view, three typical scenarios for hearing-impaired homebound individuals include (1) homebound clients who may have been evaluated and received an amplification device prior to discharge and thus require assistance with the hearing aid, orientation, and follow-up services; (2) homebound clients who are functionally impaired for a short-term basis and may be identified through a brief screening as requiring the services of the audiologist once eligible to safely leave the home; or (3) persons who are functionally impaired on a permanent basis and could benefit from assistive technology in the home to insure that the environment is safe and that health professionals can be understood by the patients. Hence, in my opinion the audiologist is peripherally involved in the delivery of services to homebound individuals. Their role is primarily ongoing education of physicians, discharge planners, nurses, home health aides, and home care professionals (especially speech-language pathologists) employed in acute care facilities regarding case finding, strategies for communicating with the hearing impaired, and tips on hearing-aid use and assistive technologies.

Case finding or the identification of individuals who need referral is made possible by hospital discharge planners, intake nurses, physicians, and other home care providers (ASHA, 1990). Audiologists working in agencies making referrals for home care should educate the staff regarding appropriate strategies for identifying individuals who may require audiologic services. The Welch Allyn Audioscope, which emits a 40 dB tone at 500, 1000, 2000, and 4000 Hz, is ideal for bedside screening for hearing impairment and can be used to identify persons with impacted cerumen who may require a referral for cerumen management. Staff should receive the training necessary to correctly screen and perform visual inspections with this simple device. Also, a brief hearing screening questionnaire, completed by the staff, can help to easily identify patients with hearing impairments. The checklist might include questions such as:

- Does the individual have the volume of the television set high?
- Does the individual ask for frequent repititions or say "what" often?
- Does the individual hear the door bell or telephone ring?
- Does the individual give incorrect answers to questions?
- Does the individual smile a lot during conversation, but fails to participate in discussions?

If the answer to any of the above questions is "yes", a referral for audiological evaluation should be considered. This checklist can be completed by a speech-language pathologist or a home health aide for homebound individuals, and placed in the patient's chart to assist in a determination of need for referral to an audiologist. The format adopted for this checklist does not require a face-to-face interview, it is based on observation of the patient over time as it is assumed that the individual completing the checklist has spent time with the patient. I do not recommend a self-assessment questionnaire as homebound individuals are more than likely focused on illnesses that may be more threatening to their lives and lifestyles than hearing impairment and thus valid responses may not be possible. I would like to emphasize that I consider that the purpose of the hearing screening should be to identify homebound individuals at risk for hearing impairment, which can interfere with safety at home and communication with formal or informal caregivers.

When a homebound older adult has recently received a hearing aid the audiologist should place in the chart maintained by the home health agency specifics about troubleshooting hearing aids, a checklist about hearing-aid care and operation, and a list of strategies to be used by the health care professional when communicating with the hearing impaired. Table 11–14 contains an example of such a list that should be included in the chart. Of course, any of the lists included in this chapter can be modified for inclusion in the chart. Finally, I urge audiologists to target marketing and educational efforts at home health agencies as they can be an important referral source. Older adults who ultimately recover and no longer need skilled home health and homemaker services are good candidates of hearing health care services.

An important aspect of home care is documentation. Record keeping must be in keeping with all agency, regulatory, and reimbursement requirements (ASHA, 1994). All entries should be legible (no corrections), accurate, and comprehensive (ASHA, 1994). All telephone contacts with the patient, family, and other members of the multidisciplinary team should be documented. Make sure to retain copies of all correspondence with or about the patient being treated (ASHA, 1994). It is important to document each visit as well as canceled or rescheduled appointments. For new hearing-aid users it is helpful to keep records of the hearing aid dispensed (e.g., serial numbers of each hearing aid), and to document limitations of the treatment process. The patient should be given all warranties pertaining to the hearing aids as well as options for insuring the units.

TABLE 11–14 Tips for Communicating with Homebound Residents to be Included in Chart

- Make sure room in which conversation takes place is well lit and noise from computers, radiators, and air conditioning is avoided.
- Face the listener directly at eye level especially for wheelchair-bound patients.
- Sit within 3 to 6 feet of the patient.
- Make sure to keep face well lit and free from shadows.
- Cue the individual when you are ready to speak.
- Speak at a moderate pace.
- Make sure to remain in the same room when speaking to the homebound individual.
- Do not cover face when speaking.
- Do not drop voice at end of sentence.
- Make sure patient is wearing hearing aid and hearing aid is turned on.
- Use an assistive listening device (e.g., hardwired system) when available.*
- Raise voice slightly when speaking.

*Hardwire devices such as the binaural amplified listener, the listenaider, the Willian Sound pocket-talker, and the sound wizard should be used when communicating with the hearing impaired. These devices are invaluable for one-to-one communication.

SPECIAL CONSIDERATION

It is important to emphasize that documentation is critical from a professional liability and risk-management perspective.

In sum, home health care is a very nontraditional setting for audiologists given the fact that Medicare does not reimburse for audiologic diagnostic or treatment services delivered to homebound individuals. However, hospitalized patients referred for home care services have a high probability of having a hearing impairment that may interfere with the delivery of services in general, and with recovery of functional health in particular. Audiologists should

SPECIAL CONSIDERATION

Audiologists should work to educate home care agencies about the importance of identifying older adults at risk for hearing impairment and about the role hearing aids and assistive-listening devices can play in the recovery process.

strive to contract with home health agencies to, at the very least, educate staff members about how best to interact with the hearing-impaired, how to identify a hearing-impaired older adult, and how to maintain hearing aids/assistive listening devices used by recipients of home care benefits. The ability to communicate should be considered an important outcome for home care beneficiaries.

SPECIAL CONSIDERATION

Home care is an integral part of the continuum of care for older adults and is likely to continue to grow in the future. At present, audiology is not a qualifying rehabilitation service under the Medicare home health benefit.

CONTROVERSIAL POINT

While home health services are required benefits under the federal Medicaid plan, audiology services are considered optional under the home health benefit. Audiologists should strive to have audiologic services considered a skilled nursing service reimbursed by Medicare and Medicaid.

CASE MANAGEMENT

Case management is a primary feature of service delivery in long-term care in general and home care in particular

(ASHA, 1990). According to Kane (1998) case management is the coordination of groups of resources and services for a specified population of individuals, in this case recipients of long-term care. The National Chronic Care Consortium (1993) defines case management as the "coordination of complex or continuous care for individuals who are vulnerable, are at risk, and have more complex problems than most individuals." Case managers, who may be any designated health professional including a physician, nurse, or social worker, link the homebound individual to the services needed at home. They are considered gatekeepers, patient advocates, and service coordinators (Glickstein, 1998). Managed care is different from case management as the former is a "system whereby an agency contracts with a provider group to deliver specific services for a set cost per enrollee" (White & Gundrum, 1996, p. 163). Managed care agencies do in fact employ case managers to manage the care of enrollees. In short, case management entails the coordination of care across areas and between agencies (White & Gundrum, 1996). Case management programs are important to audiologists in light of the components of case management. The core components of case management include case finding, multidimensional assessment, care planning, care implementation or service coordination, follow-up, and reassessment (Glickstein, 1998; White & Gundrum, 1996). Case managers carry out the case-management function and thus should be familiar with the scope of practice of audiologists so that appropriate referrals can be made. The field of expertise of case managers differs according to setting and thus audiologists must educate all health care professionals involved in case management.

The trend in health care today is to incorporate case management into all settings where health care is delivered and for the case manager to differ according to setting. In the primary care setting physicians tend to be the case managers or in a geriatric clinic for example, physicians may lead a team comprised of nurses, a social worker, and a rehabilitation therapist (White & Gundrum, 1996). Nurses assigned to specific units (e.g., oncology) tend to be case managers in acute care settings. They are typically charged with following the patient through other settings to insure continuity of care (White & Gundrum, 1996). Social workers may be the case manager in a long-term care setting, and, increasingly, home care agencies are partnering with managed-care home-care programs that use case-management teams comprising a physician, the home-health case manager, and the payer (White & Gundrum, 1996). The following organizations and agencies have been established for insuring that case management remains a viable approach to service delivery: Individual Case Management Association (ICMA) in Little Rock, Arkansas; Case Management Society of America (CMSA) in Washington, DC, and the National Association of Professional Geriatric Care Managers (GCM) in Tucson, Arizona. The latter group consists of master's-level clinicians dedicated to promoting the independence, autonomy, and quality of care delivered to frail elderly individuals. Audiologists should be counted among the ranks of social workers, nurses, and psychologists who have joined GCM (White & Gundrum, 1996). As case management is a mechanism for linking the patient to the entire continuum of care, audiologists must become more visible to case-management programs in general and to professionals assigned as case managers.

CONCLUDING REMARKS

The goal of long-term care is to enable older adults to do the most they can for themselves given their physical and mental limitations (Evashwick, 1993). Most of those who need long-term care are cared for in their homes by informal or formal networks. The majority of recipients of long-term care services are of advanced age, hence they have a high probability of having an unremediated hearing impairment. Audiologists have an important role to play in the long-term care continuum. Most important is educating payers of long-term care, including the individual, of the integral role that the ability to hear, understand, and communicate can play in the lives of individuals with chronic multifaceted problems. For this population, the goal should be the provision of amplification systems that will enable one-to-one communication, television listening, telecommunication accessibility, and safety in the home environment. As we move into the 21st century, seniors will be better educated, more vocal, and more demanding as consumers. They must come to learn that audiologists offer products and services which will enhance the quality of their prolonged lives.

Appendix A contains a list of agencies that deal with issues pertaining to aging and long-term care. Audiologists should contact some of these agencies about hearing health care services that older adults should avail themselves if to help promote their quality of life.

APPENDIX A
REFERENCE LIST OF NATIONAL ORGANIZATIONS, PROFESSIONAL ASSOCIATIONS, AND FEDERAL GOVERNMENT OFFICES*,†
National Organizations

Alzheimer's Association
  70 E. Lake Street
  Suite 600
  Chicago, IL 60601
  312-853-3060

American Association for Continuity Care
  720 Light Street
  Baltimore, MD 21230
  301-837-1600

*Numbers may have changed since printing.
†Modified from Evashwick, 1996, and Shadden and Toner, 1998.

American Association of Homes for the Aging
901 E Street, NW
Suite 500
Washington, DC 20004-2837
202-783-2242

American Association of Retired Persons (AARP)
601 E Street, NW
Washington, DC 20049
202-728-4200

American Federation for Aging Research (AFAR)
725 Park Avenue
New York, NY 10021
212-570-2090

American Geriatrics Society, Inc.
770 Lexington Avenue
Suite 300
New York, NY 10021
212-308-1414

American Health Care Association (AHCA)
1201 L Street, NW
Washington, DC 20005
202-842-4444

American Public Health Association
Gerontological Health Section
1015 15th Street, NW
Washington, DC 20005
202-789-5600

American Red Cross
National Headquarters
430 17th Street, NW
Washington, DC 20006
202-737-8300

American Society on Aging
833 Market Street
Suite 516
San Francisco, CA 94130
415-882-2910

Arthritis Foundation
1314 Spring Street
Atlanta, GA 30309
404-827-7100

Association of Gerontology in Higher Education
1001 Connecticut Avenue, NW
Suite 410
Washington, DC 20036
202-429-9277

Association of Hospital-Based Nursing Facilities
3500 Masons Mill Business Park
Suite 501-A
Huntingdon Valley, PA 19006
215-657-0228

Directory of Aging Resources Business
Publishers, Inc.
951 Pershing Drive

Silver Spring, MD 28910-4464
301-897-6300

Federation of American Health Systems
1111 19th Street, NW
Suite 402
Washington, DC 20036
202-833-3090

Foundation for Hospice and Homecare
519 C Street, NE
Stanton Park
Washington, DC 20002
202-547-6586

Gerontological Society of America
1275 K Street, NW
Suite 350
Washington, DC 20005-4006
202-842-1275

Gray Panthers
1424 16th Street, NW
Suite 602
Washington, DC 20036
202-837-3111

Healthcare Financial Management Association
1050 17th Street, NW
Suite 510
Washington, DC 20036
202-296-2920

Joint Commission on Accreditation of Healthcare
Organizations
1 Renaissance Boulevard
Oakbrook Terrace, IL 60181
708-916-5600

The Lighthouse Inc.
111 E. 59th Street
New York, NY 10022
212-821-9200

National Association for Hispanic Elderly
3325 Wilshire Boulevard
Suite 800
Los Angeles, CA 90010
213-487-1922

National Association for Home Care
519 C Street, NE
Stanton Park
Washington, DC 20002
202-547-7424

National Association for Senior Living
Industries
184 Duke of Gloucester Street
Annapolis, MD 21401-2523
301-263-0991

National Association of Area Agencies on
Aging
1112 16th Street, NW
Suite 100

Washington, DC 20036
202-296-8130

National Association of Rehabilitation Facilities
PO Box 17675
Washington, DC 20041
703-648-9300

National Association of State Units on Aging
2033 K Street, NW
Suite 304
Washington, DC 20006
202-785-0707

National Association of the Deaf
814 Thayer Avenue
Silver Spring, MD 20910
301-587-1788

National Caucus and Center on Black Aged
1424 K Street, NW
Suite 500
Washington, DC 20005
202-637-8400

National Center for Vision and Aging
The Lighthouse Inc.
111 E. 59th Street
New York, NY 10022
212-821-9200

National Chronic Care Consortium
5001 W. 80th Street
Suite 449
Bloomington, MN 55437
612-835-1915

National Citizens Coalition for Nursing Home
Reform
1224 M Street, NW
Washington, DC 20005
202-393-2018

National Clearinghouse for Aging and
Technology
College of Health and Human Services
Ohio University
Athens, OH 45701
614-448-2804

National Committee for the Prevention of
Elder Abuse
c/o Institute on Aging
The Medical Center of Central Massachusetts
119 Belmont Street
Worcester, MA 01605
508-793-6166

National Council of Senior Citizens (NCSC)
1331 F Street, NW
Washington, DC 20004-1171
202-347-8800

National Council on the Aging, Inc.
409 3rd Street, SW
2nd Floor
Washington, DC 20024
202-479-1200

National Indian Council on Aging, Inc.
6400 Uptown Boulevard
City Center
Suite 510 West
Albuquerque, NM 87110
505-888-3302

National Senior Citizens Law Center
1815 H Street, NW
Suite 700
Washington, DC 20006
202-887-5280

National Stroke Association
300 E. Hamden Avenue
Suite 240
Englewood, CO 80110-2622
303-762-9922

Older Women's League
730 11th Street, NW
Suite 300
Washington, DC 20001
202-783-6686

Senior Care Center of America
720 E. Main Street
Moorestown, NJ 08057
609-778-0624

United Seniors Health Cooperative
1331 H Street, NW
Suite 500
Washington, DC 20005
202-393-6222

Professional Associations

American Academy of Family Physicians
8880 Ward Parkway
Kansas City, MO 64114-2797
800-274-2237

American Academy of Home Care Physicians
4550 W. 77th Street
Edina, MN 55435
612-835-1973

American Academy of Physical Medicine and
Rehabilitation
122 S. Michigan Avenue
Suite 1300
Chicago, IL 60603-6107
312-922-9366

American Association for Geriatric Psychiatry
PO Box 376A

Greenbelt, MD 20786
301-220-0952

American College of General Practitioners
330 E. Algonquin Road
Arlington Heights, IL 60005
800-323-0794

American College of Healthcare Administrators
325 S. Patrick Street
Alexandria, VA 22314
703-549-5822

American College of Physicians
700 13th Street, NW
Suite 250
Washington, DC 20005
202-393-1650

American Congress of Rehabilitation Medicine
5700 Old Orchard Road
Skokie, IL 60077
708-966-0095

American Dental Association
211 E. Chicago Avenue
Chicago, IL 60611-2678
312-440-2500

American Medical Association
515 N. State Street
Chicago, IL 60610
312-464-5000

American Medical Directors Association (AMDA)
10480 Litle Patuxent Parkway
Suite 760
Columbia, MD 21044
800-321-2632

American Nurses Association (ANA)
2420 Pershing Road
Kansas City, MO 64108
816-474-5720

American Occupational Therapy Association
1383 Piccard Drive
PO Box 1725
Rockville, MD 20849-1725
301-948-9626

American Optometric Association
1505 Prince Street
Suite 300
Alexandria, VA 22314
703-739-9200

American Osteopathic Association
142 E. Ontario Street
Chicago, IL 60611-2864
312-280-5800

American Psychiatric Association
1400 K Street, NW
Washington, DC 20005
202-682-6000

American Psychological Association
1200 17th Street, NW
Washington, DC 20036
202-955-7600

American Society of Allied Health Professionals
1101 Connecticut Avenue, NW
Suite 700
Washington, DC 20036
202-857-1150

American Speech-Language-Hearing Association
10801 Rockville Pike
Rockville, MD 20852
301-897-5700

National Association of Directors of Nursing Administration in Long-Term Care (NADONA/LTC)
10999 Reed Hartman Highway
Suite 234
Cincinnati, OH 45242
800-222-0539

National Gerontological Nursing Association
3100 Homewood Parkway
Kensington, MD 20895
301-946-8349

National Rehabilitation Association
633 S. Washington Street
Alexandria, VA 22091
703-836-0850

Society for Ambulatory Care Professionals (SACP)
American Hospital Association
840 N. Lake Shore Drive
Chicago, IL 60611
312-280-6050

Federal Government Offices

Administration for Children and Families
200 Independence Avenue, SW
Washington, DC 20201
202-245-7027

Administration on Aging
330 Independence Avenue, SW
Suite 4760
Washington, DC 20201
202-619-0641

Administration on Developmental Disabilities
200 Independence Avenue, SW
Suite 349D

HHH Building
Washington, DC 20201
202-245-2890

Department of Health and Human Services
200 Independence Avenue, SW
Washington, DC 20201
202-619-0257
Surgeon General
202-245-6467
Agency for Health Policy and Research
301-277-6662
National Center for Health Statistics
301-436-7016

Department of Veterans Affairs
810 Vermont Avenue, NW
Washington, DC 20420
202-233-4000

Health Care Financing Administration
200 Independence Avenue, SW
Suite 314G
HHH Building
Washington, DC 20201
202-245-6726
1-800-683-6833—Medicare Hotline
http://www.medicare.gov

Health Resources and Services Administration
5600 Fishers Lane
Rockville, MD 20857
301-443-2216

National Institutes of Health
9000 Rockville Pike
Bethesda, MD 20891
301-496-4000
National Institutes on Aging
301-496-9265

Office of Research & Demonstrations
Division of LTC Experimentation
6401 Security Boulevard
Suite 2230
Oak Meadows Building
Baltimore, MD
410-966-6507

U.S. Senate Special Committee on Aging
Washington, DC 20510
202-224-5364
Room SD-G31

GOVERNMENT RESOURCES

Healthfinder, the consumer health and human services information Web site, is a gateway for consumer health and human services information from the U.S. government. http://www.healthfinder.gov

The Social Security Administration handles Medicare enrollment and eligibility as well as administrative concerns such as lost Medicare cards and changes of address. Their number is 800-772-1213.

The National Aging Information Center is a service of the Administration on Aging. 330 Independence Avenue, SW, Room 4656, Washington, DC 20201; 202-619-7501. http://wwwaoa.dhhs.gov/naic

A local Area Agency on Aging (AAA) may be able to provide face-to-face counseling. Call the Eldercare Locator at 800-677-1116 to get in touch with local groups.

MISCELLANEOUS ORGANIZATIONS

The following organizations provide information on managed care:

Consumers Union often directs its attention to healthcare concerns. 1666 Connecticut Avenue NW, Suite 310, Washington, DC 20009; 202-462-6262. http://www.consumersunion.org

Families USA Foundation is an advocacy organization that focuses on healthcare. 1334 G Street NW, Washington, DC 20005; (202) 628-3030. http://familiesusa.org

Medicare Survival Kit contains publications on a wide variety of Medicare topics. Available from the Medicare Rights Center, 1460 Broadway, New York, NY 10036.

HMO Flash is a definitive reference guide on Medicare HMOs. Available from the Medicare Rights Center, 1460 Broadway, New York, NY 10036.

The Medicare Rights Center, an advocacy organization, provides information and other services. 1460 Broadway, New York, NY 10036; (212) 869-3850. http://www.medicarerights.org

Data from Elizabeth Barrett, Communications Associate, Medicare Rights Center, New York, NY.

REFERENCES

Aaronson, W. (1996). Financing the continuum of care: a disintegrating past and an integrating future. In: C. Evashwick (Ed.), *The Continuum of Long-term Care: An Integrated Systems Approach.* Albany: Delmar.

Altman, B., & Walden, D. (1993). *Home Health Care: Use, Expenditures and Sources of Payment.* (AHCPR Pub. No. 93–0040). National Medical Expenditure Research Findings 15, Agency for Health Care Policy and Research. Rockville, MD.

American Speech-Language-Hearing Association. (1990). Guidelines for the delivery of speech-language-pathology and audiology services in home care. *American Speech-Language-Hearing Association,* 33 (Suppl. 5): 29–34.

———. (1994). Professional liability and risk management for the audiology and speech-language pathology professions. *American Speech-Language-Hearing Association,* 36 (Suppl. 12): 25–38.

———. (1997a). Guidelines for audiology service/delivery in nursing homes. *American Speech-Language-Hearing Association,* 39 (Suppl. 17): 15–29.

———. (1997b). *1997 Omnibus Survey Reports.* Rockville, MD: American Speech-Language-Hearing Association.

Ammentorp, W., Gossett, K., & Euchner, P. (1991). *Quality Assurance for Long-Term Care Providers.* California: Sage.

Bloom, S. (1994). Hearing care in nursing homes offers daunting challenges, special rewards. *Hearing Journal,* 47: 13–20.

Braun, E. (1996). Managed Care. *Hearing Review,* 3: 30.

Burwell, B., Crown, W., O'Shaugnessy, C., & Price, R. (1996). Financing Long-Term Care. In: C. Evashwick (Ed.), *The Continuum of Long-term Care: An Integrated Systems Approach.* Albany: Delmar.

Casey, P. (1997). Meeting the challenges of managed care *Hearing Journal,* 50: 32–34.

Evashwick, C. (1993). The continuum of long-term care services. In: S. Williams & P. Torrens (Eds.), *Introduction to Health Services,* 4th ed. Albany: Delmar.

———. (1996). *The Continuum of Long-Term Care: An Integrated Systems Approach.* Albany: Delmar.

Evashwick, C. & Langdon, B. (1996). Nursing homes. In: C. Evashwick (Ed.), *The Continuum of Long-Term Care: An Integrated Systems Approach.* Albany: Delmar.

Folstein, M., Folstein, S., & McHugh, P. (1975). "Mini Mental State": a practical method of grading the cognitive state of patients for the clinician. *Journal of Psychiatric Research,* 12: 189–198.

Garahan, M., Waller, J., Houghton, M., Tisdale, W., & Runge, C. (1992). Hearing loss prevalence and management in nursing home residents. *American Geriatrics Society,* 40: 130–134.

Glickstein, J. (1998). The continuum of care settings and service delivery models. In: B. Shadden & M. Toner (Eds.), *Aging and Communication.* Austin: Pro-ed.

Halamandaris, V. (1992). How rapidly has the home care field grown? *Basic Statistics about Home Care.* National Association of Home Care.

Hegner, B., & Caldwell, E. (1994). *Assisting in Long-Term Care,* 2d ed. Albany: Delmar.

Hing, E. (1989). Nursing home utilization by current residents: United States, 1985. *National Center for Health Statistics. Vital Health Statistics,* 13: 102.

Hughes, S. (1996). Home health. In: C. Evashwick, *The Continuum of Long-Term Care: An Integrated Systems Approach.* Albany: Delmar.

Hull, R. (1995). *Hearing in Aging.* San Diego: Singular Publishing Group.

Kane, R. (1998). Introduction. *Generations,* 12: 5.

Kane, R., Ouslander, J., & Abrass, I. (1994). *Essentials of Clinical Geriatrics,* 3d ed. New York: McGraw-Hill.

Koch, A. (1993). Financing Health Services. In: S. Williams & P. Torrens (Eds.), *Introduction to Health Services.* Albany: Delmar.

Koop, C. E. (1998). Koop on long term care. *Aging Today,* 19: 6.

Lubinski, R., & Frattali, C. (1993). Nursing home reform: the resident assessment instrument. *American Speech-Language-Hearing Association,* 35:59–62.

Mezey, A., & Lawrence, R. (1993). Ambulatory Care. In: S. Williams & P. Torrens (Eds.), *Introduction to Health Services.* Albany: Delmar.

Mulrow, C., Tuley, M., & Aguilar, C. (1991). Sustained benefits of hearing aids. *Journal of Speech and Hearing Research,* 35:1402–1405.

National Center for Health Statistics. (1985). Nursing home characteristics preliminary data from the 1985 National Nursing Home survey. Advance data from vital and health statistics. Department of Health and Human Services PHS 87–1250. Hyattsville, MD.

———. (1991). Current estimates from the National Health Interview Survey. *Vital Health Statistics,* 10.

———. (1999). Highlights Health and Aging. Available at: http://www.cdc.gov/nchswww/products/pubs/pubd/hus/charts/hus99f12.pdf. Accessed November, 1999.

National Chronic Care Consortium. (1993). Extended care pathways: working papers. In: White, M. & Gundrum, G. (1996). Case management. In: C. Evashwick (Ed.), *The Continuum of Long-Term Care: An Integrated Systems Approach.* Albany: Delmar.

National Council on Aging. (1999). The consequences of untreated hearing loss in older persons. Available at: http://www.ncoa.org. Accessed November, 1999.

National Institute on Adult Daycare. (1984). *Standards for Adult Day Care.* Washington, DC: National Council on the Aging, Inc.

Omnibus Budget Reconciliation Act. (1987). U.S. Public Law 100–203. 101 Stat. 1330. Codified at 42 U.S.C.A. Sec. 1396 (Supplement 1989).

OUSLANDER, J. (1998). The American nursing home. In: R. Tallis, H. Fillit, & J. Brocklehurst (Eds.), *Brocklehurst's Textbook of Geriatric Medicine and Gerontology.* London: Churchill Livingstone.

OUSLANDER, J., OSTERWEIL, D., & MORLEY, J. (1991). *Medical Care in the Nursing Home.* New York: McGraw-Hill.

PHILLIPS, C., HAWES, C., MOR, V., FRIES, B., & MORRIS, J. (1998). Geriatric assessment in nursing homes in the United States: Impact of a national program. *Generations,* 21: 15–21.

RICHARDSON, H. (1998). Long-term care. In: A. Kovner (Ed.), *Jonas's Health Care Delivery in the United States.* 5th ed. New York: Springer.

SCHOW, R., & NERBONNE, M. (1980). Hearing levels among elderly nursing home residents. *Journal of Speech and Hearing Research,* 45: 124–132.

SHADDEN, B., & TONER, M. (1998). *Aging and Communication.* Austin: Pro-Ed.

TEDESCO, J. (1996). Adult day care. In: C. Evashwick (Ed.), *The Continuum of Long-Term Care: An Integrated Systems Approach.* Albany: Delmar.

U.S. DEPARTMENT OF HEALTH AND HUMAN SERVICES. (1993). Home/health and hospice care. *Morbidity and Mortality Weekly Report,* 42: 42.

WHITE, M., & GUNDRUM, G. (1996). Case management. In: C. Evashwick (Ed.), *The Continuum of Long-Term Care: An Integrated Systems Approach.* Albany: Delmar.

Chapter 12

Financing Health Care

The evolution of financing and organization of health care services for older persons in the United States in the 20th century has created dilemmas as well as opportunities.

—W. Barker, 1998

LEARNING OBJECTIVES

After reading this chapter, you should be able to:

- Integrate your knowledge of Medicare and Medicaid into your practice.
- Apply the long-term care benefits under Medicare and Medicaid.
- Understand managed care and Medicare managed care.
- Explain funding of audiologic services under Medicare and managed care.

The purpose of this chapter is to provide audiologists with a brief perspective on the financing of health care, which in and of itself is a very complicated, ever-changing phenomenon. Audiologists must have an appreciation for the amount of money spent on health care, for what the money buys, and how money is paid out. More important, the government's role in health care is of critical concern to audiologists as this is key to the survival of audiology as a profession. Having this broad perspective will enable audiologists to navigate through the health care system and obtain the funding necessary for hearing health care services.

The health care industry is the largest service industry in the United States (Koch, 1993). Americans spent over $600 billion on health care in 1990, which constituted approximately 12% of the Gross National Product (GNP) (Koch, 1993). This represents approximately $2566 per year for each person. In contrast, the United Kingdom spent 65% and Sweden 9% of their gross domestic products on health care (Koch, 1993). Interestingly, prior to World War II only 4% of the U.S. GNP was devoted to health care expenditures. National health care expenditures have outpaced the GNP since the introduction of Medicare and Medicaid in the mid-1960s. Government financing of health care services, the nature of third-party reimbursement, and the growth in the proportion of older adults account in large part for the disproportionate growth in health care spending relative to the growth of the GNP (Koch, 1993).

Health care for older adults is funded in four ways: (1) private insurance, (2) Medicare, (3) Medicaid, and (4) out-of-pocket (Ouslander, 1998). As shown in Figure 12–1, private health insurance and direct patient payment finances 58% of all health care expenditures. Whereas 42% is financed publicly by federal, state, and local government agencies. Hence the government's share was approximately $283 billion (Knickman & Thorpe, 1998). It is noteworthy that in 1965, 22% of health care expenditures were financed by the public sector compared to 9% in 1929 (Knickman & Thorpe, 1998). State and local expenditures have remained the same over time ranging from 10 to 14% (Knickman & Thorpe, 1998). Hence, the significant rise in federal spending can be attributed to federally financed Medicare and Medicaid programs that are administered through the Federal Health Care Financing Administration (HCFA), a branch of the U.S. Department of Health and Human Services. HCFA's role includes (1) developing and enforcing standards that regulate quality of care, (2) monitoring compliance of local carriers that administer Medicare programs, and (3) providing guidelines to carriers on coverage and payment determinations (Craft, 1998).

PEARL

Social Security and Medicare account for 7.4% of the gross domestic product, with the proportion expected to increase to 13% by 2030.

Interestingly, spending for Medicare and Medicaid has increased more rapidly over time than national health-care expenditures. In 1990, the two programs comprised approximately 27% of the total health care bill financed by public funds as compared to 15% of the total bill in 1967. Approximately 60 million or one quarter of the total U.S. population were enrolled in either Medicare or Medicaid (Koch, 1993).

In the United States, there are essentially three categories of health insurance: voluntary health insurance (VHI), social health insurance (SHI), or public welfare. The former is funded by private insurance, either Blue Cross/Blue Shield, private or commercial insurance companies, or health

313

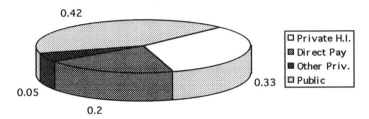

Figure 12–1 The division of the nation's health care dollar. (From Levit, Lazenby, Cowan, and Letsch, 1991.)

maintenance organizations (HMOs). SHI reflects participation in some type of government entitlement program and the public welfare health-care program primarily for persons who are low income or not gainfully employed (Koch, 1993). Medicare is the principal SHI program in the United States and Medicaid is the primary welfare medicine program. Medicare is an entitlement program, a right earned by individuals in the course of their years of employment (Koch, 1993). Funds are contributed by a payroll tax that, in the case of Social Security, is equally divided between the employee and employer (Koch, 1993). In contrast, Medicaid is a transfer payment system in which medical services are provided (instead of cash) as a welfare benefit (Koch, 1993).

The Medicare program that was enacted in 1965 represents the first entry of the federal government into the provision of SHI (Koch, 1993). Entered as Title XVIII (Medicare) of the Social Security Act, Medicare provides a range of medical care benefits to persons over 65 years of age who are recipients of Social Security beneficiaries (Knickman & Thorpe, 1998). In addition to older adults, Medicare targets disabled individuals. In 1972 benefits were extended to persons aged 65 and over who, although not meeting the criteria for Social Security benefits, were willing to pay a premium for coverage (Knickman & Thorpe, 1998). In 1993 about 13% of the total U.S. population qualified for Medicare and as of 1998 Medicare had 38 million enrollees (Burwell, Crown, O'Shaugnessy, & Price, 1996; Nichols, 1998). The Medicare program is administered at the local level by carriers, or insurance companies contracted by HCFA to process claims and pay for services (Crafat, 1998). Carriers, can be private or commercial insurance companies or Blue Cross/Blue Shield. The carriers report 10 regional HCFA offices that are ultimately responsible to HCFA. Carriers have a great deal of latitude in interpreting the HCFA guidelines concerning coverage and payment determinations, hence the differences among Medicare programs across states.

Medicare contains two parts. Part A (hospital services insurance) is available to all individuals who are eligible for Social Security benefits. It is, strictly speaking, true SHI. Part A is financed by payroll taxes collected via the Social Security system (Knickman & Thorpe, 1998). Almost everyone over age 65 is covered by Medicare. In contrast, Part B—Supplementary Medical Insurance (SMI) is a voluntary supplemental program paid in part (i.e., three quarters of the cost) by general tax revenues and in part by monthly contributions paid for by the individual subscriber. The premium for 1999 was $45.50 per month. Many older adults have also purchased a Medigap insurance policy, which is a private insurance designed to help pay Medicare cost-sharing amounts (e.g., some or all of the deductibles and coinsurance under Medicare). Medigap is a specific type of private insurance that is subject to federal and state laws. In most states, a Medigap plan must be one of ten standard plans called Plans A through to J. The advent of Medicare HMOs may obviate the need to purchase a Medigap policy, the cost of which is rising dramatically.

It is important to note that as part of the Balanced Budget Act of 1997 (BBA) a new choice was added to Medicare in the fall of 1998, moving Medicare from an insurer (fee-for-service) to a provider. Since its inception, Medicare made arrangements with hospitals, doctors, and other practitioners to provide covered services. The BBA established the Medicare + Choice program enabling Medicare to offer an array of private health-insurance plans including managed care plans (Gage, 1998). All Medicare + Choice (M+C) plans can offer whichever supplemental benefits they choose (Nichols, 1998). As part of the BBA provisions, Medicare pays each plan a fixed amount per enrollee and Medicare is responsible for managing the process by which beneficiaries choose from among the plans or from the traditional Medicare program. As of August 1999, there were 6.3 million M+C enrollees, respresenting 16% of the 39 million seniors in Medicare.

Ninety-five percent of persons over 65 are enrolled in Part A of Medicare, Hospital Insurance (HI). Part A covers care rendered in a hospital, an extended care facility, or in the home. Skilled nursing facility payments represent a minute percent (~2%) of Medicare payments. Part A finances four basic benefits including (1) ninety days of inpatient care, (2) a lifetime reserve of 60 days of inpatient care, (3) 100 days of post-hospital care in a skilled nursing facility, and (4) home health-agency visits (Koch, 1993). The Medicare beneficiary must participate in some cost sharing, which typically includes an inpatient hospital deductible in each benefit period. Coinsurance is required for the 61st through the 90th day of inpatient hospitalization and for the 21st through the 100th day of skilled nursing facility care; the coinsurance equals one-eighth of the deductible (Koch, 1993).

PEARL

Medicare will not pay for any services during a hospital stay that are not provided or arranged for by the hospital.

The majority (97%) of Part A beneficiaries are Part B—SMI enrollees. SMI complements the HI program paying for physician services, physician-ordered supplies and services, outpatient hospital services, and home health visits for persons with Part A (Koch, 1993). SMI enrollees must meet an annual deductible and pay an additional premium (Koch, 1993). Hence Part B is optional and requires a monthly premium. Physical and speech therapy services, diagnostic tests and radiographs, and prosthetics (not hearing aids) are covered services under Part B. The fixed amount of the coverage has been a subject of considerable debate. Part B covers some preventative services, including mammograms and flu shots. Medicare does not cover services essential to patient function such as eyeglasses, hearing aids, and dental care.

PEARL

Title XVIII (Medicare) of the Social Security Act pays for the medical needs of Social Security beneficiaries. Title XX provides reimbursement for social services. Medicare is a major payor of health care for older adults, with the majority of dollars spent on hospitals and doctors.

Medicare has a national fee schedule that sets fees for physicians. Fees are based on a formula known as the Resource-Based Relative Value Scale (RBRVS), which assigns relative values to services based on a number of variables. The variables include the (1) time, technical skill, and intensity it takes to provide the service, (2) overhead or practice expenses, and (3) professional liability costs (Knickman & Thorpe, 1998; ASHA, 1998). The relative value assigned for a given service is adjusted according to geography and multiplied by a national conversion factor to arrive at the dollar amount (Knickman & Thorpe, 1998). The provider can charge any amount above that stipulated according to the Table of Allowances and collect directly from the patient (Koch, 1993). The American Medical Association Current Procedural Terminal (CPT) code is level 1 of the Health Care Financing Administration Common Procedure Coding System (HCPCS) and is used almost exclusively in the RBRVS system (ASHA, 1998). The RBRVS that has been in effect for Part B physicians not employed by a health care facility also applies to nonphysicians who provide services to Medicare patients in a private practice setting or a medical clinic. Hence, audiologists who bill Medicare directly or who are employed by physicians are paid by this Medicare reimbursement system. Overall, 1998 Medicare RBRVS fees were 8.4% higher than in 1997.

The scope of coverage of audiologic services according to Section 2070.3 of the Medicare Carriers Manual (MCM) has remained the same for decades. Consistent with section 2070.3 of the MCM, independently practicing audiologists have their services covered under Medicare only through the diagnostic test benefit and such a diagnostic test continues to be covered only if it is ordered by a physician. A physician referral must be included in the patient's clini-

cal record. Each carrier has its own regulations regarding whether a written referral is required (AHSA, 1998). According to the MCM, to be reimbursed the physician must order testing to obtain additional information necessary for evaluation of the need for or appropriate type of medical or surgical treatment for a hearing deficit or a related medical problem. In certain venues for example, hearing tests can be covered for diagnosis of such conditions as cochlear deafness, sensorineural deafness, tinnitus, ear trauma, or vertigo. Under section 2070.3 there is no provision for coverage of therapeutic services performed by privately practicing audiologists or audiologists on the staff of a non–physician-directed clinic. However, audiologic rehabilitation and cerumen management are covered when rendered in a hospital inpatient setting (ASHA, 1998). Cochlear implant rehabilitation services and cerumen management are covered when rendered by an audiologist employed by a physician or a physician group (ASHA, 1999). Of course, audiology service must be performed by a "qualified audiologist," defined according to the Social Security Act. It is important to keep in mind that section 2070.3 scope of coverage is interpreted in various ways, depending upon the local carrier. Hence, as a provider, it is often important to make a case for the medical necessity of your services. Speaking to colleagues who have been successfully reimbursed by Medicare by selected services can be invaluable.

PEARL

Medicare will pay for diagnostic audiologic services when the information supplies a physician with the data necessary for medical evaluation and treatment of a hearing deficit or related medical problem (ASHA, 1998).

PITFALL

Independently practicing audiologists continue to be ineligible to receive Medicare payment for therapeutic services. Audiologic diagnostic services for screening purposes or hearing-aid evaluation are not covered by Medicare.

In contrast to fee-for-service is the capitation approach to reimbursement. With the advent of capitation, physicians formed networks known as individual practice association (IPAs). IPAs are usually organized around HMOs. Here, physicians may be assigned a capitated annual payment for each patient who uses the physician as a primary provider and this amount is designed to cover primary care and on occasion specialty care (Knickman & Thorpe, 1998). The capitation payment takes care of reimbursement for an agreed on period of time, typically one year (Koch, 1993).

Payment for hospital services is based on a prospective payment system using diagnosis related groups (DRGs).

This system is based on the classification of patient illnesses in terms of expected length of stay in the hospital (Glickstein, 1998). Under this prospective payment system, which was enacted in 1983, payment for hospital inpatient services is based on predetermined rates, with payments varying by type of case. Payments bear no direct relation to length of stay, to cost of care, or to services rendered (Koch, 1993). Under this prospective payment system, patients were classified into 23 diagnostic categories based on major body system. These diagnostic categories were further broken down into 47 diagnostic groups based on diagnosis or surgical procedure performed, age, sex, and other information (Knickman & Thorpe, 1998). Payment that a hospital receives for treating a Medicare patient in a given DRG then depends on "the DRG's cost weight multiplied by a standardized average cost for all Medicare patients" (Knickman & Thorpe, 1998, p. 286). Hence, the basis for reimbursement under the DRG systems is the diagnosis or case treated rather than individual service provided or length of stay (Knickman & Thorpe, 1998). In light of the DRG payment system, hospitalization rates and length of stays have decreased dramatically. Of course, the latter results in greater utilization of post-hospital services including home care or nursing facilities. Of course, HCFA next expanded the Medicare prospective payment system to long-term care. The case-mix system became known as RUGs (Resource Utilization Groups) wherein residents are classified according to medical condition and Activities of Daily Living dependencies (Glickstein, 1998). RUGs are used in some but not all states.

Medicaid, a welfare program that individuals qualify for depending on need and poverty level, was enacted into law in 1965 as Title XIX of the Social Security Act. It is part of the existing federal-state welfare structure to assist indigent individuals (Koch, 1993). Recipients must prove their eligibility and thus it has no entitlement feature. Each state administers its own Medicaid program and, subject to federal guidelines, determines eligibility and scope of benefits. However, according to Title XIX of the Social Security Act, every state Medicaid program must provide specific basic health services including but not limited to home health services for persons eligible for skilled nursing facility (SNF) services, SNF services for persons over 21 years of age, and physician services (Koch, 1993). Optional services include eyeglasses, hearing aids, dental care, prescribed drugs, and clinic services (Koch, 1993). Each state determines the payment rate for services provided to Medicaid recipients. Only a small proportion of persons over age 65 are enrolled in the Medicaid program (i.e., 13%). However, due in large part to high use of nursing home services, 34% of total Medicaid outlays in 1990 resulted from costs incurred by individuals over 65 years of age.

FINANCING LONG-TERM CARE

Long-term care is paid for by a variety of payors, including federal, state, local agencies, and individual families. To best appreciate some of the issues, Table 12–1 provides a context

TABLE 12–1 Facts about Long-Term Care Financing

- In 1990, the United States spent $585 billion on personal health-care expenditures.
- One half of the above amount (i.e., $256 billion) was spent on hospital care.
- Twelve percent (i.e., $105 billion) was spent on physician services.
- Nine percent (i.e., $53 billion) was spent on nursing home care.
- One percent (i.e., $6.9 billion) was spent on home care.
- Two-thirds of persons requiring long-term care are 65 or older.
- Seventy-three percent of long-term care spending is for people over 65 years of age.

Source: Evashwick, 1993; Burwell, Crown, O'Shaugnessy, and Price, 1996.

in which to view the financing of the long-term care continuum. It is clear that while the majority of persons requiring long-term care are over 65 years, the amount of money spent on acute care "dwarfs the amount spent on long-term care" (Evashwick, 1993). Payment for long-term care is primarily from individuals and states (Evashwick, 1993). Interestingly, private insurance payments for long-term care comprises less than 1% of total spending. Long-term care services are primarily funded under three parts or titles of the Social Security Act. These include Medicare; Medicaid-Title XIX; and Social Services Block Grants—Title 20 enacted in 1974. The Older Americans Act covers selected services as well. In general, Medicaid programs cover long-term care for certain categories of indigent and elderly people. Traditionally, Medicare has assumed responsibility for only a small portion of long-term care expenses. A brief review of the services covered under Medicare, Medicaid, and the Social Service Block Grants is contained in Table 12–2. Table 12–3 summarizes nursing home and home care expenditures under Medicare and Medicaid early in the decade and into the future. It is evident that Medicare pays only a small percentage of nursing home care as compared to Medicaid (less than 5% of the total Medicare budget is on nursing home expenditures) (Ouslander, 1998). In particular, Medicare primarily funds short stays in nursing facilities, skilled home care, hospice, and short-term mental health services. Medicare beneficiaries must meet stringent criteria for the Medicare skilled nursing-facility benefit.

PEARL

Unlike speech-language pathologists, audiologists can directly bill Medicare services. They may, therefore, receive payments directly as independent practitioners.

According to Evashwick (1993), in 1990, individuals paid 47% of the costs of nursing home care, which was approx-

TABLE 12–2 Federal Programs Supporting Long-Term Care Services

Federal program	Services covered	Eligibility
Medicare eligible	100 days of skilled nursing facility care; home health, hospice	All persons on Social Security and others with chronic medical conditions; voluntary enrollees 65+
Medicaid	Skilled nursing facility, intermediate care facility, home health, adult day care. Optional services vary from state to state and may include dental care, private-duty nurses, eyeglasses, hearing aids, medical transportation	Aged, blind, disabled persons, receiving cash assistance under SSI/AFDC
Title XX of Social Security Act	Various social services as defined by the state, including homemaker, home health aide, personal care, home-delivered meals	No federal requirements; states may have a means test

Source: Evashwick, 1993; Kane, Ouslander, and Abrass, 1994.

imately ten times as much as Medicare. In 1990, Medicare spent only 2.5 billion on skilled nursing-home care. Medicare is the major public payor for home care. The Medicare home health benefit will pay for services as long as a physician certifies that the individual is in need of skilled nursing services on an intermittent basis and is homebound (i.e., having a condition that restricts the ability to leave home, except with the assistance of another person or the aid of a supportive device) (Kane, Ouslander, & Abrass, 1994).

Interestingly, Medicare expenditures for home health-care services are increasing at a very rapid rate, far exceeding the rate of Medicaid spending for home care services. As of this writing, there are no limitations on the number of home health agency visits, nor are there prior hospitalization requirements, once the eligibility requirements for care are met (Glickstein, 1998). Medicare home health care has grown from 1% of Medicare expenditures in 1966 to well over 5% at the present time, encompassing more than 6129 agencies (Halamandaris, 1992). Similarly, the number of individuals served has grown tremendously from 98.5 thousand prior to the 1970s to nearly 2 million in the late 1990s. Medicare does not pay for adult day care. Medicare expenditures for home health care far exceed those of Medicaid even though Medicaid does finance some home health services (Hughes, 1996).

PEARL

Medicare is the major public payor for home care, paying only for short-term care. Home health care is the fastest-growing component of Medicare spending. Medicare Part A and Medicare Part B (supplementary insurance) both cover home health agency services without beneficiaries having to have a deductible or a coinsurance charge (Glickstein, 1998).

The financing of home health-care services under Medicaid is somewhat different from Medicare. Home health programs are steadily increasing as a proportion of Medicaid spending, however as of 1991, they remain only a small percentage of total Medicaid spending. In the mid-1990s, Medicaid paid 24.5% of the total expenditures on home health care. Under Medicaid, home health-care services are a mandatory service, and all states are required to cover home health services for certain groups of enrollees. Personal care, home, and community-based waiver services are optional; states may or may not elect to provide coverage for these services (Burwell et al, 1996). The latter services are those

TABLE 12–3 Public Expenditures on Nursing Home and Home Care

	Nursing home expenditures in billions		Home care expenditures in billions	
	1986–1990	2016–2020	1986–1990	2016–2020
Medicaid	$14.1	$46.2	$1.2	$2.4
Medicare	0.6	1.6	3.1	7.7
Patient	18.3	50.6	2.7	7.2
TOTAL	33.0	98.4	8.6	21.9

Source: National Association of Home Care—estimates by Brookings Institution. Evashwick, 1993.

services provided to individuals needing assistance with basic activities of daily living in or outside their home. The services at home include bathing, grooming, dressing, housekeeping, toileting, and other basic activities. Services outside the home include shopping or transportation. Depending on state policy, Medicaid spending on home health services can be extensive, potentially including services by nurses, home health aides, social workers, housekeepers, and various therapists. The bulk of Medicaid home care expenditures are, however, on personal care services (Burwell et al, 1996).

Unlike Medicare, the Medicaid program provides a generous package for long-term care services (Burwell et al, 1996). It is the major source of nursing home payments. Interestingly, most people entering nursing homes do not qualify for Medicaid, however they become eligible once they have depleted the resources they had in paying for their own care prior to institutionalization. The latter is known as "spend down" wherein older adults spend down their assets to pay nursing home expenditures until they become poor enough to qualify for Medicaid (Ouslander, 1998). Once elderly individuals spend down their assets, Medicaid will pay nursing home expenses. Medicaid also pays for selected social services, limited home health care, adult day care, medical transportation, and respite care. Services covered vary from state to state. In 1990, federal Medicaid paid $13.7 billion for nursing home care, and states paid a total of about $27 billion (Evashwick, 1993). Medicaid does pay for adult day care. It is the largest single payor with fees paid by families serving as the second largest source (Evashwick, 1993).

PEARL

Medicaid is a major payor for long-term care.

The third part of the Social Security legislation is Title XX administered as social services block grants. Title XX provides reimbursement for social services only. Title XX services, which are determined by the states, will provide coverage for medical care when it is integral, albeit subordinate to the provision of social services (Aaronson, 1996). This is also a welfare program, administered through state and local agencies, with states having a great deal of flexibility regarding how funds are allocated. Potential services covered include day care, home-based services, health-related services, transportation, day services, home-delivered and congregate meals (Kane, Ouslander, & Abrass, 1994). Finally the Title III of the Older Americans Act is available to all persons over age 60, regardless of income.

MANAGED CARE

Medicaid and Medicare both provide benefits through managed care as part of traditional insurance companies or as part of managed care companies that handle only Medicare and Medicaid. Managed care, an organized system of services in which financing, clinical services, and management

are combined, is becoming the predominant system for the delivery of health care in the United States (Swanson, 1998). The fundamental purposes of managed care are cost containment while assuring quality of care (Griffen & Fazen, 1993). In short, managed care organizations claim to offer two benefits in one, namely, control of health care costs and management of a patient's care. Managed health-care organizations, which take a variety of forms, provide for both the financing and the delivery of health care (Mezey & Lawrence, 1993). Recently, Medicare enrollees gained the opportunity to enter into a new health care option, namely Medicare managed care. Basically, managed care plans have contracts with the government (i.e., HCFA) to provide Medicare benefits. When individuals enroll in a Medicare managed-care plan, they select a doctor from the managed care plan's list of primary care physicians, and this individual becomes responsible for coordinating the member's health care needs. Managed care plans include HMOs and Competitive Medical Plans. Examples of managed care programs seeking to attract older adults are Medigap and Medicare Risk. Prior to discussing Medicare Managed Care, a brief overview of managed care and its features is in order.

PEARL

The term *managed care* refers to a broad array of payment, provider, and service systems that can be combined in a variety of ways (Glickstein, 1998). Over 60% of the U.S. population are in a managed care plan, with 71 million Americans in health maintenance organizations.

Managed care is an organized system of care that seeks to influence the selection and utilization of health services of enrollees and to ensure that care is provided in a high-quality and cost-effective manner (Federa & Camp, 1994). Managed care organizations truly "manage" how health care is delivered. In managed care organizations the primary care provider is the gatekeeper, who works with enrollees to determine what types, amounts, and frequency of services are appropriate or "necessary" (Swanson, 1993). In short, the primary care physician has the burden of limiting access to other health care providers and by so doing limiting health care expenses (Mezey & Lawrence, 1993). According to Klontz (1997), managed care is a system of care designed to both manage and control spending on health care by closely monitoring how providers treat their patients. Unique to all managed care organizations is that fees, rates fees, and rates that tend to be lower than the normal price of services are negotiated with selected providers and that financial incentives are offered for covered individuals to use providers and procedures covered by the managed care plan (Cornett, Klontz, & White, 1994). Managed care plans tend to offer a continuum of services with an emphasis on primary care, prevention, wellness, and health education. Under managed care, payment to providers is not based on customary charges for a particular test, rather it is based on a fixed, predetermined amount per enrollee, or a discounted

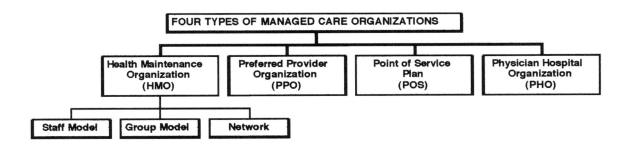

Figure 12–2 Four types of managed care organizations.

amount determined by a contractual arrangement (Cornett, Klontz, & White, 1994). For the most part, providers receive a predetermined amount of money for agreeing to care for a specified number of patients during a specified time frame. The provider receives payment irrespective of whether the patient has been treated (Glickstein, 1998). Managed care organizations prefer to work with a network of many provider practices represented by a single, centralized source (Braun, 1996). More and more hearing health-care providers are positioning themselves to become part of managed care organizations as it is clear that "this is a health care direction that is not going to go away" (Braun, 1996, p. 30).

Table 12–4 contrasts managed care plans with traditional health insurance. According to a survey conducted in the mid-1990s, only 5% of U.S. employees are enrolled in traditional rather than managed-care health plans. According to a survey conducted by the U.S. Department of Labor statistics, 12.2 million employees at companies with 20 or more employees are covered by hearing plans, which represents only 18% of the total number of workers at these companies. In 1995, only 15% of hearing instruments were fit through managed care contracts. While in 1998 approximately 18% of patients fit with hearing aids were under MCO contracts (Skafte, 1999). Dispensing audiologists fit twice as many MCO-contracted patients (24% versus 12%) as did hearing

instrument specialists (Skafte, 1999). According to Braun (1996), by the year 2005 managed-care covered fittings will represent between 25 and 55% of hearing industry sales, which translates into approximately one million hearing instruments per year. Presently, 53% of dispensing audiologists and 21% of hearing instrument specialists have contracts with managed care organizations (Strom, 1998). These contracts represented nearly one-fifth of the businesses' total revenue (Strom, 1998).

Several types of managed care organizations (MCOs) are available to consumers (Gage, 1998). Figure 12–2 describes the different types of managed care organizations in which over 160 million people are enrolled. Over half of the managed care population is enrolled in HMOs, the strictest form of MCO. The remainder are enrolled in either preferred provider organizations (PPOs), point-of-service plans (POSs), or physician hospital organizations (PHOs). Interestingly, as is shown in Table 12–5, enrollment in each type of MCO varies by state (Gage, 1998). Audiologists in different locations should be forming networks and marketing themselves accordingly.

HMOs contract to both pay for and deliver health care to enrollees (Mezey & Lawrence, 1993). HMOs control the type of client service, the billing, and the providers. There are several models of HMOs, with the primary difference being

TABLE 12–4 Managed Care Plans Versus Traditional Health Insurance

Managed care plans	Traditional health insurance
Client sees physician contracted with the plan	Client chooses any physician he/she wants
Primary care physician must make referral to a specialist. Clients who go out of network, must pay a higher percentage of the specialists bill	Client chooses which specialist to see and when a specialist is indicated
Managed care plans assume responsibility of determining whether the health care provider is qualified	Client determines the quality of the provider
Plans solicit enrollees' input about the quality of care received	Satisfaction with services is between the provider and the client
Intent of managed care plans is to improve the value of health care by managing processes to maximize health and reduce costs	Fee-for-service health plans have traditionally not been concerned with "quality of care" issues—this has been the purview of physicians and hospitals

Source: Cornett, Klontz, and White, 1994.

how the HMO relates to its participating providers. The models include (1) the staff model in which the HMO employs salaried professionals, (2) the group model in which the HMO is composed of multispecialty group practices, (3) the network model where the HMO contracts with several individual or group practices, which may be broad-based, multispecialty groups, or (4) the IPA in which the health care provider constitutes the HMO (Mezey & Lawrence, 1993; Klontz, 1997). The IPA is not included in the chart as they are considered by some as a subset of a network. In the group model, for example, any group of professionals such as audiologists would negotiate and contract with an HMO. In HMOs payment is typically a capitation fee. With capitation "the organization, be it a group practice or an individual physician, receives a monthly, prepaid, fixed fee for each covered individual or family" (Mezey & Lawrence, 1993, p. 127). Many HMOs manage the care of some Medicaid and Medicare beneficiaries (Griffen & Fazen, 1993). In fact, in 1992 New York State enacted a Medicaid Managed Care Initiative mandating that, within 5 years half of all Medicaid recipients should be enrolled in a managed care plan (Mezey & Lawrence, 1993). HMOs can be freestanding entities such as Kaiser or U.S. Healthcare, or can be owned by large commercial insurers such as Blue Cross/Blue Shield. The Blue Cross/Blue Shield Plan HMOs form a large, integrated network. Existing networks for audiologists include the National Ear Care Plan, Hear PO, Integrated Audiology Network, and Healthcare Management services (Klontz, 1997). In 1999, HEARx and Kaiser Permaneate formed an alliance to provide hearing services in southern California. Currently, audiologists contracting with managed care organizations are reimbursed in one of two ways: capitation or discounted fee for service (Klontz, 1997).

The Medicare HMO is quickly becoming commonplace, with 14 to 16% of Medicare beneficiaries enrolled in one of the 283 available plans (Gage, 1998). As is evident from

Table 12–5, enrollment varies by state. While not included in Table 12–5, it is noteworthy that New York, Pennsylvania, and Texas have a high number of enrollees (Gage, 1998). Medicare managed care is a health care option one can choose to receive Medicare benefits. In theory this type of HMO offers the full range of Medicare benefits to its enrollees in addition to extra benefits including drugs, eye care, hearing care, dental care, and preventive medicine (Table 12–6). Medicare managed care plans must provide each of the additional benefits it has agreed to provide for the money the government has agreed to pay. Oftentimes the latter benefits are provided at no charge, but on certain plans a copayment or an additional payment is required. HMOs receive a fixed monthly payment from the government for each Medicare enrollee, irrespective of the services required (Northern, 1997).

SPECIAL CONSIDERATION

Medicare managed-care plans offer a broader benefit package than the standard coverage as an incentive to attract enrollees.

Interestingly, HMOs are using hearing plans to increase enrollment in their senior plans (Casey, 1997). All Medicare managed-care plans are approved by the HCFA. About 75% of all Medicare HMOs charge no premium and all have either low or no copayments (Gage, 1998). Currently, there is at least one managed care plan available to over 75% of the Medicare population in the nation. Medicare enrollment in managed care options is on the rise such that in 1995 HMOs enrolled over 3.5 million Medicare beneficiaries (Casey, 1997). A recent HCFA report showed that 229 HMOs currently participate in the Medicare risk program. According to Northern (1997), more than 53% of dispensing audiologists provide hearing care under HMO contracts and receive 19% of their income from these services. The future appears promising for audiologists who have managed care contracts. Table 12–7 contains tips for audiologists interested in obtaining contracts with managed care agencies.

When an older adult enrolls in a Medicare managed care plan, he/she selects a physician from the managed care plan's list of approved providers and the primary care physician then coordinates the enrollee's health care needs. In

TABLE 12–5   Geographic Breakdown of MCOs

Non-Medicare MCOs
• 30% of HMO enrollees are members of HMOs based in California, Oregon, Washington, Alaska, and Hawaii
• 22% of PPO enrollees are in Illinois, Indiana, Michigan, Ohio, and Wisconsin
• 16% of PPO enrollees belong to plans based in New York, New Jersey, and Pennsylvania
• 22% of POS enrollees reside in New York, New Jersey, and Pennsylvania
Medicare MCOs
• 39% of California's older adults are enrolled
• 27% of Florida's Medicare population is enrolled
• 38% of Arizona's beneficiaries are enrolled

Source: Gage, 1998.

TABLE 12–6   Benefits Offered in Medicare Managed-Care Plans

• 97% offered routine physicals
• 83% offered eye exams
• nearly 75% offered ear exams
• more than 67% offered some type of prescription drug coverage
• In 2000, 86% of plans will have a cap on brand or generic drugs

TABLE 12–7 Tips for Audiologists in This Era of Managed Care

- Join a network of providers—the larger and more geographically extensive the network, the better. Form alliances with primary care providers, physical therapists, occupational therapists, and speech-language pathologists.
- Become an informed provider.
- Learn contract negotiation skills.
- Develop an outcome-oriented quality improvement system.
- Equip your office with professional testing and fitting equipment.
- Join a network that provides centralized contract administration, utilization data, satisfaction information, patient complaint procedures, billing, and collection of fees.
- Managed care companies value brand names that are widely recognized and respected by their members.
- Contracts should include a "no cause cancellation" clause so that the provider can "bow out" if the negotiated rate is too low for the satisfactory delivery of hearing health care.
- Market services to managed care programs and to older adults.
- Most administrators who negotiate benefits do not know about binaural advantages nor do they know a multichannel, multimemory completely-in-the-canal (CIC) from a linear CIC, hence audiologists must educate them about the differences new technology can make for hearing-impaired individuals.
- Collecting outcome data can help to justify the newer more costly technologies.

Source: Michaud, 1997; Griffen and Fazen, 1993.

order to enroll in a Medicare managed care plan the following two conditions must be met (1) the enrollee must have Medicare Part B and continue to pay Part B premiums and (2) the enrollee must live in the plan's service area. Individuals enrolled in a Medicare managed care plan can disenroll and return to the traditional Medicare fee-for-service plan. Similarly, if a patient is threatened by non-renewal of their managed care plan (a commonplace occurrence in 1999), they must remain covered through a specified date, which was December 31, 1999. Medicare benefits always remain viable even if the managed care plan leaves the medical program.

PEARL

Medicare managed-care plans do not cover custodial care and only cover skilled care for 100 days.

In PPOs, the organization contracts to provide selected health services for a set fee through the use of a predetermined group of physicians (Mezey & Lawrence, 1993). In this arrangement, the physicians agree to the fee structure of the PPO and the PPO provides them with patients. Patients can use providers outside of the PPO, but must pay the extra costs which they *will* incur. PPOs tend to be organized by providers or insurers and they do *not* have gatekeepers (Cornett, Klontz, & White, 1994). POS plans combine features of HMOs and PPOs. This hybrid plan is similar to HMOs in that the provider gets paid through a capitation or other risk-based model. It is similar to PPOs in that the member has the option to use a nonplan provider and incur the extra cost (Mezey & Lawrence, 1993). Overall, 58% of

employees surveyed in 1993 were enrolled in HMOs, PPOs, or POS plans, with the former being the most popular of the managed-care options (Mezey & Lawrence, 1993).

POSs combine features of PPOs (patient choice) and HMOs with traditional fee for service plans. In POS plans, the physician gets paid through a capitation or risk-based model as in classic HMOs, and as in PPOs the member can use network or nonnetwork providers (Mezey & Lawrence, 1993). If the enrollee chooses to go out of network, he or she will pay higher fees for the provider. Hence, the enrollee has a choice of provider but at a high cost. Finally, PSOs are organized and managed by a hospital and a community of doctors. They are typically licensed by an HMO yet they may contract with a purchaser or employer (Gage, 1998).

The typical payment for audiologic services in managed care plans is limited. Typically, health plans limit coverage to diagnostic services or they may limit coverage to illness/accident-related hearing disorders (ASHA, 1998). Some benefit packages include hearing aids, and as of this writing more and more Medicare plans are including a hearing-aid benefit, albeit small, in their package. Interestingly, major multioffice audiology corporations are being formed to respond to the new hearing-aid benefits included in many MCOs and HMOs. In short, to entice Medicare recipients to join MCOs, hearing-aid benefits are being included. Hearing-aid benefits are thus seen as a value added item (Danhauer, 1998).

CONCLUDING REMARKS

This chapter is not an exhaustive discussion of health care financing, however, it hopefully answers many of the questions audiologists have about issues pertaining to reimbursement. My goal was to include material that will not be outdated by the time the text is published and distributed. It should be clear from this chapter that health-care financing patterns are continually changing and the audiologist in private practice must keep abreast of information in this arena. The Internet is an ideal source for information on health care financing as information is constantly being updated to keep abreast with the rapid pace at which governmental regulations change.

REFERENCES

AARONSON, W. (1996). Financing the continuum of care: a disintegrating past and an integrating future. In: C. Evashwick (Ed.), *The Continuum of Long-Term Care: An Integrated Systems Approach.* Albany: Delmar.

ALTMAN, B., & WALDEN, D. (1993). *Home Health Care: Use, Expenditures and Sources of Payment* (AHCPR Pub. No. 93-0040). National Medical Expenditure Research Findings 15. Rockville, MD: Agency for Health Care Policy and Research.

AMERICAN SPEECH-LANGUAGE-HEARING ASSOCIATION. (1998). Home page. Available at: http://www.asha.org. Accessed November, 1999.

———. (1999). Home page. Available at: http://www.asha.org. Accessed November, 1999.

BARKER, W. (1998). Geriatrics in North America. In R. Tallis, H. Fillit, & J. Brockelhurst (Eds.), *Brockelhurst's Textbook of Geriatric Medicine and Gerontology,* 5th ed. London: Churchill Livingstone.

BLOOM, S. (1994). Hearing care in nursing homes offers daunting challenges, special rewards. *Hearing Journal,* 47: 13–20.

BRAUN, E. (1996). Managed Care. *Hearing Review,* 3: 30.

BURWELL, B., CROWN, W., O'SHAUGNESSY, C., & PRICE, R. (1996). Financing Long-Term Care. In: C. Evashwick (Ed.), *The Continuum of Long-Term Care: An Integrated Systems Approach.* Albany: Delmar.

CASEY, P. (1997). Meeting the challenges of managed care. *Hearing Journal,* 50: 32–34.

CORNETT, B., KLONTZ, H., & WHITE, S. (1994). Managed Care: an overview. In: *Managing Managed Care: A Practical Guide for Audiologists and Speech-Language Pathologists.* Rockville, MD: American Speech-Language-Hearing Association.

CRAFAT, R. (1998). Erasing your fears about Medicare documentation. *Therapy Student Journal,* 5: 16–20.

DANHAUER, J. (1998). Who are those major multi-office audiology groups moving in on us, and—is this town big enough for the both of us? *Audiology Today,* 10: 47–51.

EVASHWICK, C. (1993). The continuum of long-term care services. In: S. Williams & P. Torrens (Eds.), *Introduction to Health Services,* 4th ed. Albany: Delmar.

———. (1996). *The Continuum of Long-Term Care: An Integrated Systems Approach.* Albany: Delmar.

EVASHWICK, C., & LANGDON, B. (1996). Nursing homes. In: C. Evashwick, (Ed.), *The Continuum of Long-Term Care: An Integrated Systems Approach.* Albany: Delmar.

FEDERA, R., & CAMP, T. (1994). The changing managed care market. *Journal of Ambulatory Care Management,* 17: 1–7.

GAGE, B. (1998). The history and growth of medicare managed care. *Generations,* 22: 11–18.

GLICKSTEIN, J. (1998). The continuum of care settings and service delivery models. In: B. Shadden & M. Toner (Eds.), *Aging and Communication.* Austin: Pro-ed.

GRIFFIN, K., & FAZEN, M. (1993). A managed care strategy for practitioners. In: *Quality Improvement Digest.* Rockville, MD: American Speech-Language-Hearing Association, 1–7.

HALAMANDARIS, V. (1992). How rapidly has the home care field grown? *Basic Statistics about Home Care.* Washington, DC: National Association of Home Care.

HUGHES, S. (1996). Home health. In: C. Evashwick (Ed.), *The Continuum of Long-Term Care: An Integrated Systems Approach.* Albany: Delmar.

KANE, R., OUSLANDER, J., & ABRASS, I. (1994). *Essentials of Clinical Geriatrics,* 3d ed. New York: McGraw-Hill.

KLONTZ, H. (1997). Managed care 101: a primer on whats, whys, and hows. *Hearing Journal,* 50: 26–29.

KNICKMAN, J., & THORPE, K. (1998). Financing for health care. In: A. Kovner (Ed.), *Jonas's Health Care Delivery in the United States.* New York: Springer.

KOCH, A. (1993). Financing Health Services. In: S. Williams & P. Torrens (Eds.), *Introduction to Health Services.* Albany: Delmar.

LEVIT, K., LAZENBY, H., COWAN, C., & LETSCH, S. (1991). National health care expenditures, 1990. *Health Care Financing Review,* 13: 1–29.

LUBINSKI, R., & FRATTALI, C. (1993). Nursing home reform. *American Speech-Language-Hearing Association,* 35: 59–62.

MEZEY, A., & LAWRENCE, R. (1993). Ambulatory Care. In: S. Williams & P. Torrens (Eds.), *Introduction to Health Services.* Albany: Delmar.

MICHAUD, L. (1997). Gaining access to the managed care market. *Hearing Journal,* 50: 62–64.

NATIONAL INSTITUTE ON ADULT DAYCARE. (1984). *Standards for Adult Day Care.* Washington, DC: National Council on the Aging, Inc.

NICHOLS, L. (1998). Building a marketplace for elderly consumers. *Generations,* 22: 31–36.

NORTHERN, J. (1997). Quality managed care: it's not an oxymoron. *Hearing Journal,* 50: 35–40.

OMNIBUS BUDGET RECONCILIATION ACT. (1987). U.S. Public Law 100–203. 101 Stat. 1330. Codified at 42 U.S.C.A. Sec. 1396 (Supplement 1989).

OUSLANDER, J. (1998). The American nursing home. In: R. Tallis, H. Fillit, & J. Brocklehurst (Eds.), *Brocklehurst's Textbook of Geriatric Medicine and Gerontology.* London: Churchill Livingstone.

OUSLANDER, J., OSTERWEIL, D., & MORLEY, J. (1991). *Medical Care in the Nursing Home.* New York: McGraw-Hill.

PHILLIPS, C., HAWES, C., MOR, V., FRIES, B., & MORRIS, J. (1998). Geriatric assessment in nursing homes in the United States: impact of a national program. *Generations*, 21: 15–21.

SKAFTE, M. (1999). The 1998 hearing instrument market—the dispenser's perspective. *Hearing Review,* 6: 6–32.

STROM, K. (1998). A review of the 1997 hearing instrument market. *Hearing Review*, 5: 8–16, 72.

SWANSON, J. (1998). Taming managed care. *Communicator*, 27: 7.

TEDESCO, J. (1996). Adult day care. In: C. Evashwick (Ed.), *The Continuum of Long-Term Care: An Integrated Systems Approach.* Albany: Delmar.

TYE-MURRAY, N. (1998). *Foundations of Aural Rehabilitation.* San Diego: Singular Publishing Group.

U.S. DEPARTMENT OF HEALTH AND HUMAN SERVICES. (1993). Home/health and hospice care. *Morbidity and Mortality*

INDEX